T0133325

TRANSFORMING MEDICAL EDUCATION

MCGILL-QUEEN'S/ASSOCIATED MEDICAL SERVICES STUDIES
IN THE HISTORY OF MEDICINE, HEALTH, AND SOCIETY

SERIES EDITORS: J.T.H. CONNOR AND ERIKA DYCK

This series presents books in the history of medicine, health studies, and social policy, exploring interactions between the institutions, ideas, and practices of medicine and those of society as a whole. To begin to understand these complex relationships and their history is a vital step to ensuring the protection of a fundamental human right: the right to health. Volumes in this series have received financial support to assist publication from Associated Medical Services, Inc. (AMS), a Canadian charitable organization with an impressive history as a catalyst for change in Canadian healthcare. For eighty years, AMS has had a profound impact through its support of the history of medicine and the education of healthcare professionals, and by making strategic investments to address critical issues in our healthcare system. AMS has funded eight chairs in the history of medicine across Canada, is a primary sponsor of many of the country's history of medicine and nursing organizations, and offers fellowships and grants through the AMS History of Medicine and Healthcare Program (www.amshealthcare.ca).

Transforming
Medical Education

Historical Case Studies of Teaching,

Learning, and Belonging in Medicine

in Honour of Jacalyn Duffin

Edited by Delia Gavrus and Susan Lamb

McGill-Queen's University Press

Montreal & Kingston • London • Chicago

© McGill-Queen's University Press 2022

ISBN 978-0-2280-1072-2 (cloth)
ISBN 978-0-2280-1232-0 (ePDF)
ISBN 978-0-2280-1233-7 (ePUB)

Legal deposit second quarter 2022
Bibliothèque nationale du Québec

Printed in Canada on acid-free paper that is 100% ancient forest free
(100% post-consumer recycled), processed chlorine free

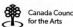

| Funded by the Government of Canada | Financé par le gouvernement du Canada | | Canada Council for the Arts | Conseil des arts du Canada |

We acknowledge the support of the Canada Council for the Arts.
Nous remercions le Conseil des arts du Canada de son soutien.

Library and Archives Canada Cataloguing in Publication

Title: Transforming medical education : historical case studies of teaching, learning, and belonging in medicine in honour of Jacalyn Duffin / edited by Delia Gavrus and Susan Lamb.

Names: Duffin, Jacalyn, honoree. | Gavrus, Delia, editor. | Lamb, S. D., 1971– editor.

Series: McGill-Queen's/Associated Medical Services studies in the history of medicine, health, and society ; 58.

Description: Series statement: McGill-Queen's/Associated Medical Services studies in the history of medicine, health, and society ; 58 | Includes bibliographical references and index.

Identifiers: Canadiana (print) 20210371196 | Canadiana (ebook) 20210371358 | ISBN 9780228010722 (cloth) | ISBN 9780228012320 (ePDF) | ISBN 9780228012337 (ePUB)

Subjects: LCSH: Medical education—History—Case studies. | LCGFT: Case studies. | LCGFT: Festschriften.

Classification: LCC R735.A5 T73 2022 | DDC 610.71—dc23

This book was typeset in Baskerville.

Contents

Contents

Tables and Figures

Acknowledgments

First and foremost, we thank our fellow historian of medicine, Jacalyn Duffin, for her mentorship and collegiality over many years. We are deeply appreciative for the opportunity to interview Jackie at her home in Kingston, Ontario. Thank you also to Jackie's husband, Robert David Wolfe, whose hospitality and conviviality made that day all the more memorable. Jackie graciously responded to a few subsequent requests to clarify factual information, and she supplied many wonderful photographs that appear in this volume.

We owe an enormous debt of gratitude to the twenty-one contributors to this volume for their exceptional scholarship, for the sustained care and professionalism they brought to our collaboration, and for responding diligently to multiple rounds of peer review and editorial suggestions.

The labour of academic peer reviewing is indispensable to vibrant epistemic communities, but it is often invisible and unremunerated. It thus gives us particular pleasure to acknowledge the time and expertise of the following reviewers of individual chapters: Domenico Bertoloni Meli, Adam Biggs, Charles Burnett, Hannah-Louise Clark, Peter Crampton, Marcos Cueto, Susan Einbinder, Nahyan Fancy, Catherine Gidney, Vivien Hamilton, Bert Hansen, John Harley Warner, Roger Jeffery, Laura Kelly, Cynthia Klestinec, David Luesink, Heather MacDougall, Paul Potter, Jonathan Reinarz, Michael Sappol, Emilie Savage-Smith, Walt Schalick, and Mindy Schwartz.

Many thanks to Kyla Madden, our editor at McGill-Queen's University Press (MQUP), who provided enthusiastic support and guidance from the moment the project sprang into existence. We are grateful to the press's anonymous reviewers and to the co-editors of the press's History of Medicine Series, Jim Connor and Erika Dyck, for their constructive input, as well as to the talented production teams at MQUP.

Delia Gavrus wishes to thank the University of Winnipeg's Chancellor's Research Chair and the Social Sciences and Humanities Research Council of Canada. While the financial support from these institutions was for her other research projects, the partial teaching release that accompanied it allowed Delia to carve out research time for the present volume as well, and for that she is deeply grateful. Susan Lamb is likewise appreciative for ongoing support from AMS Healthcare and the Department of Innovation in Medical Education (DIME) at the University of Ottawa, which enabled her to co-produce this volume of international scholarship on medical education. We also thank our student research assistants whose work supported this project: Madison Herget-Schmidt, Serina Khater, Moira Smee, Breanna Waterman, and Gayle Wong.

    Finally, the publication of this work was supported by several organizations that we have the pleasure to acknowledge and thank: AMS Healthcare, the Faculty of Medicine at the University of Ottawa, and the University of Winnipeg Research Office.

Delia Gavrus
Susan Lamb

TRANSFORMING MEDICAL EDUCATION

Introduction

Delia Gavrus and Susan Lamb

This volume brings together twenty-one case studies in the history of medical education. It has two intertwined objectives – one scholarly and the other celebratory. The first is to present readers with deeply researched, original scholarship that critically foregrounds processes of learning, teaching, and belonging in medicine, broadly defined, from different geographical and temporal contexts. In our curation, we strove to showcase a diversity of case studies from an outstanding group of international historians at various stages of their careers. Their chapters chart historical continuities and discontinuities and highlight key historiographical themes and theoretical questions. Together, the case studies examine social, cultural, political, and linguistic influences in the history of medical education; they also illuminate the diverse experiences of students, educators, and patients. This wide-ranging scholarship crystallizes around intersecting conceptual themes and critically addresses the impact of knowledge transmission, social (in)justice, identity in its myriad presentations, and the various spaces and modes of pedagogy. Individually and as a whole the chapters constitute not only an excellent scholarly resource, but also a valuable teaching aid for undergraduate and graduate education in history and medical humanities.

The second objective of this volume is to celebrate Jacalyn Duffin's outstanding contributions as an acclaimed historian and skilled clinician, as an instrumental and beloved teacher, and as a vital presence in Canadian intellectual and political life. In 2018, Dr Duffin retired from the Jason A. Hannah Chair in History of Medicine at Queen's University (Kingston, Ontario). Cross-appointed to the university's Faculties of Medicine and Arts, for three decades she worked simultaneously as a researcher, clinician, and educator, receiving innumerable awards and accolades from fellow historians and physicians. Duffin's extraordinary career and contributions are outlined below, and they are explored in detail in the final three chapters of this volume: in an homage to her medical pedagogy, an essay on her scholarship, and an original oral history interview with the honoree herself. As these final chapters make clear, the interconnectedness of medicine, history, and medical education stands out as a central theme in Duffin's research, teaching, and advocacy. Medical education, therefore, is the subject par excellence for a volume of new historical scholarship curated in her honour.

MEDICAL EDUCATION: MULTIDISCIPLINARY SCHOLARSHIP

Today, the training of health professionals faces intense scrutiny from a wide variety of disciplinary perspectives. This concern is not new. Sociologists and anthropologists, for example, have long been interested in medical education. Over the past half-century, in ethnographies and in quantitative and qualitative studies alike, these scholars have theorized and investigated the culture and processes of socialization in medical schools, the shaping of the professional self, the scientific and technical training of students, curriculum innovation and the so-called "hidden curriculum," the intricacies of the student-doctor-patient relationship, and the ways in which affect, gender, race, racialization, ethnicity, and ethics are articulated during medical education and are handled by medical curricula.[1] For example, social scientists have scrutinized how the logics of settler colonialism, as well as a lack of critical tools for unpacking those logics, continue to shape current medical education and hinder efforts to address anti-Indigenous racism in Canada.[2]

Most North American medical schools now have an interdisciplinary medical education department staffed with pedagogy researchers who hold a PhD or MD (sometimes both). Pedagogical scholarship around medical education has proliferated since the 1960s in an effort to develop assessable learning modalities, to introduce effective teaching methods, to address the legacies of toxic medical cultures, and to identify barriers to equitable access to medical training.[3] The study of historical contexts can help this endeavour by making invisible dynamics visible and tacit processes explicit. For instance, *Physicianship and the Rebirth of Medical Education*, a recent analysis produced by medical education scholars, exemplifies the productive relationship between pedagogical and historical research for medical education.[4]

In fact, historians of medicine have long made the case for the utility of their discipline to medical education.[5] David Jones, Jeremy Greene, Jacalyn Duffin, and John Harley Warner recently outlined this extensive history and made a compelling synthesis of the reasons why history of medicine belongs in the medical curriculum, "not just as a nonspecific model of fostering professionalism, but as an essential component of medical knowledge, reasoning, and practice." They argue that historical thinking "contributes essential insights to our understanding of disease, therapeutics, and institutions – things that all physicians must know in order to be effective, just as they must learn anatomy or pathophysiology."[6] Thus, history imparts not only content and context to medical students, but also an additional set of competencies rooted in historical reasoning and humanistic analysis.

The history of medical education reveals the ways in which workers across the healing professions acquired and transmitted knowledge, built epistemic foundations, developed practical skills, articulated ways of thinking and behaving, adopted moral values, and fashioned a shared (or, at times, clearly delineated) identity. At any moment in time, questions, debates, and practicalities related to these issues circumscribed a unique culture of medical education. As historians John Harley Warner, Hans Pols, and Michelle Thompson succinctly noted in a recent edited volume on the history of medical education in Southeast Asia: "Medical education has at its core the acquisition of a new culture."[7] At the same time, medical education happens *in* specific cultures and is always part of the deep social, political, and intellectual worlds in which it emerges. Its broader entanglements reveal much about economics, ideologies, policies, social inequalities, power dynamics, and ideals of health; they also expose recurring sets of tensions, such as debates about the priority of theory vs practice, skill vs knowledge, science vs art, research vs teaching.[8]

Over the past few decades, historians have explored the history of medical education from the point of view of institutional,[9] national,[10] settler-colonial,[11] regional,[12] transnational,[13] and textual[14] contexts. Historical analyses of North American medical education understandably gravitate toward the weighty consequences of educational reform early in the twentieth century, especially as codified in the 1910 Flexner Report.[15] Reforms that raised academic requirements for admission and expanded mandatory laboratory and clinical training also entrenched the profession's conservatism, elitism, sexism, and racism through exclusionary criteria for institutions and individuals.[16] Scholars have shown how, in colonial contexts, medical education illuminates the processes of translation, assimilation, interpretation, resistance, and transformation, while making visible the power imbalances that underscore these processes.[17] Other scholars, including Duffin, have highlighted economic issues, including the history of tuition fees and accessibility to medical education[18] as well as student activism that calls for more human- and community-centred medicine.[19] Studies have also investigated the influence of religion and religious guilds in physician education,[20] as well as the fraught role that the pharmaceutical industry has played in doctors' continuing education.[21] Drawing on scholarship on gender, sexuality, the history of the body, and the history of emotions, other historians have explored the ways in which medical education led doctors to fashion particular identities and specific ways of being, feeling, and performing.[22] Historians have also examined the experiences of Black,[23] Jewish,[24] Indigenous,[25] and female practitioners,[26] highlighting the explicit and systemic racism, bigotry, and sexism in the health professions and showing how colonialism (including settler colonialism) and its ideology and institutions, including teaching hospitals, impact medical education and, as a result, the delivery of health care.[27]

These more recent studies, rooted in the methods of social and cultural history and postcolonial studies, have deepened, revised, and, in some cases, critiqued earlier histories of medical education that were organized chronologically,[28] geographically,[29] or according to medical specialization.[30] The more recent historiography thus goes further to foreground questions and approaches that emphasize gender, sexuality, experience, emotion, social justice, decolonization, and anti-racism. The twenty-one historical case studies in this volume are likewise clustered around themes that resonate with these important issues that justifiably preoccupy students and teachers of history and medicine today.

MEDICAL EDUCATION FROM
FIVE CRITICAL PERSPECTIVES

The chapters in this volume are united by the common goal of offering empirically driven, methodologically sophisticated, thoroughly researched, original arguments that shed a novel light on the history of medical teaching and learning in their respective contexts. This book is not a comprehensive history of medical education, and we recognize that in important areas it falls short. At the same time, in bringing together these particular chapters in one volume, our approach is congruent with the *largo dislocare* approach used by historians of science such as Gabriela Soto Laveaga, by which familiar histories are dislocated, geographically and chronologically, with the aim of exposing the limiting effects of traditional historiographical narratives.[31] The volume thus builds upon old and new scholarship by deliberately juxtaposing studies of different geographies and eras – from medieval Japan to twentieth-century Canada, from colonial Cameroon to early Republican China, or from early modern Western Europe to Central Asia during the twelfth and thirteenth centuries. The collection also attempts to disrupt traditional historiographies of medical education by making room for schools of medicine for revolutionaries, cultural safety lessons, emotional medical students, and digital cadavers – alongside European universities, textbooks, anatomical theatres, laboratories, and MD curricula. The rich tapestry of scholarship in the volume engages as well with novel questions such as: What happens to a determined, politically engaged student when medical education is denied to her (Moore, chapter 17)? How do doctors react when they find their past textbook-based medical-school instruction to be inadequate in the face of outbreaks of epidemic disease (Jones, chapter 3)? What emotional valences are imbued in different spaces of medical education (Kelly, chapter 15)? How is the personhood of bodies used in medical education encoded into law and represented in public consciousness (Wu, chapter 9)? Collectively, by asking novel questions and producing compelling answers, this scholarship makes a powerful argument about the contextual diversity of instruction and professional identity in medicine, and it attests to the importance of scrutinizing medical teaching, learning, and belonging using the practices of history.

The chapters are organized around five themes: knowledge transmission, social (in)justice, educational spaces, professional identities, and the relationship between history and medicine. This organization facilitates both research and teaching. In addition to previewing the thematic connections and arguments of the chapters, therefore, we also discuss below how chapters in each section can help to answer broader questions related to medical education.

1. Knowledge Transmission: Text, Translation, Practical Experience

The first theme raises perennially relevant questions about how and where the dissemination of medical knowledge occurs. In their respective contexts, the authors raise compelling questions about connections between written and hands-on knowledge, about the types of texts and literature that are used for instruction, and about the sites and institutions where instructional encounters unfold. The five chapters cohere temporally around the medieval and early modern periods. Some reveal the importance of interrogating the particularities of texts – including their translations, assimilations into other traditions, and commentaries – in transcultural contexts (chapters 1, 2, and 3). Others raise and answer questions about tensions (or, at least, juxtapositions) between theoretical and practical knowledge within institutions such as the university and the hospital, as well as epistemological differences between text-based and hands-on or empirical learning. The authors show how these pressures were navigated in specific historical circumstances (chapters 3, 4, and 5).

In chapter 1, M.A. Mujeeb Khan offers a case study in the transmission of knowledge between and within cultural traditions in medieval Asia, examining the complex nature of texts that fulfilled the dual purposes of knowledge preservation and medical instruction. Khan complicates the simple, linear stories that are told about the roles medical texts played in the medieval Islamicate and Japanese traditions of medical learning. He interrogates, moreover, the relationships between form, content, authorial intent, and didactic practice; and he demonstrates the importance of the specific historical context in these relationships by contrasting the differing landscapes of the Islamicate world and medieval Japan. This case study underscores the transcultural nature of the transmission of medical knowledge in these two traditions, while foregrounding the role of translation and encyclopedias in medical instruction at the time.

In chapter 2, Sally Ragep provides an in-depth study of an influential medieval medical textbook – al-Qānūnča (*The "Little Qānūn"*) by Maḥmūd al-Jaghmīnī – as well as the commentaries and translation projects through which the knowledge within its pages was transmitted to future medical generations. Al-Jaghmīnī's *al-Qānūnča* was an abridgment of Ibn Sīnā's famous *Canon*, which was a staple of medical education throughout the post-classical world. In addition to a critical new appraisal of where al-Jaghmīnī's *Little Canon* and its commentaries fit within the Arabic-Islamic educational world, Ragep offers examples that challenge standard narratives on the uses of scientific and medical texts in madrasas and other Islamic institutions of learning. Significantly, Ragep supplies a major new contribution to the field by dating the medical treatise decisively, and by producing a revised lineage chart for all extant works derived from al-Jaghmīnī's *Little Canon* and the locations of many of these manuscripts.

Lori Jones, in chapter 3, similarly scrutinizes a highly specialized textual genre used to impart and disseminate medical knowledge: the plague tract. She shows how European physicians in the late medieval and early modern periods struggled to reconcile received knowledge from their medical education, which was based on traditional textbook learning, with the reality of plague as they observed it first-hand. This tension between past authority and direct observation was negotiated and resolved by doctors in different ways: whereas some decided to give more weight to the former, others preferred the latter. Jones argues that while historically we can observe a transition from a preference for relying on formal education and past medical authority to a preference for direct observation and experience, the line between these two was never stark. Rather, the constant dialectic between education and practical experience is present at all times, and at any given time, it mirrors broader intellectual, social, and cultural contexts.

Michael Stolberg (chapter 4) focuses on universities as privileged and sought-after sites of sixteenth- and early-seventeenth-century knowledge transmission in medical education. Using the notebooks of medical students who attended university at either Padua or Montpellier, he demonstrates that despite some differences, the two schools stood on the brink of an important shift in medical education in the sixteenth century: an increased focus on empiricism and practical education in the form of bedside teaching, anatomically grounded surgery, and pharmaceutically oriented botany.

The perceived importance of practical knowledge for successful future medical practice altered the university as a site of medical instruction in early modern Europe.

Maria Pia Donato (chapter 5) provides new perspectives on surgical education in Rome during an equally transformative period: 1650 to 1750. Donato investigates the hospital as a site of knowledge transmission for surgeons by combining newly investigated archival sources (hospital records, printed texts, and student notebooks) with records from Italian universities. Her chapter shows how surgeons who trained in hospitals and physicians who learned medicine in university faculties – groups typically treated as foes in the history of European medicine – relied on shared medical treatises, pedagogical methods, and clinical practices in this period. This educational development led to the expansion of surgeons' domain to include internal conditions and prescribed therapies that had been traditionally the domain of physicians. Donato also shows how this expansion contributed to the intensification of theoretical tensions between the traditional humoral-Galenic framework and emerging corpuscular theories. Teaching hospitals, she emphasizes, became sites where practical bedside experience and the study of medical texts were combined to create a new standard of surgical knowledge and training.

2. Social (In)Justice: Racism, Inequities, (De)Colonization

The next four chapters coalesce around historical questions about medical education within the context of unjust social realities such as class oppression, racism, and colonialism. They also document reactions to such injustices through movements for civil rights and decolonization. Their authors show how, in diverse cultural settings across the nineteenth and twentieth centuries, systemic social and political factors profoundly shaped not only medical education (chapters 6, 7, 8) but also its perception among oppressed populations and the public (chapter 9). This section includes scholarship that draws attention to current concerns in medical schools, such as the lack of socioeconomic diversity in medicine, by scrutinizing injustices that continue to cast a long shadow on the profession (chapters 6, 7, 9, and 10). As Jethro Hernández Berrones observes in chapter 8, for example, the work of historians who recover these troubling episodes from the archives is itself a political act of social justice and a tribute to those who campaigned for equitable access to medical education and health care.

In their analysis of the history of medical education in India between 1880 and 1956, Anna Ruddock and Pratik Chakrabarti (chapter 6) illustrate how the larger fight for civil rights profoundly influenced colonial-era medical education. Indian doctors, such as the influential Dr Jivraj N. Mehta, denounced the racist, discriminatory policies of the colonial administration and demanded representation in medical schools and in medical practice. By looking at the establishment of the All India Institute of Medical Sciences (AIIMS) in the early post-colonial period, the authors examine the rhetorical role that an appeal to science and technology had in the process of nation-building. Ultimately, Ruddock and Chakrabarti argue, the history of AIIMS and the role that this institution played in medical education showcase a persistent tension between economic growth, social welfare, and politics of medicine that can be better understood in light of the legacy of colonialism.

In his innovative case study of colonial medical education in twentieth-century Cameroon, Jean Baptiste Nzogue (chapter 7) delivers new findings on the specific conditions that shaped the creation, recruitment, and training of medical "assistants" from the region's Autochthonous populations. He also offers a critical comparative analysis of analogous auxiliary medical personnel in other colonialized contexts. Nzogue identifies the key structural effects of successive training models enacted by French colonial officials to produce "African doctors" who were deemed capable of treating regional diseases and improving health conditions for local populations – initially informal apprenticeship models, and later, formalized and professionalized medical education. His critical approach demonstrates how colonial structures and mentalities persist today in integrated systems of medical education, accreditation, and licensing in Cameroon and beyond.

In Chapter 8, Jethro Hernández Berrones examines in depth the history of free schools, which emerged in the context of the Mexican Revolution as private institutions providing inexpensive training in medicine, nursing, and midwifery. Hernández Berrones argues that this type of school constituted a transitional model of medical education. On the one hand, like their government-funded counterparts did in the 1930s, free schools exemplified the ideals of socialized medicine with its emphasis on public health and the delivery of health care to poor, working-class, and rural Mexicans in the 1920s. On the other hand, free schools were in tension with the state and with state-run medical schools: unlike the latter, free schools included homeopathy in their curricula, eschewed government funding and surveillance, and were deemed by bureaucrats to be sub-par. Despite the essential services that free schools provided to underserved people, the state fought these schools on multiple fronts, for instance by refusing to recognize their graduates' diplomas. By the 1940s, the government succeeded in closing most but not all of the free schools. Novel in its approach and content, Hernández Berrones's analysis illuminates in new ways the heterogeneity of models of medical education in the early twentieth century during a time of political upheaval.

Harry Yi-Jui Wu, in chapter 9, documents the changing status and treatment of human bodies used in anatomy education in Taiwan under different political regimes over the past century and a quarter. During the colonial period in which Japan controlled the island, the racialized bodies of Chinese and Indigenous peoples were exploited by both anthropologists and anatomists trained in the racist science of the late nineteenth century. In the postwar period, the state affirmed its authority over unclaimed deceased bodies and the bodies of executed political prisoners and distributed them to medical schools for anatomical dissections. In 1984, a major shift occurred: dead bodies were granted the status of personhood, and both family members and the medical profession acquired more power at the expense of the state. Finally, Wu recounts how, after the intervention of Buddhist organizations in the 1990s, the ways in which deceased bodies were used in medical education emphasized commemoration, empathy, and the remembrance of and gratitude to the unique individual whose body became a "silent mentor" for doctors-to-be. Wu argues that this respectful treatment and decolonization process led to more donations of bodies for the purpose of education, influenced similar changes in other countries as well, and led to an emphasis on humility in contemporary medical education.

In chapter 10, Geoffrey L. Hudson and Marion Maar recount the recent history of a world first in medical education: a mandatory medical school placement in Indigenous communities in Northern Canada. Other medical curricula have implemented cultural immersion as a means of raising consciousness, countering racism and implicit bias, and showing how cultural safety is an integral part of health care delivery – all of which this new program does as well. However, the Northern Ontario School of Medicine (NOSM) was the first to make this approach mandatory for all medical students. When the school rolled out its pilot program in 2005 – as the authors document – the learning curve was much steeper than official accounts depicted it at the time. Nevertheless, the school persisted. Working in partnership with Indigenous communities and with the help of community coordinators, NOSM continues to evaluate the effectiveness of this unique placement program in educating physicians to better serve Indigenous communities.

Hudson and Maar's chapter brings us close to the present, a time in which many countries, including Canada, are responding to reports and calls for action from Truth and Reconciliation Commissions. As the chapters in this section amply demonstrate, the history of medical education can make an important contribution to these conversations and to future social equity. Physicians are confronted by social disparities and health inequities in their work every day. Social justice, moreover, is recognized as the shared characteristic of the many disciplinary perspectives that contribute to the burgeoning discipline of health humanities.[32] By tracing the roots of medical education to its political historical pasts, the scholarship in this section shines a powerful light on persistent problems and inequalities still present in medical schools and professional medicine today.

3. Educational Spaces: Architectural, Gendered, Marginal, Digital

Specialized spaces have played essential roles in the development of medical education. The four chapters in this section foreground space as a medium and catalyst of both learning and teaching medicine. Objects of study include specialty hospitals, medical school buildings, and laboratories that connect to important changes in medical education, such as novel instructive technologies and new public health policies. While some explore the role that gender or marginality play in medical training (chapters 11 and 12), others foreground the issue of spatial organization and specialized "ways of seeing" within contexts of technological and curricular change (chapters 13 and 14).

Kim Girouard rediscovers in chapter 11 the suppressed history of a medical college for women founded in China in 1899. Her careful examination of the origins of Hackett Medical College for Women makes clear that female physicians, both North American and Chinese, were founding architects of science-based medical education in South China in the twentieth century. She shows how this teaching hospital designed to train and treat women – long disregarded and thereby able to flourish unaffected by enduring political turmoil – emerged as the premium site of medical education for men as well in the influential Guangdong province after World War I. Girouard's chapter provides a vital new gendered perspective on histories of medical education in China, and shows how cultural, medical, and professional concerns specific to women did so much to forge the character of Chinese medical education in the twentieth century.

In chapter 12, Heini Hakosalo investigates the intersection between tuberculosis (TB) sanatoria and medical education in Finland across three distinctive periods over the course of the twentieth century. She argues that several factors made sanatoria a popular and productive place for the training of future doctors, despite the fact that, at first glance, sanatoria appeared marginal both medically and geographically. These factors included government-led public health policy; the particular features of Finnish medical education, specialization, and certification; and changes in medical technology and medication that made medical skills related to TB care more widely applicable.

In a richly illustrated chapter, Annmarie Adams (chapter 13) offers an in-depth "reading of" and "looking at" two iconic buildings for medicine at McGill University – the neo-classical Strathcona and the modernist McIntyre. Adams explores how each of these very different buildings emerged from its own distinctive historical context. The Strathcona was built in the era of the Flexner Report (1910) and accommodated spaces such as anatomy laboratories and lecture halls equipped with permanent didactic illustrations. The McIntyre was designed in the 1960s, the era of the Hall Commission Report, as an internationally oriented tower that facilitated the connection between medical research and teaching. By illustrating how architecture shaped medical learning and experience, Adams makes a powerful case for the centrality of architecture as a way to understand critical aspects of medical education at two moments in time, as well as for the epistemic value of visual evidence.

Jenna Healey (chapter 14) also studies a highly distinctive teaching space in twentieth-century medicine: the digital anatomy laboratory. Healey's research shows how, in response to "curricular bloat" and looming cuts to teaching hours after World War II, many anatomy departments in North America introduced experimental educational technologies – new digital methods of viewing and evaluating anatomical knowledge – that threatened to undermine traditional cadaver-based teaching. Novel technologies and modes of instruction have disrupted and powered medical education for centuries. By identifying continuous and discontinuous pedagogical lines from human cadavers to video screens to algorithms, Healey's analysis adds a new late-twentieth-century perspective to historiographies of medical technology and training.

These chapters exemplify how historical perspectives on novel technological, instructional, or spatial interventions shed constructive light on contemporary issues in education in the health professions, including the use of self-directed learning technologies to address curricular overload, as well as programs that buckle under the weight of constant innovation without adequate assessment or maintenance of pedagogical methods. Focusing on educational spaces as an investigatory and analytical tool allows both historians and contemporary medical educators to understand and engage with these central issues.

4. *Professional Identities: Gender, Emotions, Performance*

The chapters in the fourth section all foreground processes by which individuals create professional and personal identities, particularly in relation to existing cultures of medicine. Scholars have shown that gender, emotions, and performance have all played decisive roles in determining who does (and who does not) enter the medical profession, as well as how one becomes (or is prevented from becoming) a physician. The authors make innovative use of fascinating primary sources – from fictional accounts of medical education (chapter 16) to memoirs and letters (chapters 15, 17, and 18) – in order to piece together ways in which gender and cultural expectations, personal and professional goals, happiness and anxieties, barriers and opportunities have influenced the lives and identities of those who sought to belong in the medical profession.

Laura Kelly, in chapter 15, shows how Irish medical students and their professors in the nineteenth and early twentieth centuries created a common culture and a collective identity through shared emotions. Public and private memoirs of medical students identified key sites – such as the dissection room and the hospital – that elicited strong and often shared emotions such as fear, anxiety, and happiness. Meanwhile, professors repeatedly emphasized the importance of empathy in the doctor-patient encounter as well as the necessity for diligence and hard work in attaining happiness. Thus, Kelly demonstrates how useful the history of emotions can be to the history of medical education.

In chapter 16, Jonathan Reinarz looks at medical education through a fictional lens – the work of the novelist Francis Brett Young, who attended medical school in early-twentieth-century Birmingham, England, and then went on to draw extensively from his real-life experiences to craft his autobiographical novels. By cross-checking fictional details with archival material, Reinarz demonstrates the potential utility of fiction in revealing not only the general social and cultural milieu in which medicine exists, but specific aspects of the history of medical education, such as a shared medical culture and professional identity in the making.

In chapter 17, Diana Moore shows how gender and politics interacted to shape the identity and eventful life of Jessie White Mario, a British woman who joined the Italian nationalist cause in the mid-nineteenth century. Determined to have an education in the healing professions, she turned to nursing in the aftermath of her rejection by British medical schools. Moore shows that White Mario's motivations were less medical and more political: she used nursing care as a means to enact her political goal of participating in the fight for Italian unification and republicanism led by Giuseppe Garibaldi and Giuseppe Mazzini. With her path to medical education blocked by a sexist and exclusionary establishment, she was prevented from becoming a physician. As Moore keenly detects in this analysis of *not belonging* in medicine, White Mario overcame the temporary pain of being barred from medical training to nevertheless achieve her political objectives.

In a Canadian context, Whitney Wood's case study (chapter 18) examines a critical shift in medical education in which obstetrics moved from being marginal to a significant set of skills in professionalized medicine by the end of the nineteenth century. Wood shows that medical students and early-career physicians considered obstetrics to be an increasingly important aspect of general physicians' professional identity, and thus sought out formalized clinical instruction and bedside experience in both obstetrics and gynecological examinations. This included post-graduate education beyond a young doctor's local Canadian contexts. Wood's work expands existing scholarship on men's medical education at the end of the nineteenth century, as well as the professionalization of medicine and its stringent hierarchies between physician and patient that subsequently undermined women's own expertise and knowledge of childbirth. By knitting together gender and sociological analyses, this chapter shows how constructions of maleness, medical authority, and professional identity coalesced in the experiences of young physicians at a critical moment: when obstetrics gained prominence in medical education and changed relations between men and women, physician and patient in the birthing room.

5. History Matters: Medical Practice and Historical Thinking

The final three chapters use the work and experiences of Jacalyn Duffin to explore relationships between history and medicine. They consider the rationale for incorporating the history of medicine into medical training, an area of medical pedagogy to which Duffin has devoted considerable efforts in her research and teaching. These chapters illuminate in more detail the significance of her contributions to her discipline, students, and peers. The sobering disruption of the COVID-19 pandemic, with its myriad contexts and complex political and cultural dimensions, has reaffirmed that historical analyses and thinking matter more than ever to those who train and teach in health care professions.

Frank Huisman (chapter 19) describes recent efforts by him and his colleagues in the Netherlands to integrate the history of medicine into the medical curriculum. Medical historians working in clinical settings, Huisman emphasizes, must pay attention to Jacalyn Duffin's observation: without a handbook or textbook (long considered to be an essential teaching tool in basic sciences and clinical specialties) neither medical students nor curriculum committees take our discipline seriously. Influenced and inspired by Duffin's infiltrative and determined strategies, Huisman explains the didactic and thematic choices that his team made in producing *Leerboek medische geschiedenis* (*Handbook of Medical History*) for Dutch medical schools.

In chapter 20, Susan Lamb explores and celebrates various dimensions of Jacalyn Duffin's scholarly life and corpus. Blending biographical and historiographical insights, she puts Duffin's expansive and diverse body of work into the context of her dual practices of history and medicine, and shows some of the ways Duffin successfully bridged disciplinary boundaries in research, teaching, and advocacy. Reading across her corpus as well as her academic choices, Lamb concludes, makes Duffin's character as a humanist scholar unmistakable: disciplined, curious, critical, freethinking, and always attuned to the constructed nature of the knowledge she analyzes, creates, translates, and applies.

The final chapter, chapter 21, curated by Delia Gavrus and Susan Lamb, takes the form of a wide-ranging interview with Jacalyn Duffin. This original oral history illuminates not only Duffin's personal journeys to becoming a physician and historian, but also the educational contexts of the professions of medicine and history in late-twentieth-century North America and France. Together with the essays by Huisman and Lamb, Duffin's testimony makes a powerful case for the value of history to medical education and of historical thinking to medical practice.

A TRIBUTE TO JACALYN DUFFIN

A wide call for original, innovative histories of medical learning and teaching seemed a fitting tribute for an exceptional scholar, physician, teacher, mentor, and activist in whose work medical education has featured so prominently. The overwhelming response from historians to our call for papers indicates both current scholarly interest in the subject and the desire to celebrate Jackie, as she is widely and warmly known. Jackie Duffin has advanced the history of medicine with exemplary research and service, and she has demonstrated how history helps medical trainees become better doctors. She has made it a lifelong practice to uplift students and colleagues, both intellectually and professionally, and she continues to do all of this unabated by her voluntary move to emerita status at age sixty-five.

Jackie Duffin graduated in medicine from the University of Toronto in the 1970s and trained in internal medicine and hematology. As she explains in the oral history interview (chapter 21), she then earned a doctorate in the philosophy and history of science from the Sorbonne under the direction of the well-known scholar Mirko Grmek. In 1988, she was appointed Hannah Chair in the History of Medicine at Queen's University, one of a handful of distinguished professorships established by AMS Healthcare. At the same time, as a fellow of the Royal College of Physicians and Surgeons of Canada, she practised and taught hematology at Queen's. Duffin wielded this unique interdisciplinary position to enrich the history of medicine as well as generations of future doctors.

Her original contributions to knowledge are so many, and so varied, and her achievements and honours so numerous, that they can only be highlighted here briefly. She is the author of four historical monographs and two outstanding biographies, including the award-winning *To See with a Better Eye: A Life of R.T.H. Laennec*.[33] Her peer-reviewed studies in humanities and science journals number over one hundred.[34] In addition, Duffin has edited two scholarly volumes, and, most recently, the memoirs of a female scientist and Holocaust survivor.[35] Her intellectual orientation combines multi-disciplinary approaches with an abiding interest in conceptualizations of disease, diagnostic semiology, the nature of scientific evidence, medical technology, health policy, and religion and medicine.

The originality and excellence of her historical research is recognized internationally, as reflected in a steady stream of invitations from around the world to deliver keynote addresses. At home, she is a fellow of the Canadian Academy of Health Sciences and the Royal Society of Canada for her substantial contributions to knowledge. She has recently been appointed to the Order of Canada for "her leadership as an academic and mentor in the field of medical history."[36] Duffin has remained in constant service to the discipline of the history of medicine in North America; this includes her leadership as president of both the Canadian Society for the History of Medicine–Société canadienne d'histoire de la médecine (CSHM-SCHM) and the American Society for the History of Medicine (AAHM). Remarkably, though not surprisingly, within the space of a few weeks in the spring of 2019, she accepted the AAHM's Genevieve Miller Lifetime Achievement Award from fellow historians and was inducted into the Canadian Medical Hall of Fame by her peers in medicine. Shortly thereafter we had the pleasure of interviewing her for this book.

The inspiration for the focus of this celebratory volume was Jackie Duffin's transformative contributions to medical education through the teaching and practice of history. She has modelled her educational approach on the self-described goal of infiltrating the medical curriculum with the lessons and tools of history.[37] At Queen's University, she successfully mapped over twenty hours of history teaching onto corresponding disciplinary areas in the medical curriculum such as anatomy, physiology, obstetrics, pharmacology, and of course her own specialty, hematology. Her textbook, *History of Medicine: A Scandalously Short Introduction*, is now in its third edition and is treasured by readers globally.[38]

According to Duffin, history of medicine prepares medical students for their future medical practice in several ways. First, it makes them question the durability and unassailability of what they are taught in medical school, and therefore readies them to adapt to the changes in medical knowledge and ethics that will inevitably occur during their careers. Second, her students learn that history's utility is not in memorizing events or dates, but in integrating historical analysis as a valuable component of clinical reasoning.[39] Duffin's innovative historical research on medical education has led to greater awareness of social injustices within medical education. She has examined the covert use of discriminatory admission quotas in North American medical schools that limited places for Jewish and female physicians, for example, and has demonstrated that tuition fees fluctuated based on external political influences that reduced many students' accessibility to medical training.[40] Just as historical evidence motivates Duffin's own advocacy on behalf of patients and Canada's universal health care system, her teaching in the faculties of Health Sciences (medicine and nursing), Law, Education, and Arts and Sciences (philosophy and history) has equipped countless health care providers and policy-makers with tools to effect just and lasting change.[41]

This volume's scholarship, like its honoree, is original, provocative, and energized by activism. These historical case studies of what it means to teach, learn, and belong in medicine, past and present, are warmly dedicated to Jackie in celebration of *her* outstanding contributions to medicine, the history of medicine, and medical education.

NOTES

1   Brosnan and Turner, eds., *Handbook of the Sociology of Medical Education*; Prentice, *Bodies in Formation*; Wendland, *A Heart for the Work*; Geer et al., *Boys in White*; Merton, Reader, and Kendal, eds., *The Student-Physician*.

2   See Sylvestre et al., "The Tools at Their Fingertips."

3   See, for example, Sam, Hameed, and Meeran, "Medical Students Are the Physician's Apprentices"; Batlle, "Professionalism from the Apprentice's Perspective"; Brooks, "Medical Education and the Tyranny of Competency"; Chen, "The Hidden Curriculum of Medical School."

4   Boudreau, Cassell, and Fuks, *Physicianship and the Rebirth of Medical Education*.

5   See Jones et al., "Making the Case for History in Medical Education"; Ludmerer, "The History of Medicine in Medical Education"; Arrizabalaga, "Does History Matter?"; Chowkwanyun, "The Seat at the Table Problem"; Metcalfe and Stuart, "A Short History of Providing Medical History"; Duffin, "Infiltrating the Curriculum"; Duffin, "Editorial: Why History of Medicine in the Undergraduate Curriculum"; Warner, "The Humanising Power of Medical History"; Duffin, "On Humanities in Medical Education"; Duffin, "Infiltrating the Curriculum"; Duffin and Weisberg, "Evoking the Moral Imagination"; Bylebyl, ed., *Teaching the History of Medicine at a Medical Center*; Galdston, *On the Utility of Medical History*.

6   Jones et al., "Making the Case for History in Medical Education," 626.

7   Warner, Pols, and Thompson, "Introduction," 1.

8   Nutton and Porter, "Introduction," 13. For an exploration of some of these tensions, see the essays in the latter volume.

9   Abraham, "Psychiatry in American Medical Education; Brazelton, "Western Medical Education on Trial"; Solberg, *Reforming Medical Education*; Rosner, *Medical Education in the Age of Improvement*.

10   Miller and Weiss, "Medical Education Reform"; Fedunkiw, *Rockefeller Foundation Funding*; Heaman, *St. Mary's*; Waddington, *Medical Education at St*

Bartholomew's Hospital; Ludmerer, *Time to Heal*; Lawrence, *Charitable Knowledge*;
Nutton and Porter, eds., *The History of Medical Education in Britain*; McPhedran,
Canadian Medical Schools; Barzansky and Gevitz, eds., *Beyond Flexner*; Ludmerer,
Learning to Heal; Ludmerer, *Let Me Heal*.

11 There is a growing historical literature that critically analyzes the role medicine has played, and continues to play, in settler colonialism, especially on the
topics of unethical and racist medical research and experimentation,
Indigenous health history, health policies, and the delivery of health care.
There is a problematic dearth of scholarship, however, specifically on the history of physicians' education from this critical perspective. Scholars have
written about the education of nurses and midwives, including Indigenous
nurses, in settler colonial contexts. See McCallum, *Indigenous Women, Work, and
History*; Charbonneau-Dahlen and Crow, "A Brief Overview of the History of
American Indian Nurses"; Meijer Drees, "Training Aboriginal Nurses." On
self-determination of Indigenous communities in the context of nursing education, see Gregory et al., "Self-Determination and the Swampy Cree Tribal
Council." More generally on settler colonialism and medicine see Anderson,
"The Colonial Medicine of Settler States"; McCallum, "Starvation,
Experimentation, Segregation, and Trauma."

12 Chen, Reich, and Ryan, eds., *Medical Education in East Asia*; Pols, Thompson, and
Warner, eds., *Translating the Body*; Duffin, "Salerno, Saints, and Sutton's Law."

13 Bonner, *Becoming a Physician*.

14 Horstmanshoff, *Hippocrates and Medical Education*.

15 Flexner, *Medical Education*.

16 Bonner, "Abraham Flexner and the Historians"; Carroll, "Creating the
Modern Physician"; Duffin, "Did Abraham Flexner Spark the Founding of
CMAJ?"; Dyhouse, "Driving Ambitions"; Gevitz, "From Flexner to Elliott";
Kruse Thomas, *Deluxe Jim Crow*; Ludmerer, *Learning to Heal*; Markowitz and
Rosner, "Doctors in Crisis"; Moehling et al., "Shut Down and Shut Out";
Penney, "Marked For Slaughter"; Steinecke, "Progress for Whose Future?";
Ward, *Black Physicians*; Weiss and Miller, "The Social Transformation of
American Medical Education"; Wheatley, *Politics of Philanthropy*.

17 Warner, Pols, and Thompson, "Introduction," 2–3. On medical education in
the context of colonialism and empire, see also Hochmuth, "Patterns of
Medical Culture in Colonial Bengal"; Verma, "Western Medicine,
Indigenous Doctors and Colonial Medical Education"; Haynes,
"Fit to Practice."

18 Duffin, "What Goes Around, Comes Around."

19 Bates, "Yesterday's Doctors."

20 Martucci, "Religion, Medicine, and Politics"; Golden and Abel, "Modern
Medical Science and the Divine Providence of God."

21   Greene and Podolsky, "Keeping Modern in Medicine."

22   Kelly, *Irish Medical Education*; Poirier, *Doctors in the Making*; Warner and
     Edmonson, *Dissection*; Poirier, "Medical Education and the Embodied
     Physician"; Geer et al., *Boys in White*.

23   Wangui, "'Something Wasn't Clean'"; Ward, *Black Physicians in the Jim Crow
     South*; Savitt, "Money versus Mission"; Savitt, "Four African-American
     Proprietary Medical Colleges."

24   Duffin, "The Queen's Jews"; Halperin, "The Jewish Problem in U.S. Medical
     Education."

25   Hamilton, "Canada's First Indigenous Physician?"; Verma, "Western
     Medicine, Indigenous Doctors and Colonial Medical Education." More his-
     torical research has been done on the experience of Indigenous nurses; see
     for instance McCallum, *Indigenous Women, Work, and History*; Meijer Drees,
     "Indian Hospitals and Aboriginal Nurses."

26   Appel, "Writing Women into Medical History in the 1930s"; Duffin and
     Stuart, "Feminization of Canadian Medicine"; More, Fee, and Parry, eds.,
     Women Physicians and the Cultures of Medicine; Tuchman, *Science Has No Sex*;
     Duffin, "CSHM/SCHM Presidential Address: The Quota"; Wear, ed., *Women in
     Medical Education*; Bonner, *To the Ends of the Earth*; Apple, ed., *Women, Health, and
     Medicine in America*; Ludmerer, "Seeking Parity for Women in Academic
     Medicine: A Historical Perspective."

27   Hogarth, *Medicalizing Blackness*; Lux, *Separate Beds*; McCallum and Perry,
     Structures of Indifference.

28   Puschmann, *A History of Medical Education*.

29   Norwood, *Medical Education in the United States*; O'Malley, *The History of Medical
     Education*.

30   Numbers, ed., *The Education of American Physicians*.

31   Soto Laveaga, "Largo Dislocare."

32   Klugman and Lamb, eds., *Research Methods in Health Humanities*.

33   Duffin, *Langstaff*; Duffin, *To See with a Better Eye*; Duffin, *Lovers and Livers*; Duffin,
     Medical Miracles; Duffin, *Medical Saints*; Duffin, *Stanley's Dream*.

34   The research themes of Duffin's impressive body of journal publications
     are discussed in chapter 20. At the time this volume was printed, Jacalyn
     Duffin's complete bibliography was available on her website: http://www.
     jacalynduffin.ca.

35   Duffin, ed., *Clio in the Clinic*; Duffin and Sweetman, eds., *SARS in Context*;
     Robinson, *Heaven, Hell, and Purgatory*.

36   "Governor General Announces 61 New Appointments to the Order of
     Canada – December 30, 2020," https://www.gg.ca/en/activities/2020/
     governor-general-announces-61-new-appointments-order-canada.

37   Duffin, "Infiltrating the Curriculum."

38   Duffin, *History of Medicine: A Scandalously Short Introduction.*
39   Duffin, "A Hippocratic Triangle."
40   Duffin, "The Queen's Jews"; Duffin, "CSHM/SCHM Presidential Address: The
      Quota"; Duffin, "What Goes Around, Comes Around."
41   Duffin and Weisberg, "Evoking the Moral Imagination."

BIBLIOGRAPHY

Abraham, Tara H. "Psychiatry in American Medical Education: The Case of
    Harvard's Medical School, 1900–1945." *Canadian Bulletin of Medical History* 35,
    no. 1 (2018): 63–93.
Anderson, Warwick. "The Colonial Medicine of Settler States: Comparing Histories
    · of Indigenous Health." *Health and History* 9, no. 2 (2007): 144–54.
Appel, Toby A. "Writing Women into Medical History in the 1930s: Kate Campbell
    Hurd-Mead and 'Medical Women' of the Past and Present." *Bulletin of the History
    of Medicine* 88, no. 3 (2014): 457–92.
Apple, Rima, ed. *Women, Health, and Medicine in America: A Historical Handbook.* New
    Brunswick, NJ: Rutgers University Press, 1992.
Arrizabalaga, Jon. "Does History Matter? Commentary on 'Making the Case for
    History in Medical Education.'" *Journal of the History of Medicine and Allied Sciences*
    70, no. 4 (2015): 653–5.
Barzansky, Barbara, and Norman Gevitz, eds. *Beyond Flexner: Medical Education in the
    Twentieth Century.* New York: Greenwood Press, 1992.
Bates, Victoria. "Yesterday's Doctors: The Human Aspects of Medical Education in
    Britain, 1957–93." *Medical History* 61, no. 1 (2017): 48–65.
Batlle, Juan Carlos. "Professionalism from the Apprentice's Perspective." *The American
    Journal of Bioethics* 4, no. 2 (2004): W11–12.
Bonner, Thomas Neville. *Becoming a Physician: Medical Education in Britain, France,
    Germany, and the United States, 1750–1945.* Oxford, UK: Oxford University Press,
    1995.
– *To the Ends of the Earth: Women's Search for Education in Medicine.* Cambridge, MA:
    Harvard University Press, 1992.
– "Abraham Flexner and the Historians." *Journal of the History of Medicine and Allied
    Sciences* 45, no. 1 (1990): 3–10.
Boudreau, J. Donald, Eric Cassell, and Abraham Fuks. *Physicianship and the Rebirth of
    Medical Education.* Oxford, UK: Oxford University Press, 2018.
Brazelton, Mary Augusta. "Western Medical Education on Trial: The Endurance of
    Peking Union Medical College, 1949–1985." *Twentieth-Century China* 40, no. 2
    (2015): 126–45.
Brooks, M.A. "Medical Education and the Tyranny of Competency." *Perspectives in
    Biology and Medicine* 52, no. 1 (2009): 90–102.

Bylebyl, Jerome, ed. *Teaching the History of Medicine at a Medical Center.* Baltimore, MD: Johns Hopkins University Press, 1982.

Caragh, Brosnan, and Bryan S. Turner, eds. *Handbook of the Sociology of Medical Education.* New York: Routledge, 2009.

Carroll, Katherine. "Creating the Modern Physician: The Architecture of American Medical Schools in the Era of Medical Education Reform." *Journal of the Society of Architectural Historians* 75, no. 1 (2016): 48–73.

Charbonneau-Dahlen, B., and K. Crow. "A Brief Overview of the History of American Indian Nurses." *Journal of Cultural Diversity* 23, no. 3 (2016): 79–90.

Chen, Lincoln, Michael Reich, and Jennifer Ryan, eds. *Medical Education in East Asia: Past and Future.* Bloomington: Indiana University Press, 2017.

Chen, Pauline W. "The Hidden Curriculum of Medical School." *New York Times*, 29 January 2009. https://nyti.ms/2mnUxna.

Chowkwanyun, Merlin. "The Seat at the Table Problem: Broadening Reception for Historians of Medicine and Public Health." *Journal of the History of Medicine and Allied Sciences* 70, no. 4 (2015): 661–6.

Czajkowska Robinson, Halina Maria. *Heaven, Hell, and Purgatory: A Canadian Memoir of a Happy Polish Childhood, Nazi Horror, and Swedish Refuge.* Edited by Jacalyn Duffin. Toronto: Poison Spindle Press, 2020.

Duffin, Jacalyn, ed. *Clio in the Clinic: History in Medical Practice.* Toronto: University of Toronto Press, 2005.

– "CSHM/SCHM Presidential Address: The Quota: 'An Equally Serious Problem' for Us All." *Canadian Bulletin of Medical History* 19, no. 2 (2002): 327–50.

– "Editorial: Why History of Medicine in the Undergraduate Curriculum." *University of Toronto Medical Journal* 88, no. 3 (2011): 127–8.

– "A Hippocratic Triangle: History, Clinician-Historians, and Future Doctors." In *Locating Medical History: The Stories and Their Meanings*, edited by Frank Huisman and John Harley Warner, 432–49. Baltimore, MD: Johns Hopkins University Press, 2014.

– *History of Medicine: A Scandalously Short Introduction.* Toronto: University of Toronto Press, 1999.

– "Infiltrating the Curriculum: An Integrative Approach to History for Medical Students." *Journal of Medical Humanities* 16, no. 3 (1995): 155–74.

– "Infiltrating the Curriculum: Triumphs and Disasters in Bringing History to Future Doctors." In *Students Matter: The Rewards of University Teaching*, edited by J. Kevin Dorsey and P.K. Rangachari, 74–92. Springfield: Southern Illinois University School of Medicine, 2012.

– *Langstaff: A Nineteenth-Century Medical Life.* Toronto: University of Toronto, 1993.

– *Lovers and Livers: Disease Concepts in History.* Toronto: University of Toronto Press, 2005.

– *Medical Miracles: Doctors, Saints, and Healing in the Modern World.* New York: Oxford University Press, 2009.

– *Medical Saints: Cosmas and Damian in a Postmodern World.* New York: Oxford University Press, 2013.

– "On Humanities in Medical Education." *Dermanities* 4, no. 1 (2003): a2.

– "Salerno, Saints, and Sutton's Law: On the Origin of Europe's 'First' Medical School." *Medical Hypotheses* 73 (2009): 265–7.

– *Stanley's Dream: The Medical Expedition to Easter Island.* Montreal, QC, and Kingston, ON: McGill-Queen's University Press, 2019.

– *To See with a Better Eye: A Life of R.T.H. Laennec.* Princeton, NJ: Princeton University Press, 1998.

– "The Queen's Jews: Religion, Race, and Change in Twentieth-Century Canada." *Canadian Journal of History* 49, no. 3 (December 2014): 369.

– "What Goes Around, Comes Around: A History of Medical Tuition." *Canadian Medical Association Journal* 164, no. 1 (2001): 50–6.

Duffin, Jacalyn, and Meryn Stuart. "Feminization of Canadian Medicine: Voices from the Second Wave." *Canadian Bulletin of Medical History* 29, no. 1 (2012): 83–100.

Duffin, Jacalyn, and Arthur Sweetman, eds. *SARS in Context: Memory, History, Policy.* Montreal, QC, and Kingston, ON: McGill-Queen's University Press, 2006.

Duffin, Jacalyn, and Mark Weisberg. "Evoking the Moral Imagination: Using Stories to Teach Ethics and Professionalism to Nursing, Medical, and Law Students." *Change, The Magazine of Higher Learning* 27, no. 1 (1995): 20–7 (also published in *Journal of Medical Humanities* 16, no. 4: 247–63).

Dyhouse, Carol. "Driving Ambitions: Women in Pursuit of a Medical Education, 1890–1939." *Women's History Review* 7, no. 3 (1998): 321–43.

Fedunkiw, Marianne P. *Rockefeller Foundation Funding and Medical Education in Toronto, Montreal and Halifax.* Montreal, QC, and Kingston, ON: McGill-Queen's University Press, 2005.

Flexner, Abraham. *Medical Education in the United States and Canada.* New York: Carnegie Foundation for the Advancement of Teaching, 1910.

Galdston, Iago. *On the Utility of Medical History.* New York: International Universities Press, 1957.

Geer, Blanche, et al. *Boys in White: Student Culture in Medical School.* Chicago, IL: University of Chicago Press, 1961.

Gevitz, Norman. "From Flexner to Elliott: The Educational Survey Movement and the Health Professions." *Pharmacy in History* 30, no. 3 (1988): 120–8.

Golden, Janet, and Emily K. Abel. "Modern Medical Science and the Divine Providence of God: Rethinking the Place of Religion in Postwar U.S. Medical History." *Journal of the History of Medicine and Allied Sciences* 69, no. 4 (2014): 580–603.

Greene, Jeremy A., and Scott H. Podolsky. "Keeping Modern in Medicine: Pharmaceutical Promotion and Physician Education in Postwar America." *Bulletin of the History of Medicine* 83, no. 2 (2009): 331–77.

Gregory, David, Mary Jane McCallum, Brenda Elias, and Karen Grant. "Self-Determination and the Swampy Cree Tribal Council: A Case Study Involving Nursing Education in Northern Manitoba." *The Canadian Journal of Nursing Research* 40, no. 2 (2008): 132–49.

Halperin, Edward C. "The Jewish Problem in U.S. Medical Education, 1920–1955." *Journal of the History of Medicine and Allied Sciences* 56, no. 2 (2001): 140–67.

Hamilton, Michelle A. "Canada's First Indigenous Physician? The Story of Dr. O (1841–1907)." *Canadian Journal of Surgery* 60, no. 1 (2017): 8–10.

Haynes, Douglas Melvin. *Fit to Practice: Empire, Race, Gender, and the Making of British Medicine, 1850–1980.* Rochester, NY: University of Rochester Press, 2017.

Heaman, Elspeth. *St. Mary's: The History of a London Teaching Hospital.* Montreal, QC, and Kingston, ON: McGill-Queen's University Press, 2003.

Hochmuth, Christian. "Patterns of Medical Culture in Colonial Bengal, 1835–1880." *Bulletin of the History of Medicine* 80, no. 1 (2006): 39–72.

Hogarth, Rana A. *Medicalizing Blackness: Making Racial Difference in the Atlantic World, 1780–1840.* Chapel Hill, NC: University of North Carolina Press, 2017.

Horstmanshoff, Manfred, ed. *Hippocrates and Medical Education.* Leiden, Netherlands: Brill, 2010.

Jones, David S., Jeremy A. Greene, Jacalyn Duffin, and John Harley Warner. "Making the Case for History in Medical Education." *Journal of the History of Medicine and Allied Sciences* 70, no. 4 (2015): 165–94.

Kelly, Laura. *Irish Medical Education and Student Culture, c. 1850–1950.* Liverpool, UK: University of Liverpool University Press, 2017.

Klugman, Craig M., and Erin Gentry Lamb, eds. *Research Methods in Health Humanities.* Oxford, UK: Oxford University Press, 2019.

Kruse Thomas, Karen. *Deluxe Jim Crow: Civil Rights and American Health Policy, 1935–1954.* Athens, GA: University of Georgia Press, 2011.

Lawrence, Susan. *Charitable Knowledge: Hospital Pupils and Practitioners in Eighteenth-Century London.* Cambridge: Cambridge University Press, 1996.

Ludmerer, Kenneth M. "The History of Medicine in Medical Education." *Journal of the History of Medicine and Allied Sciences* 70, no. 4 (2015): 656–60.

– *Time to Heal: American Medical Education from the Turn of the Century to the Era of Managed Care.* New York: Oxford University Press, 1999.

– *Learning to Heal: The Development of American Medical Education.* New York: Basic Books, 1985.

– *Let Me Heal: The Opportunity to Preserve Excellence in American Medicine.* New York: Oxford University Press, 2015.

– "Seeking Parity for Women in Academic Medicine: A Historical Perspective."
    Academic Medicine 95, no. 10 (2020): 1485–87.

Lux, Maureen K. *Separate Beds: A History of Indian Hospitals in Canada, 1920s–1980s.*
    Toronto: University of Toronto Press, 2016.

Markowitz, Gerald E., and David Karl Rosner. "Doctors in Crisis: A Study of the
    Use of Medical Education Reform to Establish Modern Professional Elitism in
    Medicine." *American Quarterly* 25, no. 1 (1973): 83–107.

Martucci, Jessica. "Religion, Medicine, and Politics: Catholic Physicians' Guilds in
    America, 1909–32." *Bulletin of the History of Medicine* 92, no. 2 (2018): 287–316.

McCallum, Mary Jane Logan. *Indigenous Women, Work, and History, 1940–1980.*
    Winnipeg: University of Manitoba Press, 2014.

– "Starvation, Experimentation, Segregation, and Trauma: Words for Reading
    Indigenous Health History." *Canadian Historical Review* 98, no. 1 (2017): 96–113.

McCallum, Mary Jane Logan, and Adele Perry. *Structures of Indifference: An Indigenous
    Life and Death in a Canadian City.* Winnipeg: University of Manitoba Press, 2018.

McPhedran, N. Tait. *Canadian Medical Schools: Two Centuries of Medical History, 1822–
    1992.* Montreal, QC: Harvest House, 1993.

Meijer Drees, Laurie. "Indian Hospitals and Aboriginal Nurses: Canada and
    Alaska." *Canadian Bulletin of Medical History* 27, no. 1 (2010): 139–61.

– "Training Aboriginal Nurses: The Indian Health Services in Northwestern
    Canada, 1939–75." In *Caregiving on the Periphery: Historical Perspectives on Nursing and
    Midwifery in Canada*, edited by Myra Rutherdale, 181–209. Montreal, QC, and
    Kingston, ON: McGill-Queen's University Press, 2010.

Miller, Lynn E., and Richard M. Weiss. "Medical Education Reform Efforts and
    Failures of U.S. Medical Schools, 1870–1930." *Journal of the History of Medicine
    and Allied Sciences* 63, no. 3 (2008): 348–87.

Merton, Robert K., George G. Reader, and Patricia L. Kendal, eds. *The Student-
    Physician: Introductory Studies in the Sociology of Medical Education.* Cambridge, MA:
    Harvard University Press, 1957.

Metcalfe, N.H., and E. Stuart. "A Short History of Providing Medical History within
    the British Medical Undergraduate Curriculum." *Medical Humanities* 4, no. 1
    (2014): 31–7.

Moehling, Carolyn M., Gregory T. Niemesh, and Melissa A. Thomasson. "Shut
    Down and Shut Out: Women Physicians in the Era of Medical Education Reform."
    Ostrom Workshop Working Paper, 2019. https://ostromworkshop.indiana.edu/
    pdf/piep2019/moehling-niemesh-thomasson.pdf.

More, Ellen S., Elizabeth Fee, and Manon Parry, eds. *Women Physicians and the Cultures
    of Medicine.* Baltimore, MD: Johns Hopkins University Press, 2012.

Norwood, William Frederick. *Medical Education in the United States before the Civil War.*
    Philadelphia, PA: University of Philadelphia Press, 1944.

Numbers, Ronald, ed. *The Education of American Physicians: Historical Essays.* Berkeley,
  CA: University of California Press, 1980.
Nutton, Vivian, and Roy Porter, eds. *The History of Medical Education in Britain.*
  Amsterdam: Rodopi, 1995.
O'Malley, C.D. *The History of Medical Education.* Berkeley, CA: University of California
  Press, 1970.
Penney, S.M. "'Marked for Slaughter': The Halifax Medical College and the Wrong
  Kind of Reform, 1868–1910." *Acadiensis* 19, no. 1 (1989): 27–51.
Pols, Hans Thompson, C. Michelle, and John Harley Warner, eds. *Translating the Body:
  Medical Education in Southeast Asia.* Singapore: National University of Singapore
  Press, 2017.
Poirier, Suzanne. *Doctors in the Making: Memoirs and Medical Education.* Iowa City, IA:
  University of Iowa Press, 2009.
– "Medical Education and the Embodied Physician." *Literature and Medicine* 25, no. 2
  (2006): 522–52.
Prentice, Rachel. *Bodies in Formation: An Ethnography of Anatomy and Surgery Education.*
  Durham, NC: Duke University Press, 2013.
Puschmann, Theodor. *A History of Medical Education: From the Most Remote to the Most
  Recent Times.* Translated by Evan H. Hare. London: H.K. Lewis, 1891.
Rosner, Lisa. *Medical Education in the Age of Improvement: Edinburgh Students and Apprentices,
  1760–1826.* Edinburgh: Edinburgh University Press, 1991.
Rothstein, William G. *American Medical Schools and the Practice of Medicine.* Oxford, UK:
  Oxford University Press, 1987.
Sam, Amire H., Saira Hameed, and Karim Meeran. "Medical Students Are the
  Physician's Apprentices." *BMJ: British Medical Journal* 351 (30 Nov. 2015–6 Dec.
  2015): h5671.
Savitt, Todd L. *Race and Medicine in Nineteenth- and Early-Twentieth-Century America.* Kent,
  OH: Kent State University Press, 2007.
– "Four African-American Proprietary Medical Colleges: 1888–1923." *Journal of the
  History of Medicine and Allied Sciences* 55, no. 3 (2000): 203–55.
– "Money versus Mission at an African-American Medical School: Knoxville College
  Medical Department, 1895–1900." *Bulletin of the History of Medicine* 75, no. 4
  (2001): 680–716.
Solberg, Winton U. *Reforming Medical Education: The University of Illinois College of
  Medicine, 1880–1920.* Urbana, IL: University of Illinois Press, 2009.
Soto Laveaga, Gabriela. "Largo Dislocare: Connecting Microhistories to Remap and
  Recenter Histories of Science." *History and Technology* 34, no. 1 (2018): 21–30.
Steinecke, A., and C. Terrell. "Progress for Whose Future? The Impact of the
  Flexner Report on Medical Education in the Era of Medical Education Reform."
  Academic Medicine 85, no. 2 (2010): 236–45.

Sylvestre, Paul, Heather Castleden, Jeff Denis, Debbie Martin, and Amy Bombay. "The Tools at Their Fingertips: How Settler Colonial Geographies Shape Medical Educators' Strategies for Grappling with Anti-Indigenous Racism." *Social Science and Medicine* 235 (2019): 112363.

Tuchman, Arleen Marcia. *Science Has No Sex: The Life of Marie Zakrzewska, M.D.* Studies in Social Medicine. Chapel Hill, NC: University of North Carolina Press, 2006.

Verma, Rupalee. "Western Medicine, Indigenous Doctors and Colonial Medical Education: A Case of Desire for 'Hegemony' in Conflict with Demands of 'Colonial Partiality.'" *Itinerario* 19, no. 3 (1995): 130–41.

Waddington, Keir. *Medical Education at St Bartholomew's Hospital, 1123–1995.* Woodbridge, UK: Boydell Press, 2003.

Wangui, Muigai. "'Something Wasn't Clean': Black Midwifery, Birth, and Postwar Medical Education in *All My Babies.*" *Bulletin of the History of Medicine* 93, no. 1 (2019): 82–113.

Ward Jr., Thomas J. *Black Physicians in the Jim Crow South.* Fayetteville, AR: University of Arkansas Press, 2003.

Warner, John Harley. "The Humanising Power of Medical History: Responses to Biomedicine in the 20th Century United States." *Medical Humanities* 37 (2011): 91–6.

Warner, John Harley, and James M. Edmonson. *Dissection: Photographs of a Rite of Passage in American Medicine 1880–1930.* New York: Blast Books, 2009.

Wear, Delese, ed. *Women in Medical Education: An Anthology of Experience.* Albany: SUNY Press, 1996.

Weiss, Richard, and Lynn E. Miller. "The Social Transformation of American Medical Education: Class, Status, and Party Influences on Occupational Closure, 1902–1919." *The Sociological Quarterly* 51, no. 4 (2010): 550–75.

Wendland, Claire L. *A Heart for the Work: Journey through an African Medical School.* Chicago, IL: University of Chicago Press, 2010.

Wheatley, Steven C. *The Politics of Philanthropy: Abraham Flexner and Medical Education.* Madison: University of Wisconsin Press, 1989.

PART ONE

Knowledge Transmission: Text, Translation, Practical Experience

1

Knowing and Transposing: Text, Medicine, and Learning in the Medieval Non-West

M.A. Mujeeb Khan

This chapter examines the place of text within and between traditions of medical education. Texts are often considered to be a means to disseminate information or a mode of transmission, but their agency along with that of their authors is lost in favour of an assumed but abstract continuum of knowledge. How then do texts function in the history of medical knowledge and its transmission? Linear trajectories are often inevitable when constructing long histories of knowledge, but historians should complicate this artificial linearity. This chapter takes medical education as a case study to demonstrate how texts were utilized in the medieval world for learning. It focuses on the medieval Islamicate and Japanese medical traditions to explore how foreign and local texts were incorporated into education. To understand the dynamics between text and learning in medical education, it surveys a range of texts created and repurposed for didactic objectives, including the doxographical encyclopedic works of the tenth-century medical writers Abū Bakr al-Rāzī (864–925/932) and Tanba no Yasuyori (912–95). The examination will consist in a case study of each culture's medical texts to understand how texts and textual expository style changed in the context of medical education within each tradition. A comparative examination will allow greater insights into the broader features of text and medical education within medieval non-Western cultures.

MEDIEVAL MEDICAL CULTURES AND TRANSPOSITION

Both early Islamicate and Japanese medicine developed in a period clearly demarcated as "medieval" in the study of world history. Historiographically, pre-modern medicine is often divided into the ancient, medieval, and early modern periods, whereas so-called "non-Western" medicine is identified as "Eastern," "traditional," or simply "non-Western." Shifting away from these traditional historiographical approaches to non-Western medical history, this chapter premises the study of Islamic and Japanese medical literary traditions as both inextricably connected to their origins in neighbouring traditions and uniquely local to their socio-cultural landscapes in each respective region. In other words, rather than a study of Greek medicine in the Islamicate world or Chinese medicine in Japan, this study is an examination of medicine in the Islamicate world and Japan. Both the early Islamicate world and early Japan, as new cultures, fully appropriated their neighbouring traditions. This inevitably led to the essentialization of these earlier traditions in their new cultural homes as medical writers in both cultures participated in the newly appropriated traditions. Foreign works, which possessed an individuality in their original traditions as each represented a new contribution to a developing tradition, were ascribed specific interpretations when they were appropriated because the creative process in the original tradition was replaced with a recreative process in the receiving tradition that necessarily required clear meanings rather than interpretative ambiguity. This delimiting of interpretive freedom due to the transposition of each tradition's medical literature into a new cultural environment represented the invisible driving force behind the essentialization of these foreign works in both the Islamicate world and early Japan.[1]

The Islamicate world and Japan are important case studies due to their similar acts of tradition-building. A close study of these traditions discloses how knowledge was transmitted within medieval Asia while conveying greater detail of the ambiguous relationship between text and learning. For this reason, this chapter examines medical writers participating in the production of knowledge within the Islamic and Japanese medical literary traditions. For the Islamicate world, the chapter considers medical education in conjunction with the introductory works of Ḥunayn ibn Isḥāq (Lat. Johannitius, 808–873) and the Alexandrian Summa of Galen with the encyclopedic works of Abū Bakr al-Rāzī (Lat. Rhazes) and Ibn Sīnā (Lat. Avicenna, 980–1037); and for Japan, the examination concentrates on connecting education with the works of Tanba no Yasuyori 丹波康頼 and Tanba no Masatada 丹波雅忠 (1021–1088), as well as earlier continental medical works. As al-Rāzī's name implies, he was from the city of Ray, where he worked as a physician before moving to Baghdad and becoming famous as a clinician there. A prolific medical writer, he also composed philosophical works. In contrast, records show that Yasuyori held a position in the state medical bureaucracy, where he held a leadership position in the acupuncture department.

Through an examination of medical history, this chapter will demonstrate how medical texts that were explicitly styled as repositories of knowledge also functioned as teachable treatises. It will also underscore the trends observable in medical writing in each medical literary tradition. The medieval world was a period of development, empire, and transformation throughout Eurasia.

A combination of these three factors led to the rise of new intellectual traditions in the Islamicate world and Japan.[2] Both civilizations had cultural exposure to neighbouring societies through trade and other forms of interaction. Thereafter, each culture proactively appropriated its neighbouring traditions in an endeavour that resulted in what historians would consider a nascent medical tradition. The complex socio-cultural background that supported each culture's eventual acquisition of these larger cross-cultural traditions requires a separate examination, as the basis for these developments shifts the discussion away from an analysis of how these cross-cultural medical traditions were consumed in their new home cultures.[3]

Such a comparison could be misleading as it draws into focus the comparability of the two cultures while distancing important differences. A large comparison considering trends and trajectories necessarily centres on this aspect of comparability, despite how pronounced these differences can be. For example, the decentralized nature of education in the geographically expansive Islamicate world contrasts with an established state medical curriculum in Japan. Even so, the use of Arabic disconnected the Islamicate world from a living Greco-Roman tradition, although this did not preclude translation into Arabic or interaction with the latter. In contrast, literary Chinese, the language of the East Asian medical tradition, was employed by local Japanese scholars, thus connecting the geographically distant cultures linguistically.[4] On initial consideration, the Japanese and Islamicate traditions might appear incomparable due to a vast difference in culture, size, and language, but, as the preceding paragraph demonstrates, their situations were similar, and this comparison positions itself to examine their negotiation of their neighbouring traditions not simply at the outset (i.e. the period of reception) but also in the establishment of tradition. The comparative aspect of this chapter will incorporate these similarities and differences to provide deeper insights into the role of texts in each tradition that would remain indiscernible through individual case studies.

In all cultures, education is an important facet of establishing tradition. Medical education covers a broad range of subjects but, as the aforementioned discussion has noted, the focus of this study is an investigation into the role of texts within education. The larger process of appropriating these medical traditions from their neighbouring civilizations led to the importation not only of medical knowledge but also of its practice. In other words, in addition to the medical knowledge required to function as a medical professional, foreign medical practice was also emulated, a process that included medical training, medical licensure, the creation of hospitals, and other broader social developments.[5]

The medieval medical cultures of the Islamicate world and Japan share the period of their development and their roots in foreign cultures, but less obvious is the fact that both cultures were transcultural in nature. The cross-cultural nature of their inherited traditions, namely Greco-Roman in the Islamicate world and Sino-Korean in Japan, remains the most salient feature of the study of each medical culture. In addition to these cross-cultural traditions, both medical cultures include characteristics and knowledge from other cross-cultural medical cultures. For example, both include elements of Indian medicine, philosophical knowledge, and locally developed principles of medicine. These additional features identify transculturality as another salient feature of these medieval medical cultures.[6] In particular, the combination of these cross-cultural and transcultural features in each tradition presents an interesting conundrum: an inevitable focus on the varying traditions intersecting within each tradition emphasizes the larger cross-cultural traditions rather than the transcultural framework within which they were consumed as a coherent single tradition known simply as medicine. The way in which a specific historical instance is examined directly affects the results of its examination, so the results cannot be identified as universal.

The outcome of each culture's acquisition of foreign traditions necessarily resulted in new conceptualizations of what they had appropriated. However, in both cultures, no writer imagined their participation in a new tradition, but rather regarded their work as an extension of the older tradition or even a new version of it. How writers approached the medical tradition was often defined by their engagement with it. Before an analysis of this engagement is understood, a critical examination of our approach to its historicization must be undertaken. A revealing distinction between contemporary realities and historicized realities is the lasting designation of Galen (c. 129–210 CE) as the interpreter of Hippocrates (corpus c. 4th c. BCE).[7] Galen's influence on the Greek, Roman, Islamicate, and Latin medical traditions is undeniable.[8] In his contemporary intellectual marketplace, Galen was not *the* interpreter of Hippocrates but rather simply *an* interpreter, yet the historicized Galen is the interpreter of Hippocrates. During the second century, Galen functioned as an interpreter in an intellectual milieu with various interlocutors.[9] The historicized Galen is the received Galen and arguably different in each period of history. Recent studies of ancient medicine have transformed how early medicine should be understood by disavowing linearity in medical history and removing the methodological hold of Galen over the Hippocratic corpus.[10] The Islamicate world's relationship with Galen is no different.

The role of Galen in the Islamicate world is easily understood by considering the Alexandrian Summa of Galen. The Alexandria Summa, a collection of epitomes, were sixteen books attributed to Galen. Despite their origins in Alexandria as interpretations of Galen, they were treated in Islamicate medical culture as the works of Galen himself. That is, these reworked Galenic treatises and systematized ideas were believed to have been written by Galen himself and functioned as key introductory texts to the medical art. For example, Abū Bakr al-Rāzī's *Kitāb al-shukūk 'alā jālīnūs* (*The Book of Criticism against Galen*) includes tracts that critique Galen's approach to medicine, wherein he cites the Alexandrian Summa as quotations from Galen's statements.[11]

In a similar manner, the following case studies of the Islamicate world and Japan will explore what types of treatises were used in medical education with a short introduction to the doxographical encyclopedias of Abū Bakr al-Rāzī and Tanba no Yasuyori, whose respective works were both sources for education and repositories of knowledge.

THE ISLAMICATE WORLD

The rise of medical literature in the Islamicate world was a product of the translation movement, recent studies of which have historiographically focused on Greco-(Syriac-)Arabic translation. Centuries of translation resulted in refined medical works that were localized into Arabic.[12] The most significant aspect of the translation movement in the Islamicate world, like the transposition of knowledge in any other culture, was the immediate access of writers and compilers to a complete foreign tradition. In the case of the Islamicate world, this included access not only to the Greco-Roman tradition itself but also to its reformulation into an easily teachable format by the early medieval Alexandrians.[13] This discussion will therefore consider the works from the ninth through eleventh centuries. As medical education in the Islamicate world drew heavily on the Greco-Roman medical tradition, the translation movement was instrumental in facilitating access to these texts. In addition to translation, there were two other modes of transposing Greco-Roman medical knowledge into the Islamicate world. The first was the reformulation of medical knowledge by translators and early medical writers. The second was the development of an encyclopedic tradition.[14]

Those involved in the initial reformulation of medical knowledge were early Arabic medical writers (that is, those writing in Arabic) who were also translators. Their access to the traditions they were translating promoted the recreation and reformulation of this knowledge for practical purposes ranging from organization for clarity to systematization for educating students. In fact, the intentional reformulation of the Alexandrian epitomes of Galen was an example of how these reformulations had already been created before the rise of the translation movement in the Islamicate world.

The educational aspect of the recreative process is evident in the straightforward non-narrative style of the Alexandrian texts. For example, Galen's *al-Ṣinā'a al-ṣaghīra* (*The Small Art*) begins with an introduction to the methods of instruction.[15] The treatise consists of twenty-eight chapters that cover the definitions of medicine, signs of health and disease, and temperaments. The purpose of the text is clearly visible in its standard didactic approach. Although the Summa were an interpretation of Galen, by being treated as original works in their use as educational tools, they ostensibly taught students Galen's original medicine. These epitomes were a part of a medical literary corpus drawing on a historicized Greco-Roman tradition. In this translated corpus were included works spanning a thousand years of Greco-Roman medicine, from early Greek works like the *Aphorisms* of Hippocrates to later Roman works from centuries after Galen with translations of the works of Paul of Aegina (625–90) and Oribasius (c. 329–403).

Among the translators who rendered the Greco-Roman tradition into Arabic, Ḥunayn ibn Isḥāq remains the most famous, so much so that numerous later and anonymous translations would often be attributed to Ḥunayn, including the Alexandrian Summa.[16] In addition to being a translator, Ḥunayn was also a medical writer, having produced introductory treatises such as *al-Madkhal* (*The Introduction*) and *Masāʾil fī al-ṭibb* (*Questions on Medicine*).[17] His *Masāʾil*, written in question-answer format, is an introductory work detailing the fundamental principles of medicine. His work on the eyes is also presented in question-answer format. An examination of the *Masāʾil* quickly reveals Ḥunayn's intentions in composing a didactic treatise to aide in the comprehension of basic medical concepts.

The early works, both the translations and reformulations, functioned explicitly as didactic treatises for use by students of the medical art. The translated source texts were reformulations themselves and the translation process sometimes resulted in unintentional conceptual changes, leading to a difference in understanding between the original Greco-Roman tradition and the tradition that existed in Arabic translation within the Islamicate world. The significance of these accidental cognitive misconstruals cannot be overemphasized. For example, Manfred Ullmann discusses such a point in the context of ʿAlī ibn al-ʿAbbās al-Majūsī (930–994). Al-Majūsī, whose name reveals his Zoroastrian background though he himself was a Muslim, was an important medical encyclopedist whose influence is observable in the lasting use of his works in the Islamicate world and even in medieval Europe. Ullmann's examination of al-Majūsī's *Kitāb kāmil al-ṣināʿa al-ṭibbiyya* (*The Complete Book on the Medical Art*) revealed how the "vital spirit" (Gr. πνευμα ζοτικον) became the "animal spirit" (Ar. *rūḥ ḥayawānī*) due to a mistranslation.[18] Ullmann notes this in reference to how such issues were observable in the translation movement, but the emphasis of such a perspective is necessarily on the source tradition, Greco-Roman medicine, rather than on what was produced through its translation into Arabic, the medicine of the Islamicate world. For medical students in the Islamicate world, this was not a mistranslation; the animal spirit was a fact, one that was incorporated throughout the Islamicate tradition. The terminological difference did not change its meaning, only its semantic representation as "animal spirit" in Arabic, because its usage in the Islamicate medical literary tradition followed its Greco-Roman predecessors. Therefore, Ullmann's comment is significant in the context of translation, which is where he discusses it, but not in its employment to represent a misunderstanding of the vital spirit in the Islamicate tradition.[19]

Subsequent trends in writing following the translation movement, however, were not limited to the recreation of earlier works. Increased systematization and encyclopedism led to the creation of new types of works. Peter Pormann identifies the process of systematization as *diairesis*, dating to the Roman medical compilers.[20] The Alexandrian epitomes and the early introductory treatises of the Islamicate world demonstrate that diairesis was an important aspect of presenting information to readers.[21] While it is unlikely that medical compilers of the Islamicate world were intentionally coopting a Roman practice of compilation, the presence of these similarities indicates that writers of the Islamicate world incorporated these practices for different reasons. The rise of encyclopedism resulting from that diairesis was due in part to a move towards systematization within and between disciplines. These works would often be titled *kunnāsh* (compilation or pandect, pl. *kanānīsh*), a term that appears to have originated with the Syriac *kenāshā* (collection).[22] The nature of the *kunnāsh* genre can be described as a genre of diairesis. Ya'qūb al-Kashkarī's (fl. 10th c.) *Kunnāsh fī al-ṭibb (Pandect on Medicine)* is one example of this, with its clearly divided sections and quotations from earlier writers, especially Galen.[23] Moreover, in contrast to the early reformulations and translations, these later encyclopedic works were not constructed in a visibly didactic manner. Put another way, encyclopedic medical texts were not simply understood as systematizations of medical knowledge by different writers, but were also consumed as textbooks through their inclusion in educational curricula.

Examining education also requires an investigation into the history of people and their lives. In the Islamicate world, numerous 'biographical' dictionaries were composed to assess and identify important individuals in various fields, with the medical field producing many such works. In particular, the biographical dictionaries of Ibn Abī Uṣaybi'a (1203–1270) and al-Qifṭī (1172–1248) provide a concrete outline for the history of medicine in the Islamicate world, but these biographical histories place an emphasis on compilers by enumerating their works.[24] Instead of a close analysis of textual content, the histories list works written, with an occasional discussion of more famous treatises. An examination of the actual use of the texts must be found elsewhere. For example, al-Samarqandī (1250–1310) includes in his *Chahār Maqāla (Four Treatises)* a discussion of what works should be studied in medicine as follows:

On the science of medicine, the student should procure and read the
Fuṣūl of Hippocrates, the *Masāʾil* of Ḥunayn ibn Isḥāq, the *Murshid* of
Muḥammad ibn Zakariyyā [al-Rāzī], and the Commentary of Nīlī, who
has made abstracts of these. After he has carefully read these works with a
kind and congenial master, he should diligently study with a sympathetic
teacher and following intermediate works, to wit, the *Dhakhīra* of Thābit
ibn Qurra, the *Manṣūrī* of Muḥammad ibn Zakariyyā of Rayy; the *Hidāya*
of Abū Bakr Ajwīnī, or the *Kifāya* of Aḥmad ibn Faraj and the *Aghrād*
of al-Sayyid Ismaʿīl al-Jurjānī. Then he should take up one of the more
detailed treatises, such as the *Sitta ʿashar* [Alexandrian Summa] of Galen,
or the *Ḥāwī* of Muḥammad ibn Zakariyyā, or the *Kāmil al-ṣināʿa*, or the *Ṣad
Bāb* [al-Miʾa fī al-ṣināʿa al-ṭibbiyya] of Abū Sahl al-Masīḥī, or the *Qānūn* of Ibn
Sīnā, or the *Dhakhīra-i Khwārazm-shāhī*,[25] and read it in his leisure moments;
or, if he desires to be independent of other works, he may content himself
with the *Qānūn*.[26]

Although al-Samarqandī's work dates to a period even later than the biographical dictionaries and was composed in Persian, his list demonstrates that in the
thirteenth century the encyclopedic works of the *kunnāsh* genre were considered texts for use in medical education just like Ḥunayn's *Masāʾil* and other
introductory counterparts.

In addition to the introductory didactic works discussed above, he includes
larger tomes like the works of al-Rāzī, al-Majūsī, and Ibn Sīnā.[27] While the
former two held important positions in the local and foreign medical literary
traditions, Ibn Sīnā's corpus is considered to be even more substantial. A self-
claimed autodidact, his medical and philosophical works influenced each field
significantly. His name can be considered synonymous with medicine both in
the Islamicate world and in Europe.

Al-Rāzī's *Kitāb al-manṣūrī fī al-ṭibb* (*The Manṣūrī in Medicine*) was a work intend-
ing to outline medicine, dedicated to the governor of Ray, Abū Ṣāliḥ Manṣūr
(d. 915, governed 902–15). Its organization and clarity made it an effective
source of information. Al-Majūsī's *Kitāb kāmil al-ṣināʿa al-ṭibbiyya* (*The Complete
Book of the Medical Art*), the subject of the Ullmann study identified above, had
a similarly clear expository style. In contrast, Abū Sahl al-Masīḥī's (c. 970–
1010) *al-Miʾa fī al-ṣināʿa al-ṭibbiyya* (*Hundred Questions on the Medical Art*), known
as *Ṣād Bāb* in Persian, was also a large tome but constructed like Ḥunayn's
Masāʾil in question-answer format. Al-Rāzī's and al-Majūsī's works were systematic encyclopedias in an expository style different from that of al-Masīḥī.
It is Ibn Sīnā, purportedly a pupil of al-Masīḥī, whose expository style would
dominate through his *Qānūn fī al-ṭibb* (*Canon of Medicine*).[28]

Al-Rāzī also composed a different type of encyclopedia, much larger than his other works. This work, titled *Kitāb al-ḥāwī fī al-ṭibb* (*The Comprehensive Book on Medicine*), was referred to by al-Rāzī as *al-Jāmiʿ al-kabīr* (*The Large Compendium*).[29] Its unique place in al-Rāzī's oeuvre is due to its comprehensiveness as a doxographical work on medicine. In the *Ḥāwī*, he included his own experiences and opinions along with those of his predecessors. Doxographical works were not unique in the field of medicine, as demonstrated by the translator Thābit ibn Qurra (826–901), who wrote *al-Dhakhīra fī ʿilm al-ṭibb* (*The Repository for the Science of Medicine*), which like the *Ḥāwī* was composed of quotations.[30] Besides this style of incorporating the statements and opinions of predecessors, however, the texts differ greatly. Al-Rāzī provides numerous opinions and his work spans twenty-five volumes, whereas Thābit's *Dhakhīra* at one volume is not nearly as large.

In the case of the medical arts, the nature of medical education and medical compilation created a space for texts to function simultaneously in an educational and rhetorical capacity.[31] Both Thābit's and al-Rāzī's works are found in al-Samarqandī's list of works to be studied by medical students. The *Ḥāwī*'s use as an educational tool, therefore, is in conjunction with its role as a doxographical treatise and as a comprehensive medical encyclopedia. The notable distinction between the earlier, shorter works and later, larger tomes is that the latter consisted in a systematization of medical knowledge coupled with an exhaustive analysis of the knowledge under consideration. On the other hand, the earlier works were systematized specifically for introductory purposes, as is evidenced by the way in which the texts presented medical knowledge in didactic form and not through discursive methods to argue particular points of view.[32] These earlier works were compiled in a straightforward manner with clear answers and without discussion of alternatives or proofs.[33] Their simple presentation format also facilitated memorization.

The afterlife of these larger encyclopedic texts differed, and encyclopedism was eventually replaced by a new form of commentary writing that was equally encyclopedic.[34] However, what is clear is that the texts utilized in Islamicate medical education drew upon translated literature, reformulations of translated knowledge, and later textual compositions. It is within this cultural context that the rise of encyclopedic writing led to a highly organized form of medical literature, but the repurposing of these texts also made them an integral part of medical education as well.

JAPAN

The locally developed Japanese tradition of medical compilations began following Japan's large-scale exposure to the cross-cultural medical literary tradition of East Asia. This exposure was first in the form of its reception of continental medical texts from continental East Asia, primarily through the Korean peninsula.[35] Its eventual appropriation of the continental tradition was a result of Japan's proactive participation in the cross-cultural network of East Asia.[36] The nature of medical education in Japan is therefore a consideration of medical education within the Sinitic cultural sphere, with Sinitic often called "literary Chinese" 文言文 (Ch. *wenyanwen*) in China and "Chinese-style writing" 漢文 (Kr. *hanmun*, Jp. *kanbun*) in other regions.[37] In examining the medical education of early Japan, this section will consider the state of medical works from those in the early Japanese medical curriculum, which were foreign works, through to the eleventh-century Tanba no Masatada's locally composed compilation.

Early Japan's appropriation of the continental medical literary tradition was not a linear process. Through missions to China during the Sui and Tang dynasties, Japan acquired texts from various disciplines and even accommodated visiting teachers. Some of these overseas travellers were invited to be installed in positions within the developing culture, including Jian Zhen 鑑真 (Jp. *Ganjin*, 688–763), a Buddhist priest who was called to Tōdai Temple 東大寺 and later established the Tōshōdai Temple 唐招提寺 in Nara.[38] Medical knowledge also travelled with these movements of people, which can be seen, for example, in the list of medical formularies attributed to Jian Zhen.[39] The Japanese acquisition of the continental medical literary tradition, however, did not involve translating a corpus of texts. As a language, Sinitic had already been appropriated as the intellectual lingua franca of Japan, a move that was modelled after Korean practices.[40] In fact, Sinitic was an intellectual lingua franca throughout cultural China's neighbouring regions, including Vietnam.[41]

In Japan, Chinese medical works from the continent constituted the core of medical bureaucracy. Early Japanese culture emulated continental institutions, with medicine being no exception. The Medical Bureau 典薬寮 (Jp. *ten'yakuryō*) was the seat of medical bureaucracy in early Japan, where teaching and other official medical activities were conducted.[42] The Medical Bureau was designed to emulate the bureaucracies of the Sui and Tang dynasties. For example, medical leadership positions in the bureau included Erudite of Medicine 醫博士 (Jp. *i hakase*), Erudite of Acupuncture 針博士 (Jp. *hari hakase*), Erudite of [Therapeutic] Massage 按摩博士 (Jp. *anma hakase*), and Erudite of Incantation 呪文博士 (Jp. *jugon hakase*).[43]

Each department of the Medical Bureau had its own protocols for teaching. The medical curricula that were taught followed their Sui- and Tang-period counterparts. The *Engishiki* 延喜式 (*Protocols of the Engi [Era]*) enumerates the medical works that early Japan employed as textbooks in training future medical practitioners; all were standard Chinese texts.[44] The following table is a list of the works that *Engishiki* identifies as textbooks for students, divided into the works used by medical students 醫生 (Jp. *isei*) and acupuncture students 鍼生 (Jp. *harisei*), for whom the Medical Bureau had different curricula.

Table 1.1 | Textbooks identified in the *Engishiki*

Medical students	Acupuncture students
Classic of ABCs 甲乙經 (Ch. *Jiayi jing*, Jp. *Kōotsu kyō*)	*Simple Questions* 素問 (Ch. *Suwen*, Jp. *Somon*)
Classic of the Pulse 脈經 (Ch. *Maijing*, Jp. *Myakuketsu*)	*Yellow Emperor's Classic of Acupuncture* 黃帝鍼經 (Ch. *Huangdi zhenjing*, Jp. *Kōtei shinkyō*)
Newly Revised Materia Medica 新修本草 (Ch. *Xinxiu bencao*, Jp. *Shinshū honzō*)	*Mingtang* 明堂 (Jp. *Meidō*)
Simple Formularies 小品方 (Ch. *Xiaopin fang*, Jp. *Shōhinhō*)	*Pulse Poem* 脈訣 (Ch. *Maijue*, Jp. *Myakuketsu*)
Collected Effective Formularies 集驗方 (Ch. *Jiyan fang*, Jp. *Shūken hō*)	*Classic of Chiniao* 赤鳥經 (Ch. *Chiniao jing*, Jp. *Sekiu kyō*)

Set of works for medical students and acupuncture students (Hattori, *Heian jidai*, 114–15)..

The clearest difference between the two sets of works is the focus of medical students on formularies and materia medica. The set for acupuncture students instead concentrates on acupuncture works, including the standard medieval text *Mingtang*. In both cases, the base of medical knowledge was defined by continental medical works. Both medical students and acupuncture students invested heavily in early Chinese classics, such as the *Classic of ABCs* and the *Simple Questions*, but also included medieval works as seen in *Newly Revised Materia Medica* and *Mingtang*.

Engishiki's list is not exhaustive, in that it only includes the texts required for study in the medical curricula of the Medical Bureau. Fujiwara no Sukeyo's 藤原佐世 (847–97) *Nihonkoku genzaisho mokuroku* 日本国見在書目録 (*Catalogue of Books Extant in Japan*) provides evidence of what works students and practitioners might have had access to in the ninth century. Sukeyo structured his catalogue as a list of works available in Japan during the ninth century and divided the list by genre. Sukeyo's list reveals that numerous works of every genre composed in Sinitic were available in Heian Japan.[45] Numerous texts from the Sinitic medical literary tradition of China and Korea can be found in this list, including in subheadings other than medicine.[46]

In this list can be found Chao Yuanfang's 巢元方 (fl. 7th c.) *Zhubing yuanhou lun* 諸病源候論 (*Treatise on the Origins and Symptoms of Diseases*) and Sun Simiao's 孫思邈 (581–682) *Qianjin yao fang* 千金要方 (*Formularies Worth a Thousand in Gold*).[47] Both texts were composed during the Sui and early Tang dynasties. While both individuals had a relationship with the imperial courts of their time, Sun Simiao was also itinerant and interacted with the common people.

Earlier continental works had already incorporated a systematic explicative style, like the *Simple Questions*, which was composed in a question-answer format. However, a new genre of encyclopedic texts called *leishu* 類書 (Jp. *ruisho*) developed in the early medieval period that often consisted of excerpts from texts of a genre, in effect combining large amounts of knowledge in a clear expository style. Early compilers attempted to incorporate all types of knowledge within their treatises.[48] Eventually, medical writers also composed works in the *leishu* and broadly encyclopedic styles. In the context of encyclopedic works, Chao Yuanfang's *Bingyuan*, as it is often called in medieval texts, became a standard theoretical text on pathology with some therapeutic information also included. Sun Simiao's work similarly became a standard text for its collection of formularies. Even so, being Sui- and Tang-period texts, neither was a part of the Sui and Tang medical curriculums that early Japanese bureaucrats had incorporated into the Medical Bureau. Texts in the medical curriculum like *Simple Formularies* and *Collected Effective Formularies* were older texts but collections of formularies nonetheless. Their inclusion in the curriculum demonstrates the importance placed on teaching formularies as therapeutic methods for medical students. Therefore, the exclusion of Sun Simiao's *Qianjin yao fang* and Chao Yuanfang's *Bingyuan* was not a result of preference but an indication of the period in which the original curricula had been created. The integration of these later works into medical education is evidenced in Japan's earliest extant medical work, Tanba no Yasuyori's *Ishinpō* 醫心方 (*Essential Medical Methods*).

Yasuyori was a medical bureaucrat in service to the Heian court. His official position was Erudite of Acupuncture in the Medical Bureau, meaning he was closely affiliated with medical education.[49] His *Ishinpō* is doxographical in nature, made up almost entirely of excerpts from continental medical works. In addition to extensive citation of *Bingyuan* as a theoretical source, he includes numerous quotations from *Qianjin yao fang* and other medieval texts. For this reason, it is clear that both *Qianjin yao fang* and *Bingyuan* played an important role in education besides the earlier texts identified in the standard medical curriculum.

The highly organized style of these medieval texts is also observable in Yasuyori's *Ishinpō*, which totalled thirty volumes. As a work of medicine, it covers areas from medical ethics, acupuncture, and various diseases to obstetrics, gynecology, life cultivation, and materia medica. It is possible that Yasuyori compiled *Ishinpō* together with his colleagues and students at the Medical Bureau. The vast number of texts cited in *Ishinpō* is due in part to the broad subjects covered in the text, but it also speaks to the access that Yasuyori and, presumably, his colleagues had during the tenth century. Historically, *Ishinpō* does not appear to have circulated widely, but a copy was kept in the Medical Bureau.[50] Thus, it is highly likely that Yasuyori's contemporaries and subsequent medical bureaucrats had access to the text, at least those working under the Erudite of Acupuncture, if not the whole Medical Bureau.

Ishinpō also reveals a different approach to medical education in Japan through its act of excerption. Earlier continental texts that were being utilized for education in the Medical Bureau, such as *Collected Effective Formularies*, demonstrate that it was already a common practice to collate effective prescriptions and systematize knowledge. While not explicitly quotations, the act of collecting and organizing earlier knowledge was not limited to the *leishu* genre. Sukeyo's catalogue is proof of an influx of numerous continental texts, but the presence of these texts in early Japan facilitated opportunities for local intellectuals to engage with them. As part of this process, Japanese compilers created a genre of texts that were composed of excerpts of earlier texts, especially the continental texts. These texts often included the character 抄 (Jp. *shō*) or some variation of it, indicating that they were summaries of other texts or synopses of genres. Texts of this nature were observable earlier in the Sino-Korean classical tradition, considered to be synopses 抄書 (Ch. *chaoshu*, Jp. *shōsho*).[51] Yasuyori's *Ishinpō* is not a synopsis, but his collation of excerpts resembles the approach that some authors took when composing these synopses. In fact, Yasuyori's great-grandson Tanba no Masatada composed such a work, titled *Iryakushō* 醫略抄 (*Redaction and Synopsis of Medicine*). Masatada's *Iryakushō* is not only a synopsis of medicine but also a redaction of *Ishinpō*, such that the "medicine" in *Iryakushō*'s title can be reconstrued as "a redaction and synopsis of *Essential Medical Methods*." The significance of this is twofold. First, being a part of the Medical Bureau, Masatada's access to Yasuyori's work indicates that *Ishinpō* was also accessible to members of the Tanba family in addition to medical bureaucrats.[52] Second, it also reveals that *Ishinpō* was used as a reference by Masatada as a practical work or a didactic treatise.

In early Japan, the Medical Bureau replicated the continental medical curriculum, leading to a reliance on earlier texts. However, the medical bureau also facilitated access to numerous works not listed in the curriculum, such as collections and encyclopedias, as seen in the excerpts found in *Ishinpō*. The larger continental works and the locally compiled *Ishinpō* both demonstrate that encyclopedic works were repurposed for educational purposes either directly, as in the case of the texts found in educational curricula, or indirectly, as evidenced through excerption.

COMPARING TRAJECTORIES

The early Islamicate and Japanese societies both incorporated foreign medical knowledge into their educational curricula. The development of literature utilized for medical education in both societies had a similar trajectory. For example, encyclopedic works were appropriated as a form of educational literature in each society. Even so, there were also significant differences such as how this foreign medical knowledge was introduced into each society.

On the transposition of knowledge, Islamicate societies first encountered texts in Greek, Syriac, Persian, and Sanskrit, from west to east. Through the translation movement this knowledge was localized into Arabic, a process that involved various forms of interpretation, intentional or not, that resulted in clarifications, specification, and mistranslations. The early medieval Islamicate medical scholars writing in Arabic necessarily interpreted the texts to which they had access, but the access they obtained was provided through the interpretive lenses of the translators. All these factors led to the creation of early teachable texts. In contrast, Japan's encounter with Sinitic medical literature did not require initial linguistic intermediaries to localize the knowledge into Japanese, as the intellectuals of early Japan had already been using Sinitic as their lingua franca. Unlike the two levels of interpretation that existed in the Islamicate world, in Japan, then, the interpretation of texts remained primarily the job of the intellectuals without an intermediary in the form of translators. Educational texts in Japan were, therefore, primarily continental texts.

On the development of literature, both shared the appropriation of original texts as well as of reworked and reformulated texts. Not only did each culture appropriate reformulations, but both incorporated them into medical education as well. It is unclear whether the new acquisitions were always understood to be reformulations and epitomes. In the case of the Islamicate world, works like the Alexandrian Summa of Galen and Ḥunayn's *Masāʾil* were considered a part of standard medical education. Written in Arabic, Ḥunayn's *Masāʾil* was appropriately understood as having reworked knowledge for didactic purposes. However, the epitomes from Alexandria were often considered to be Galen's own words. In fact, this was attested to by al-Rāzī, who related a story to his contemporaries about a Chinese individual who came to study under him and eventually asked to learn the Summa from him and his students.[53] In the case of early Japan, reformulations are not as clear. *The Classic of ABCs* was a reworking of earlier knowledge from the *Huangdi* tradition but stood on its own as a standard medical text. The origins of the work lie in *Huangdi neijing* 黃帝內經 (*Yellow Emperor's Classic of Medicine*), whose earliest works date to at least the Mawangdui tombs. The *Huangdi* corpus functioned like the Hippocratic corpus in forming the early foundations of medical knowledge. Texts such as *The Classic of ABCs, Simple Questions, Yellow Emperor's Classic of Acupuncture*, and *Mingtang* are all part of the *Huangdi* tradition.[54]

The reorganization of medical knowledge differed between the larger cross-cultural traditions that each culture had appropriated. The Alexandrian Summa, extensively used in the Islamicate tradition, were composed explicitly for didactic purposes later in the Greco-Roman tradition, while the *Huangdi* treatises were highly organized but not reworked into smaller treatises. In both cases, these earlier texts were used for medical education, but the number of medical treatises locally developed in each culture through to the end of the eleventh century was vastly different. The most obvious reason for this is the inordinate difference in geographical size between the Islamicate world and Japan.

Moreover, *leishu* and other forms of encyclopedism in East Asia resemble the style of diairesis developed in the Greco-Roman tradition, not in an absolute sense but rather in the trend towards increasingly organized and encyclopedic works. Both Japan and the Islamicate world continued these traditions that had developed in the medical literary cultures they had appropriated. In both cultures, these encyclopedic works were also repurposed for teaching and education. Their use in education indicates the importance of highly organized and comprehensive works in teaching that moved beyond introductory texts. The doxographical and encyclopedic works of al-Rāzī's *Ḥāwī* and Yasuyori's *Ishinpō* are a more salient example of convergence in each culture's medical education. The use of these two doxographical works for educational purposes signifies the importance placed on earlier medical opinions. In the traditions themselves, al-Rāzī's *Ḥāwī* includes his own opinions, whereas in *Ishinpō* Yasuyori rarely includes such explicit observations.[55] Al-Samarqandī's citation of *Ḥāwī* and Masatada's redaction of *Ishinpō* both reveal how these observations continued to be important for later generations, despite differences in medical literary development.

These two doxographical encyclopedias also reveal a shared historical reality both cultures experienced. The almost instantaneous transposition of the thousand-year corpora of the Greco-Roman and Sino-Korean medical literary traditions into the Islamicate world and Japan respectively means that both cultures had access to a wide range of literature without having experienced the historical progression that the source traditions had experienced. Therefore, in the case of the Islamicate world, early texts of the Greco-Roman tradition were used in tandem with later Roman works and the Alexandrian reformulations. Al-Rāzī's *Ḥāwī* is the culmination of this transposition. The wide variation in historical period of texts incorporated into medical education was shared by early Japan, whose medical curricula were shaped by its continental counterpart. Members of early Japan's Medical Bureau not only studied established textbooks as students, but also had exposure to centuries of medical literature, as evidenced by Sukeyo's list and Yasuyori's *Ishinpō*.

The nature of texts involved in education did differ between both cultures. In the case of the Islamic world, there were far shorter introductory treatises incorporated in teaching, contrasted with the use of only larger works in the medical curriculum of Japan. In addition, the doxographical medical encyclopedias of al-Rāzī and Yasuyori reveal in the first instance a shared historical reality and the importance of opinions, but upon further inspection also indicate that the range of works studied extended beyond traditionally understood introductory works.

CONCLUSION

The Islamicate and Japanese medical literary traditions were composite if seen from the standpoint of their heritage in their neighbouring traditions. To privilege the transmissive aspect of writing over its literary aspect – that is, how the nature of its content is defined by its form – leads to a misrepresentation of facts when examining anything but the text's transmission. This same perspective holds true when considering medical texts meant to articulate certain approaches to knowledge together with those explicitly composed for didactic purposes. Liba Taub's recent *Science Writing in Greco-Roman Antiquity* is perhaps the only wholesome study of science writing to focus on writing rather than transmission or the assertion of a specific set of ideas.[56] History of science, medicine, and technology studies have failed to investigate this historical aspect of inquiry. Taub's work is perhaps the first examination of form in intellectual writing of the ancient period that seriously considers the nature of form. This chapter has shown that different forms of writing existed in the medical literary corpora of Islamicate and Japanese medicine, but to understand their incorporation into medical education requires transcending the strict form of writing.

At the same time, form cannot be abandoned to such a degree that the intentionality of an author is lost. Early reformulations and translations of the Alexandrian Summa in Islamicate medicine and smaller treatises in the Japanese tradition were clearly designed with educational objectives in mind. In this context, al-Rāzī's and Yasuyori's doxographical encyclopedias are of particular note as they function as collections of opinions and highly organized texts, two facets that distinguish them from their later utilization for explicitly educational purposes. The use of these encyclopedias in some form therefore evidences the repurposing of treatises for medical education in addition to the functioning of encyclopedias as works for advanced study. It must be noted that the medical literature included in this examination of medical education was standard educational material and works popular within the Islamicate world and early Japan. The purpose of the examination was to understand the relationship between text and education, not the nature of instruction. A text can have many functions, often unrelated to the reasons of their composition – like the educational texts discussed here that were not explicitly composed for students.

The differences between medical education in these two traditions derives from their historical circumstances. The Islamicate world's translation movement would imply that the development of local encyclopedism and large-scale textual production was due to linguistic barriers not seen in early Japan, which had adopted the language of its neighbouring tradition. Instead, it was the existence of highly organized encyclopedias like *Qianjin yao fang* extant in the Chinese tradition that were includable as more advanced studies in early Japan. This is not to say that Roman medical writers did not produce highly organized works, but rather to suggest that their inclusion as didactic works was not in accord with the needs of the Islamicate medical tradition. In other words, obvious differences are not necessarily the deciding factors of historical trends, nor is linearity an adequate explanation. On account of this, it is hoped that the observations of this chapter will be instructive for scholars working on medical education and those focusing on non-European, non-Western, and Asian medical traditions in their own explorations of non-European medical traditions.

NOTES

1   For a study of this in respect to Chinese medical knowledge in Japan, see Khan, "Critique in Early Japan."

2   See Hodgson, *The Venture of Islam.*

3   For the best examination of the Greco-Arabic translation movement's sociocultural factors, see Gutas, *Greek Thought.* For a study of Japan's proactive engagement with the continent, see Sugimoto and Swain, *Science and Culture,* and for a study of the Japanese missions to China, see Tōno, *Kentōshi.*

4   For an exhaustive examination of this phenomenon, and the first such detailed study known to this author in a Western language, see Kornicki, *Languages.*

5   For a broad introduction to social aspects of medicine with respect to the Islamicate world, see Pormann and Savage-Smith, *Medieval Islamic Medicine.* For a study of the social and institutional aspects of medicine in early Japan,

see Hattori, *Heian jidai*. Hattori's work on the earlier Nara period is also a useful guide: Hattori, *Nara jidai*.

6   For a list of non-Greco-Roman sources in al-Rāzī's work on the Islamicate side, see the introduction to Kahl, *The Sanskrit, Syriac and Persian Sources*. For a study of non-Chinese sources in Yasuyori's work on the Japanese side, see ch. 5 in Khan, "Early Japan."

7   Nutton, "The Fatal Embrace," 111–21.

8   See Temkin's lectures: Temkin, *Galenism*.

9   Mattern, *The Prince of Medicine*.

10 Nutton, "Fatal Embrace."

11 The *shukūk* (criticism) tradition in Arabic is not unique to al-Rāzī's work, to which the Andalusian Abū ʿAlāʾ ibn Zuhr (fl. 11th c.) wrote a response; see Ibn Abī Uṣaybiʿa, *ʿUyūn al-anbāʾ*, 519. A massive project to translate this treatise was recently completed and is also available online through Oxford University Press. Its physical reference is Ibn Abi Usaybiʿah, *Anecdotes and Antidotes*.

12 Gutas, *Greek Thought*.

13 See Iskandar, "An Attempted Reconstruction."

14 Khan, "Transposing Knowledge: Beyond Translation." The distinction between early medical writers who composed original texts and the encyclopedic works of later works is the style of composition.

15 Walbridge, *The Alexandrian Epitomes*, 50–6.

16 For a recent case study of this issue, see Barry, "Was Ḥunayn," 457–65.

17 For a critical edition of the *Masāʾil*, see Ibn Isḥāq al-ʿIbādī, *Masaʾil*.

18 Ullmann, *Islamic Medicine*, 28.

19 I would be remiss were I not to mention Shakespeare here:
>   What's in a name? that which we call a rose
>   By any other name would smell as sweet;
>   So Romeo would, were he not Romeo call'd,
>   Retain that dear perfection which he owes
>   Without that title. Romeo, doff thy name …

Romeo and Juliet (2.2.47–51). Shakespeare's words spoken through Juliet identify precisely why a mistranslation of "vital spirit" as "animal spirit" is meaningless if the concept itself remains the same.

20 Pormann, "Medical Education," 429.

21 Khan, "The Two Ibn Sīnās," 5–6.

22 Meyerhof, "The Book of Treasure," 55.

23 His work can be found in Yaʿqūb al-Kashkarī, *Kitāb kunnāsh fī al-ṭibb*, reproduced in al-Kashkarī, *Book on Medicine*. He is recorded as a historical writer in Debié and Taylor, "Syriac and Syro-Arabic," 175.

24 Ibn al-Qifṭī's work can be found as Ibn al-Qifṭī, *Tārīkh*.

25 Shihadeh, "A Post-Ghazalian Critic," 148. This enormous text, described by Shihadeh as "the most important encyclopaedia in Persian," was composed in Persian by the same al-Jurjānī cited earlier in the passage, but was also later translated into Arabic by al-Jurjānī himself.

26 Browne, *Chahār*, 78–9. The translation from Persian here is Browne's but has been edited to remove the translations of the titles and to Arabicize the pronunciation of titles, except when they were distinctly Persian. For a brief discussion in relation to introductory treatises, see Khan, "Two Ibn Sīnās," 5.

27 For a discussion of these texts from a structural point of view, see Khan, "Transposing Knowledge: Beyond Translation."

28 See for example Siraisi, *Avicenna*.

29 Savage-Smith, "The Working Files." In particular, see 179–80 for her final comments on the issue.

30 Meyerhof, "The Book of Treasure," 55–76. Meyerhof translates the title as *Book of Treasure*, as "treasure" and "treasury" share etymological origins, but the former's contemporary usage no longer implies the meaning of storage or repository.

31 Brentjes, *Teaching and Learning*, 247–9.

32 Khan, "Two Ibn Sīnās," 22–3.

33 This discussion excludes short discursive treatises that should be considered advanced works focused on specialized topics.

34 For a discussion in the medical context, see Khan, "Transposing Knowledge: Beyond Translation." For a review of this trend in all disciplines, see el-Rouayheb, *Islamic Intellectual History*.

35 For example, see Kosoto, *Chūgoku igaku koten*. His study examines the relationship between these classical texts and Japan.

36 For an exhaustive examination of this literary cross-cultural network, see Kornicki, *Languages*.

37 For a thorough study of Sinitic practices in East Asia, see Kin, *Kanbun*.

38 For an extended discussion, see Tōno, *Kentōshi*.

39 Khan, "Early Japan," 30–1.

40 Kin, *Kanbun*. See especially ch. 1.

41 Kornicki, *Languages*, 25–41.

42 Medical activities were not solely conducted in these official capacities. For example, Buddhist temples were also places to receive medical treatment. Extant works from later Buddhist medical writers such as Koremune Tomotoshi 惟宗具俊 (d. 13th c.) and Kajiwara Shōzen 梶原性全 (1266–1337) survive.

43 Khan, "Early Japan," 17.

44 For an introduction, see Tōno, *Kentōshi*, 146–54.

45   Yajima, *Nihonkoku*.

46   Khan, "Early Japan," ch. 5.

47   Yajima, *Nihonkoku*, 189, 201.

48   Zurndorfer, "The Passion to Collect," 509.

49   For more information on positions in the Medical Bureau, see Hattori, *Heian jidai*, 106–12.

50   Sugitatsu, *Ishinpō*, 32–3.

51   Tian, "Literary Learning," 143.

52   Sugitatsu, *Ishinpō*, 32–3.

53   There are numerous references to this story in contemporary works on the history of science, in English, for example by Needham, *Science and Civilisation*, 219. For the original, see Ibn al-Nadīm, *Kitāb al-fihrist*, 39–40.

54   Sivin, "Huang ti," 196–215.

55   There are exceptions to this, the most notable being the introduction to its volume 2 on acupuncture and moxibustion, wherein Yasuyori states his reasoning for organizing the volume in the way that he did and for selecting *Mingtang* as a source.

56   Taub, *Science Writing*.

BIBLIOGRAPHY

Barry, Samuel C. "Was Ḥunayn ibn Isḥāq the Author of the Arabic Translation of Paul of Aegina's *Pragmateia*? Evidence from the Arabic Translations of the Hippocratic *Aphorisms* and the Syriac Lexicons of Bar Bahlul and Bar ʿAli." *Journal of Semitic Studies* 63, no. 2 (2018): 457–65.

Brentjes, Sonja. *Teaching and Learning the Sciences in Islamicate Societies (800–1700)*. Turnhout, Belgium: Brepols Publishers, 2018.

Debié, Muriel, and David Taylor. "Syriac and Syro-Arabic Historical Writing, c. 500–c. 1400." In *The Oxford History of Historical Writing: Volume 2: 400–1400*, edited by Sarah Foot and Chase F. Robinson, 155–79. Oxford, UK: Oxford University Press, 2012.

Gutas, Dimitri. *Greek Thought, Arabic Culture: The Graeco-Arabic Translation Movement in Baghdad and Early ʿAbbāsid Society (2nd–4th/8th–10th Centuries)*. London: Routledge, 1998.

Hattori Toshirō 服部敏郎. *Heian jidai igakushi no kenkyū* 平安時代医学史の研究. Tokyo: Yoshikawa kōbunkan, 1955.

– *Nara jidai igakushi no kenkyū* 奈良時代医学史の研究. Tokyo: Yoshikawa kōbunkan, 1984.

Hodgson, Marshall G.S. *The Venture of Islam*, vol. 1. Chicago, IL: University of Chicago Press, 1974.

– *The Venture of Islam*, vol. 2. Chicago, IL: University of Chicago Press, 1977.

Ibn al-Qifṭī. *Tārīkh al-ḥukamāʾ*. Edited by Fuad Sezgin. Frankfurt, Germany: Institute for the History of Arabic-Islamic Science, 1999.

Ibn Abī Uṣaybiʿa. *ʿUyūn al-anbāʾ fī ṭabaqāt al-aṭibbāʾ*. Beirut: Dār Maktabat al-Hayāʾ, 1965.

Ibn Abi Usaybiʿah. *Anecdotes and Antidotes A Medieval Arabic History of Physicians. A New Translation*. Edited by Henrietta Sharp Cockrell. Oxford, UK: Oxford World's Classics, 2020.

Ḥunayn ibn Isḥāq al-ʿIbādī. *Masaʾil fi al-ṭibb*. Edited by Muḥammad ʿAli Abū Rayyān. Cairo: Dar al-Jamiʿat al-Miṣriyya, 1978.

Ibn al-Nadīm. *Kitāb al-fihrist*, vol. 1. Edited by Ayman Fuʾād Sayyid. London: Al-Furqan Islamic Heritage, 2009.

Iskandar, A.Z. "An Attempted Reconstruction of the Late Alexandrian Medical Curriculum." *Medical History* 20 (1976): 235–58.

Kahl, Oliver. *The Sanskrit, Syriac and Persian Sources in the* Comprehensive Book *of Rhazes*. Leiden, Netherlands: Brill, 2015.

Yaʿqūb al-Kashkarī. *Book on Medicine: Kunnāsh, Series Publications of the Institute for the History of Arabic-Islamic Science, vol. 17*. Edited by Fuat Sezgin. Frankfurt, Germany: Institut für Geschichte der Arabisch-Islamischen Wissenschaften, 1985.

Khan, M.A. Mujeeb. "Early Japan and the Continental Medical Literary Tradition: Tanba no Yasuyori's Conceptualization of Medicine in *Ishinpō*." PhD diss. Cambridge: University of Cambridge, 2016.

– "Critique in Early Japan: *Ishinpō* as a Case Study on How to Read a Text." *New Ideas in East Asian Studies Special Edition* (2017): 56–61.

– "Transposing Knowledge: Beyond Translation in the Medieval Islamic and Japanese Medical Literary Traditions." In *Knowledge in Translation: Global Patterns of Scientific Exchange, 1000–1800 CE*, edited by Patrick Manning and Abigail Owen, 191–205. Pittsburgh, PA: University of Pittsburgh Press, 2018.

– "The Two Ibn Sīnās: Negotiating Traditions." *Journal for the Intellectual History of the Islamicate World* 6, no. 1–2 (2018): 1–26.

Kin Bunkyō [Mungyŏng] 金文京. *Kanbun to higashi ajia: Kundoku no bunkaken* 漢文と東アジア―訓読の文化圏. Tokyo: Iwanami shoten, 2010.

Kornicki, Peter Francis. *Languages, Scripts, and Chinese Texts in East Asia*. Oxford, UK: Oxford University Press, 2018.

Kosoto Hiroshi 小曽戸洋. *Chūgoku igaku koten to nihon: shoshi to denshō* 中国医学古典と日本: 書誌と伝承. Tokyo: Hanawa shobō, 1996.

Mattern, Susan P. *The Prince of Medicine: Galen in the Roman Empire*. Oxford, UK: Oxford University Press, 2013.

Meyerhof, Max. "The 'Book of Treasure,' an Early Arabic Treatise on Medicine." *Isis* 14, no. 1 (1930): 55–76.

Needham, Joseph. *Science and Civilisation in China. Vol. 1: Introductory Orientations.* Cambridge: Cambridge University Press, 1965.

Nutton, Vivian. "The Fatal Embrace: Galen and the History of Ancient Medicine." *Science in Context* 18, no. 1 (2005): 111–21.

Pormann, Peter E., and Emilie Savage-Smith. *Medieval Islamic Medicine.* Edinburgh: Edinburgh University Press, 2007.

Pormann, Peter E. "Medical Education in Late Antiquity: From Alexandria to Montpellier." In *Hippocrates and Medical Education*, edited by Manfred Horstmanshoff, 419–41. Leiden, Netherlands: Brill, 2010.

El-Rouayheb, Khaled. *Islamic Intellectual History in the Seventeenth-Century: Scholarly Currents in the Ottoman Empire and the Maghreb.* Cambridge: Cambridge University Press, 2015.

Savage-Smith, Emilie. "The Working Files of Rhazes: Are the *Jāmiʿ* and the *Ḥāwī* Identical?" In *Medieval Arabic Thought: Essays in Honour of Fritz Zimmerman*, edited by Rotraud Hansberger, M. Afifi al-Akiti, and Charles Burnett, 163–80. London: The Warburg Institute, 2012.

Shihadeh, Ayman. "A Post-Ghazalian Critic of Avicenna: Ibn Ghaylān al-Balkhī on the Materia Medica of the *Canon of Medicine.*" *Journal of Islamic Studies* 24, no. 2 (2013): 135–74.

Siraisi, Nancy. *Avicenna in Renaissance Italy: The* Canon *and Medical Teaching in Italian Universities after 1500.* Princeton, NJ: Princeton University Press, 1981.

Sivin, Nathan. "Huang ti nei ching 黃帝內經." In *Early Chinese Texts: A Bibliographical Guide*, edited Michael Loewe, 196–215. Berkeley, CA: University of California Press, 1993.

Sugimoto Masayoshi and David Swain. *Science and Culture in Traditional Japan: A.D. 600–1854.* Cambridge, MA: MIT Press, 1978.

Sugitatsu Yoshikazu 杉立義一. *Ishinpō no denrai* 医心方の伝来. Kyoto, Japan: Shibunkaku shuppan, 1991.

Taub, Liba. *Science Writing in Greco-Roman Antiquity.* Cambridge: Cambridge University Press, 2017.

Temkin, Owsei. *Galenism: Rise and Decline of a Medical Philosophy.* Ithaca, NY: Cornell University Press, 1973.

Tian, Xiaofei. "Literary Learning: Encyclopedias and Epitomes." In *The Oxford Handbook of Classical Chinese Literature (1000 BCE–900 CE)*, edited by Wiebke Denecke, Wai-Yee Li, and Xiaofei Tian, 132–46. Oxford, UK: Oxford University Press, 2017.

Tōno Haruyuki 東野治之. *Kentōshi* 遣唐使. Tokyo: Iwanami shoten, 2007.

Ullmann, Manfred. *Islamic Medicine.* Edinburgh: Edinburgh University Press, 1997.

Walbridge, John, trans. *The Alexandrian Epitomes of Galen, Volume 1.* Provo, UT: Brigham Young University Press, 2014.

Yajima Genryō 矢島玄亮. *Nihonkoku genzaisho mokuroku: shūshō to kenkyū* 日本国見在書目録—集証と研究. Tokyo: Kyūko shoin, 1984.

Zurndorfer, Harriet T. "The Passion to Collect, Select, and Protect: Fifteen Hundred Years of the Chinese Encyclopaedia." In *Encyclopaedism from Antiquity to the Renaissance*, edited by Jason König and Greg Woolf, 505–28. Cambridge: Cambridge University Press, 2013.

2

Jaghmīnī's *Qānūnča*:
A Popular Abridgement of Avicenna's *Canon*

Sally P. Ragep

Modern histories of Islamic medicine tend to emphasize new discoveries, prominent individuals, and transmission to medieval and early modern Europe.[1] Much less attention has been paid to the importance of transmission of medical knowledge within Islamic lands and the textbook tradition that was an integral component of this transmission. This chapter focuses on one important medical textbook that played a prominent part in medical education and, most likely, provided knowledge of learned medicine to a lay public.

Maḥmūd al-Jaghmīnī (fl. 1200) wrote multiple scientific works on astronomy, arithmetic, astrology, and medicine.[2] These books, all in Arabic, were composed in Central Asia under the auspices of the Khwārizm-Shāhs (r. 1077–1231), a period often erroneously considered one of scientific stagnation within Islamic lands. Two of his works became extremely popular teaching textbooks: an introduction to Ptolemaic theoretical astronomy entitled *al-Mulakhkhaṣ fī ʿilm al-hayʾa* (*Epitome on the Science of Astronomy*) and his medical treatise, *al-Qānūnča* (*The "Little Qānūn"*[3]), the focus of this chapter, which is an abridgement of Ibn Sīnā's [Avicenna's] (d. 1037) medical compendium (the *Qānūn* or *Canon*).[4] It is well known that abridgements and commentaries on Ibn Sīnā's *Qānūn* played an important role in a medical education in various traditions; and the *Qānūnča*, from its original composition in early-thirteenth-century Khwārizm, endured to the extent that it is included in the list of required reading in the curriculum of institutions under British rule in twentieth-century India.[5] Moreover, readership notes attest that this medical primer and its various derivatives were read in hospitals and also religious institutions.[6] Indeed, many Muslim religious authorities (the *ʿulamāʾ*) considered the practice of medicine (meaning Galenic/Avicennian medicine) a kind of religious activity, in this case healing the body as a prerequisite for healing the soul. And the nobility of the medical profession found support in an oft-cited verse from the Qurʾān (V.35): "And if any one saved a life, it would be as if he saved the life of the whole people."[7]

The fact remains, however, that the *Qānūnča*, though recognized, has received little modern scholarly attention despite its impact and tenacity as a teaching textbook. This chapter is a preliminary attempt to rectify this by contextualizing the teaching of the *Qānūnča*. Broadly speaking, this consists of: (1) situating the *Qānūnča* within the textual tradition of Ibn Sīnā's *Qānūn*; (2) providing the *Qānūnča*'s table of contents (to give a sense of chosen topics); (3) definitively establishing Jaghmīnī's floruit date (since most sources get it wrong), allowing us to investigate the target audience, patronage, and the network of scholars actively engaged in developing a scientific education during this period; and (4) documenting the influence of the work's extensive commentary tradition and translations (via Table 2.1 below).

Al-Qānūn fī al-ṭibb (*Canon medicinae*) was described by William Osler (d. 1919) as "the most famous medical text-book ever written. It is safe to say that the 'Canon' was a medical bible for a longer period than any other work."[8] This is high praise indeed, considering that Ibn Sīnā was only one of several renowned authors who composed works (originally in Arabic) that influenced the medical tradition of Western Europe in their Latin renditions well into the seventeenth century.[9]

Avicenna's *Canon* stands out as a major influence that helped integrate Greek medicine into various traditions. And some hundred and fifty years after Ibn Sīnā completed his massive five-volume compendium in 1024,[10] Gerard of Cremona (d. 1187) translated it into Latin; the *Canon* was subsequently used in western European universities. According to Nancy Siraisi, "between 1500 and 1674 at least sixty editions of the complete or partial text of the *Canon* in Latin were printed and a substantial body of new commentary was composed."[11] Its influence outside the universities "may be seen in citations of Avicenna in vernacular medical treatises as well as in the existence of vernacular medical compendia purportedly based on Avicenna's work."[12] Furthermore, in 1593 the *Canon* was one of five Arabic scientific texts selected for publication in the original Arabic by the Medici Oriental Press under the direction of Giovanni Battista Raimondi in Rome.[13]

Not surprisingly, Ibn Sīnā's *al-Qānūn fī al-ṭibb* has also been a seminal influence on medical learning within Islamic lands, South Asia, and elsewhere.[14] The proliferation of copies of the work and its various derivatives (whose copies number in the tens of thousands) span over nine centuries.[15] Despite its enormous influence, the *Qānūn* did incur its share of detractors. Medieval Andalusian scholars in particular did not greet medical knowledge received from "eastern authorities," such as Ibn Sīnā, with much enthusiasm.[16] And in more recent times, what we might call the tradition of the *Qānūn* – its commentaries, glosses, and abridgements – has been criticized for being mostly descriptive and lacking any intellectual merit.[17] In a way, nineteenth- and

twentieth-century medical historians have often followed the view articulated
by the eleventh-century Egyptian physician Ibn Riḍwān (d. 1067) that "works
should be studied in the original without a commentary … and that shortcuts
to medical education hurt the profession, for they allow ignorant men to practice medicine."[18] Ibn Riḍwān's stance, however, should be tempered in light
of the fact that he himself composed some hundred medical works, many of
which were short treatises on various medical topics.[19]

In fact, commentaries were recognized by premodern actors as a means
to introduce new ideas as well as clarify obscure points. Ibn al-Haytham
[Alhazen] (d. c. 1040), renowned for his work in optics, mathematics, and
astronomy, makes this point explicitly in the introduction to his commentary
on Ptolemy's *Almagest*.[20] And Ibn Sīnā tells us in his autobiography how he
rejoiced in finding a commentary in the marketplace by al-Fārābī (tenth century) that clarified obscure points and helped him comprehend the content
of Aristotle's *Metaphysics*.[21] Therefore, it is somewhat ironic that Ibn Sīnā
claims in his introduction to Book One (*On General Principles of Medicine*) of
the *Qānūn* that his work alone sufficiently provides a physician the minimum
indispensable amount of information needed to master the general and particular principles of both theoretical and practical aspects of medicine, and
in a "concise" manner.[22]

Ibn Sīnā's notion of "brevity," however, is a matter of opinion.[23] His idea of
a concise work for Book One of the *Qānūn* consists of four parts: Part One: six
lessons (contained in 92 sections); Part Two: three lessons (contained in 99 sections); Part Three: five lessons (contained in 42 sections); and Part Four: one
lesson (contained in 31 sections) – 264 sections in total.[24] Clearly, the unwield-
iness of the compendium's size made it understandable (if not inevitable) that
a growing demand would emerge for works that could elucidate the content
and make it readily accessible; these would take the form of commentaries,
glosses, translations, and abridgements.[25]

We are thus led back to the *Qānūnča*. Jaghmīnī states in the introduction that
it contains the "choicest parts" from "books of the Ancients"; but based on
preliminary evidence, he relied principally on Ibn Sīnā's Book One (*On General
Principles of Medicine*). In order to get a sense of the range of medical topics
Jaghmīnī covers, as well as an idea of what constituted the "choicest parts,"
the following is the table of contents.[26] The *Qānūnča* is divided into ten parts
(containing 94 sections). Part One (in five sections) deals with natural matters
(*al-umūr al-ṭabīʿiyya*), these being the underlying principles of medicine. Part
Two (in seven sections) deals with anatomy (of various organs). Part Three
(in five sections) deals with conditions of the human body, their causes and
symptoms. Part Four (in six sections) deals with the pulse and urine (and stool).
Part Five (in ten sections) deals with regimens for health and treatments of

diseases. Part Six (in thirteen sections) deals with diseases of the head. Part Seven (in eighteen sections) deals with other diseases of the body from the chest to the bottom of the navel. Part Eight (in nine sections) deals with diseases affecting the remaining parts of the body. Part Nine (in eight sections) deals with manifest deformities on the exterior of the body and with fevers. Part Ten (in thirteen sections) deals with the efficacy of foods and drinks.

According to an early-fifteenth-century *Qānūnča* commentator, Ḥusayn ibn Muḥammad ibn ʿAlī al-Āstarabādhī, Jaghmīnī's "abridgement" was "currently used in all countries, and, indeed, students were as familiar with it as with the midday sun."[27] This assertion is indicative of the importance of the *Qānūnča* as a teaching textbook. It also seemingly affirms that Jaghmīnī managed to scale down Ibn Sīnā's general principles of medicine rather successfully into a relatively manageable size, concise enough to meet the needs of a broad readership. The extent of its readership is borne out by the fact that the base text and its ensuing commentaries and translations (Persian, Turkish, Urdu, Punjabi) continued to be studied and reproduced extensively into the twentieth century throughout Anatolia as well as Central and South Asia.[28] The proliferation of copies of Jaghmīnī's *Qānūnča* is in fact emblematic of the efforts made by the British in the late eighteenth century to promote the study of selected works in the original language and in translation in both Britain and India.[29] Thus it is not surprising that among the hundreds of extant copies and lithographs of these works (currently located in repositories worldwide),[30] one finds an anonymous English rendition of Jaghmīnī's *Qānūnča*, based on a fifteenth-century Persian translation from the original Arabic, printed in eighteenth-century Calcutta.[31] Also interesting is an extant copy of the *Qānūnča* transliterated into Hebrew characters (see table 2.1 at end of chapter, no. [44]).[32]

It could be that the *Qānūnča* has been overshadowed due to the plethora of abridgements of Ibn Sīnā's *Qānūn*; there are at least eleven others.[33] Among them, two especially stand out. One is by Ibn Sīnā's student Muḥammad ibn Yūsuf Īlāqī (d. 1048), who composed an epitome entitled *al-Fuṣūl Īlāqiyya* or *Ikhtiṣār Kitāb al-Qānūn*.[34] The other is by Ibn al-Nafīs (d. 1288), whose *Mūjaz min al-Qānūn* rivals Jaghmīnī's *Qānūnča*; the *Mūjaz*'s dissemination and "popularity was such that the text and its commentaries were still being published in Urdu at the turn of the twentieth century in India."[35] Despite its rivals, it is noteworthy that the neglect of the *Qānūnča* has meant there is little (if any) research on the remarkable existence of six *Qānūnča* commentaries dedicated to the Ottoman Sultan Bayezid II (r. 1481–1512);[36] their existence raises intriguing questions related to the identity of these commentators, why so many were composed at this time and place, and so on. However, the number of copies of the *Qānūnča* and its commentaries amount to less than 2 per cent of all medical titles listed in Bayezid II's Topkapı Palace library collection, according to the inventory of the collection prepared in 1502–03 in Istanbul by the chief librarian Khayr al-Dīn ʿAṭūfī (d. 1541).[37]

In addition, little was known, until recently, about Jaghmīnī, including the date for his floruit; hence questions about the kind of society that produced such a scholar and his target audience received little attention and remained unaddressed.[38] Most reference sources in the field of Islamic studies, including some of the most reputable and widely used, misdate the *Qānūnča* to the fourteenth century.[39] Moreover, this error occurs in both Western and non-Western sources.[40] Some reference two Jaghmīnīs, distinguishing between an early-thirteenth-century astronomer/mathematician (d. 1221–22) who authored the *Mulakhkhaṣ* and a fourteenth-century physician (d. 1344–45) who wrote the *Qānūnča*.[41]

Since it is important to establish a definitive date for a single Jaghmīnī who composed in essence a corpus of elementary scientific textbooks during this formative period of the late twelfth and early thirteenth centuries (i.e., not the fourteenth), let me briefly summarize how this misdating and bifurcation originated, and how they were ultimately resolved. It originated with a reliance on a specious marginal note in a *Qānūnča* copy stating that Jaghmīnī died in 745 H [1344–45 CE] (Gotha, Forschungsbibliothek, MS orient. A 1930, folio 1b);[42] and this error continued to be perpetuated for several basic reasons: 1) there was an over-reliance on authority (in this case Heinrich Suter, d. 1922) that led to an initial mistake being perpetuated for over a century; 2) commentaries on Jaghmīnī's scientific works did not emerge until roughly the mid-fourteenth century, making it seem that Jaghmīnī was later than he was; and 3) modifications by later commentators to Jaghmīnī's *Mulakhkhaṣ* made it appear that he was dependent on later sources.[43]

Ultimately, it was possible to establish a single, earlier Jaghmīnī based upon extant *Qānūnča* and *Mulakhkhaṣ* manuscripts bearing thirteenth-century copy dates (the earliest one being of the *Qānūnča* dated 1205 in Konya),[44] in conjunction with internal textual evidence that included the names of two dedicatees whose dates could be established. All placed Jaghmīnī as flourishing in the late twelfth and early thirteenth centuries, most likely in the environs of Merv in Central Asia during the reigns of the Khwārizm-Shāhs ʿAlāʾ al-Dīn Tekish (r. 1172–1200) and ʿAlāʾ al-Dīn Muḥammad (r. 1200–20).

Jaghmīnī's two dedicatees not only allowed for a determination of his dates, but they also provided insights into the social, political, and religious milieu of the period that indicated the increasing importance of a scientific education. Jaghmīnī dedicates his introduction to Ptolemaic astronomy (the *Mulakhkhaṣ*) and a treatise on planetary sizes and distances to a certain Imām Badr al-Dīn al-Qalānisī,[45] a scholar recognized not for astronomy, but for his pharmaceutical treatise (in forty-nine chapters) entitled *Aqrābādhīn al-Qalānisī* (composed

c. 1194).[46] The life of Badr al-Dīn is not well known,[47] but the *Aqrābādhīn* is full of quotations that "attest to [Qalānisī's] wide reading in the field; besides Ibn Sīnā, a whole range of authors, of whom al-Bīrūnī is the latest datable one, is represented."[48] Badr al-Dīn exemplifies why twelfth-century Central Asia has been depicted as "remarkable for the development of a vernacular medical and scientific literature of which only scanty traces are found in earlier times."[49] Although several sources also misdate Badr al-Dīn (like Jaghmīnī) as flourishing in the early fourteenth century,[50] a substantial number of medical sources reference Qalānisī,[51] several stemming from the thirteenth century. One is the pharmacological treatise by Najīb al-Samarqandī (d. 1222, Herat);[52] another the work on remedies of al-Suwaydī (1204–1292, Damascus),[53] who was a student of the Andalusian Ibn al-Bayṭār [Ebenbitar] (d. 1248, Damascus),[54] and a contemporary of the physician and bio-bibliographer Ibn Abī Uṣaybiʿa (d. 1270, Damascus).[55]

The network of scholarly pipelines between the regions of Syria and Central Asia is striking (and certainly not limited to these regions alone). It is significant that Badr al-Dīn, who apparently lived in Central Asia, hailed from a prominent Damascene family with members who were prominent government bureaucrats, scholars, and religious judges (*qāḍī*s). The Qalānisīs played an important role in "professionalizing" the Islamic religious scholars (the *ʿulamā*), where professionalization included standardizing their educational textbooks.[56] Remarkably, these textbooks were not limited to law and ancillary subjects (although this has, until recently, been the standard view regarding madrasa education). Thus Badr al-Dīn's connection with Jaghmīnī, and the latter's writing of scientific textbooks, may not be coincidental and may well indicate the professionalization role of the Qalānisī family in Central Asia as well as Syria. As for medical professionalization, we know of three thirteenth-century madrasas in Damascus designated specifically for the study of medicine that presumably required medical textbooks.[57] And it is reported that the Nūrī hospital, also in Damascus (est. c. 1174), was considered a major centre of medical activity in the thirteenth century and continued to function into the nineteenth century, influencing hospital practice in other regions, such as at the Manṣūrī hospital in Cairo (est. 1284–85), which also thrived into the nineteenth century.[58] It is not incidental that there is a note appended to a copy of a *Qānūnča* commentary (dated 1760–61) by a certain senior physician named Muḥammad at the Manṣūrī hospital, explicitly stating that the *Qānūnča* was taught there.[59]

There is evidence that not only were Jaghmīnī's textbooks taught in Islamic institutions, but this may well have been their intended use. Support for this comes from primary and secondary sources related to his second dedicatee, Shihāb al-Dīn al-Khiwaqī, an eminent scholar[60] to whom Jaghmīnī dedicated an astrological work and a treatise on Euclid's *Elements*. Shihāb al-Dīn was a trusted advisor (*wakīl*) to the Khwārizm-Shāh ʿAlāʾ al-Dīn Muḥammad, who "consulted [Shihāb al-Dīn] in all serious circumstances and yielded to his decision in important matters."[61] That prominent scholars often used their positions with governmental connections to promote scholarly activities is relevant here. It is reported that Shihāb al-Dīn was directly responsible for establishing numerous Islamic institutions throughout the region and filling their libraries with extensive collections. Furthermore, he was charged with teaching in five madrasas, and is alleged to have built a library in a Shāfiʿī mosque in Khwārizm that had no equal "either before or since."[62] This would mean that Shihāb al-Dīn's library would have surpassed Yāqūt al-Ḥamawī's citing of 12,000 volumes (in one library alone) among the multitude of scholarly books he scouted that were located throughout Merv during this time.[63] (Perhaps copies of the *Qānūnča* made up more than 2 per cent of his medical collection!)

The scientific activities of the twelfth and early thirteenth centuries underscore the point that this was a formative period for the development of a scientific educational program in the Islamic world. Many of the initiatives that standardized scientific textbooks on Greek science (and other topics), laying the foundations for the institutional structures in which they could be taught, occurred at this time.[64] That science in Islam stretched over well-nigh a millennium is, among other things, testament to how entrenched the scientific textual tradition had become.

The enduring textual tradition of Ibn Sīnā's *al-Qānūn* and its Arabic, Persian, and Urdu derivatives is certainly impressive and encourages a view of the continuity of Greek medicine within Islam.[65] In this chapter, I have sought to emphasize this continuity by focusing on the long-lived tradition of Jaghmīnī's *Qānūnča*. In doing so, I have, due to limitations of space and time, underplayed the importance of the local, whether defined by geography or time period.[66] Another reason to pay attention to a tradition of *longue durée* is to counter a tendency in microhistory to emphasize exceptions and idiosyncratic individuals. But there is no reason we should not be able to bridge the divide between tradition and the local.

The first step, of course, is to acknowledge difference within a tradition. The social, political, and historical realities that influenced a medical education under the Ottomans[67] differs from that of Egypt or Iran or South Asia; in the latter region, treatises on Avicennian medicine continued to constitute a sizable body of medical literature during the Mughal (1526–1857)[68] and Colonial (1858–1947) periods. And the continuing relevance of Unani (i.e., Avicennian medicine) in South Asia, despite its diminished significance in much of the rest of the Islamic world, calls for a "local" explanation. Here we can do little more than point to such an explanation. In the late nineteenth and early twentieth centuries, as a result of rising nationalist and religious sentiment to counter the British Raj, the hakims of South Asia, exemplified by Hakim Ajmal Khan (d. 1928, Delhi), attempted to revive the tradition of studying Greek medicine and defend its approach as a scientific discipline.[69] Given that Unani is currently practised in various parts of the world, and especially thriving in South Asia,[70] it is not farfetched to believe that the *Qānūnča* is still being read today, not as a historical relic or as a way to identify with Muslim culture,[71] but as an alternative source of healing.

Table 2.1 Works derivative from the *Qānūnča*

Author	Description: Title
	Notes and Bibliography

A. Commentaries, Glosses, etc. (Arabic) [26]

1 Tāj al-Dīn Ḥasan al-Ṭabīb [Ḥakīm zāde]   Commentary: *Sharḥ al-Qānūnča*
[1] (fl. 14th century)
Cited in the *Sharḥ al-Qānūnča* by al-Fāḍil al-Baghdādī (Berlin, Stabi, Wetzstein II MS 1187, f. 2a); see [2].
Istanbul: TSMK, A. MS 1983, copied by Niẓām ibn ʿAbd Allāh ibn Muḥammad al-Tabrīzī, 773/1371–72; see Karatay, 3:826, no. 7274 and Şeşen et al., 186.

2 [Yūsuf] al-Fāḍil al-Baghdādī   Commentary: *Sharḥ al-Qānūnča*
[2] (fl. after 710/1311)
Lived post-710/1311 based on references to a *Qānūn* commentary by Quṭb al-Dīn al-Shīrāzī (d. 1311). Also mentioned are Ibn al-Nafīs (d. 1288) and the physician Tāj al-Dīn Ḥasan ([1]).
Berlin: Stabi, Wetzstein II MS 1187, ff. 1a–193a, copied 1122/1710–11 (Ahlwardt, 5:556–8, no. 6294). See also *Fankhā*, 24:743(1) (=*DENA*, 6:909; 4 copies in Iran); *GAL* 1:457(aa) [=598(aa)]; Perwāz, 305(m); Rahman, no. 43.

3 Ḥusayn ibn Muḥammad ibn ʿAlī al-   Commentary: *Sharḥ al-Qānūnča*
[3] Āstarabādhī (fl. 830/1426–27)
Dedicated to Bayezid II (r. 1481–1512); composed Thursday, 17 Ramaḍān 831/30 June 1428 in Herat for Amīr Sayyid al-Murtaḍā (d. 837/1433).
Cambridge, UK: Or. 6 (copy contains some Persian interlinear glosses) (Browne, *Suppl.*, 151, no. 914). Istanbul: IU, MS 6163; SK, Ayasofya MS 3676, copied 976/1569; TSMK, A. MS 1979, copied 901/1496, contains Bayezid II's seal

Table 2.1 Works derivative from the *Qānūnča* (continued)

(Karatay, 3:826–7, no. 7275 and Şeşen et al., 186). Kütahya: Vahid Paşa Library, MS 804. London: WMS, Or. 132, copied 897/1491–92 (f. 189a) (Iskandar, 56–7, 64, 184). Oxford: Bodleian, Arab. e. 178, copied end of Shaʿbān 999/June 1591 by Aḥmad ibn ʿAbd Allāh (Savage-Smith, 310–12, no. 69). Rampur: Riḍā Lib., copied 1150/1737 (Arshi, 5:272–3, no. 3980, 4477 M.). See also Buonazia, 236, no. 95; *Fankhā*, 24:743(2) (=*DENA*, 6:909–10; 29 copies in Iran); *GAL* 1:457(bb) [=598(bb)]; *GAL* suppl., 1:826(bb); Hameed-Bari, 8(a); Loth, 297, no. 1041, III, ff. 164–253; Rahman, no. 55. Perwāz, 304(a) also lists a Persian *Sharḥ Qānūnča* attributed to him (306(2)), but most likely this is another copy of the Arabic work.

| 4 | Mullā Yaḥyā Nīsābūrī Fattāḥī | Commentary: *Sharḥ al-Qānūnča* |

[4] (d. 832/1448)

Peshawar Univ., 1626. See *GAL* suppl., 1:826(oo); Perwāz, 305(j); Rahman, no. 53.

5   ʿAlī ibn Kamāl al-Dīn Maḥmūd al-   Commentary: *Sharḥ al-Qānūnča*

[5] Āstarābādhī al-Makkī (fl. c. 884/1480)

Dedicated to Bayezid II (r. 1481–1512). The author calls himself *mutarjim* (interpreter). A contemporary of al-Miṣrī [no. 7]. He is also the copyist of a commentary by Aqsarāʾī on the *Mūjaz* of Ibn al-Nafīs (d. 1288) dated 22 Shawwāl 884/6 Jan. 1480; see LJS 444 (f. 240b) (Black, 82–3), http://dla.library.upenn. edu/dla/medren/detail.html?id=MEDREN_9959031653503681. Gotha 1930, copied 949/1542 (Pertsch, 3/3:468–70). London: WMS, Or. 26, copied Friday, 24 Shawwāl 1174/29 May 1761 by Muḥammad Ṭāhir (f. 97a). The end of this copy contains a note by a certain senior physician named Muḥammad stating the *Qānūnča* was taught at the *Dār al-shifāʾ* [lit., house of healing], i.e., the Manṣūrī hospital in Cairo (est. 1284–85) (f. 99b). See Iskandar, 56, 58–63, 184–5 (esp. for his analysis on the misattribution of Gotha 1930 to al-Miṣrī). Oxford: Bodleian, Or. 421.2. Parts 5–10 have been transcribed by Henry Wild in the 18th c. Listed as anonymous, the table of contents Wild provides is identical to WMS, Or. 26 (Savage-Smith, 314–18, no. 71).

6   ʿAlī ibn Aḥmad al-Lāhjānī (d. 901/1496)   Commentary: *Sharḥ al-Qānūnča*

[6] Dedicated to Bayezid II (r. 1481–1512)

Istanbul: TSMK, A. MS 1977, copied 901/1495–96 by Muṣṭafā, contains Bayezid II's seal; see Karatay, 3:827, no. 7276; Şeşen et al., 186.

7   Muḥammad ibn Muḥammad   Commentary: *Sharḥ al-Qānūnča*

[7] al-Ṭabīb al-Miṣrī (c. 915/1510)

Dedicated to Bayezid II (r. 1481–1512). He calls himself *al-mutaṭabbib ibn al-mutaṭabbib* (physician, son of a physician) and claims his is the first commentary (Chester Beatty, MS 4006, f. 2a); however, there are earlier ones.

Table 2.1 Works derivative from the *Qānūnča* (continued)

Dublin: Chester Beatty, MS 4006, autograph copy dated 15 Jumādā I 915/31 Aug. 1509 (Arberry, 5:3, no. 4006). See *Fankhā*, 24:743(4) (=*DENA*, 6:910; 1 copy in Iran); *GAL* 1:457(cc) [=598(cc)]; Iskandar, 57–9; *Osmanlı Tıbbi*, 96, no. 55; Perwāz, 305(n).

8   'Abd al-Bāsiṭ ibn Khalīl ibn Shāhīn   Commentary: *Sharḥ al-Qānūnča*
[8]   al-Malaṭī al-Ḥanafī [Ibn al-Wazīr]
(844–920/1440–1514)
Composed Friday, 14 Shawwāl 884/29 Dec. 1479. 'Abd al-Bāsiṭ was a physician and the son of a Mamluk Wazir to Sultan Barsbay (r. 1422–38); died 872/1468. Istanbul: BSL, Veliyüddin Efendi MS 251 (Şeşen et al., 187). Manchester, UK: John Rylands Lib., Crawford MS 621, copied 890/1485, contains ownership marks dated 18th and 19th cc. (Mingana, cols. 513–15, no. 331). See *GAL* suppl., 1:826(mm); Perwāz, 305(h); Rahman, no. 65. For 'Abd al-Bāsiṭ, see Brunschvig, 7; Massoud, 67–9.

9   Ḥusayn al-Ḥusaynī 'Unṣurī al-Jīlī   Commentary: *Sharḥ al-Qānūnča*
[9]   (al-Jīlānī) al-Mutaṭabbib (c. 919/1513)
Composed 903/1498; dedicated to Bayezid II (r. 1481–1512). Istanbul: TSMK, A. MS 1987 (Karatay, 3:828, no. 7278); SK, Hafid Efendi MS 268, copied by Ḥasan ibn Walī al-Jīlī (no. [10]). See *Osmanlı astronomi*, 73, no. 40; Şeşen et al., 186–7.

10   Ḥasan ibn Walī Khān al-Shifā'ī   Commentary: *Sharḥ al-Qānūnča*
[10]   al-Jīlānī (al-Jīlī) (al-Jabalī)
(fl. late 15th/early 16th centuries)
According to the Riḍā Library catalogue (Rampur), Ḥasan ibn Walī dedicated the work to Kār Kiyā Mīrzā 'Alī, a ruler who flourished in the late 15th and early 16th centuries in Lāhīdjān, a province of Jīlān. Hyderabad: Salar Jung, Tibb 41 (Ashraf, 8:91–2, no. 2312). Leiden: Or. 718, copied 983/1575–76; Rampur: Riḍā Lib., copied 11th/17th c. (Arshi, 5:272–3, no. 3979, 4476 M.). See *Fankhā*, 24:743(3) (=*DENA*, 6:910–11; 2 copies in Iran); *GAL* suppl., 1:826(nn); Hameed-Bari, 8(g); Perwāz, 305(i); Rahman, no. 51. *GAL* 1:457(dd) [=598(dd)] and 3 catalogue entries for Leiden, Or. 718 (f. 89a) give Ḥalabī (Aleppine) [sic], i.e., not Jīlānī for the nisba: CCO, 3:241, no. 1324; Voorhoeve, 264; and Witkam, 1:299 (Or. 718).

11   Rūḥ Allāh ibn Akhī al-Mutaṭabbib   Listed as *Sharḥ tashrīḥ*
[11]   [Ibn al-Mutaṭabbib]   *al-Qānūnča* and *Sharḥ kulliyyāt al-Qānūnča*
(fl. 915/1509 or earlier)
Dedicated to Bayezid II (r. 1481–1512). Istanbul: TSMK, A. MS 2051, copied Jumādā I 915/Aug.–Sept. 1509, contains Bayezid II's seal; see Karatay, 3:827, no. 7277; Şeşen et al., 187.

Table 2.1 Works derivative from the *Qānūnča* (continued)

12   'Abd al-Fattāḥ ibn 'Ubayd Allāh   Commentary: *Sharḥ al-Qānūnča*
[12] al-Qazwīnī (fl. first half of 16th century)
      Istanbul: SK, MS Fatih 3577, copied 934/1527–28, Mecca (Şeşen et al., 187).
      See *GAL* suppl., 1:826(pp); Rahman, no. 80 ('Abd al-Fattāḥ Qazwīnī).

13   'Abd al-Fattāḥ ibn Sayyid Ismāʿīl   *Qānūnča* commentary also entitled
[13] al-Ḥusaynī al-Lāhūrī   *al-Fattāḥī*
      (fl. late 15th and first half of 16th centuries)
      Composed 945/1539. This 'Abd al-Fattāḥ flourished during the Mughal period in
      India. He also composed an epitome of Ibn Sīnā's *Qānūn* in Persian and a
      pharmacological work in Persian entitled *Bustān-i afrūz*.
      Hyderabad: Āṣafiyya, 928, nos. 20, 236, the former copied 1088/1677. Oxford:
      Bodleian, Ind. Inst. Arab 10, unsigned and undated (opening identical to
      Patna copy) (Savage-Smith, 312–14, no. 70). Patna: Khuda Bakhsh, vol. 4, no. 52.
      Rampur: Riḍā Lib., entitled *al-Fattāḥī*, copied 1094/1683 (Arshi, 5:272–3, no.
      3981, 1318 D.). See *GAL* suppl., 1:826(gg); Hameed-Bari, 8(c); Perwāz, 304(d);
      Rahman, no. 68; Rahman-Hāshimī, 154–5; Speziale, *Culture persane*, 48.

14   ʿImād al-Dīn Maḥmūd ibn Masʿūd   Commentary: *Sharḥ al-Qānūnča*
[14] ibn Maḥmūd al-Ḥusaynī al-Shīrāzī al-Ṭabīb
      (d. c. 1000/1591–92)
      Muḥammad ibn Maḥmūd Shīrāzī is the abbreviated name given in *GAL*,
      Hameed-Bari, and Perwāz, all of whom cite only the Rampur copy. Arshi provides
      the full name and death date in his listing for a *Qānūn* commentary by the same
      author (5:234, no. 3923). Arshi states that the Rampur copy of the *Qānūnča*
      commentary is unique.
      Rampur: Riḍā Lib. (Arshi, 5:274–5, no. 3982). See *GAL* suppl., 1:826(ee);
      Hameed-Bari, 8(b); Perwāz, 304(b).

15   Anonymous (16th century)   Commentary: *Sharḥ al-Qānūnča*
[15] Istanbul: IU, MS 518 (Şeşen et al., 187).

16   [Abū Ṣalāḥ] Madyan ibn 'Abd   *Qānūnča* commentary entitled *al-Miṣbāḥ*
[16] al-Raḥmān al- Qūsūnī [Qawṣūnī]   *al-munīr ʿalā al-Qānūn al-ṣaghīr*
      (d. after 1044/1634)
      Fl. late 16th to early 17th centuries. In his *Qānūnča* commentary, he states that he
      was a physician at *Dār al-shifāʾ* in Cairo. It is also stated in a reader's note that "Abū
      Ṣalāḥ Madyan ibn 'Abd al-Raḥmān al-Ṭabīb" read in the hospital between 1020
      and 1025 [1611–17] a 15th-c. commentary on a 15th-c. medical treatise (*al-
      Lamḥa*) by al-ʿAfīf, a chief physician of Cairo (Princeton Univ. Lib., Garrett, MS
      570H, f. 293a–b).
      Leipzig: Leipzig Univ. Lib., Vollers, DC 198 (247–8, no. 764).
      Rabat: Al-Khizāna al-Malakiyya (Royal Palace), MS 5374, copied 14 Rabīʿ II
      1309/17 Nov. 1891. See *GAL* suppl., 1:826(ff); *Osmanlı Tıbbi*, 231, no. 143.3;
      Pewāz, 304(c); Rahman, no. 43.

Table 2.1 Works derivative from the *Qānūnča* (continued)

17 Qiwām al-Dīn Muḥammad al-Ḥasanī   Versification of the *Qānūnča* entitled
[17] (d. c. 1150/1738)   *al-Mufriḥ fī ʿilm al-ṭibb*. Also called:
                                                     al-Mufriḥ al-Qiwāmī; *Mufriḥ al-Qiwām*;
                                                     Qānūnča manẓūm

Completed 1106/1694; *Fankhā* gives this date but lists his name as Muḥammad ibn Muḥammad Mahdī Ḥusaynī Sayfī. He also composed (1132/1711) five poems, collectively entitled *al-Khamsa al-Qazwīniyya* (NLM Microfilm Reel: FILM 48–129, no. 3).
Fankhā, 24:743(7) (=*DENA*, 9:1084; 14 copies); GAL suppl., 1:826(pp); Perwāz, 305(l). See also *Islamic Medical Manuscripts:* https://www.nlm.nih.gov/hmd/arabic/bioQ.html#qiwam.

18 Junayd Allāh Ḥādhiq Harawī [Heravi]   *Qānūnča* commentary also entitled
[18] (d. 1259/1844); east Azerbaijan   *Taḥqīq al-qawāʿid*
     Fankhā, 24:743(9)

19 Abū al-Qāsim ibn Jaʿfar Sulṭān   *Qānūnča* commentary entitled *al-Tuḥfa*
[19] al-ḥukamāʾ (1245–1322/1830–1905)   *al-nāṣiriyya*
     Fankhā, 24:743(10) (=*DENA*, 2:1008; 1 copy in Iran)

20 [Ḥakīm] ʿAbd al-Mājid   *Qānūnča* commentary
[20] Printed in Calcutta in 1872. See GAL suppl., 1:826(ii); Hameed-Bari, 8(d); Perwāz, 304(e); Rahman, no. 105.

21 Aḥmad al-Dīn Lāhūrī   *Qānūnča* commentary
[21]   entitled *Tarwīḥ al-arwāḥ*
Printed in Lahore in 1907. See GAL suppl., 1:826(kk); Hameed-Bari, 8(e); Perwāz, 305(f).

22 ʿAbd Allāh ibn Dāʾūd Panjābī   *Qānūnča* commentary
[22] Printed in Delhi in 1908 and in Lucknow in 1909. See GAL suppl., 1:826(ll); Hameed-Bari, 8(f); Perwāz, 305(g); Rahman, no. 121 (listed as Ali bin Daud Panjabi).

23 Muḥammad ibn Mūsā Ḥusaynī Hamdānī   *Qānūnča* commentary
[23] (d. 1349/1941)
     Fankhā, 24:743(11).

24 Abū al-Ḥusayn ibn Muḥammad   *Qānūnča* commentary entitled *Zubdat*
[24] Hādī ʿUlawī Shīrāzī   *al-nikāt fī sharḥ al-kulliyyāt*
     Fankhā, 24:743(12) (=*DENA*, 5:1230; 1 copy in Iran).

25 ʿAbd al-Rasūl ibn Zayn al-ʿĀbidīn   *Qānūnča* commentary entitled
[25] [Ṭabīb Ḥusaynī]   *Farāʾid al-kalām*
     Fankhā, 24:743(14).

Table 2.1 Works derivative from the *Qānūnča* (continued)

26   Shaykh Muḥammad Muʾmin Jazarī   *Qānūnča* commentary
[26] Rahman, no. 79.

B. Commentaries and Translations (Persian) [11]

1   Maḥmūd ibn Muḥammad Khwārizmī   Persian translation of the *Qānūnča*
[27] (d. 745/1334-35)
Printed in Lahore in 1330/1911. See Hameed-Bari, 8(c); Perwāz, 306(5);
Rahman, no. 131.

2   [Masīḥ al-Dīn] Abū al-Fatḥ Jīlānī   Persian commentary of the *Qānūnča*
[28] (d. 1589)   entitled *Fattāḥī*
Appointed *ṣadr* (head of religious affairs and land grants) of various Mughal
provinces. He also translated into Persian the first book of the *Qānūn* in 1593
(see Speziale). This Persian work may be related to ʿAbd al-Fattāḥ's Arabic *Qānūnča*
commentary bearing the same name (see [13]), but this needs to be checked.
Rahman, no. 133 (Hakim Abu al-Fatah Gilani); Speziale, "India xxxiii."
See also Alavi, 35-6; Rahman-Hāshimī, 147.

3   Iskandar ibn Mīr Fayḍ al-Ṭabīb   Persian commentary of the *Qānūnča*
[29] (fl. 17th century)
Fankhā, 24:743(8) (=*DENA*, 6:910; 1 copy in Iran).

4   Shāh Arzānī: Muḥammad Akbar   Persian translation of the *Qānūnča*.
[30] ibn Mīr Ḥājjī Muḥammad Muqīm
(d. 1134/1722, Delhi)
Lived in India; travelled to Shiraz in 1115/1703.
Fankhā, 24:743(5); Hameed-Bari, 8(a). Note that Storey does not list this
translation (see 269-71, no. 465).

5   Shāh Arzānī (same as 4 [30])   Persian commentary on the *Qānūnča*
[31]   entitled *Mufarriḥ al-qulūb*
According to Speziale, this commentary "became the most diffused Indo-Persian
commentary on the *Qānūnča*."
London: WMS, Persian: MSS 221, 401, 520, 521, 522, 597 B. (Keshavarz, 57-9,
135, no. 34). Published by Nawal Kishore, Lucknow in 1886. See *Fankhā*,
24:743(6) (=*DENA*, 9:1083-4) [15 copies listed]; Rahman, no. 139; Storey,
219-20, no. 377(g) and 269, no. 465(5). See also Speziale, "Arzānī."

6   Shams ibn Ḥasan Munajjim   Persian translation of the *Qānūnča*
[32] *Fankhā*, 24:743(13); Perwāz, 306(4); Storey, 219, no. 377(d).

Table 2.1 Works derivative from the *Qānūnča* (continued)

7 'Alī Akbar ibn Muḥammad Labīb   Persian translation of the *Qānūnča*
[33] (fl. 18th century)   entitled *Tarjamah-i Suhrābī*
According to the preface, this was translated from Arabic at the request of
Nawāb 'Alī Qulī Khān Bahādur Suhrāb-Jang, son of Mirzā 'Alī Khān Bahādur
Dilāwar-Jang (c. 1691–1765).
Calcutta: Būhar Lib. (Hasir Radavi, 1:183–4, no. 232). See Storey, 219, no. 377(b).

8 Ḥakīm 'Abd al-Mughnī Ramaḍān Purī   Translation of the *Qānūnča*
[34] (d. 1218/1803)   [Persian or Urdu?]
Printed in Lucknow in 1893. Hameed-Bari, 8(b).

9 Anonymous   Persian translation of the *Qānūnča*
[35]   entitled *Wāfiyah*
Cambridge, UK: Add. 3518 (Browne, *Hand-list*, 310–11, no. 1392). London: WMS,
Persian: MSS 27, 568, 569. According to the preface of MS 568 (f. 2a), this copy
was translated after 850/1446 (Keshavarz, 146–8, no. 42 and Storey, 219, no.
377(a), (c)). Rahman, no. 132, lists an author and title (Abdu Allah bin Haj,
"Wa-fiyya") that may be this work.

10 Ḥakīm Mirzā Hādī Shīrāzī   Persian commentary on the *Qānūnča*
[36] Rahman, no. 138. This may be [no. 24], who wrote the Arabic *Qānūnča*
commentary.

11 Ḥakīm Aḥmad Dīn Lāhūrī   A Persian gloss on the *Qānūnča*
[37]   (*Ḥall-i Qānūnča*, also entitled *Kashf al-Rumūz*)

Rahman, no. 152.

C. Commentaries and Translations (Turkish) [2]

1 Aḥī Çelebi Mehmed (Ahmed)   Turkish commentary on the *Qānūnča*
[38] ibn Kemal al-Shirwānī
(d. 930/1524)
Head of physicians during the time of Bayezid II (r. 1481–1512) and
Selīm I (1512–20).
Istanbul: NO, MS 3529, copied 2 Dhū al-Ḥijja 982/15 March 1575).
See *Osmanlı Tıbbi*, 108, no. 66.5.

2 'Abd al-Wahhāb al-Mārdānī: Turkish translation of the *Qānūnča*
[39] 'Abd al-Wahhāb ibn al-Shaykh Jamāl
al-Dīn Yūsuf ibn Aḥmad al-Mārdānī
(c. 823/1420)
For copies of the treatise and references, see *Osmanlı Tıbbi*, cxviii, clxix, 35–6,
no. 14.2; Şeşen et al., 339.

Table 2.1 Works derivative from the *Qānūnča* (continued)

D. Commentaries and Translations (Urdu) [3]

1 Ḥakīm Tāj Muḥammad Khān [40] Rahman, no. 171.	Urdu commentary on the *Qānūnča*

2 Ḥakīm Ghulām Ḥusayn Kantūrī   Urdu translation of the *Qānūnča*
[41] Published by Nawal Kishore, Lucknow in 1889 (with Arabic text).
See Hameed-Bari, 8(d); Rahman, no. 162.

3 Ḥakīm ʿAbd al-Ghānī   Urdu translation of the *Qānūnča*
[42] Rahman, no. 165.

E. Translation (Punjabi) [1]

1 Ḥakīm Muḥammad al-Dīn   Punjabi translation of the *Qānūnča*
[43] Rahman, no. 181.

F. Transcriptions (Hebrew) [3]

1 Anonymous   Judeo-Arabic transcription of
[44]   the *Qānūnča*
According to Langermann, the spelling is phonetic, indicating that the work may
have been read aloud to the copyist.
New York: JTS, Mic 2651, ff. 2a–47b. See Langermann, "Arabic Writings," 148.

2 Anonymous   Judeo-Arabic transcription of
[45]   the *Qānūnča*
New York: JTS, Mic 2658.

3 Anonymous   Judeo-Arabic transcription of
[46]   the *Qānūnča*
A 17th-c. fragment that may be part of the *Qānūnča*.
St Petersburg: The National Lib. of Russia, MS EVR ARAB II 2190
(NLI film no. F 6016).

Abbreviations used in table 2.1
Berlin: Stabi = Staatsbibliothek zu Berlin
Cambridge, UK = University Library, Cambridge University
Gotha = Forschungsbibliothek, MS orient. A 1930
Hyderabad: Āṣafiyya = Oriental MSS Lib. and Research Institute
Hyderabad: Salar Jung = Salar Jung Museum and Library
Istanbul: BSL = Bayazit State Library
Istanbul: IU = Istanbul University Library
Istanbul: NO = Nuruosmaniye Library

Table 2.1 Works derivative from the *Qānūnča* (continued)

Istanbul: SK = Süleymaniye Library
Istanbul: TSMK = Topkapı Sarayı Museum Library
London: WMS = Wellcome Medical Library
LJS = Philadelphia, University of Pennsylvania, Lawrence J. Schoenberg Collection
New York: JTS = Jewish Theological Seminary of America

Sources

Ahlwardt: Ahlwardt, *Die Handschriften-Verzeichnisse der Königlichen Bibliothek zu Berlin*, vol. 5.

Alavi: Alavi, *Islam and Healing.*

Arberry: Arberry, *The Chester Beatty Library*, vol. 5.

Arshi: Arshi, *Catalogue of the Arabic Manuscripts in Raza Library, Rampur*, vol. 5, *Mathematics, Medicine, Natural Science, Agriculture, Occult Sciences, Ethics & Politics, Education & Military Science.*

Āṣafiyya: *Fihrist-i kutub-i makhṭūṭāt 'Arabī, Fārsī va Urdū makhzūnah-yi Kutub Khānah Āṣafiyya Sarkār-i 'Ālī.* Catalogue of Urdu, Arabic and Persian manuscripts.

Ashraf: Ashraf, *A Concise Descriptive Catalogue of the Arabic Manuscripts in the Salar Jung Museum & Library*, vol. 8, *Mathematics, Astronomy, Astrology, Medicine, Natural History and Alchemy.*

Black: Black, ed., *Transformation of Knowledge: Early Manuscripts from the Collection of Lawrence J. Schoenberg.*

Browne, *Hand-list*: Browne, *A Hand-list of the Muhammadan Manuscripts: including all those written in the Arabic character, preserved in the Library of the University of Cambridge.*

Browne, *Suppl.*: Browne, *A Supplementary Hand-List of the Muhammadan Manuscripts.*

Brunschvig: Brunschvig, "Deux Récits de Voyage inédits en Afrique du Nord au XVᵉ siècle."

Buonazia: Buonazia, *Catalogo dei Codici Arabi della Biblioteca Nazionale di Napoli.*

CCO: Jong and de Goeje, *Catalogus Codicum Orientalium*, vol. 3.

DENA: Dirāyatī, *Fihristvārah-i dastnivisht'hā-yi Īrān*, 12 vols.

Fankhā: Dirāyatī, *Fihristgān*, vol. 24.

GAL: Brockelmann, *Geschichte der arabischen Litteratur*, 2 vols. plus 3 supplements. Reprint reference in square brackets.

Hameed-Bari: Hameed and Hakim, "Impact of Ibn Sina's Medical Works in India."

Hasir Radavi: Hasir Radavi, *Catalogue Raisonné of the Buhar Library*, vol. 1, *Catalogue of the Persian Manuscripts in the Buhar Library.*

Iskandar: Iskandar, *A Catalogue of Arabic Manuscripts on Medicine and Science in the Wellcome Historical Medical Library.*

Karatay: Karatay, *Topkapı Sarayı Müzesi Kütüphanesi Arapça Yazmalar Kataloğu*, vol. 3.

Keshavarz: Keshavarz, *A Descriptive and Analytical Catalogue of Persian Manuscripts in the Library of the Wellcome Institute for the History of Medicine.*

Khuda Bakhsh: Khudā Bakhsh Oriyanṭal Pablik Lā'ibrerī, *Catalogue of the Arabic and Persian Manuscripts in the Khuda Bakhsh Oriental Public Library*, vol. 4, *Medical Works: Arabic.*

Langermann: Langermann, "Arabic Writings in Hebrew Manuscripts."

Loth: Loth, *A Catalogue of Arabic Manuscripts in the Library of the India Office.*

Massoud: Massoud, *The Chronicles and Annalistic Sources of the Early Mamluk Circassian Period.*

Mingana: Mingana, *Catalogue of the Arabic Manuscripts in the John Rylands Library Manchester.*

Table 2.1 Works derivative from the *Qānūnča* (continued)

Osmanlı Astronomi: İhsanoğlu et al., *Osmanlı Astronomi Literatürü Tarihi* (History of Astronomy Literature during the Ottoman Period).

Osmanlı Tıbbi: İhsanoğlu et al., *Osmanlı Tıbbi Bilimler Literatürü Tarihi* (History of the Literature of Medical Sciences during the Ottoman Period).

Pertsch: Pertsch, *Die orientalischen Handschriften der Herzoglichen Bibliothek zu Gotha*, vol. 3, part 3.

Perwāz: Perwāz, "Ibn Sīnā's Medical Works."

Rahman: Rahman, "Commentators and Translators of Ibn Sina's Canon of Medicine."

Rahman-Hāshimī: Rahman, *Qānūn-i Ibn Sīnā, Sharḥān va Mutarjimān-i ān*. Translated into Persian by ʿAbd al-Qādir Hāshimī.

Savage-Smith: Savage-Smith, *A New Catalogue of Arabic Manuscripts in the Bodleian Library, University of Oxford*, vol. 1, *Medicine*.

Şeşen et al.: Şeşen et al., *Catalogue of Islamic Medical Manuscripts [in Arabic, Turkish & Persian] in the Libraries of Turkey*.

Speziale, "Arzānī": Speziale, "Arzānī, Moḥammad Akbar." *Encyclopædia Iranica*. http://www.iranicaonline.org/articles/mohammad-akbar-arzani.

Speziale, "India": Speziale, "India xxxiii. Indo-Muslim Physicians." *Encyclopædia Iranica*. http://www.iranicaonline.org/articles/india-xxxiii-indo-muslim-physicians.

Speziale, *Culture persane*: Speziale, *Culture persane et médecine ayurvédique en Asie du Sud*.

Storey: Storey, *Persian Literature: A Bio-Bibliographical Survey*, vol. 2, part 2, E. Medicine.

Vollers: Vollers, *Katalog der islamischen, christlich-orientalischen, jüdischen und samaritanischen Handschriften der Universitäts-Bibliothek zu Leipzig*.

Voorhoeve: *Handlist of Arabic Manuscripts in the Library of the University of Leiden and Other Collections in The Netherlands*.

Witkam: Witkam, *Inventory of the Oriental Manuscripts of the Library of the University of Leiden*, vol. 1.

ACKNOWLEDGMENTS

I wish to thank Jamil Ragep for his careful read of this chapter and his insightful comments. I also wish to express my appreciation to the editors of this volume, Delia Gavrus and Susan Lamb, for their comments and support, and to Emilie Savage-Smith, for a number of helpful suggestions and additional references.

NOTES

1   Although overviews on medical theory, practices, and writings within the Islamic tradition reference selected individuals and works (see, for example, Pormann and Savage-Smith, *Medieval Islamic Medicine*, and Savage-Smith, "Medicine in Medieval Islam"), far more research is needed on the works themselves and their influence.

2 See S.P. Ragep, "al-Jaghmīnī," 2. "Works by al-Jaghmīnī."

3 Jaghmīnī's choice of *Qānūnča* for the title is interesting, since the medical treatise is written in Arabic, but the diminutive suffix "*ča*" is used in Persian. As far
as I know, Jaghmīnī never wrote scientific texts in Persian, but the title may be
an indication of Jaghmīnī's background, have something to do with his
patrons, or perhaps be some playful tribute by him acknowledging the wealth
of medical literature written in Persian during the twelfth century.

,4 See S.P. Ragep, *Jaghmīnī's Mulakhkhaṣ*. On the *Qānūnča*, see vii–viii, 6, 10,
12–14, 19–20, 25, 283.

5 See Sufi, *Al-minhāj*, 108, 124.

6 For examples of readership notes stating that the *Qānūnča* was used by a physician in a Cairo hospital in the eighteenth century, and that it was studied by a
Qurʾān teacher in sixteenth-century Syria, see, respectively, London, WMS, Or
26, f. 99b (see Table 2.1, no. [5]) and Oxford, Bodleian, Huntington 502,
f. 264b (cited in Savage-Smith, *A New Catalogue*, 1:309–10 [entry 68B]).

7 See Metcalf, "The Madrasa at Deoband," 119. Regarding the idea that
"Science is twofold: Theology and Medicine," see Browne, *Arabian Medicine*, vi;
and Sufi, *Al-minhāj*, 38.

8 Osler, *The Evolution of Modern Medicine*, 98.

9 See Hasse, *Success and Suppression*, 317–407 ("Appendix: The Availability of
Arabic Authors in Latin Editions of the Renaissance"). See also Leclerc,
Histoire de la médecine arabe; Pormann and Savage-Smith, *Medieval Islamic
Medicine*; and Thorndike and Kibre, *A Catalogue of Incipits*.

10 Ibn Sīnā composed the *Qānūn* between 1012 and 1024 in the cities of Jurjān,
Rayy, and Hamadān; see Gohlman, *The Life of Ibn Sīnā*, 154 ("Chronological
Order of Ibn Sīnā's Works").

11 See Siraisi, *Avicenna in Renaissance Italy*, 3, 361–6 ("Appendix I: Latin Editions
of the *Canon* Published after 1500"), 367–76 ("Appendix 2: Latin
Commentaries on the *Canon* Written after ca. 1500"). See also Hasse, *Success
and Suppression*, 360–4; Leclerc, *Histoire de la médecine arabe*, 2:498–500; and
Siraisi, *Medieval and Early Renaissance Medicine*.

12 Siraisi, *Avicenna in Renaissance Italy*, 47.

13 See ibid., 143–4, 146–53; and Jones, "The Medici Oriental Press (Rome
1584–1614)," 88, 95–6.

14 To get a sense of the extent of the work's influence and the numbers involved,
see Rahman's list of 207 "Commentators and Translators of Ibn Sina's
Canon of Medicine." His breakdown of derivative works is: 129 in Arabic;
26 in Persian; 5 in Turkish; 20 in Urdu; 1 in Punjabi; 8 in Latin; 4 in
German; 2 in French; 1 in Russian; 1 in Uzbek; 1 in Japanese; 2 in Hebrew;
4 in English; 1 in Italian; 1 in Catalan; and 1 in Chinese.

15 For more on the *Qānūn* and its commentaries, see Hameed and Bari, "Impact
    of Ibn Sina's Medical Works in India"; İhsanoğlu et al., *Osmanlı Tıbbi Bilimler
    Literatürü Tarihi*; Iskandar, *A Catalogue of Arabic Manuscripts*, 26–64, 156–70,
    180–5, 221–2; Perwāz, "Ibn Sīnā's Medical Works"; and Savage-Smith, *A
    New Catalogue*, 220–318 (entries 54–71).

16 See Pormann and Savage-Smith, *Medieval Islamic Medicine*, 70–1, 85; and
    Savage-Smith, "Medicine in Medieval Islam," 147. For an example of
    Andalusian criticism related to Book Two of Ibn Sīnā's *Qānūn* (which is
    devoted to simple drugs), see F.J. Ragep and Wallis, eds., *The* Herbal *of
    al-Ghāfiqī*, 6, 13, 54.

17 Nahyan Fancy has ardently challenged the notion that the medical commen-
    taries and summaries composed post-1100 are little more than a sign of intel-
    lectual stagnation and verification of the source text. See Fancy, "Medical
    Commentaries" and "Post-Avicennan Physics in the Medical Commentaries
    of the Mamluk Period." See also Pormann and Savage-Smith, *Medieval Islamic
    Medicine*, 180.

18 Ibn Riḍwān, *Medieval Islamic Medicine*, 29, 62–3. See also Iskandar, "An
    Attempted Reconstruction," esp. 241–4 (on "Causes of the Decline of
    Medicine").

19 See Ibn Abī Uṣaybiʿa, *ʿUyūn al-anbāʾ*, ed. Müller, 2:99–105. For an English
    translation of a list of Ibn Riḍwan's works, see Savage-Smith et al., *A Literary
    History of Medicine*, 14.25.9.

20 "Most commentators on the *Almagest*, Ibn al-Haytham says in the introduction
    [to his *Almagest* commentary], were more interested in proposing alternative
    techniques of computation than in clarifying obscure points for the beginner";
    see Sabra, "Ibn al-Haytham," 6:199.

21 Dimitri Gutas analyzes this passage from Ibn Sīnā's autobiography, highlight-
    ing the importance of commentaries for clarifying issues considered problem-
    atic, in this case the purpose of the *Metaphysics* (*Avicenna and the Aristotelian
    Tradition*, 16–17 [nos. 8–9], 270–5); cf. Gohlman, *The Life of Ibn Sīnā*, 31–5.

22 See Ibn Sīnā, *Al-Qānūn fi'l-Ṭibb*, Preface, xvii, xviii.

23 According to Savage-Smith, "It appears that, having achieved a high level of
    exhaustive systemization, an awareness set in that these compendia were too
    large to be really useful for ready reference" ("Medicine in Medieval Islam,"
    148).

24 See *Al-Qānūn fi'l-Ṭibb*, i–xii (Contents Book I).

25 "Numerous abridgements and explanatory commentaries on parts of the
    Canon of Ibn Sīnā were composed … it was not until the late twelfth century
    that a serious need was perceived for aids to understand it … it was this
    industry of glossing and condensing the *Canon* that assured the encyclopedia

its preeminent position in medieval medicine"; see Savage-Smith, "Medicine in Medieval Islam," 150.

26   The English translation of the table of contents is mine.

27   Iskandar, *A Catalogue of Arabic Manuscripts*, 56–7.

28   In an interview in which he discussed his life and education (in Turkish), Muhammad Mustafa Al-Azami, a leading scholar on *ḥadīth* (sayings attributed to the Prophet and his Companions) told of how he studied a commentary on Jaghmīnī's *Mulakhkhaṣ* (on astronomy) at the Deoband madrasa in India in the 1950s before completing his PhD at the University of Cambridge (1966). Given that medicine was also part of the curriculum there, he may have read the *Qānūnča* as well. See "Bir Hadis Aliminin İlim Yolculuğu: Mustafa el-A'zami" (The Intellectual Journey of a Hadith Scholar: Mustafa el-A'zami), an interview of Muhammad Mustafa Al-Azami (in Turkish) by Prof. Dr Recep Şentürk, 18 December 2009, https://www.sonpeygamber.info/bir-hadis-aliminin-ilim-yolculugu-mustafa-el-azami. See also Metcalf, "The Madrasa at Deoband," 119–20.

29   "Established in 1777, Calcutta's presses became renowned from the mid-1780s onwards for printing in dual language Persian, as well as Hindi and some Sanskrit, classics of history, law, literature and language previously known from manuscripts only." Apparently, the translators of these works varied, and consequently so did the quality of the translations. See Teissier, "Texts from the Persian in Late Eighteenth-Century India and Britain," 135–7.

30   On the *Qānūnča*, see Şeşen et al., *Catalogue of Islamic Medical Manuscripts*, 184–7, 339; and Dirāyatī, *Fihristgān (Fankhā)*, 24:732–54. See also Hameed and Bari, "Impact of Ibn Sina's Medical Works in India," 5, 8; Iskandar, *A Catalogue of Arabic Manuscripts*, 56–64, 166–70; Perwāz, "Ibn Sīnā's Medical Works," 301, 304–5; Savage-Smith, *A New Catalogue*, 306–18, entries 68–71; and Storey, *Persian Literature*, E. Medicine, 2/2:219–20, 269–70.

31   See al-Jaghmīnī, *Terjuma Cannonché*.

32   Langermann, "Arabic Writings in Hebrew Manuscripts," 148.

33   See Perwāz for a list of twelve titles of *Qānūn* abridgements ("Ibn Sīnā's Medical Works," 301–2). See also Hameed and Bari, "Impact of Ibn Sina's Medical Works in India," 5 (nos. 1–7); Iskandar, *A Catalogue of Arabic Manuscripts*, 51–63 (1–4).

34   On the abridgement by Īlāqī, see Hameed and Bari, "Impact of Ibn Sina's Medical Works in India," 5 (no. 1); Iskandar, *A Catalogue of Arabic Manuscripts*, 51–2 (1); and Perwāz, "Ibn Sīnā's Medical Works," 301 (1), 303–4.

35   On Ibn al-Nafīs's *Mūjaz*, see Fancy, "Medical Commentaries," 528. See also Hameed and Bari, "Impact of Ibn Sina's Medical Works in India," 5 (no. 2), 7, 9; Iskandar, *A Catalogue of Arabic Manuscripts*, 52–5 (3); Perwāz, "Ibn Sīnā's

Medical Works," 301 (2), 304; and Savage-Smith, *A New Catalogue*, 269–306 (64–7).

36 The six commentaries dedicated to the Ottoman Sultan Bayezid II (r. 1481–1512) are nos. [3], [5], [6], [7], [9], and [11] in Table 2.1.

37 See ʿAṭūfī, *Asmāʾ al-kutub al-khizāna al-ʿāmira*, MS Török F 59. For the section on books on medicine (*kutub al-ṭibb*), see 151–72, which includes four copies of the *Qānūnča* (153, line 16; 159, lines 3–5) and three of its commentaries (159, lines 11–12). For a facsimile of MS Török F 59, see Necipoğlu, Kafadar, and Fleischer, eds., *Treasures of Knowledge: An Inventory of the Ottoman Palace Library (1502/3–1503/4)*, vol. 2, appendix.

38 For more details on definitively dating Jaghmīnī, and why it matters, see S.P. Ragep, *Jaghmīnī's Mulakhkhaṣ*, vii, 5–26.

39 Prominent sources that incorrectly date Jaghmīnī to the fourteenth century include (listed chronologically): Suter, "al-Djaghmīnī," 1038 [1913]; Suter (rev. Vernet), "al-Djaghmīnī," 2:378 [1965]; Iskandar, *A Catalogue of Arabic Manuscripts*, 56 [1967]; Sezgin, "Maḥmūd b. Muḥammad b. ʿUmar AL-ĠAĠMĪNĪ (probably 745/1345)," vol. 5, *Mathematik*, 115 (no. 56) [1974]; Keshavarz, *A Descriptive and Analytical Catalogue of Persian Manuscripts in the Library of the Wellcome Institute*, 57, 147 [1986]; Savage-Smith, *A New Catalogue of Arabic Manuscripts in the Bodleian Library*, 306 [2011]; and a 2012 edition of Jaghmīnī's *Qānūnča fī al-ṭibb* with the date 751 H [!] on the book cover *and* 745 H on the inside title page (see al-Jaghmīnī, *Qānūnča*).

40 Examples of the latter include: The Majlis Library Catalogue, 10/1:512 [Tehran 1968/9]; İnalcık's *The Ottoman Empire*, 176n* [1973]; and Qurbānī's *Zindagī'nāmah-ʾi riyāżī'dānān-i dawrah-ʾi Islāmī*, 219–20 (no. 69) [Tehran 1986].

41 See Brockelmann, *GAL* 1:473 (no. 5) [=624–5] for Jaghmīnī on astronomy (where his death date is given as after 618 H/1221 CE); and *GAL* 1:457 [=598] for Jaghmīnī on medicine (where his date is given as 745 H/1344 CE). Brockelmann repeats this bifurcation in suppl. 1:826, 865. After Brockelmann, other prominent sources followed suit, such as: the *Islamic Medical Manuscripts at the National Library of Medicine* (http://www.nlm.nih.gov/hmd/arabic/bioJ.html, accessed 27 June 2020); Richter-Bernburg, "Jaġmini, Maḥmud," *Encyclopædia Iranica*, 14/4:373 (http://www.iranicaonline.org/articles/jagmini-mahmud, accessed 27 June 2020); and Necipoğlu, Kafadar, and Fleischer, eds., *Treasures of Knowledge* (2019), 1:539 (26b), 1015[20] (d. 1344 for the *Qānūnča*) and 1:178, 242, 380n75, 799, 834 (fl. 1221 for the *Mulakhkhaṣ*).

42 Heinrich Suter claimed that "with near certainty" Jaghmīnī flourished in the "first half of the eighth century H" (fourteenth century CE), relying on the 1881 Gotha Library catalogue description ("Zur Frage über die Lebenszeit des Verfassers des Mulaḫḫaṣ fiʾl-heiʾa, Maḥmûd b. Muḥ. b. ʿOmar

al-Ġaġmînî," 539–40 [no. 2]). In 1971, Storey refers to the marginal note on folio 1b in Gotha MS 1930 listed in Pertsch's catalogue as the basis for dating Jaghmīnī in "745/1344–5" (*Persian Literature, E. Medicine*, 2/2:219). Cf. Pertsch, *Die orientalischen Handschriften der Herzoglichen Bibliothek zu Gotha*, 3/3:468–9 (no. 1928), 469–70 (no. 1930).

43   See F.J. Ragep, "On Dating Jaghmīnī and His *Mulakhkhaṣ*."

44   See Istanbul, Süleymaniye Library, Ayasofya MS 3735, f. 25a. This manuscript of the *Qānūnča* states that it was copied in Konya (in Anatolia) in 601 [1205]. For more details on dating the *Qānūnča*, see S.P. Ragep, *Jaghmīnī's Mulakhkhaṣ*, 19–20.

45   The *Mulakhkhaṣ* also contains a dedicatory poem to Badr al-Dīn al-Qalānisī in the original version; see S.P. Ragep, *Jaghmīnī's Mulakhkhaṣ*, 16–17, 281.

46   For the German translation of Qalānisī's pharmaceutical work, see Fellmann, *Das Aqrābāḏīn al-Qalānisī*.

47   The paucity of information on the life of "Mohammed ben Bahram ben Mohammed Bedr eddin el Calanisy Essamarcandy" was expressed by Leclerc (*Histoire de la médecine arabe*, 2:128); and a century later by Fellmann in her introduction to *Das Aqrābāḏīn al-Qalānisī*, 1.

48   Richter-Bernburg, "Medical and Veterinary Sciences, Part One: Medicine, Pharmacology and Veterinary Science in Islamic Eastern Iran and Central Asia," 310.

49   Browne, *Arabian Medicine*, Lecture IV, 98.

50   Examples include: Kaḥḥāla, *Muʿjam al-muʾallifīn*, 9:122; and Arshi, *Catalogue of the Arabic Manuscripts in Raza Library, Rampur*, 5:394.

51   In addition to the ones already mentioned, see Brockelman, *GAL* 1:489 (no. 23) [=644]; suppl. 1:893 (no. 23); Iskandar, *A Catalogue of Arabic Manuscripts on Medicine and Science*, 79–80; and Ullmann, *Die Medizin im Islam*, 307.

52   Iskandar points out that the marginal notes to two medical works by Najīb al-Samarqandī contain quotes attributed to Qalānisī; see codex Coll. 1062, MS. Ar. 73 [= UCLA Ar. 73] ("A Study of Al-Samarqandī's Medical Writings," 452, esp. fn7).

53   Badr al-Dīn al-Qalānisī was among the sources cited by Abū Isḥāq Ibrāhīm ibn Muḥammad ʿIzz al-Dīn ibn Ṭarkhān al-Suwaydī in his medical treatise on remedies entitled *al-Tadhkira al-hādiya* (Leclerc, *Histoire de la médecine arabe*, 2:128, 199–202 [on "Soueidy"]).

54   For Latin translations, see Hasse, *Success and Suppression*, 366–7.

55   See Ibn Abī Uṣaybiʿa, *ʿUyūn al-anbāʾ fī ṭabaqāt al-aṭibbāʾ* (ed. Müller), 2:31. See also Ibn Abī Uṣaybiʿa, *ʿUyūn al-anbāʾ fī ṭabaqāt al-aṭibbāʾ*, ed. N. Riḍā, 472. For an English translation, see Savage-Smith et al., *A Literary History of Medicine*, 11.22 ("Badr al-Dīn Muḥammad ibn Bahrām ibn Muḥammad al-Qalānisī al-Samarqandī").

56   Joan E. Gilbert provides valuable information about the Banū Qalānisī resid-
     ing in Damascus between 1076 and 1335 in "The Ulama of Medieval
     Damascus and the International World of Islamic Scholarship." See also
     Gilbert, "Institutionalization of Muslim Scholarship and Professionalization
     of the 'Ulamā' in Medieval Damascus."

57   The three Damascene madrasas were: (1) al-Madrasa al-Dakhwariyya,
     founded in 621 H/1224 CE; (2) al-Madrasa al-Dunaysiriyya, founded by the
     Shāfiʿī jurisconsult-physician ʿImād al-Dīn al-Dunaysirī (d. 686 H/1287 CE);
     and (3) al-Madrasa al-Lubūdiyya al-Najmiyya, founded in 664 H/1266 CE
     by Najm al-Dīn al-Lubūdī. The latter was the author of a work on medicine
     "according to the scholastic method of jurisconsults"; see Makdisi, *The Rise of
     Colleges*, 313, fn38.

58   See Pormann and Savage-Smith, *Medieval Islamic Medicine*, 98–9. See also
     Ragab, *The Medieval Islamic Hospital*, and Fancy's "Essay Review" of Ragab's
     book.

59   See London, Wellcome Collection, WMS. Or. 26, f. 99b; and Iskandar, *A
     Catalogue of Arabic Manuscripts on Medicine and Science*, 56, 184–5. See also Table
     2.1, no. [5].

60   In his biography of the Khwārizm Shāh Jalāl al-Dīn (r. 1220–32), Nasawī (fl.
     1241) informs us that "[r]egarding the science of law, [Shihāb al-Dīn] com-
     bined knowledge of lexicography, medicine, and dialectic, and other sciences.
     Eloquent and versed in various languages, he was also a man of good counsel.
     Mars had bought happiness from him, Mercury had benefited from his les-
     sons, the finest man was the slave of his wisdom and the greatest thinker was
     the servant of his ideas." See Nasawī, *Sīrat al-Sulṭān Jalāl al-Dīn*, 109 (=French
     trans. Houdas, *Histoire du sultan*, 82).

61   Nasawī, *Sīrat al-Sulṭān Jalāl al-Dīn*, 109 (=Houdas, *Histoire du sultan*, 82). The
     position of *wakīl* meant that he "was by no means a subordinate official whose
     function was literally to carry the decision of the sultan to the chancery … it is
     obvious that it was an honorary duty attributed to high-ranking courtiers."
     See Stern, "Petitions from the Ayyūbid Period," 15–16.

62   Nasawī, *Sīrat al-Sulṭān Jalāl al-Dīn*, 109–10 (=Houdas, *Histoire du sultan*, 83,
     84).

63   See Yāqūt al-Ḥamawī (d. 1229), who was in Merv just prior to its destruction
     (616 H/1220 CE) and reports on the extensive endowed libraries and collec-
     tions of the city (*Muʿjam al-buldān*, 5:114). Soucek provides an English trans-
     lation of these relevant passages in *A History of Inner Asia*, 114–15.

64   These initiatives have often been associated with scholars working under the
     Mongol Īlkhānid dynasty from the later thirteenth and early fourteenth cen-
     turies. But these scholars, working in Marāgha and Tabrīz in northwest Iran,
     should more correctly be seen as reviving or resuscitating their

twelfth-century predecessors, whose works and pedagogical innovations might have otherwise been lost as a result of the Mongol invasions. One of the major figures in this later revival project was Naṣīr al-Dīn al-Ṭūsī (d. 1274), who was engaged in a monumental undertaking (that spanned almost twenty years) of providing a body of textbooks, with commentary, of the Greek classics and early Islamic scientific works. See F.J. Ragep, "Naṣīr al-Dīn al-Ṭūsī," 3321–3.

65 Attewell challenges the conception of Unani *tibb* "as a seamless continuation of Galenic and later West Asian 'Islamic' elaborations" revolving around "a coherent body of knowledge and practice," in "Authority, Knowledge and Practice in Unani Ṭibb in India, c. 1890–1930," 2, 20–8.

66 For a discussion on the role locality plays "in situating the tradition of Arabic science with reference both to the place that the tradition occupies in the general history of science and to its place in civilization where it emerged and developed," see Sabra, "Situating Arabic Science: Locality versus Essence," 655.

67 The central administration of the Ottomans standardized educational reforms and sanctioned the teaching of the mathematical sciences within their institutions, which were dispersed throughout three continents from the fifteenth to twentieth centuries. However, the number of hospitals with teaching schools attached may have been relatively few. See Shefer-Mossensohn, who lists only two hospitals in Asia Minor with attached medical schools that were founded between 1154 and 1845: Gevher Nesibe (est. c. 1206 in Kayseri, Central Anatolia) and Kanuni Sultan Süleyman (est. c. 1555 in Istanbul) (*Ottoman Medicine: Healing and Medical Institutions 1500–1700*, 198).

68 Fabrizio Speziale points out that "Iranian scholars rose to important positions in the Mughal administration and gave a fundamental impulse to the translation and commentary of Avicenna's *Qānūn* in India" ("India xxxiii. Indo-Muslim Physicians," *Encyclopædia Iranica*, https://iranicaonline.org/articles/india-xxxiii-indo-muslim-physicians).
See also Speziale, "Les traités persans sur les sciences indiennes," 404; Speziale, ed., *Hospitals in Iran and India, 1500–1950s*, esp. 1–4 (on "The Hospital and Other Muslim Institutions"); and Speziale, *Culture persane et médecine ayurvédique en Asie du Sud*.

69 See Liebeskind, "Arguing Science: Unani *tibb*, Hakims and Biomedicine in India, 1900–50," esp. 63–7. See also Liebeskind, "Unani Medicine of the Subcontinent"; and Metcalf, "Nationalist Muslims in British India."

70 According to a report by the Central Council for Research in Unani Medicine (CCRUM; est. 1978), there are 46 teaching institutions that offer Unani medical education training set up by the Central Government of India, 1,491 Unani hospitals and dispensaries, and plans for establishing an All India

Institute of Unani Medicine (AIIUM) at Ghaziabad, Uttar Pradesh (see "Unani Medicine in India – An Overview," 5, 6, 101, 103, 117). The Hamdard Foundation Pakistan (est. 1969) also actively promotes Unani medicine through various publications (among which is a quarterly *Journal for Science and Medicine* [*Hamdard Medicus*], and the English translation of Ibn Sīnā's *Qānūn al-ṭibb* cited above). In addition, they support international conferences and associations, such as the Pakistan Association of Eastern Medicine (PAEM) and the International Association for Unani Medicine (IAUM).

71 See Metcalf, "The Madrasa at Deoband," 132.

BIBLIOGRAPHY

Ahlwardt, Wilhelm. *Die Handschriften-Verzeichnisse der Königlichen Bibliothek zu Berlin. Verzeichniss der arabischen Handschriften*, vol. 5. Berlin: Asher & Co., 1893.

Alavi, Seema. *Islam and Healing: Loss and Recovery of an Indo-Muslim Medical Tradition, 1600–1900*. Houndmills, UK: Palgrave Macmillan, 2008.

Arberry, Arthur J. *The Chester Beatty Library. A Handlist of the Arabic Manuscripts. Volume V. MSS. 4001–4500*. Dublin: Hodges, Figgis & Co., Ltd., 1962.

Arshi, L.A. *Catalogue of the Arabic Manuscripts in Raza Library, Rampur*, vol. 5, *Mathematics, Medicine, Natural Science, Agriculture, Occult Sciences, Ethics & Politics, Education & Military Science*. Rampur, India: Published under the auspices of the Ministry of Education, Government of India, 1975.

Ashraf, Maulānā al-Ḥājj Muḥammad. *A Concise Descriptive Catalogue of the Arabic Manuscripts in the Salar Jung Museum & Library*, vol. 8, *Mathematics, Astronomy, Astrology, Medicine, Natural History and Alchemy*. Hyderabad, India: Salar Jung Museum and Library, 2000.

Attewell, Guy Nicolas Anthony. "Authority, Knowledge and Practice in Unani Ṭibb in India, c. 1890–1930." PhD diss. London: School of Oriental and African Studies, University of London, 2004. ProQuest (10673235).

Black, Crofton, ed. *Transformation of Knowledge: Early Manuscripts from the Collection of Lawrence J. Schoenberg*. London: Paul Holberton, 2006.

Brockelmann, Carl. *Geschichte der arabischen Litteratur* [*GAL*], 2 vols. plus 3 supplements. Weimar, Germany: Verlag von Emil Felber (vol. 1 [1898]); Berlin: Verlag von Emil Felber (vol. 2 [1902]); Leiden, Netherlands: E.J. Brill (suppl. 1 [1937]; suppl. 2 [1938]; suppl. 3 [1942]). Reprinted with a new introduction by Jan Just Witkam. Leiden, Netherlands: E.J. Brill, 1996 (referenced in square brackets).

Browne, Edward G. *Arabian Medicine, Being the Fitzpatrick Lectures Delivered at the College of Physicians in November 1919 and November 1920*. Cambridge: Cambridge University Press, 1921.

– *A Hand-list of the Muḥammadan Manuscripts, including all those written in the Arabic character, preserved in the Library of the University of Cambridge.* Cambridge: Cambridge University Press, 1900.

– *A Supplementary Hand-List of the Muḥammadan Manuscripts, including all those written in the Arabic character preserved in the libraries of the University and Colleges of Cambridge.* Cambridge: Cambridge University Press, 1922.

Brunschvig, Robert. "Deux Récits de Voyage inédits en Afrique du Nord au XVᵉ siècle: ʿAbdalbāsiṭ b. Ḥalīl et Adorne." PhD diss. Paris: University of Paris, 1936.

Buonazia, Lupo. *Catalogo dei Codici Arabi della Biblioteca Nazionale di Napoli.* Naples, Italy: 1880.

Central Council for Research in Unani Medicine. "Unani Medicine in India – An Overview." New Delhi: Ministry of AYUSH, Government of India, June 2016.

Dirāyatī, Muṣṭafā. *Fihristgān: nuskhah'hā-yi khaṭṭī-i Īrān (Fankhā),* vol. 24. Tehran, 2012.

– *Fihristvārah-i dastnivisht'hā-yi Īrān (DENA).* 12 vols. Tehran, 2010.

Fancy, Nahyan. "Essay Review: Ahmed Ragab, *The Medieval Islamic Hospital: Medicine, Religion, and Charity.* New York: Cambridge University Press, 2015." *Naẓariyat, Journal for the History of Islamic Philosophy and Sciences* 3, no. 1 (2016): 137–46.

– "Medical Commentaries: A Preliminary Examination of Ibn al-Nafīs's *Shurūḥ,* the *Mūjaz* and Subsequent Commentaries on the *Mūjaz.*" *Oriens* 41 (2013): 525–45.

– "Post-Avicennan Physics in the Medical Commentaries of the Mamluk Period." *Intellectual History of the Islamicate World* 6 (2018): 55–81.

Fihrist-i kutub-i makhṭūṭāt ʿArabī, Fārsī va Urdū makhzūnah-yi Kutub Khānah Āṣafiyya Sarkār-i ʿAlī. Catalogue of Urdu, Arabic and Persian manuscripts. Hyderabad, India, 1332 H./1913–14.

Fellmann, Irene. *Das Aqrābādīn al-Qalānisī: Quellenkritische und begriffsanalytische Untersuchungen zur arabisch-pharmazeutischen Literatur.* Beirut: Orient-Institut der Deutschen Morgenländischen Gesellschaft. Wiesbaden, Germany: In Kommission bei F. Steiner, 1986.

Gilbert, Joan Elizabeth. "Institutionalization of Muslim Scholarship and Professionalization of the ʿUlamā' in Medieval Damascus." *Studia Islamica* 52 (1980): 105–34.

– "The Ulama of Medieval Damascus and the International World of Islamic Scholarship." PhD diss. Berkeley, CA: University of California, 1977. ProQuest (7812573).

Gohlman, William E. *The Life of Ibn Sīnā: A Critical Edition and Annotated Translation.* Albany: State University of New York Press, 1974.

Gutas, Dimitri. *Avicenna and the Aristotelian Tradition: Introduction to Reading Avicenna's Philosophical Works.* Leiden, Netherlands: Brill, 2014.

Hameed, Hakim Abdul, and Hakim Abdul Bari. "Impact of Ibn Sina's Medical Works in India." *Studies in History of Medicine* 8, nos. 1–2 (1984): 1–12.

Hasir Radavi, Maulavi Qasim. *Catalogue Raisonné of the Būhar Library*. Vol. 1, *Catalogue of the Persian Manuscripts in the Būhar Library*. Revised and completed by Maulavi 'Abd-ul-Muqtadir. Calcutta, India: Imperial Library, 1921.

Hasse, Dag Nikolaus. *Success and Suppression: Arabic Sciences and Philosophy in the Renaissance*. Cambridge, MA: Harvard University Press, 2016.

Ibn Abī Uṣaybiʿa. *ʿUyūn al-anbāʾ fī ṭabaqāt al-aṭibbāʾ*. Edited by August Müller. 2 vols. plus corrections. Cairo: al-Maṭbaʿa al-Wahabiyya, 1299/1882; Königsberg, Germany: Selbstverlag, 1884.

– *ʿUyūn al-anbāʾ fī ṭabaqāt al-aṭibbāʾ*. Edited by Nizār Riḍā. Beirut: Dār maktabat al-ḥayāh, 1965.

Ibn Riḍwān. *Medieval Islamic Medicine: Ibn Riḍwān's Treatise, "On the Prevention of Bodily Ills in Egypt."* Translation and introduction by Michael W. Dols. Arabic text edited by Adil S. Gamal. Berkeley, CA, and London: University of California Press, 1984.

Ibn Sīnā. *Al-Qānūn fiʾl-Ṭibb*. *Al-Shaikh al-Raʾīs Abū ʿAlī al-Ḥusain bin ʿAbdullāh bin Sīnā*. Book I, *General Principles of Medicine Assessment, Regimen in Health and Disease*. English translation of the critical Arabic text by a team of scholars at Hamdard University, India, Department of Islamic Studies. New Delhi: Jamia Hamdard, 1993.

İhsanoğlu, Ekmeleddin, Ramazan Şeşen, and Cevat Izgi. *Osmanlı Astronomi Literatürü Tarihi (History of Astronomy Literature during the Ottoman Period)*. 2 vols. Istanbul: IRCICA, 1997.

İhsanoğlu, Ekmeleddin, et al. *Osmanlı Tıbbi Bilimler Literatürü Tarihi (History of the Literature of Medical Sciences during the Ottoman Period)*. Edited by Ekmeleddin İhsanoğlu, Ramazan Şeşen, M. Serdar Bekar, Gülcan Gündüz, and Veysel Bulut. General editor Ekmeleddin İhsanoğlu. Istanbul: IRCICA, 2008.

İnalcık, Halil. *The Ottoman Empire: The Classical Age 1300–1600*. Translated by Norman Itzkowitz and Colin Imber. London: Weidenfeld and Nicolson, 1973.

Iskandar, A.Z. "An Attempted Reconstruction of the Late Alexandrian Medical Curriculum." *Medical History* 20, no. 3 (1976): 235–58.

– *A Catalogue of Arabic Manuscripts on Medicine and Science in the Wellcome Historical Medical Library*. London: The Wellcome Historical Medical Library, 1967.

– "A Study of Al-Samarqandī's Medical Writings." *Le Muséon Revue d'Études Orientales* 85 (1972): 451–79.

Islamic Medical Manuscripts at the National Library of Medicine: Project of the History of Medicine Division of the National Library of Medicine. Text by Emilie Savage-Smith. Oxford, UK: The Oriental Institute, Oxford University. https://www.nlm.nih.gov/hmd/arabic/bioJ.html.

al-Jaghmīnī. *Qānūnča fī al-ṭibb*. Edition and Persian translation by Ismāʿīl Nāzim. Tehran: Tehran University of Medical Sciences, 2012.

– *Terjuma Cannonché Mahmood Cheghmeny der Elm Tebb*. (*Short Canons of the Art of Physic. Being a compendium, both of Theory and Practice. Written originally in Arabic; by Mahmood Cheghmeny.*) Calcutta, India: Printed by B. Messink, 1782.

Jones, Robert. "The Medici Oriental Press (Rome 1584–1614) and the Impact of Its Arabic Publications on Northern Europe." In *The 'Arabick' Interest of the Natural Philosophers in Seventeenth-Century England*, edited by G.A. Russell, 88–108. Leiden, Netherlands: E.J. Brill, 1994.

de Jong, P., and M.J. de Goeje. *Catalogus Codicum Orientalium: Bibliothecae Academiae Lugduno Batavae* [CCO], vol. 3. Leiden, Netherlands: E.J. Brill, 1865.

Kaḥḥāla, ʿUmar Riḍā. *Muʿjam al-muʾallifīn: tarājim muṣannifī al-kutub al-ʿArabiyya*, vol. 9. Beirut: Dār iḥyāʾ al-turāth al-ʿarabī, 1980.

Karatay, Fehmi Edhem. *Topkapı Sarayı Müzesi Kütüphanesi Arapça Yazmalar Kataloğu.* 3 vols. Istanbul: Topkapı Sarayı Müzesi, 1962–66.

Keshavarz, Fateme. *A Descriptive and Analytical Catalogue of Persian Manuscripts in the Library of the Wellcome Institute for the History of Medicine.* London: The Wellcome Historical Medical Library, 1986.

Khudā Bakhsh Oriyanṭal Pablik Lāʾibrerī. *Catalogue of the Arabic and Persian Manuscripts in the Khuda Bakhsh Oriental Public Library*, vol. 4, *Medical Works: Arabic.* Patna, India: The Library, 1970.

Langermann, Y. Tzvi. "Arabic Writings in Hebrew Manuscripts: A Preliminary Relisting." *Arabic Sciences and Philosophy* 6 (1996): 137–60.

Leclerc, Lucien. *Histoire de la médecine arabe: exposé complet des traductions du grec; Les sciences en Orient, leur transmission à l'Occident par les traductions latines.* 2 vols. Paris: E. Leroux, 1876.

Liebeskind, Claudia. "Arguing Science: Unani *tibb*, Hakims and Biomedicine in India, 1900–50." In *Plural Medicine, Tradition and Modernity, 1800–2000*, edited by Waltraud Ernst, 58–75. Studies in the Social History of Medicine. London and New York: Routledge, 2002.

– "Unani Medicine of the Subcontinent." In *Oriental Medicine: An Illustrated Guide to the Asian Arts of Healing*, edited by Jan van Alphen and A. Aris, 39–65. Boston, MA: Shambhala, 1996.

Loth, Otto. *A Catalogue of Arabic Manuscripts in the Library of the India Office.* London: Stephen Austin and Sons, 1877.

Majlis Library Catalogue (*Fihrist-i Kitābkhānah-i Majlis-i Shūrā-yi Millī, kutub-i khaṭṭī*), vol. 10, part 1. Tehran 1347 H. Sh./1968–69.

Makdisi, George. *The Rise of Colleges: Institutions of Learning in Islam and the West.* Edinburgh: Edinburgh University Press, 1981.

Massoud, Sami G. *The Chronicles and Annalistic Sources of the Early Mamluk Circassian Period.* Leiden, Netherlands: Brill, 2007.

Metcalf, Barbara D. "The Madrasa at Deoband: A Model for Religious Education in Modern India." *Modern Asian Studies* 12, no. 1 (1978): 111–34.

– "Nationalist Muslims in British India: The Case of Hakim Ajmal Khan." *Modern Asian Studies* 19, no. 1 (1985): 1–28.

Mingana, A. *Catalogue of the Arabic Manuscripts in the John Rylands Library Manchester*, Sections 7–12. Manchester, UK: The Manchester University Press, 1934.

al-Nasawī, Muḥammad ibn Aḥmad. *Histoire du sultan Djelal ed-Din Mankobirti, prince du Kharezm par Mohammed en-Nesawi.* Translated into French from the Arabic by Octave Houdas. Paris: E. Leroux, 1895.

– *Sīrat al-Sulṭān Jalāl al-Dīn Mankubirtī li-Muḥammad ibn Aḥmad al-Nasawī.* Edited by Ḥāfiẓ Aḥmad Ḥamdī. Cairo: Dār al-fikr al-ʿarabī, 1953.

Necipoğlu, Gülru, Cemal Kafadar, and Cornell H. Fleischer, eds. *Treasures of Knowledge: An Inventory of the Ottoman Palace Library (1502/3–1503/4).* Studies and Sources in Islamic Art and Architecture. 2 vols. Leiden, Netherlands, and Boston, MA: Brill, 2019.

Osler, William. *The Evolution of Modern Medicine. A Series of Lectures Delivered at Yale University on the Silliman Foundation in April, 1913.* New Haven, CT: Yale University Press, 1921.

Pertsch, Wilhelm. *Die orientalischen Handschriften der Herzoglichen Bibliothek zu Gotha*, vol. 3, part 3. Gotha, Germany: Friedrich Andreas Perthes, 1881.

Perwāz, Sayed Riaz ʿAli. "Ibn Sīnā's Medical Works." *Indian Journal of History of Science* 21, no. 4 (1986): 297–314.

Pormann, Peter E., and Emilie Savage-Smith. *Medieval Islamic Medicine.* Washington, DC: Georgetown University Press, 2007.

Qurbānī, Abū al-Qāsim. *Zindagī'nāmah-'i rīyāẓī'dānān-i dawrah-'i Islāmī.* Tehran: Markaz-i Nashr-i Dānishgāhī, 1986.

Ragab, Ahmed. *The Medieval Islamic Hospital: Medicine, Religion, and Charity.* New York: Cambridge University Press, 2015.

Ragep, F. Jamil. "Naṣīr al-Dīn al-Ṭūsī." In *Encyclopaedia of the History of Science, Technology, and Medicine in Non-Western Cultures*, 3rd ed., edited by Helaine Selin, 3321–3. Dordrecht, Netherlands: Springer, 2016.

– "On Dating Jaghmīnī and His *Mulakhkhas.*" In *Essays in Honour of Ekmeleddin İhsanoğlu*, edited by Mustafa Kaçar and Zeynep Durukal, 461–6. Istanbul: IRCICA, 2006.

Ragep, F. Jamil, and Faith Wallis, eds., with Pamela Miller and Adam Gacek. *The Herbal of al-Ghāfiqī.* Montreal, QC: McGill-Queen's University Press, 2014.

Ragep, Sally P. "al-Jaghmīnī." In *Encyclopaedia of Islam THREE*, edited by Kate Fleet, Gudrun Krämer, Denis Matringe, John Nawas, and Everett Rowson. First published online 2020. http://dx.doi.org/10.1163/1573-3912_ei3_COM_32689 (accessed 26 June 2020).

– *Jaghmīnī's Mulakhkhaṣ: An Islamic Introduction to Ptolemaic Astronomy.* New York: Springer, 2016.

Rahman, Hakim Syed Zillur. "Commentators and Translators of Ibn Sina's Canon of Medicine." Translated into English by Zakaria Virk. Aligarh, India: Ibn Sina Academy, Aligarh Muslim University, Tijara House, Dodhpur, 1986 (Urdu); 2012 (2nd ed., Urdu and English).

– *Qānūn-i Ibn Sīnā, shārḥān va mutarjimān-i ān.* Translated into Persian by ʿAbd al-Qādir Hāshimī. Tehran: Anjuman-i Āsār va Mafākhir-i Farhangī, 1383 H. Sh./2004.

Richter-Bernburg, Lutz. "Jaḡmini, Maḥmud." *Encyclopædia Iranica*, vol. 14, fasc. 4, 373. Originally published 15 December 2008; last updated 10 April 2012. http://www.iranicaonline.org/articles/jagmini-mahmud.

– "Medical and Veterinary Sciences. Part One: Medicine, Pharmacology and Veterinary Science in Islamic Eastern Iran and Central Asia." In *History of Civilizations of Central Asia*, vol. 4, *The Age of Achievement: A.D. 750 to the End of the Fifteenth Century. Part Two: The Achievements*, edited by C. Edmund Bosworth and M.S. Asimov, 299–317. Paris: UNESCO Publ., 2000.

Sabra, A.I. "Ibn al-Haytham, Abū ʿAlī Al-Ḥasan ibn al-Ḥasan." In *Dictionary of Scientific Biography*, edited by Charles Coulston Gillispie, 6:189–210. New York: Charles Scribner's Sons, 1972.

– "Situating Arabic Science: Locality versus Essence." *Isis* 87, no. 4 (1996): 654–70.

Savage-Smith, Emilie. "Medicine in Medieval Islam." In *The Cambridge History of Science*, vol. 2, *Medieval Science*, edited by David C. Lindberg and Michael H. Shank, 139–67. Cambridge: Cambridge University Press, 2013.

– *A New Catalogue of Arabic Manuscripts in the Bodleian Library, University of Oxford*, vol. 1, *Medicine*. Oxford, UK: Oxford University Press, 2011.

Savage-Smith, Emilie, Simon Swain, and G.J.H. van Gelder, eds. *A Literary History of Medicine: The ʿUyūn al-anbāʾ fī ṭabaqāt al-aṭibbāʾ of Ibn Abī Uṣaybiʿah.* Leiden, Netherlands: Brill, 2020. https://brill.com/view/db/lhom.

Şeşen et al. *Catalogue of Islamic Medical Manuscripts [in Arabic, Turkish & Persian] in the Libraries of Turkey.* Prepared by Ramazan Şeşen, Cemil Akpınar, and Cevat İzgi. General editor Ekmeleddin İhsanoğlu. Istanbul: IRCICA, 1984.

Sezgin, Fuat. "Maḥmūd b. Muḥammad b. ʿUmar AL-ǦAǦMĪNĪ (probably 745/1345)." *Geschichte des arabischen Schrifttums*, vol. 5, *Mathematik*, 115 (no. 56). Leiden, Netherlands: E.J. Brill, 1974.

Shefer-Mossensohn, Miri. *Ottoman Medicine: Healing and Medical Institutions 1500–1700.* Albany: SUNY Press, 2009.

Siraisi, Nancy G. *Avicenna in Renaissance Italy: The Canon and Medical Teaching in Italian Universities after 1500.* Princeton, NJ: Princeton University Press, 1987.

– *Medieval and Early Renaissance Medicine: An Introduction to Knowledge.* Chicago, IL: The University of Chicago, 1990.

Soucek, Svat. *A History of Inner Asia.* Cambridge: Cambridge University Press, 2000.

Speziale, Fabrizio. "Arzānī, Moḥammad Akbar." *Encyclopædia Iranica.* Last updated 16 August 2011. http://www.iranicaonline.org/articles/mohammad-akbar-arzani.

– *Culture persane et médecine ayurvédique en Asie du Sud.* Leiden, Netherlands: Brill, 2018.

– ed. *Hospitals in Iran and India, 1500–1950s.* Leiden, Netherlands: Brill, 2012.

– "India xxxiii. Indo-Muslim Physicians." *Encyclopædia Iranica*. Originally published
15 July 2009; last updated 31 August 2011. https://iranicaonline.org/articles/
india-xxxiii-indo-muslim-physicians.

– "Les traités persans sur les sciences indiennes: médecine, zoologie, alchimie."
In *Muslim Cultures in the Indo-Iranian World during the Early-Modern and Modern Periods*,
edited by Denis Hermann and Fabrizio Speziale, 403–47. Berlin: Institut français
de recherche en Iran – Klaus Schwarz Verlag, 2010.

Stern, S.M. "Petitions from the Ayyūbid Period." *Bulletin of the School of Oriental and
African Studies, University of London* 27, no. 1 (1964): 1–32.

Storey, Charles A. *Persian Literature: A Bio-Bibliographical Survey*, vol. 2, part 2, E.
Medicine. London: Luzac and Co., 1971.

Sufi, G.M.D. *Al-minhāj, Being the Evolution of Curriculum in the Muslim Educational
Institutions of India*. Delhi: Idarah-i Adabiyat-i Delli, 1977.

Suter, Heinrich. "al-Djaghmīnī." In *Encyclopaedia of Islam, First Edition*, vol. 1, edited
by M.Th. Houtsma, T.W. Arnold, and R. Basset, 1038. Leiden, Netherlands: E.J.
Brill, 1913.

– "Zur Frage über die Lebenszeit des Verfassers des Mulaḫḫaṣ fi'l-hei'a, Maḥmûd b.
Muḥ. b. ʿOmar al-Ġaġmînî." *Zeitschrift der Deutschen Morgenländischen Gesellschaft* 53
(1899): 539–40. Reprinted in *Islamic Mathematics and Astronomy*, edited by Fuat
Sezgin, vol. 77, *Miscellaneous Texts and Studies on Islamic Mathematics and Astronomy*, II,
305–6. Frankfurt am Main, Germany: Institut für Geschichte der Arabisch-
Islamischen Wissenschaften, 1998.

Suter, Heinrich, and rev. J. Vernet. "al-Djaghmīnī." In *Encyclopaedia of Islam*, 2nd ed.,
edited by B. Lewis, Ch. Pellat, and J. Schacht, 2:378. Leiden, Netherlands: E.J.
Brill, 1965.

Teissier, Beatrice. "Texts from the Persian in Late Eighteenth-Century India and
Britain: Culture or Construct?" *Iran* 47 (2009): 133–47.

Thorndike, Lynn, and Pearl Kibre. *A Catalogue of Incipits of Mediaeval Scientific Writings
in Latin*. London: The Mediaeval Academy of America Publication no. 29, 1963.

Ullmann, Manfred. *Die Medizin im Islam*. Handbuch der Orientalistik. Leiden,
Netherlands: E.J. Brill, 1970.

Vollers, K. *Katalog der islamischen, christlich-orientalischen, jüdischen und samaritanischen
Handschriften der Universitäts-Bibliothek zu Leipzig*. Leipzig, Germany: Otto
Harrassowitz, 1906.

Voorhoeve, P. *Handlist of Arabic Manuscripts in the Library of the University of Leiden and
Other Collections in The Netherlands*. Codices Manuscripti VII. Leiden, Netherlands:
Bibliotheca Universitatis, 1957.

Witkam, Jan Just. *Inventory of the Oriental Manuscripts of the Library of the University of
Leiden*, vol. 1, *Manuscripts Or. 1–Or. 1000: Acquisitions in the Period between 1609 and*

1665. Mainly the Collections of Jacobus Golius (1629), Josephus Justus Scaliger (1609), and Part of the Collection of Levinus Warner (1665). Leiden, Netherlands: Ter Lugt Press, 2007.

Yāqūt ibn ʿAbd Allāh al-Ḥamawī. *Muʿjam al-buldān li-l-Shaykh al-imām Shihāb al-Dīn Abī ʿAbd Allāh Yāqūt ibn ʿAbd Allāh al-Ḥamawī al-Rūmī al-Baghdādī*, vol. 5. Beirut: Dār Ṣādir, 1957.

3

Experience over Education or Education over Experience? Pre-modern Medical Writing on Plague

Lori Jones

MEDICAL EDUCATION, KNOWLEDGE TRANSMISSION, AND PLAGUE

On 18 October 1720, Monsieur D.M. Pons, a physician in Montpellier's Faculty of Medicine, wrote to Monsieur de Bon, president of the Societé royale des sciences, to describe the early months of Marseille's plague epidemic. The previous week, de Bon had asked Pons to go to Marseille and report back on the nature of the city's widespread illness and how it could be addressed. In his responding letter, Pons recalled having learned about plague while getting his own medical education at Montpellier some decades earlier, between 1688 and 1691. But, he contended, what he was taught about the disease – and hence the training that he now offered to his own students – was based solely on inherited tradition and presumption. Indeed, Pons lamented, his university medical education, like those of his contemporaries, had been provided by "professors [who] had never actually seen the plague."[1]

This lack of direct, personal knowledge of the disease was problematic: because neither he nor his university professors had ever seen a real case of plague, Pons had graduated from medical school – and conducted his own teaching of future physicians – firmly believing that *la Peste* did not even exist. Instead, he was inclined to believe that the authoritative texts that underlay his medical education were inherently misguided on the subject, even if they purportedly drew from the personal observations of earlier medical practitioners. For Pons, buboes, carbuncles, and other "efflorescences qu'on observe dans la Peste" were not in fact the markers of any specific disease; rather, they were nothing more than the manifested result of medical prejudice against using phlebotomy and purging to release the body's accumulated impurities.[2] Now, in Marseille, he was conflicted: what he witnessed first-hand in 1720 challenged everything that he had learned at university decades before. His textbooks were failing him, and he could not reconcile the received knowledge that he had acquired formally at university with the reality that he observed at his patients' bedsides. To use modern parlance, his continuing medical education entirely upended his formal medical education.

This chapter explores how and under what circumstances plague tracts reflect physicians' struggles to reconcile, on the one hand, the received canonical knowledge that underscored their university medical education and, on the other hand, their personal and cumulative experience with the disease between the mid-fourteenth and mid-eighteenth centuries. It also touches on how plague literature influenced medical education in the medieval and early modern eras. Medical education was, of course, not limited to the university and university-trained physicians, who in any event were only a small minority of medical practitioners throughout the pre-modern era. Especially after the early sixteenth century, the occupations of plague tract writers also expanded considerably to include medical practitioners of all kinds, clerics, civil administrators, and lay "professional" writers. I focus here on university-trained physicians, however, to trace continuities and changes in plague writing by one identifiable group of authors. I take this approach assuming, as Jon Arrizabalaga does, that these "practitioners' perceptions and reactions constitute a historical reality in themselves."[3]

Plague tracts first emerged in response to the massive epidemic that historians call the Black Death (1346–53), the beginning of the multi-century Second Plague Pandemic that affected Eurasia and North (and possibly Sub-Saharan) Africa. The treatises were largely formulaic, typically organized into three distinct sections: causes and signs of the disease, prevention, and treatment. Their authors used a novel format that combined the existing genres of the *regimina sanitatis* (health and its preservation) and the *consilia* (case studies outlining the causes of and treatments for disease) to organize their thinking and advice. As devastating outbreaks recurred frequently and regularly over the following centuries, plague treatises appeared and circulated in large numbers throughout Europe and the Middle East, as original, copied, translated, or adapted versions in manuscript and then in print. They varied in length: some, devoted largely to offering prevention and treatment advice, were short and concise (one to five pages), while others provided extended and often detailed philosophical-medical discussions of the meaning, nature, and cause of the disease. Drawing heavily from the canonical sources that marked pre-modern medical education, these latter tracts could run to hundreds of pages. Whatever their length or focus, the tract genre's long-term popularity was maintained by the medical optimism and familiar remedies they offered against the threat that plague continually posed to personal and community health.[4]

Pons's conundrum, the apparent dissonance between his formal medical education and his personal observation of plague, certainly was not new to late medieval and early modern medical practitioners and writers. Nor was his turn to his direct experience over his education in medical writing unusual. Medical knowledge transmission and acquisition took many forms, and all medical practitioners learned their craft from a variety of sources that crossed a wide spectrum, from the generational passing-down of skills to hands-on apprenticeship to the university classroom. Before the Black Death, though, a formally trained physician's experience was not expected to openly contradict his textual learning. Indeed, medieval medical education focused on teaching students the Galenic principles of inductive reasoning: "proceeding by way of the more obvious causes and effects to the hidden causes of disease."[5] Experiment and experience, dialectic and debate, all were meant to confirm the theory taught in the medical faculty, not to refute it. The first Hippocratic aphorism, after all, was that experience alone – empiricism – was deceptive, and written accounts of hands-on experience typically cited the ancient authorities for support, veracity, and validity. Book learning through formal medical education thus distinguished the medieval learned physician from "the mere empiric."[6] Even when accounts of personal observation and experience became increasingly common in early modern medical texts, as physicians faced a growing number of "new" ailments, the tension between medical education and personal observation remained.[7]

Certainly university-educated physicians struggled to fit what they learned through their training with what they observed on the ground during plague epidemics, whether first-hand while treating patients, by conducting autopsies on the plague dead, or even vicariously through the reports of their contemporaries. For those who wrote plague tracts, the challenge could be stark. Whether they sought to explain the disease, or simply to recommend suitable preventatives and therapies, there was little in the classical medical canon to prepare them for the visual and medical reality of plague. Through their tracts, and across the centuries, physicians drew from the numerous authoritative medical figures – such as Hippocrates, Galen, Avicenna, Rhazes, and even Aristotle – whose works and theories underlay their education as they attempted to explain the causes of plague, urged personal and environmental prophylactic measures, and recommended therapies and cures for those who fell ill. The tracts were thus seemingly predicated on long-standing medical education and wisdom. Yet these physician-authors also grappled increasingly boldly with the reality of their personal plague experiences – both observational and evaluative – that seemed to contradict, or at least not accord with, what they had learned from their books. Some sought to reconcile the differences, some ultimately rejected ancient medical authority in favour of experience, and still others remained almost absurdly attached to recycling inherited wisdom.

The authors' personal, empirical interpolations became a key component of the tracts' long-term appeal amongst a growing non- and less-formally medically trained readership: references to everyday knowledge and successful practice, rather than only theoretical learning, met their audience's desire for practical texts that provided useful explanations and recommendations. Even as academic medical education evolved and expanded over the centuries to incorporate ever more practically oriented training and the weighted experience of physicians' hands-on learning about plague, though, the disease itself remained problematic and nosologically contested.[8] When the number of large-scale epidemics declined in Western Europe after the mid-seventeenth century, fewer and fewer physicians could draw on direct experience and had to rely once again on their medical books and their education for knowledge about the disease.[9] But not all found these to be satisfactory.

When their university training proved insufficient to explain what they were seeing, how did physicians incorporate their direct experience with plague? When could experience override received knowledge learned through university training? What kinds of experience mattered and carried weight? Under what circumstances could the long-standing medical theory that was a core part of the medical education curriculum prevail, even when it was observably useless in practice? What about those physicians who wrote about the disease, but had never actually seen a plague patient (alive or dead): how did they blend the purported observations made by others with what they had learned themselves during their formal training? Teasing out these tensions of education versus personal experience helps to further bridge two aspects of historical medicine: formal medical education versus its perceived applicability on the ground in times of epidemic crisis.[10] I argue that although a general transition from reliance on formal medical education to preference for personal experience can be observed in the tracts, at no point was there a definitive dichotomy between the two. Nor was there a marked divide between those tracts that were a product of university circles and those that emerged from public or private medical practice. Instead, what we see in the tracts is the constant recalibration of the respective value assigned to medical education and personal experience, reflecting the evolution both of medical education itself – in response to the long centuries of plague outbreaks – and of larger cultural and intellectual phenomena.

THE BLACK DEATH AND THE FIRST PLAGUE TRACT WRITERS

The earliest plague tract authors hastily penned their explanations and advice in reaction to the first wave of the Second Plague Pandemic known as the Black Death (c. 1346–53). They faced an incredibly difficult situation. Some, such as Jacme d'Agramont, chair in medicine at the University in Lleida (Lérida), and Pierre de Damouzy, former regent of the Paris Faculty of Medicine, wrote in early 1348 before plague had even reached their respective cities (Damouzy was in Reims); these men had to fit the horrors of what they were only hearing about through second- or third-hand rumour and news with their own classical medical training and previous teaching. At the request of France's King Philip VI, leading representatives of the Paris Faculty of Medicine produced their own tract later that same year. By then, the epidemic was already causing high mortality in surrounding regions, but, like Agramont and Damouzy, the Paris Faculty members had neither direct experience with nor knowledge of anything like plague. Others early tract writers, such as Gentile da Foligno, professor and doctor of medicine at the University of Perugia, Giovanni della Penna, lecturer in the Naples medical faculty, Johannes von Göttingen, professor of medicine at Montpellier, and five local physicians in Strasbourg, wrote their tracts while or shortly after the disease actually affected their respective communities; as such, they were able to consider both the canonical authorities and their first-hand challenges in treating plague victims. Only a minority, such as Foligno, prolifically listed the authorities on whom their theories were based but gave preference to their own experience. Between 1348 and 1350, as many as thirty plague tracts appeared, many written by physicians who held high-level appointments in university medical faculties and/or who actively practised as private or public physicians.[11]

Whether they were writing with or without direct knowledge of plague, these mid-fourteenth-century physicians' assessments of the disease's signs, symptoms, and effects did not easily reflect anything that they had learned. The canon on which their medical education and teaching curricula were based – such as the collection known as the *Ars medicine* that brought together works by the ancient and early medieval writers Hippocrates, Galen, Johannitius, Theophilus, and Philaretus, as well as standardized collections of commentaries – included medical theory and disease classifications that did not correspond to the catastrophic mortality that they now witnessed.[12] The medical canon did not include reference to the First Plague Pandemic of the mid-sixth to mid-eighth centuries, and in fact authoritative medical texts written during the latter stages of the First Pandemic, such as Isidore of Seville's *On Medicine* and *De natura rerum*, provide no sense of the disease's devastation or its scope; certainly nothing like the Black Death existed in the medical education curriculum of the mid-fourteenth century. Historian Melissa Chase has noted that "[c]ollections of symptoms were given names [in the medieval medical canon] and were written about as though they were distinct entities," and so the lack of canonical precedent for the Black Death's specific signs and symptoms meant that it had no name and could not be identified readily in the existing medical literature.[13] Practical educational learning on anatomy and surgery likewise offered nothing concrete that could be used to explain plague. None of the earliest tract authors provided detailed descriptions of the signs of plague, and the bubo was rarely presented as a potentially unique and distinctive marker of the disease. The medical canon certainly had addressed painful apostemes or swellings, fevers, and stinking putrid matter, but not in this dramatic form. Some writers, including the renowned Paris Medical Faculty, made no mention at all of buboes or any other direct signs that might point to the particular disease that they were attempting to explain.[14]

This reticence to offer observations that did not accord with the authoritative canon can be explained, in part, by the fact that medieval society was governed to a large extent by custom, traditional authority, and historical precedent. Medical writing was little different in the sense that it too was a textual tradition predicated on long-standing authority and consistency, in which ancient deliberations ruled contemporary understanding and interpretation of health, illness, and disease. Tradition and authority thus typically overrode physicians' personal observations that might have contradicted accepted canonical knowledge; as a result, many early tract writers were unable (or perhaps unwilling) to conceive that they were facing a phenomenon unexplained by, and thus untreatable through, ancient knowledge. Even when they offered elaborate discussions of the disease's causes and attempted to construct somewhat novel explications, tract authors drew largely from very traditional medical, astrological, and religious knowledge to make sense of what they were seeing.[15]

Notably, tract authors relied on long-standing tradition that explained disease as the result of imbalanced humours. Stretching this explanation, which was most applicable to sick individuals, to a widespread epidemic required a universal precipitating cause. Plague was thus explained as the result of adverse astrological conjunctions, earthquakes, or other similar events that had produced evil vapours and corrupted the air. The infected air was then spread widely by the wind. To explain why some people in a community became sick and died while others did not, recourse was made to variations in individual humoral balances, which rendered some people more susceptible to the infected air. Some writers also emphasized human-to-human transmission, which could occur via the breath, skin perspiration, or gaze. Physicians then suggested preventive measures that aimed to identify places that were or that could be protected from infected air, that corrected or purified the infected air, and that kept the body resistant to infection. Perhaps most important was avoiding contact with infected people.[16] Therapeutic remedies included management of the six non-naturals, and the use of plasters, cold electuaries and cordials, theriac, herbs mixed with wine, phlebotomy, and lancing buboes.[17]

Yet alongside their efforts to stretch existing knowledge to account for the disease's inexplicable eruption and spread, some authors acknowledged the need to incorporate "modern" experts' opinions. The Paris Medical Faculty asserted that although the "ancients, notably Hippocrates ... [and] numerous wise men who are still remembered with respect" were aware of the climatic, astrological, and terrestrial signs that foretold a local epidemic, they had neither direct experience with nor personal knowledge of the kind of widespread outbreak that now faced humankind. Traditional medicine could only go so far to explain the great mortality's cause or provide appropriate treatments for it. The opinions and conclusions of modern experts also left "room for considerable uncertainty," though, since they too were dealing with something that seemed to be unheralded.[18]

POST–BLACK DEATH TRACT WRITERS AND THE TURN TO "MODERN" EXPERIENCE

Beginning in the early 1360s, the next generations of tract writers, who had gained first-hand knowledge of and experience with plague, more comfortably argued that their medical education could not always be relied upon to provide answers for "modern" diseases. While Sigismund Albicus (physician to the king of Bohemia, c. 1406) noted that the ancients could only have written about the diseases of their own time, for John of Burgundy, a Liège-based physician, this signalled the need to rely on modern expertise. "I make bold to say," he wrote around 1365, "not in criticism of past authorities, but out of long experience in the matter, that modern masters are more experienced in treating pestilential epidemic diseases than all the doctors from Hippocrates downward ... Galen, Dioscorides, Rhazes, Damascenus, Geber, Mesue, Copho, Constantine, Serapion, Avicenna, Algazel and all their successors never saw a general or long-lasting epidemic, or tested their cures by long experience although they draw on the sayings of Hippocrates to discuss many things concerning epidemics."[19] Ancient masters had relied on their own observations and experiences to describe and treat the diseases that were prevalent in their times. John and his colleagues had already survived at least one plague outbreak by virtue of their newly acquired skills treating this unique epidemic, and thus they alone were the experts. Even so, not all modern physicians were reliable either: "there are many masters in the art of medicine who are admirable scholars, well-versed in theories and hypotheses," John cautioned, "but who are too little experienced in the practicalities and are entirely ignorant" of the best means and methods of appropriate medical practice.[20] Claiming that he had read and studied everything that the ancients had written about epidemic diseases, Raymond Chalin de Vinario, a physician at the Avignon court writing in the early 1380s, likewise asserted that the ancient medical authorities had only "transmitted incomplete and superficial explanations" of large-scale epidemics "because they knew neither what caused the disease nor what action to take." As a result, he argued, it was necessary to "look [instead] to the writings of various modern doctors" who taught at Paris, Montpellier, and Avignon.[21] Blasius of Barcelona, an early-fifteenth-century royal physician in Aragon, concurred, noting that the ancient authors could not have written about plague because it did not exist in their time.

Although these tract authors and numerous others claimed that the authoritative medical canon that was part of their education was no longer sufficient on its own, their apparent turn to personal experience over their education was incomplete, and they failed to completely escape their reliance on tradition. The papal physician Guy de Chauliac suggested that he had saved himself from death during the second wave of plague epidemics (early 1360s) when his own "external apostemes were brought to a head with figs and cooked onions mixed with yeast and butter; then they were opened and treated as ulcers. The tumors were cupped, scarified, and cauterised."[22] Alongside this direct therapy, he recommended that the best preventatives were "to purge oneself with pills, to diminish the blood by phlebotomy, to purify the air with fire, and to strengthen the heart with tyriac [sic], fruits, and good-smelling things; to fortify the humors with Armenian *bolus*, and to resist decay with sharp[-tasting] things. For a cure men tried bleedings and evacuations, electuaries and cordial syrups." Chauliac then provided the recipe for an electuary of his own making, drawn "from the teachings of Master Arnald of Villanova [c. 1240–1311] and of the masters of Montpellier and Paris." Johannes Jacobi, a chancellor at Montpellier's medical faculty around the same time, claimed to have survived plague by relying on traditional dietary advice. Blasius of Barcelona claimed to have survived his buboes some years earlier by having them cut open and evacuated, as recommended by Albucasis and Avicenna but, more importantly, proven by his own hand and witnessed through decades of experience. All three had, in other words, survived plague by relying on traditional treatment practices offered up as something not just new but also personally verified.

Despite their efforts, physicians faced bitter and often satirical commentary about their apparent inability – and hence that of long-established medical education, theory, and practice – to halt the epidemic. Shortly after the Black Death, Boccaccio had noted in his novella *Decameron* that "it seemed that all the advice of physicians and all the power of medicine were profitless and unavailing." The Florentine chronicler Matteo Villani likewise complained that "[t]o gain money some [doctors] went visiting and dispensing their remedies, but these only demonstrated through their patients' death that their art was nonsense and false."[23] Some tract authors, such as the early-fifteenth-century physician Theobaldus Loneti from Besançon, even acknowledged that physicians were arguing among themselves about whether plague was treatable and curable; he took issue with the assumption made by some of his colleagues (and by the public) that there were no remedies at all for the disease simply because the ancient authorities had not specifically provided them. Loneti relied instead on many personal experiences (including his own affliction) to recommend a blend of remedies and therapies that, although little more than repackaged traditional therapeutics, he offered as "well-proved for the plague" through private test and trial. Criticism and disdain, then, did not shake physicians' tendency to turn to their traditional medical education for answers, although it may have pushed them to balance it with direct observation and experimentation. The popularity of plague tracts that offered long-standing remedial advice against plague certainly did not suffer.

Loneti and his contemporaries used the tract genre to engage in debates and discussions, frequently condemning the theories and techniques of their colleagues and of non-university-trained practitioners.[24] They also attempted to build on the apparent limitations of their university education. Among the later-fourteenth-century tract authors associated with the University of Montpellier, for example, two distinct groups emerged: some, such as Chauliac and Johannes de Tornamira (Johannes Jacobi's competitor for the medical faculty chancellorship), considered plague to be an apostemic disease, while others such as Jacobi considered it to be a pestilential fever.[25] The difference mattered, as it pointed to the predominance of celestial causes of disease, in the first instance, or terrestrial ones in the second. Another Montpellier physician, Vinario, introduced a third disease category: pestilential disease. All three approaches drew heavily from the Greek and Islamicate medical canon that had underscored the physicians' education, but adjusted the prevailing theories to account for direct "modern" observation. In the process of assimilating their own experiences into existing medical theory, these writers devised new explanatory models that were carried forward into the medical education environments of subsequent centuries.

EARLY MODERN REORIENTATION OF THE EDUCATION-VERSUS-EXPERIENCE CONUNDRUM

Socio-cultural and technological changes in the later fifteenth and sixteenth centuries generated another set of changes to the education-experience balance in the tracts over time. A renewed reliance on traditional authorities is evident, although this did not stop authors from promoting their own experience and success (perhaps more muted now). Also evident are a significant re-orientation to practical advice in the place of theory and, towards the end of this period, a different style of writing. Samuel Cohn attributes this reversion to authority to physicians' loss of self-confidence in their ability to manage the disease, but it was more a reaction to the combined influences of increased literacy and the emergence of print (which brought a vastly broader audience with a different set of needs), the rise and spread of humanism (which encouraged, if not demanded, both a renewed study and appreciation of the works of classical antiquity and the use of literary narrative), and a decided move toward the vernacular in plague writing.[26]

From the mid-fourteenth century, plague tract authors typically claimed to have written their texts for the benefit of the general public, people who had no access to a learned physician but who nevertheless sought medical information. The largely theoretical nature, and Latin language, of most early tracts belied this claim. Peter Murray Jones has noted that already by the early fifteenth century, though, "written information came to be of increasing value ... for practical purposes."[27] There was a significant increase in the production of practically oriented texts written in the vernacular that addressed scientific and medical subjects, including plague treatises that provided everyday therapies and remedies to combat the disease. The more theoretical treatises no longer met readers' needs and expectations. Instead, the tracts of the fifteenth and early sixteenth centuries were to a large extent "practical manuals of traditional wisdom" written to aid personal and public preservation and treatment as outbreaks unfolded.[28] Eric A. Heinrichs has recently noted that because of the early prevalence of the printing press in German-speaking towns, vernacular tract authors there in particular walked "a fine line between establishing their learned authority through scholarly discussion, on the one hand, and appealing to the practical interests of [their] audience, on the other."[29] In this context, it is easy to understand why some tract writers, such as an anonymous German author of 1493, sought to emphasize their combined learning and personal "extensive experience against this disease."[30]

Medical training and practice at the beginning of the early modern era was complicated and engaged a fraught blend of Latin scholastic tradition, a humanist turn to recently available ancient Greek medical texts, and the constant threat of plague and other diseases.[31] At the same time, the expansion of the curricula in numerous medical faculties to include more practical matters and empirical experiences reshaped both the learning experience and student expectations.[32] Trained and teaching in this newly synthetic medical environment, learned physicians offered tracts that heavily relied once again on the medical theories of their formal university training; by now, though, more works from Hippocrates and Galen were available, which added renewed vigour to their authority and standing as respected and influential medical texts.[33]

Not all tract writers appreciated this re-engagement with the ancient masters. Writing in the first decade of the sixteenth century, the Cologne physician Johann Vochs criticized contemporary medical education and its "slavish devotion" to ancient and modern texts that were suited only to conditions around the Mediterranean. An ardent national patriot, Vochs instead urged his contemporaries to rely on their own direct observations, "since the bodies and *materia medica* of northern Europe were best known through experience."[34] His tract explicitly ignored much of the then-current thinking about plague, since such learning was based on inherited tradition, not on actual – and local – experience: "[F]ew physicians are found," he argued, "who practice in many plagues or in great cities. And for this reason they are able to write or teach nothing about their own experience, but [simply] glorify the writings of others."[35]

Despite their erudite university training, lack of or little previous experience with plague could be seriously problematic for some physicians, as the case of the physician Girolamo Mercuriale demonstrates. Mercuriale may have been present during the 1555–56 plague outbreak in Venice, where he received his doctorate after studying in Padua. In 1576, Venetian officials called upon Mercuriale and his colleague Capodivacco to confirm if a local outbreak was plague, as the Board of Health believed to be the case; upon investigating, the two men decided that the disease in question was not plague and insisted that preventative measures such as quarantines and moving the sick to lazarettos not be put into place. Unfortunately for them, and for the city's residents, they were wrong. Some fifty thousand people died, and Mercuriale's critics blamed him and his staff for spreading the disease as they moved about the city.

In a series of lectures given early the following year, and in his subsequent plague treatise, Mercuriale turned not to his medical education, to traditional medical authority, nor even to previous experience to explain his misjudgment. Instead, he recalled the records of long-past epidemics taken from the accounts of "all the historians," such as Thucydides, Procopius, and Evagrius, who (according to Mercuriale) had demonstrated that some epidemics were outbreaks of "true plague" while others were not. This historical "fact" apparently vindicated Mercuriale's complete misreading of Venice's outbreak, since he now claimed that when he was consulted, the epidemic had not yet turned into "true plague."[36] To explain how the disease spread, though, he drew heavily from Girolamo Fractastoro's theory of contagion-by-"seed"; and in providing therapeutic recommendations for the future, he fell back on his conservative, Galenic university training: moderation, phlebotomy (judiciously applied), and proper diet. Despite his unfortunate misreading of the epidemic in 1576, Mercuriale nevertheless emphasized that "he alone possesse[d] the experience and learning to judge what plague is, and when (and how) to intervene."[37] Perhaps luckily for him, this failure limited his career but did not greatly damage it.[38]

The Tours physician Nicolas de Nancel also downplayed physicians' lack of success in treating plague victims, but instead advanced the general wisdom of late-sixteenth-century humanists: return to the traditional sources. For Nancel, closely following the sacrosanct teachings of the ancient masters studied in university was more beneficial than relying on the empiric trials and errors of modern apothecaries who "muddle[d] innumerable Arabic words, and pervert[ed] in a number of places the intent of the good Greek authors whom [they] neither read, nor followed, nor understood."[39]

Most sixteenth- and seventeenth-century tract writers took a middle road: questioning traditional medicine while simultaneously paying tribute to accumulated learned wisdom, adding contemporary experts to the list of revered authorities (Fracastoro, Jean Fernel, Paracelsus, Marsilio Ficino, Montanus, and even Mercuriale himself), and allowing space for personal observation. Heinrichs's examination of experiments undertaken to assess the validity and efficacy of the so-called live chicken treatment for buboes demonstrates that many doctors both offered new ideas for the long-standing practice attributed to one of the fathers of the medical canon (Avicenna), and reinterpreted its value and place in "modern" medicine on the basis of their own experience with it.[40] What set these tract authors apart from their fourteenth-century predecessors was their willingness to engage more whole-heartedly with the medical tradition, albeit in its newly discovered and more complete form.

Most tracts by the seventeenth century thus included both references to what "many noble & most excellent learned men have in times past worthely considered" and "the best learned Physitions in this age," alongside their authors' own observations.[41] The exiled physician Simone Simoni, who like Mercuriale had graduated from Padua, wrote his tract after facing criticism during an outbreak in Leipzig. Unlike Mercuriale's, Simoni's tract focused heavily on the classical and medieval authorities, although he argued that much of the traditional approach to addressing plague was flawed. He openly dismissed "large parts of the standard discussions of plague as irrelevant to the practical advice" that he offered. Instead, he contended that his stance sprung from "the fruit of a long and successful tradition of [humoral] healing" that he blended with Fractastoro's theories to "create his own 'skilful and scientific' method of effective treatment."[42] Simoni was not actually in Leipzig during the outbreak, having fled the city, and could not offer any real hands-on experience to demonstrate the efficaciousness of his recommendations. Nevertheless, he claimed, accusations that physicians had done little to help plague victims were unfair, since "learned advice is not always easy to follow," and patients typically preferred the simpler remedies offered by "quacks, unlearned charlatans, and travelling salesmen."[43]

Other tract authors were just as keen to validate their own authority and combined their experiences with narrative (and sometimes long-winded) accounts of what they had learned formally or through others.[44] The Parisian physician Pierre Drouet noted that six years before writing his tract in 1572, he had experienced an outbreak in Lyon where he saw "men fell downe dead to the grounde, eue[n] as they were going in the streets."[45] He claimed that his knowledge about plague was gained not only through that first-hand experience, but also through prodigious reading (and rereading) of the works of Hippocrates and Galen, deep questions posed to him "and other professours of Phisick" by his patron (Lorde Vidam Chartres, Prince of Chabanoys), and "conference with the best learned Phisitions both in England, Germanie, and many other places." His tract refers to many learned writings about plague and to the varied medical treatments that he had observed during his travels.[46] For Drouet, the continuing medical education that he had gained by studying a range of treatments first-hand with famous medical men such as Jacques Houllier and Leonard Fuchs, and with a great many other "verye well learned" physicians, surgeons, and apothecaries in Rouen, Antwerp, England, and Germany, was an integral addition to his formal university training and helped him to better understand and address what he was seeing on the ground. That luminaries such as Ficino, Ambroise Paré, and George Agricola had endorsed such treatments only added to their authenticity.

The third-generation London physician Stephen Bradwell, who studied at Cambridge but did not complete his degree, likewise offered through his two plague tracts knowledge that he had acquired "both by *Reading* & *Experience*."[47] His first tract, published in 1625, was "Collected out of the best authors, mixed with auncient experience, and moulded into a new and most plaine method." Bradwell wrote in that work that he "may not take upon me to cure the Sicke, because I meddle not with the Sicknesse (for to practise on the *Plague* now, would prove a plague to my Practise hereafter)."[48] Clearly he did take it upon himself to treat the ill, and realized through that encounter that he had much to learn. By 1636, when his second tract appeared, he claimed that there were very few physicians still alive who, like himself, had remained in the city and gained "experience of the last great Sicknesse." But because he had stayed and treated patients against his original intention – and had spent much time since then learning as much as he could about the disease "out of the Choycest Authors" – Bradwell argued that he was now especially well placed to "prescribe a course of *Physicke*, such as both my much reading, and also my manifest Experience in the last great *Visitation*, have preferred to my best approbation."[49]

Thirty years later, in 1666, English physician George Thomson instead railed against traditional medical approaches and their ineffectiveness against plague. Thomson rejected Galenic explanations and treatments in particular, insisting that "the *First-fruits* of my *Difficult Labours*" – referring to the autopsy that he had performed on a plague corpse the previous year – had plainly proved the errors of traditional medical assumptions and practices.[50] Thomson also claimed to have risked his own life to save those of his fellow citizens, both by treating the sick and by accidentally cutting himself while conducting the autopsy to better understand the bodily effects of plague. Thomson was an ardent follower of the new Helmontian medicine that combined medical, chemical, and moral theories and therapies that stood in stark contrast to the traditional humoral approaches of Galenism; he had become attracted to Helmontism following his study of medicine in Leyden in the late 1640s. For him, the benefits of the dissection lay not solely in the immediate medical knowledge that it generated and that could be used to counter traditional medical education: they also revealed the value of "undertak[ing] any dangerous and difficult design, [so] that a particular Countrey, Nation, yea, the whole World may be meliorated in its condition, and enjoy some comfort therefrom."[51] In this case, the new empiricism based on clinical observation and inductive reasoning served as a counterpoint to traditional Galenism and deductive epistemologies, and demonstrated a "contempt for mere academic learning" that, alone, could never prepare a physician to adequately treat plague victims.[52]

EIGHTEENTH-CENTURY RECONSIDERATIONS
OF TRADITIONAL MEDICAL KNOWLEDGE

On travelling to Marseille in 1720, Monsieur D.M. Pons quickly realised the insufficiency of his traditional medical education. He saw with surprise that the city was, in fact, afflicted with "the true Plague, described by all the Authors who have written about it, and accompanied by all the most essential symptoms."[53] Real-life experience contradicted his formal university medical education, and showed him that there was no longer any "reason to doubt that the Plague is a real and existing disease." Even though he was convinced of the reality of plague, however, Pons's traditional educational training did not make it easy for him to understand its character and nature; in some ways, he reasoned, the disease was similar to smallpox (*Petite Verole*): it spread from country to country, successively infecting one city or village after another, and it appeared to infect people just once. But beyond suggesting that plague was likely the result of some kind of airborne *Seminium pestis*, Pons forbore from speculating about its causes, preferring to leave such theorizing to Monsieur de Bon's "sçavans Professeurs."[54]

After providing a detailed description of the various stages of signs and symptoms through which he had seen Marseille's plague-afflicted patients suffer, Pons offered a short commentary on his experience using various remedies, suggesting which were most suitable for which stage of the disease. He had first tried antimonial emetics and purgatives, but with little success: by the third or fourth day, all his patients had died. He had then tried using emetics alone on patients who had been ill for twenty-four hours or less, along with light cordials of various traditional ingredients (theriac, Armenian bole, diaphoretic antimony, powder of viper, bezoar, and others). His greatest success, though, came from opening the suppurating buboes of hundreds of hospital patients who had survived to the fifth or sixth day; through this method, he said, plague victims were most likely to recover.[55]

Although he ultimately relied on remedial therapies long recommended by his predecessors in their tracts, Pons allowed his personal observation that plague was a "real" disease to challenge and override what he felt that his formal medical training had taught him. His experience using various therapeutic practices permitted him to test what he had read against the real conditions of plague. He acknowledged that the ideas that he provided might appear to be extraordinary, not only because they were to some extent "new," but also because they directly contradicted what he and others apparently had learned at the university. Yet, he hoped that his remarks would assist other physicians who also had never seen the disease before, in case they too were tasked with treating it.[56] Many of course were, as the outbreak continued into 1722.

Writing from the safety of London around the same time, the English Leyden- and Padua-trained physician Richard Mead sought to explain what caused this still-fearsome disease. He claimed, based on what he called the evidence of "the Natural History of several Countries" and the observations of "the ancientist and best Authors of Physick," that underlying the outbreak were specific topographical and environmental features. Mead's early-eighteenth-century turn to modern "Reason" also caused him to reject what he considered to be the past's misguided efforts to manage the disease. New approaches, he argued, needed to reflect current knowledge rather than old errors and misunderstandings: "proper Directions should be drawn up to defend our selves from such a Calamity ... [including] some new Regulations."[57]

Unlike Pons, though, Mead and his London colleagues had no opportunity to test either their education or their assumptions: plague did not reach London. But this did not stop them from engaging in a heated debate about the relative merits and reliability of Mead's "new" ideas that plague spread through infected commercial trade goods against theories "Founded upon the Experience of those who were Practitioners when [plague last] raged." These "most learned Physicians of [earlier] Times" had actually observed plague first-hand and could therefore speak with some authority on the subject. They should not, most eighteenth-century English writers argued, be dismissed quite so readily.[58] As Richard Brookes passionately stated: "Whoever writes with any tolerable Success upon the *Plague*, must found his Opinions upon the Observations and Experience of his Predecessors; for they alone are able to inform us of the different Fortune of a various Practice ... However specious or conclusive the Reasonings of some may be, yet they satisfy us no farther than they have *Experience* for their *Foundation*."[59] It was clear to most that the experiences of their predecessors mattered more than book learning alone for truthful discussions about plague.

Like Pons's work, French plague tracts of the early 1720s focused almost exclusively on the authors' personal observations about, encounters with, and reflections on the Marseille outbreak. Treating a large number of infected people daily over a short period of time and "opening and dissecting many cadavers" offered them, as Pons had noted, a unique and timely opportunity to test their formal university medical education against "a certain number of evident and incontestable facts" of a real-life disease outbreak.[60] What this contrast made clear to them was that the high plague mortality in Marseille could be traced, at least in part, to physicians' and surgeons' lack of experience with and insufficient training – "novices dans ce fait" – for a disease that had caught them all by surprise.[61]

CONCLUSION

The majority of university-educated physicians who penned plague tracts between the mid-fourteenth and early eighteenth centuries relied on their formal medical education and canonical medical theory inherited from the ancient Greeks and Romans to help them make sense of the plague epidemics that they encountered. For the most part, the discourse found in tracts before the early sixteenth century was rooted in a universal system of ideas about the causes of and cures for plague. Personal observations added to some tracts typically served to validate or expand upon that education; their purpose was largely to enable the authors to promote their experience – and thus their authority – to speak about plague. Centuries of accumulated wisdom about and familiarity with the disease thus augmented but were not meant to entirely replace formal medical education. Medical knowledge could be acquired in various ways, but book learning remained paramount.

Yet many tract authors found that their personal experience with plague did not accurately reflect what they had been taught. In these cases, where they blended their personal observations with reference to their university-based learning, the writers did so not only to demonstrate their erudition and authority through experience, but also to point to the need to rethink the canon that underscored their education. The Munich city physician Alexander Seitz, for example, argued in his tract that blind recourse to long-standing therapeutic bloodletting as a plague treatment was dangerous, having been improperly understood from ancient practice and thus poorly taught.[62]

This sense of discordance between education and experience with plague can be read in many tracts, and it increased during and after the sixteenth century, as emerging approaches to medicine and medical training competed for prominence alongside the humanist turn to original sources and the rise of print. The seventeenth century's emphasis on empiricism and experimentation at the expense of authority – a critical component of the "scientific revolution" – further pushed tract writers to question their formal medical education when it did not match what they were seeing with their own eyes.[63] Even when they did rely to a large extent on the existing canon, physicians perceived the inadequacies of their formal training, and some attempted to contribute to continuing medical education and learning by teaching others about plague through the pages of their treatises. Their success in doing so is evidenced by the incorporation of some of the more erudite writers into the updated medical curriculum itself.

Plague tracts were full of medical debates about the nature and cause of plague, predicated on different learned theories of its cause, but in the end, actual experience with the disease could not entirely override book learning and formal medical education. For most of those tract writers who struggled with outbreak in Marseille in 1720–22, whether directly and in the city itself or vicariously and from afar, the inclination to turn for advice to the hands-on experiences of their predecessors prevailed, as long as it was read in the context of accepted theory.

What I hope to have shown here is that physicians were not rigidly guided either by the medical canon – as they learned it in university medical faculties – or by experience; instead, there was a constant, dynamic interplay of both factors in their ongoing attempts to grapple with the challenges of plague. Different physicians occupied different places on the experience versus education spectrum, and sometimes the same physician – such as Pons – moved from one side to another. While tract authors walked a tightrope between education and experience, and while the balance sometimes tipped one way or the other, seeing a clear dichotomy between the two tells us more about how we think about medieval and early modern medicine than how these university-trained physicians thought about it themselves.

NOTES

1   "C'est la doctrine qu'on nous a enseignée à Montpellier en 1688. 1689. 1690. & 1691. pendant que j'y faisois mes études ... Mais cette doctrine n'etoit fondée que sur la simple presomption, Mrs. les Professeurs de ce tems là n'ayant jamais vû de Peste." D.M. Pons's full letter is included in Boecler, *Recueil des observations*, 12–21. The quote is on p. 15.

2   "... j'étois dans la prévention qu'il n'y avoit jamais eu de Peste dans la Nature; que ce, qui avoit été qualifié de ce nom par nos Autheurs , n'étoit qu'une suite de leurs prejugés à ne point saigner ni purger ... [dont] il arrivoit des Parotides, des Bubons, des Charbons , des Éxanthémes , & toutes les autres efflorescences qu'on observe dans la Peste." Ibid., 14.

3   Arrizabalaga, "Facing the Black Death," 237–88.

4   I offer a much more detailed and comparative examination of plague treatises and their contents in Jones, *Patterns of Plague*.

5   Talbot, "Medical Education in the Middle Ages," 74.

6   Getz, "Medical Education," 78. Although Galen's works encompassed both rational and empirical medicine, and even "set a high value on evidence derived from personal observation and experience," there was a long-standing battle between those who advocated for empirically based medical practice and those who insisted on the superiority of book learning and formal education. Ultimately, the institutionalization of medical education, and the university curricula itself, "systematized the transmission and reinforced the authority of a body of medical books, concepts, and techniques" whose adoption marked the intellectual supremacy of formally educated physicians. Siraisi, *Medieval and Early Renaissance Medicine*, 5, 48. This battle, which stretched into the early modern era, is beyond the scope of this chapter, but Siraisi's book provides an excellent overview. What constitutes "experience" is of course a cultural construct that changed over time. Numerous medieval medical recipes, for example, invoked *experimentum* as the basis of their authority; in this case, *experimentum* meant personal experience (either the scribe's own or someone else's). Occasionally it also meant "experiment," always in the sense that the scribe had tried it rather than the modern meaning of the word. Heinrichs, "Live Chicken Treatment," provides an excellent example of an *experimentum* that continued over several centuries.

7   This is discussed in more detail below; see also Siraisi, "'Remarkable' Diseases," 226–52.

8   On the expansion of medical education to include practical matters, see Stolberg, "Training Future Practitioners," ch. 4 in this volume.

9   Plague was largely absent in official English records after 1665–66, but the autumnal mortality spike associated with the disease did not disappear from

around London until the late 1720s; see Cummins, Kelly, and Ó Gráda, "Living Standards," 5. In France, the number and extent of officially recorded plague outbreaks declined considerably between the mid-seventeenth century and 1720, but annual outbreaks continued (albeit largely unnoticed) until at least 1770; see Jones, "Plague and Its Metaphors," 99. The last large outbreak in Central Europe was in 1708–13; see Christensen, "Copenhagen 1711." Sporadic epidemics persisted in Southern and Eastern Europe for another century, and devastated North Africa and the Russian and Ottoman Empires well into the nineteenth century.

10 On the interaction between early modern medical education and practice more broadly, see among others Wear, *Knowledge & Practice*; Brockliss and Jones, *Medical World*; and Lindemann, *Medicine and Society*. On new medical theories and practices and their incorporation into medical education, see Debus, *French Paracelsians*; Debus, *English Paracelsians*.

11 Well-known non-Christian writers of the earliest tracts, such as Ibn al-Khaṭīb, Ibn Khātimah, and al-Shaqūrī, Islamicate scholars in Andalusia, and Abraham Caslari, a Jewish physician practising in Girona and Besalú (Catalonia), absorbed the university medical curriculum via translation, personal relationships, and/or personalized study, but were never part of the formal university system. I thank Susan Einbinder and Justin Stearns for discussing these cases with me.

12 For the main canonical texts of medieval medical training, see (in general) Talbot, "Medical Education in the Middle Ages"; for Paris, see O'Boyle, *Art of Medicine*; for Italy, see Siraisi, *Medicine and the Italian Universities*; for Cambridge and Oxford, see Jones, "Reading Medicine," and Getz, "Medical Education."

13 Chase, "Fevers, Poisons, and Apostemes," 153. It is important to note here that the term "Black Death" was not used until much later, and is not a contemporary term.

14 On descriptions and representations of the plague's physical signs, see Jones, "'Apostumes, Carbuncles, and Botches.'"

15 For a more detailed discussion of traditional medical theory and training and its use in the earliest plague tracts, see Arrizabalaga, "Facing the Black Death," and Chase, "Fevers, Poisons, and Apostemes."

16 Arrizabalaga, "Facing the Black Death"; Stearns, *Infectious Ideas*, 69.

17 The six non-naturals were the controllable physiological, psychological, and environmental elements that affected health: exercise/rest, food/drink, repletion/excretion, sleep/wakefulness, air, and passions/emotions. Rectifying imbalances in the non-naturals was central to the university medical curriculum.

18 "Report of the Paris Medical Faculty," 161–2, 158.

19 "Treatise of John of Burgundy," 192. The list of authorities varies from one version of the tract to another. For more detailed discussions of John of Burgundy and his work, see Jones, "Itineraries," and Honkapohja and Jones, "From *Practica Phisicalia*."

20 "Treatise of John of Burgundy," 185. The practicalities that John referred to here were preparing and administering medicines at astrologically appropriate times.

21 "Antiqui siquidem in causis talium morborum diminute et superficialiter tran-siuerunt ... vel quia causas illorum vel modos actionis causarum ignoraverunt quia morbus est incognitus suis non cognitis causis vel modus actionis eorum ... Postquam itaque vidi dicta antiquorum super morbis epidimicis tractancium, aspexi etiam tractatus diuersos doctorum modernorum." Vinario, "Raïmundüs de Peste," 37–8.

22 Chauliac, "Bubonic Plague," 774.

23 Boccaccio, *Decameron*, 7; Villani quoted in Aberth, *Black Death*, 37.

24 Inter-professional strife often played out in medical texts. See Amundsen, *Medicine, Society, and Faith*.

25 Chase, "Fevers, Poisons, and Apostemes."

26 Cohn, *Cultures of Plague*, 13. Humanism was a Western European cultural movement of the fourteenth through sixteenth centuries that involved, among other things, a return to the study of classical antiquity to recover the cultural and literary legacy, moral philosophy, and engaged citizenry of that earlier period. Humanists sought to eliminate what they perceived to be the corrupting influences of Arabic and medieval translations by studying ancient texts (such as the works of Hippocrates and Galen) in their original form; see Nauert, *Humanism and the Culture of Renaissance Europe*. On humanist medicine, see Bylebyl, "The School of Padua," and Wear, French, and Lonie, eds., *Medical Renaissance of the Sixteenth Century*.

27 Jones, "Information and Science," 100.

28 Carmichael, "Last Past Plague," 158.

29 Heinrichs, *Plague, Print, and the Reformation*, 23.

30 "Hab ich. N. aus vil unde mancher doctorum un lerer in der artzney erfaren schrifftum, disz buchlin ausgetzogen unde tzu samen getragen, nicht anders in diesem buchelin beschriben hab dan alleyn wasz ich durch lange erfarung wider diese kranckheyt dyenen vor anderen erkanth hab." Anonymous, *Arznei wider die Pestilenz*, quoted in Fabbri, "Continuity and Change," 41–2.

31 Siraisi, "'Remarkable' Diseases," 228.

32 See Stolberg, "Training Future Practitioners," ch. 4 in this volume.

33 The "more or less" complete Hippocratic corpus became readily available, for example, only after its publication in Latin in the early 1500s, while the

complete works of Galen (in Greek) appeared only in 1525. Siraisi, *History, Medicine, Traditions*, 15; Wear, *Knowledge & Practice*, 35.

34 Heinrichs, *Plague, Print, and the Reformation*, 53–4. As Heinrichs notes, "Somewhat paradoxically, Vochs supported his ideas about German medicine with Hippocrates's teachings on locality and environment, using them to challenge physicians' systemic neglect of the particular characteristics of northern Europe."

35 Vochs, *De pestilentia*, F5^r, quoted in Heinrichs, *Plague, Print, and the Reformation*, 64.

36 Siraisi, *History, Medicine, Traditions*, 102–5. See also Palmer, "Girolamo Mercuriale and the Plague of Venice."

37 Nutton, "With Benefit of Hindsight," 11, 17.

38 Laughran, "Body, Public Health and Social Control," 219–20. I thank Susan Einbinder for sharing this source.

39 "... a suyui la descriptio[n] des Arabes, com[m]e il fait partout, broüillant infinis mots Arabiques, & peruertissant en plusieurs endroits l'inte[n]tion des bons autheurs Grecs: lesquels il n'a ni leu, ni suyui, ni entendu." Nancel, *Discours tresample*, 164.

40 Heinrichs, "Live Chicken Treatment."

41 Phayer, *Goodly Bryefe Treatyse*, 5; Thayre, *Excellent and Best Approoued*, title page.

42 Nutton, "With Benefit of Hindsight," 7, 12–13, 15.

43 Ibid., 10.

44 On the shift to narrative, and especially its impact on visual descriptions of the disease, see Jones, "'Apostumes, Carbuncles, and Botches.'" On the use of personal experience as a broader authorial trend, see Einbinder, "Poetry, Prose and Pestilence."

45 Drouet, *New Counsell*, 14. The tract was first published as *Consilium novum de pestilentia*.

46 On early modern medical learning and travel, see Grell, Cunningham, and Arrizabalaga, eds., *Centres of Medical Excellence?*

47 Bradwell, *Physick for the Sicknesse*, A2^v.

48 Bradwell, *Watch-man for the Pest*, title page, A1^v. Emphasis in the original.

49 Bradwell, *Physick for the Sicknesse*, A3^v, title page, B3^r.

50 Thomson, *Loimotomia*, A4. Thomson was a leading figure in the ultimately unsuccessful creation of a College of Chemical Physicians.

51 Ibid., 107.

52 Cook, *Decline of the Old Medical Regime*, 154. On the shift to empiricism and experimentation in seventeenth-century England, see also Carvallo, "The Empirical Turn of Medicine in England," and Barry, "'Compleat Physician' and Experimentation."

53   "la Maladie dont cette Ville est affligée, étoit la veritable Peste, décrite
     par tous les Autheurs qui en ont traité, & accompagnée de tous les
     Symptomes les plus essentiels ; en sorte qu'il n'y a plus lieu de douter , que
     la Peste ne soit une Maladie réelle & existente." Pons, in Boecler, *Recueil des
     observations*, 15.

54   Ibid., 16.

55   "j'ay plus de 250 Malades [à un Hôpital]; & je trouve qu'avec cette Methode
     les Malades le portent plus loin , & qu'il en réchapé devantage." Ibid., 20.

56   "l'idée que j'en donne paroitra extraordinaire , parce qu'elle est nouvelle, mais
     j'espere qu'elle servira aux Medecins qui n'ont pas vû ce Mal , en cas qu'ils
     soient obligez de traiter des Pestiferez." Ibid., 21.

57   Mead, *Short Discourse*, 2–3, A2^v–A3^r.

58   Brookes, *History*, title page; Browne, *Practical Treatise*, title page.

59   Brookes, *History*, 5, 7. Emphasis in the original.

60   "Les experienees réiterées que nous avons eu occasion de faire , dans l'espace
     de neuf mois , pendant lesquels nous avons traité journellement un grand
     nombre de Pestiferez, ouvert plusieurs cadavres, & fait des dissections ...
     certain nombre de faits évidens & incontestables." Chicoyneau, Verny, and
     Soulier, *Observations et reflexions*, 6, 26.

61   "D'autres circonfiances devoient encore concourir à augmenter la mortalité
     dans Marseille ; la surprise , le peu d'experience des Médecins & des
     Chirurgiens, & les causes dispositives qui particulierement s'y trouvoient."
     Baux, *Traité de la peste*, 10.

62   Heinrichs, *Plague, Print, and the Reformation*, 85.

63   Shapin, *Scientific Revolution*; Webster, *Great Instauration*.

BIBLIOGRAPHY

Amundsen, Darrel W. *Medicine, Society, and Faith in the Ancient and Medieval Worlds.*
    Baltimore, MD: Johns Hopkins University Press, 1996.
Arrizabalaga, Jon. "Facing the Black Death: Perceptions and Reactions of University
    Medical Practitioners." In *Practical Medicine from Salerno to the Black Death*, edited by
    Luis García-Ballester, Roger French, Jon Arrizabalaga, and Andrew Cunningham,
    237–88. Cambridge: Cambridge University Press, 1994.
Barry, Jonathan. "'Compleat Physician' and Experimentation in Medicines: Everard
    Maynwaring (c. 1629–1713) and the Restoration Debate on Medical Practice in
    London." *Medical History* 62, no. 2 (2018): 155–76.
Baux, Pierre. *Traité de la peste.* Toulouse, France: Jean Guillemette, 1722.
Boccaccio, Giovanni. *Decameron*, 2nd ed. Translated by G.H. McWilliam.
    Harmondsworth, UK: Penguin Classics, 2003.

Boecler, Johann. *Recueil des observations qui ont étées faites sur la maladie de Marseille.* Strasbourg, France: Jean Regnauld Doulssecker, 1721.

Bradwell, Stephen. *Physick for the Sicknesse, Commonly Called the Plague.* London: for Benjamin Fisher, 1636.

– *A Watch-man for the Pest.* London: John Dawson, 1625.

Brockliss, Laurence, and Colin Jones. *The Medical World of Early Modern France.* Oxford, UK: Clarendon Press, 1997.

Brookes, Richard. *A History of the Most Remarkable Pestilential Distempers that have Appeared in Europe for Three Hundred Years Last Past.* London: A. Corbett, 1721.

Browne, Joseph. *A Practical Treatise of the Plague and All Pestilential Infections that have Happen'd in this Island for the Last Century*, 2nd ed. London: for J. Wilcox, 1720.

Bylebyl, Jerome J. "The School of Padua: Humanistic Medicine in the Sixteenth Century." In *Health, Medicine and Mortality in the Sixteenth Century*, edited by Charles Webster, 335–70. Cambridge: Cambridge University Press, 1979.

Carmichael, Ann G. "The Last Past Plague: The Uses of Memory in Renaissance Epidemics." *Journal of the History of Medicine and Allied Sciences* 53, no. 2 (1998): 132–60.

Carvallo, Sarah. "The Empirical Turn of Medicine in England, 1660–1690." *Archives Internationales d'Histoire des Sciences* 67, no. 178 (2017): 75–112.

Chase, Melissa P. "Fevers, Poisons, and Apostemes: Authority and Experience in Montpellier Plague Treatises." *Annals of the New York Academy of Sciences* 441, no. 1 (1985): 153–70.

Chauliac, Guy de. "Bubonic Plague." In *A Source Book in Medieval Science*, vol. 1, edited by Edward Grant, 773–4. Boston, MA: Harvard University Press, 1974.

Chicoyneau, François, François Verny, and Jean Soulier. *Observations et reflexions touchant la nature, les evenemens, et le traitement de la peste de Marseille.* Toulouse, France: Claude-Gilles Lecamus, 1720.

Christensen, Peter. "Copenhagen 1711: Danish Authorities Facing the Plague." In *Body and City: Histories of Urban Public Health*, edited by Sally Sheard and Helen Power, 50–8. Aldershot, UK: Ashgate, 2000.

Cohn, Samuel K., Jr. *Cultures of Plague: Medical Thinking at the End of the Renaissance.* Oxford, UK: Oxford University Press, 2010.

Cook, Harold J. *The Decline of the Old Medical Regime in Stuart London.* Ithaca, NY: Cornell University Press, 1986.

Cummins, Neil, Morgan Kelly, and Cormac Ó Gráda. "Living Standards and Plague in London, 1560–1665." *Economic History Review*, 69, no. 1 (2016): 3–34.

Debus, Allen G. *The English Paracelsians.* New York: F. Watts, 1966.

– *The French Paracelsians: The Chemical Challenge to Medical and Scientific Tradition in Early Modern France.* Cambridge: Cambridge University Press, 1991.

Drouet, Pierre. *A New Counsell Against the Pestilence Declaring What Kinde of Disease it is, of*

What Cause it Procedeth, the Signes and Tokens Thereof: With the Order of Curing the Same.
Translated by Thomas Twine. London: John Charlewood, 1578.

Einbinder, Susan L. "Poetry, Prose and Pestilence: Joseph Concio and Jewish
Responses to the 1630 Italian Plague." In *Song of Deborah: A Gift of Friendship and
Appreciation to Professor Dvora Bregman*, edited by Haviva Ishai, 73–101. Beer-Sheva,
Israel: Ben-Gurion University Press, 2018.

Fabbri, Christiane Nockels. "Continuity and Change in Late Medieval Plague
Medicine: A Survey of 152 Plague Tracts from 1348 to 1599." PhD diss. New
Haven, CT: Yale University, 2006.

Getz, Faye. "Medical Education in Later Medieval England." In *The History of
Medical Education in Britain*, edited by Vivian Nutton and Roy Porter, 76–93.
Amsterdam: Rodopi, 1995.

Grell, Ole Peter, Andrew Cunningham, and Jon Arrizabala, eds. *Centres of Medical
Excellence? Medical Travel and Education in Europe, 1500–1789*. Aldershot, UK:
Ashgate, 2010.

Heinrichs, Erik A. "The Live Chicken Treatment for Buboes: Trying a Plague Cure
in Medieval and Early Modern Europe." *Bulletin of the History of Medicine* 91, no. 2
(2017): 210–32.

– *Plague, Print, and the Reformation: The German Reform of Healing, 1473–1573*. London:
Routledge, 2018.

Honkapohja, Alpo, and Lori Jones. "From *Practica Phisicalia* to *Mandeville's Travels*:
Untangling the Misattributed Identities and Writings of John of Burgundy." *Notes
and Queries* 67, no. 1 (2020): 18–27.

Jones, Colin. "Plague and Its Metaphors in Early Modern France." *Representations* 53
(1996): 97–127.

Jones, Lori. "'Apostumes, Carbuncles, and Botches': Visualizing the Plague in Late
Medieval and Early Modern Medical Treatises." In *Asclepius, the Paintbrush, and the
Pen: Representations of Disease in Medieval and Early Modern European Art and Literature*,
edited by Rinaldo Canalis and Massimo Ciavolella, 173–200. Turnhout, Belgium:
Brepols, 2021.

– "Itineraries and Transformations: John of Burgundy's Plague Treatise." *Bulletin of
the History of Medicine* 95, no. 3 (2021): 277–314.

– *Patterns of Plague: Changing Ideas about Plague in England and France, 1348–1750*.
Montreal, QC, and Kingston, ON: McGill-Queen's University Press, 2022.

Jones, Peter Murray. "Information and Science." In *Fifteenth-Century Attitudes:
Perceptions of Society in Late Medieval England*, edited by Rosemary Horrox, 97–111.
Cambridge: Cambridge University Press, 1994.

– "Reading Medicine in Tudor Cambridge." In *The History of Medical Education in
Britain*, edited by Vivian Nutton and Roy Porter, 153–83. Amsterdam: Rodopi,
1995.

Laughran, Michelle Anne. "The Body, Public Health and Social Control in
    Sixteenth-Century Venice." PhD diss. Storrs, CT: University of Connecticut,
    1998.
Lindemann, Mary. *Medicine and Society in Early Modern Europe.* Cambridge: Cambridge
    University Press, 1999.
Mead, Richard. *A Short Discourse Concerning Pestilential Contagion and the Methods Used to
    Prevent It.* London: Sam. Buckley and Ralph Smith, 1720.
Nancel, Nicolas de. *Discours tresample de la Peste.* Paris: Denis du Val, 1581.
Nauert, Charles Garfield. *Humanism and the Culture of Renaissance Europe.* Cambridge:
    Cambridge University Press, 2006.
Nutton, Vivian. "With Benefit of Hindsight: Girolamo Mercuriale and Simone
    Simoni on Plague." *Medicina & Storia* 6, no. 11 (2006): 5–19.
O'Boyle, Cornelius. *The Art of Medicine: Medical Training at the University of Paris, 1250–
    1400.* Leiden, Netherlands: Brill, 1998.
Palmer, Richard. "Girolamo Mercuriale and the Plague of Venice." In *Girolamo
    Mercuriale : medicina e cultura nell'Europa del Cinquecento : atti del convegno Girolamo
    Mercuriale e lo spazio scientifico e culturale del Cinquecento : Forlì, 8–11 novembre 2006,*
    edited by Vivian Nutton and Alessandro Arcangeli, 51–65. Florence, Italy: Leo S.
    Olschki, 2008.
Phayer, Thomas. "Here beginneth a goodly bryefe tretise of the Pestilence." In *The
    Kegiment* [sic] *of Life.* London: Edward Whitchurche, 1546.
"Report of the Paris Medical Faculty, October 1348." In *The Black Death,* translated
    and edited by Rosemary Horrox, 158–63. Manchester, UK: Manchester
    University Press, 1994.
Shapin, Steven. *The Scientific Revolution.* Chicago, IL: University of Chicago Press,
    1996.
Siraisi, Nancy. *History, Medicine, and the Traditions of Renaissance Learning.* Ann Arbor, MI:
    The University of Michigan Press, 2007.
– *Medicine and the Italian Universities: 1250-1600.* Leiden, Netherlands: Brill, 2001.
– *Medieval and Early Renaissance Medicine: An Introduction to Knowledge and Practice.*
    Chicago, il: University of Chicago Press, 1990.
– "'Remarkable' Diseases, 'Remarkable' Cures, and Personal Experience in
    Renaissance Medical Texts." In *Medicine and the Italian Universities: 1250–1600,*
    226–52. Leiden, Netherlands: Brill, 2001.
Stearns, Justin K. *Infectious Ideas: Contagion in Premodern Islamic and Christian Thought in
    the Western Mediterranean.* Baltimore, MD: The Johns Hopkins University Press,
    2011.
Stolberg, Michael. "Training Future Practitioners: Medical Education in Sixteenth-
    and Early-Seventeenth-Century Padua and Montpellier from the Students'
    Perspective." In *Transforming Medical Education: Historical Case Studies of Teaching,*

Learning, and Belonging in Medicine, edited by Delia Gavrus and Susan Lamb, 112–35. Montreal, QC, and Kingston, ON: McGill-Queen's University Press, 2022.

Talbot, Charles. "Medical Education in the Middle Ages." In *The History of Medical Education: An International Symposium Held February 5–9, 1968,* edited by C.D. O'Malley, 73–88. Berkeley, CA: University of California Press, 1970.

"The Treatise of John of Burgundy." In *The Black Death,* translated and edited by Rosemary Horrox, 184–93. Manchester, UK: Manchester University Press, 1994.

Thomson, George. *Loimotomia, or, the Pest Anatomized.* London: for Nathaniel Crouch, 1666.

Villani, Mateo. *Cronica,* 2 vols. Edited by Giuseppe Porta. Parma, Italy: Fondazione Pietro Bembo, 1995.

Vinario, Raymond Chalin de. "Raïmundüs de Peste." In Karl Sudhoff, "Pestschriften aus den ersten 150 Jahren nach der Epidemie des „schwarzen Todes" 1348. XVIII. Pestschriften aus Frankreich, Spanien und England." *Archiv für Geschichte der Medizin* Bd. 17, H. 1/3 (May 1925): 37–8.

Wear, Andrew. *Knowledge & Practice in English Medicine, 1550–1680.* Cambridge: Cambridge University Press, 2000.

Wear, Andrew, Roger French, and Ian M. Lonie, eds. *The Medical Renaissance of the Sixteenth Century.* Cambridge: Cambridge University Press, 1985.

Webster, Charles. *The Great Instauration: Science, Medicine and Reform 1626–1660.* London: Duckworth, 1977.

4

Training Future Practitioners: Medical Education in Sixteenth- and Early-Seventeenth-Century Padua and Montpellier from the Students' Perspective

Michael Stolberg

The acquisition of practical skills plays a crucial role in medical education today. It has become hard to imagine a medical curriculum that does not give ample space to clinical instruction and bedside teaching, to ward rounds and case discussions for students, to skills labs and practice-oriented courses on how to interview and examine patients and on how to arrive at a diagnosis and a suitable treatment.

Medical education did not always attribute such great importance to imparting the skills that future physicians would require in their daily practice. Quite to the contrary, for many centuries medical education was profoundly bookish. The major means by which medical knowledge was imparted in universities all over Europe was the *lectura*, the lecture, in an often quite literal sense: the professor would read passages from a work by Hippocrates, Galen, Avicenna, or another authority and comment on it, sometimes dictating his lecture to the students word by word.

In many universities, lectures on the works of ancient and (increasingly) recent authorities remained at the centre of medical education throughout the early modern period. However, as I will argue in this chapter, medical training in some of the most prestigious universities of the time started to change profoundly in the sixteenth century. Universities in France and Northern Italy inaugurated a shift towards the more practical and empirical aspects of medicine which was to prove pivotal for the future development of medical education in the West.

In what follows, I will look at the most renowned institutions that promoted this trend in Italy and France respectively, namely Padua and Montpellier.[1] Both universities have been extensively studied by generations of medical historians[2] but our knowledge of what the students could actually learn there is still quite sketchy. It comes primarily from normative sources such as statutes, administrative records, and official lists of authoritative texts on which the professors had to lecture. In this chapter, I will take a distinctly different approach. I will draw on sources that reflect the students' actual experience, and above all, on a remarkably underused source: student notebooks. They have come down to us in considerable numbers from the sixteenth century, but so far have largely escaped the attention of historians. As we will see, they not only provide a different perspective; they also offer a much richer and more nuanced account of what medical students actually learnt, and they show just how marked the shift in medical education was, from theory to a focus on useful, practical knowledge and skills.

INSTITUTIONAL CONTEXT

Medical students and young physicians from all over Europe came to Padua and Montpellier in the sixteenth and seventeenth centuries. Between twenty and fifty foreign medical students arrived at each of them every year,[3] at a time when many medical faculties north of the Alps only had a handful of medical students.[4] Contemporaries praised the cost of living as bearable in both places.[5] Moreover, although Padua, which was on Venetian territory, was decidedly Catholic and Montpellier became Huguenot in 1561, both places offered a relatively high degree of religious tolerance, at least when it came to foreigners – certainly when compared to staunchly Catholic or Protestant universities, such as Cologne, Ingolstadt, Strasbourg, or Wittenberg. It was, above all, the outstanding reputation of both universities and their professors that attracted the students, however. A doctoral degree obtained in Padua or Montpellier carried considerable prestige and could help ensure the student's future professional career, for example, when they applied for a position as a town physician.[6] In France, moreover, only physicians who had obtained their doctorate in Paris or Montpellier had the licence to practise wherever they wanted, without having to pass additional exams.

Yet, obtaining a doctoral title seems to have been of somewhat secondary importance, certainly to many of the foreign students. A fair number of them already came with a doctoral title and many more eventually opted for a less demanding and expensive doctoral degree elsewhere.[7] Avignon, Orange, and Valence were popular in this respect in Southern France.[8] For students from Padua, nearby Ferrara offered a welcome alternative, and by the late sixteenth century, it was above all Basel, where many German students, a particularly large group among those who studied in Montpellier and Padua, received their doctorate.[9] It was thus clearly not just the prestigious degree that made students from all over Europe flock to Montpellier and Padua. They came because they sought the best medical education that was available at the time, and more precisely, I would argue, a training that would prepare them for a successful future medical practice.

ANATOMY

A major and often-cited reason why many medical students and young physicians opted for Montpellier, Padua, and a handful of other universities in Northern Italy was the superior quality of anatomical teaching. Above all, the future physician should hear the professor of anatomy, Hieronymus Besler advised in his *Ratio progrediendi in studio medico*. He should study anatomical illustrations and learn from frequent dissections.[10] Students at universities north of the Alps could rarely attend anatomical demonstrations. The sheer range of opportunities in the south for acquiring anatomical knowledge directly at the dissection table was truly impressive by comparison, especially in Padua. It was much more impressive, in fact, than historians have for a long time assumed.[11] Traditionally, historical research has focused on the large, public anatomies.[12] Even in Padua, these tended to take place only once or twice per academic year, and there were years without a single public dissection of an entire human body. As their notebooks show, however, students in Padua could also participate in numerous private anatomies for a smaller circle, on patients in the hospital and in private homes, and sometimes even in pharmacies or in the anatomist's house. By the end of the sixteenth century, in the period when the famous permanent anatomical theatre was established in Padua, Konrad Zinn, a German student from Öhringen, recorded, in just one winter, more than a dozen anatomical demonstrations. By that time, many of these anatomical demonstrations were devoted to a specific, particularly complex part or structure of the body, such as the brain, the nerves, or the uterus. The students not only learnt about the form and structure of the various parts, but also about their functions and their uses. In the 1550s, Gabrielle Falloppia routinely complemented the dissection of human cadavers with that of various animals, and we find the same for Girolamo Fabrizi d'Acquapendente and Giulio Casseri, who taught generations of medical students in late-sixteenth- and early-seventeenth-century Padua.[13]

In sixteenth-century Montpellier, anatomical instruction at the dissection table appears to have been somewhat less intense than in Padua, but still far surpassed what could be found north of the Alps. Between 1529 and 1534, the *Liber procuratoris studiosorum* recorded at least eight anatomical demonstrations by various professors, with a barber-surgeon doing the actual manual work of cutting up the corpse. The *procurator*, a kind of student rector, worked hard to get hold of suitable cadavers. In October 1532, he learnt, for example, that

someone had been sentenced to die on the cross. He deemed the body particularly suitable for an anatomical demonstration and succeeded in obtaining
it. The corpses of two women who had drowned – one of them, perhaps by
suicidal intent, in a well – were also dissected in 1532, and in 1534 further
corpses came from the local Hôtel Dieu and from the hospital.[14]

It is not entirely clear where these early dissections took place in Montpellier,
but it seems that some kind of permanent anatomical theatre had been established by the 1520s, in the garden of the *collegium*. It may well have been
the first of its kind in Europe.[15] In 1530, the *Liber procuratoris* mentioned a
corpse that had just been "acquired" and was brought "ad locum anatomiae"
– which thus clearly could not have been established specifically for that occasion. From 1532, we find repeated references to a "theatrum anatomiae" in
the context of the entrance fee that the students had to pay, and to the cost
of cleaning the "theatrum anatomiae."[16] In 1552, Felix Platter, a medical
student from Basel who was to become a famous anatomist himself, witnessed
a dissection in the "old theatre" ("im alten theatro"), contrasting it against
the new theatre, which was inaugurated in 1556 in a building that houses the
École de Pharmacie today.[17]

Platter's detailed account of his student years in 1550s Montpellier shows
that anatomical dissections continued to take place frequently. He saw, among
others, the typical changes in the pregnant uterus of a woman who died
during birth and in that of a maid who was executed for infanticide and dissected afterwards.[18] He also participated in animal anatomies.[19] Still, Platter
and some of his fellow students were not content. They dissected dogs on their
own[20] and robbed corpses from graveyards in the surrounding countryside to
perform secret dissections of their own.[21]

The importance of anatomy and the desire of students to acquire detailed
anatomical knowledge may seem to contradict, at first glance, my claim that
the attraction Padua and Montpellier held for medical students all over Europe
was due, in particular, to their interest in medical practice. After all, as Roger
French and other historians have pointed out, it is by no means obvious why
anatomy should have been perceived as relevant for the practising physician
in the era of humoral pathology.[22] As the student notes and other sources
reveal, however,[23] the anatomists consistently highlighted the importance of
anatomical knowledge for the diagnosis and treatment of diseases. Even more
importantly, dissections were not limited to the corpses of (usually young and
healthy) convicted criminals. Students also witnessed autopsies of deceased
patients and saw different types of pathology on these occasions. Shortly after
his arrival in Montpellier, Platter participated in two dissections of young men,
for example, who had died of pleurisy or chest disease.[24] With his teacher,
Guillaume Rondelet, he also saw the liver and spleen of a monkey that were

both full of cysts.[25] From his experience in Padua, Hieronymus Besler explicitly recommended that the medical student should constantly read and compare what he found in three or four works on medical practice by famous authors such as Jean Fernel, Jacques Houllier, and Guillaume Rondelet with what he learnt and saw on the dissection table.[26] Historians have tended to downplay the importance and value of post-mortems on deceased patients because the results often seemed of little relevance in the eyes of the modern pathologist. Renaissance anatomists frequently found pathological changes, however, that made sense to them, such as a hardened or enlarged liver or spleen, tumours, obstructions of the gastro-intestinal pathways, and kidney- or bladder-stones. From the perspective of contemporary medical students and physicians, anatomical dissections and post-mortems held a great promise. With their help, physicians could hope to arrive at a better understanding of the physiological and pathological processes inside the body, which, in turn, would enable them to fight diseases at their very roots.[27]

BOTANY AND SIMPLES

For good reasons, virtually all leading botanists in sixteenth- and seventeenth-century Europe had medical training. Botany was largely synonymous, at the time, with studying the "simples," individual substances of medicinal value. The ability to identify and distinguish medicinal plants and to assess their efficacy, depending also on the state of the specimen, was a crucial skill for any practising physician. Even Antonio Musa Brasavola in Ferrara, a highly renowned medical humanist, undertook extensive botanical research and criticized those who wanted to leave the study of the simples to the pharmacists.[28] A good knowledge of the simples and the ability to identify them correctly was essential for the successful treatment of patients. It also protected the physician against the embarrassing experience of proving unable to identify plants that patients or other lay people showed him and knew well themselves. Last but not least, botanical expertise was indispensable for town physicians, who were usually expected to inspect the local pharmacies and to examine the quality of their stock at regular intervals.

The history of sixteenth-century botany, of its protagonists and their publications and illustrations, has been studied by numerous scholars. We know much less, by contrast, about the teaching of botany in the medical schools.[29] Again, students' notebooks and accounts prove particularly enlightening. For obvious reasons, lectures could offer a useful overview but were ultimately of limited value. The students had to learn to identify and distinguish different types of plants and their various parts and stages of development. Doing so just from descriptions, without using actual plants or at least dried specimens or illustrations, was virtually impossible. Contemporaries were well aware of this problem and found some ingenious solutions, with Padua and Montpellier once more at the vanguard. They were among the very first universities that offered students hands-on training in medical botany.

The best-known and often-praised devices for this purpose were botanical gardens, where students could go and look at the plants in all their variety and, over time, at different stages of development. The one that was established in Pisa, in 1543–44, on the initiative of Luca Ghini, was probably the first of its kind,[30] but soon, in 1545, the one in Padua followed.[31] In Montpellier, it was only in 1593 that a botanical garden was officially established.[32] However, a long time before that, in 1550, the Grand Jours de Béziers, a kind of regional parliament, had already demanded an annual botanical course that included the demonstration of plants. As a matter of fact, Guillaume Rondelet not only showed plants to his students but also cultivated a little garden for that purpose next to the university building.[33] Carolus Clusius and Johann Bauhin, who later acquired great fame as botanists, were among his students.[34]

As the notebooks and other writings of medical students show, they appreciated and took ample advantage of the opportunities that botanical gardens offered. In Padua in the 1550s, Georg Handsch, a student from Leipa near Prague, filled about ten pages in his notebook just with entries on all the different plants that his professors, among them Antonio Fracanzano and Gabrielle Falloppia, and his fellow students showed and explained to him.[35]

The students also took advantage of a range of other opportunities, however, for observing and studying plants. Botanical excursions were one of them. The area around Montpellier was, in Johann Stefan Strobelberger's words, nothing else but a lovely garden, with fields, vineyards, olive trees, with woods, mountains, hills, rivers, lagoons, and the sea, with all kinds of plants and flowers.[36] Felix Platter described how he and his fellow students went botanizing in the area.[37] Carolus Clusius and Leonhard Rauwolf[38] did the same, in their time. Maybe due to more intensive agricultural use, the area around Padua did not receive similar praise as a destination for botanical excursions. During his time in Padua, Georg Handsch did mention going into the fields ("in agro"), however, where he saw some of the plants he had learnt to recognize in the botanical garden.[39]

There was another site where medical students and young physicians could acquire extensive knowledge about medicinal plants, one to which historians have so far paid much less attention, namely local pharmacies. Pharmacists usually had not studied at a university but the better ones among them were quite learned and possessed great knowledge and skills. After all, medicinal plants were the principal objects of their trade. They constantly dealt with them and their professional and economic success depended on their ability to

identify the nature and quality of the plants and plant specimens they bought
and sold. Just by visiting the pharmacies and talking with the pharmacists
about different plants and watching them prepare medicines, students could
thus learn a great deal. In Padua, Georg Handsch took notes on the various
plants and medicinal substances he saw in the pharmacy, on his own. Even
his professor, Antonio Fracanzano, sometimes went with his students into a
pharmacy to demonstrate simples and composite medicines.[40]

Writing from his own experience in Padua, Hieronymus Besler, in his *Ratio
progrediendi in studio medico*, therefore had very clear advice for the future medical student. He should not only visit the *hortus medicorum* in Padua but also seek
to become acquainted with scholars who knew something about the simples,
and above all with the pharmacists and those who worked for them. If there
was a very learned pharmacist somewhere, the student should try to obtain
food and lodging with him, even if that cost more than usual. In the pharmacist's workshop, he would be able to see all the simples that physicians used,
plants as well as minerals and animal matter. By close and constant practice
("exercitatione"), he would learn how to distinguish good, pure simples from
adulterated ones and fresh ones from old ones. Last but not least, he would
witness the preparation of composite remedies and could lend a hand himself,
an exercise that was "extremely useful and most necessary for the physician."[41]

This was exactly what Felix Platter did in Montpellier. When he learnt,
upon his arrival in 1552, that a student from Strasbourg had died who had
lodged with the pharmacist Catalan, he urged his father to enable him to live
in Catalan's house. There he found ample opportunities to watch the daily
work.[42] Years later, when he himself lectured in Basel, he still drew on the
pharmaceutical knowledge he had acquired in Montpellier.[43] Around 1600,
Strobelberger likewise praised the "perfect demonstration" he witnessed there
in public and in private, with "most learned pharmacists," of the whole *materia
medica*, including exotic plants and the preparation of theriac, mythridate, and
other complex medicines.[44]

MEDICAL PRACTICE AND BEDSIDE TEACHING

Anatomical and botanical teaching were considered important and useful
for medical practice, but students from all over Europe came to Padua and
Montpellier also, if not above all, because of the quality of teaching in medical practice.[45] Both universities counted some of the most eminent medical
practitioners of the time among their professors: men such as Laurent Jou-
bert, André du Laurens, François Ranchin, Guillaume Rondelet, and Jean
Varanda in Montpellier,[46] and Giovanni Battista da Monte, Girolamo Capi-
vaccia, Vettore Trincavella, Ercole Sassonia, and Girolamo Mercuriale in

Padua.[47] Furthermore, both universities, though Padua possibly even more than Montpellier, offered exceptionally good opportunities for the acquisition of practical skills.

Padua has often been described as the place where, for the first time in the history of Western medicine, clinical bedside training was introduced. In the 1540s, Giovanni Battista da Monte started teaching his students in the Ospedale di San Francesco, a model that was later copied successfully in Leiden by students who had witnessed it in Padua. Some authors have expressed doubts because Da Monte did not hold an official appointment at San Francesco, but the evidence from printed and published students' notes is overwhelming.[48] They show, among other things, that Da Monte and his students paid at least ten visits to a patient in the hospital with consumption and empyema and six visits to a boy who suffered from dropsy.[49] Da Monte also seems to have linked his bedside teaching to his lectures. Discussing two cases of pseudo-tertian fever during a hospital visit in 1543, he announced that he would "connect what we have taught today in cathedra with what appears in the sick."[50]

Bedside teaching in the hospital gave students a chance to see a fair number of patients with different diseases and symptoms during one and the same visit and to follow the course of diseases and the effects of treatment during repeat visits over extended periods of time. Da Monte was not alone in offering this kind of teaching. Other professors in Padua also took their students with them when they visited patients in the hospital. In his notebooks, Georg Handsch mentioned more than thirty patients he saw in the hospital with Antonio Fracanzano in the early 1550s, and it is very likely that there were even more on whom he did not take notes. Just like Da Monte, Fracanzano also used these visits as an opportunity for teaching. When they saw a patient, for example, with asthma and a coarse, strident voice who believed he had been bewitched, Fracanzano talked at length about the power of incantations, about people who could stop nosebleeds, and about evil women who employed dried menstrual blood to harm others.[51]

Historians of medical education have tended to focus on bedside teaching in San Francesco,[52] presumably because they valued it as the first major step towards establishing what remains the standard approach to medical training to this day. As the student notes make clear even for Padua, however, the hospital was not the only and, in fact, probably not even the principal site of bedside teaching. Professors also frequently took smaller groups of students with them on their numerous visits to patients in private homes. Georg Handsch took notes, for example, on various visits he made, together with Gabrielle Falloppia and several fellow students, to a child who had drunk poison and to a patient with the "French disease," and he also mentioned a visit one of his teachers made to a young man with a head injury.[53] As his notes show,

these patient visits also offered an opportunity to discuss the cases with the
professor on their way to or from the patient's house.[54] In the early 1550s,
Handsch recorded some of these cases in considerable detail under the heading "observationes" – a term that was to become synonymous with one of
the most popular genres of medical writing, collections of *observationes medicae*,
which quite likely originated from such personal note-taking practices.[55]
Bedside teaching in the patients' private homes is likewise documented, even
before 1550, for other Northern Italian universities, in Bologna with Elideo
Padoani and in Ferrara with Musa Brasavola and other local physicians.[56]

Patient visits not only taught students how to apply their theoretical knowledge to the individual case, how to identify the true causes of the disease,
and how to choose the best treatment, taking the patient's temperament and
general state into due consideration. Students could also acquire a range of
concrete practical skills.[57] They learnt how to take a patient's history and how
to ask the right questions, and they became proficient in the most important
diagnostic method of the time: uroscopy. "We inspected the urine," Johann
Brünsterer from Nürnberg wrote in 1547, for example, describing a visit that
he undertook together with his professor, Alvise Bellocati, to a patient with a
fever. The first day, the urine was turbid and reddish; the second day, it was
greenish and some very crude matter could be seen at the bottom. When the
urine eventually started looking less turbid, this was taken as a sign that Nature
had successfully evacuated the morbid matter over the previous days.[58] The
students also inspected the patients' stools, sputum, and other excrements,
together with their professors,[59] and they learnt how to identify pathological
changes from a careful examination of the patient's blood in the bloodletting
bowl. In his notes, Handsch described, for example, how one of his professors,
Comes de Monte aka Pamfilio Monti from Vicenza, poured off the watery
parts of the blood, pointed out some yellow foam on the remaining black
mass, which he identified as yellow bile, and eventually divided that black mass
to show some "melancholic humor" in its centre.[60]

Last but not least, the students acquired manual skills. They were introduced
into the difficult art of feeling the pulse – after uroscopy, the most important
diagnostic method of the time.[61] Moreover, the students could practise the
manual examination of the patient's abdomen. This may come as a surprise.
After all, generations of historians have claimed that early modern physicians
abstained from touching their patients, other than for feeling the pulse.[62]
Already in the 1550s, however, Georg Handsch mentioned many patients on
whom his professors performed a physical examination, and in some cases he
explicitly also described how he himself felt for pathological changes in the
spleen or the liver.[63] At one point, he even remarked that palpating a patient's
abdomen was the "custom" ("ut mos est").[64]

In addition to bedside teaching, Padua also developed and cultivated a highly original approach to medical teaching in the patient's absence. It might offer a useful didactic tool for medical education still today. In the so-called *collegia*, a group of professors discussed the case of a patient in front of a student audience, based on a written account by a consulting physician ("exhibita charta") or on an oral presentation by one of the participating professors ("audivistis historiam"). Then the professors, one after the other, discussed the case and offered their diagnostic and therapeutic conclusions, frequently contradicting each other to some degree. The students valued these *collegia* highly. They took extensive notes[65] and some student notes were later published in print, though sometimes somewhat confusingly mixed with *consultationes* or *consilia* in the conventional sense, i.e. with epistolary advice on a specific case that a physician wrote on the request of a distant patient or his or her physician.[66]

Regarding the quality of practical medical training in sixteenth- and seventeenth-century France, Lawrence Brockliss has arrived at a much more negative assessment. Even in Montpellier, he claimed, "few gained any knowledge of actual patient care."[67] It was only in 1634, he found, that the statutes demanded that the bachelors and licentiates in medicine visit patients in the hospital, twice a month. As is so often the case, however, statutes do not offer the full picture. A closer look at sources that reflect the actual teaching and the experience of medical students suggests that practical training at the bedside had a prominent place in sixteenth-century Montpellier, too. This was due, in particular, to the same common practice of allowing medical students to accompany their professors to visits in the patients' homes that we find in Northern Italy. The practice was probably facilitated by a custom that was peculiar to Montpellier: when medical students arrived in Montpellier, they were asked to choose a "godfather" among the professors, a "parrain," or indeed as it was sometimes called a "father" ("parens"; "pater").[68] Moreover, before taking their final exams, medical students in Montpellier were expected to do a kind of internship with a physician in the area, and many of them did.[69] In the early seventeenth century, Strobelberger could thus praise Montpellier for the many opportunities for visiting patients in the town, in the palaces, and in the hospitals, for taking their history, inspecting their urine, and feeling their pulse.[70]

The prominent place accorded to practical training in Montpellier is underlined by the prominent place of diagnostic and therapeutic knowledge and skills in medical exams. Discussing altogether ten different diseases was a core feature of the four examinations per intentionem, for the licentiate, and of the six examinations during the so-called triduanes, which the future doctor had to pass and which lasted over three mornings and three afternoons.[71] By the early seventeenth century, the candidates for the licentiate even had to go and see four professors, each of whom would present them with the case of a specific patient. For example, when Stephan Geiger obtained his licentiate in 1606, François Ranchin made him discuss a patient with intermittent tertian fever, Petrus Dortoman confronted him with a case of pleurisy in an ageing man, Jean Varanda examined him on a pregnant woman with abdominal cramps and the consequent risk of a miscarriage, and Jean Schyron tested him on a feverish young man who was sweating so profusely that he was about to faint.[72] Similarly, Wilhelm Reh, in 1617, was examined about the cases of a little child with measles, on the treatment of a young man who suffered from severe insomnia, on a fifty-year-old hypochondriac who had accumulated earthy, blackish, melancholical humours in his abdomen, and on a thirty-year-old man with fever, headaches, loss of appetite, and cardialgia.[73]

We so far only have anecdotal evidence, in this respect, for Padua: in 1533, Girolamo Amalteo recorded a "case that was proposed to me in my examination," the case of a (presumably fictive) patient with intense fever occasioned by a "cold cause," together with his own quite detailed answers on how he would deal with it.[74]

LECTURES

As we have seen, Montpellier and Padua offered a wide range of opportunities for the acquisition of the knowledge and skills that future physicians would need for a successful practice. Nevertheless, even in Padua and Montpellier, formal lectures remained the backbone of medical education.[75] When Felix Platter began his studies in Montpellier, he attended two or three lectures in the morning, and another three in the afternoon. Dozens of lecture notes or indeed transcripts – some possibly based on dictation – have survived from both institutions, some in print, others in manuscript.[76] They suggest that the approach to teaching medicine in the Padua and Montpellier was, in many respects, not fundamentally different from that in other universities. Lecturers commonly read out and commented on a major work by an authority. Hippocrates and Galen were the principal authors.[77]

Although even lectures on *medicina practica* tended to be quite theoretical,[78] the reliance on formal lectures and learned commentary must not be misinterpreted as indicating a lack of interest in the demands of medical practice. Many of the works of Hippocrates and Galen discussed concrete practical matters of medicine, such as fevers, tumours, the *methodus medendi*, dietetics, and prognosis. Moreover, while writings of Avicenna, Rhazes, and other Arabic authors lost the outstanding place in medical education they had previously held, Avicenna's *Canon* and the ninth book of Rhazes's *Liber ad Almansorem* remained important points of reference – precisely, it seems, because they dealt extensively with practical matters, with different kinds of diseases and their treatment. This goes for Padua even more than for Montpellier, where the "Arabic" writers no longer had their recognized place in medical training from the 1550s onwards.[79] In Padua in the 1570s and 1580s, students still attended lectures on Avicenna's *Canon* as well as on the Hippocratic *Aphorisms* and *Prognostics*,[80] and in the 1590s, we find Konrad Zinn taking notes on Alessandro Massaria's commentary on Avicenna's writings on fevers.[81]

Moreover, professors sometimes integrated casuistic approaches into their lectures and courses, even using fictive cases at times. According to Georg Handsch's notes, Vettore Trincavella, for example, in his lectures on diseases of the head, presented various cases and introduced them with words such as: "Let us propose a case. Let there be someone," followed, for example, by "who has lost sensation and motion in a certain part, not preceded by a blow or a dislocation but by a life of idleness and gluttony."[82] In Konrad Zinn's notes on a "cursus practicus" by Alessandro Massaria, we find cases in which the patient's name is rendered as "Socrates." Since revealing a patient's real name was common practice in published case histories at the time, this suggests that Massaria combined fictive cases with "real" ones – such as the one that Zinn recorded under the heading "historia curati hydropici" – in order to familiarize his students with pathologies such as paralysis, epilepsy, pleurisy, dropsy, dysentery, or an obstructed liver.[83]

Even more importantly, themed lectures that dealt with a specific topic rather than a certain text acquired growing importance, especially private lectures, outside of the official syllabus. They were devoted, in particular, to hitherto marginal or new fields such as women's diseases and pediatrics, which came to be seen as important areas for which the future physicians required particular expertise.[84] In Padua, students could learn about such matters from prominent professors including Massaria and Sassonia.[85] From Montpellier, we have Johann Mattenberg's neat copy of notes on Guillaume Rondelet's lectures on the diseases of women.[86] Another new and popular topic of private lectures was the "French disease," on which the ancients had little to say, of course, but which was of great relevance to medical practice.[87]

Both universities even offered some surgical education. Few learned physicians north of the Alps would practise surgery themselves in the course of their professional lives, but patients would expect them to give them advice on surgical matters, such as tumours and ulcers, and to guide and supervise the work of barber-surgeons. Interest in surgery was supported by a considerable overlap between surgery and anatomy within the university. The leading Paduan anatomists of the second half of the sixteenth century – Falloppia, Casseri, and Fabrizi – all also practised and taught surgery. Falloppia explained and discussed surgical issues and therapies such as paracentesis, herniotomy, and the operation of cataracts in his anatomy lectures.[88] Fabrizi devoted a whole series of lectures just to surgery.[89] In Montpellier, too, students could watch experienced surgeons perform major operations such as paracentesis, the removal of bladder stones, and trepanations.[90]

CONCLUSIONS

There were some important differences between the universities in Padua and Montpellier, which helped make Padua ultimately the more prestigious institution. Medical students who came to Padua felt no need to defend their choice as Strobelberger did for Montpellier.[91] Until the 1590s, when two new chairs for anatomy, surgery, and botany were established, Montpellier only had four medical professors, with some additional teaching done by ordinary physicians and, from the early seventeenth century, by two salaried *docteurs aggregés*. In theory, new professors were to be chosen competitively by means of a *concours*, but the rule was rarely enforced, allowing for some clientelism.[92] In Padua, by contrast, the same medical subject area was often taught by three professors and the first two lectured in explicit and intentional competition with each other, at the same time of the day. They had to give their best if they wanted to attract students.[93] Padua was also close to and governed by Venice, one of the largest and richest cities in Europe. The university was able to offer generous salaries and, on top of that, professors could supplement their income through private practice among the city's most affluent families. Since physicians from Padua were not eligible for professorships, the university was compelled to look further afield, and succeeded in attracting some of the most famous medical writers, teachers, and practitioners of the time from outside.

Moreover, Padua successfully combined a marked shift towards a more practical and empirical approach with unprecedented epistemological sophistication. The peculiar institutional framework helped. There was no separate medical faculty. Medical professors taught in the arts faculty and interacted closely with some of the leading philosophers of the time. Medical students in Padua thus continued to be exposed to Aristotelian natural philosophy and logic as part of their medical training.[94] An important result of these close links between medicine and philosophy was the prominent place of "method" in medical education in Padua – in the sense of a suitable didactic organization of knowledge and as a tool for the production of knowledge about the human body, in general, and individual patients, in particular.[95] Students attended special lectures not only on the *methodus medendi* but also on the *methodus consultandi*[96] and even on the *methodus anatomica*.[97] Most importantly in our context, the analytical method, the "methodus resolutiva," also served as the basis for the highly systematic and analytical approach to medical diagnosis for which

Giovanni Battista da Monte was famous and which profoundly influenced generations of future physicians all over Europe.[98]

When it comes to medical teaching and to the knowledge and skills medical students could acquire, both institutions had much more in common, however, than what set them apart. As we have seen, both universities were at the vanguard of a major shift, a reorientation of medical training towards the needs of practice. They offered casuistic and bedside teaching, botanical gardens, anatomical demonstrations that connected anatomical findings with physiological and pathological matters, and topical lectures on fields such as women's and children's diseases or the "French disease," which had acquired major importance in ordinary medical practice.[99]

This shift towards practice was not an obvious choice, at the time. After all, the bookish scholarly habitus of the medieval physician had proved instrumental in the rise of the academic physician as the privileged medical caregiver of kings and princes and of the upper classes in general. For good reasons, medical doctors in the sixteenth century self-fashioned themselves as learned humanists. Their learned habitus highlighted the cultural background they shared with their preferred – educated and affluent – patients and served to distinguish them from their numerous less-learned competitors who had no academic training.

Future research will have to identify the various driving forces that, in spite of all this, may have been behind this shift towards practice in medical education. I would like to underline one major driving force, however, which, I would argue, may well have been the most important and powerful one. From the late fifteenth century, the place of the academic physician in the medical marketplace underwent a gradual but profound and pervasive change, certainly in many areas north of the Alps. With the rising cultural and economic importance of towns and cities and the growing appreciation for learning among the upper classes, medicine became an attractive career option for many who came from a relatively modest background. The number of young men who graduated from the universities grew rapidly. Their professional and economic prospects were generally quite good, all the more so because many towns created salaried positions as a town physician or hospital physician and allowed the incumbent to work in private practice as well, and to treat patients who paid for his services. In many places, the physician faced tough competition, however, especially when he was still young and inexperienced. He had to hold his own against other physicians, barber-surgeons, and countless lay healers. After all, patients had a choice. When they were not satisfied with the physician's diagnosis, advice, or treatment, they were quick to turn to someone else. What ultimately counted in this situation was that the learned physician was perceived as particularly skillful in his diagnosis and successful in his treatment. A thorough acquaintance with the works of Hippocrates, Aristotle, Galen, and Avicenna remained helpful for this purpose but it was no longer considered sufficient. In order to secure superior outcomes and to establish a successful practice, physicians had to be better at recognizing and treating patients than their competitors. They needed detailed and sophisticated practical knowledge and skills – and it was with these that Montpellier and Padua promised to equip them.

NOTES

1 I am very grateful to Nathalie Vienne-Guerrin, Jean-Pierre Schandeler, and the staff of the Institut de Recherche sur la Renaissance, l'Âge Classique et les Lumières (IRCL) for the generous hospitality they offered me during my sabbatical in Montpellier in the summer of 2017, which enabled me to examine the relevant local sources.

2 For Montpellier see, in particular, Astruc, *Mémoires*; Germain, *L'école de médecine*; Dulieu, *La médecine à Montpellier*, vol. 2: *La Renaissance* and vol. 3: *L'époque classique*; for Padua see Tomasini, *Gymnasium patavinum*; Facciolati, *Fasti gymnasii patavini*; Bylebyl, "School of Padua," 335–70; Ongaro, "La medicina"; Klestinec, "Medical Education in Padua."

3 O'Malley, "Medical Education"; for Montpellier see Gouron, *Matricule*; Germain, "Les pèlerins de la science"; Berlan, *Faire sa médecine*, 105.

4 Nauck, "Die Zahl der Medizinstudenten."

5 Brugi, *Gli scolari*, 12.

6 Schlegelmilch, "Promoting a Good Physician."

7 In Montpellier, students had to pass sixteen major exams altogether to obtain the title of a bachelor, licentiate, and finally doctor in medicine; cf. Astruc, *Mémoires*, 84–8; James Primrose, "Academia monspeliensis," 11.

8 Ecoiffier, *Recherches historiques*; Vidor-Borricand, *Une université méconnue*; Nadal, *Histoire de l'université de Valence*; Basset, *Histoire de la faculté de médecine de Valence*.

9 Maclean, "Trois facultés," 355.

10 Universitätsbibliothek Erlangen, Ms. 1150, foll. 93r–94r.

11 Stolberg, "Teaching Anatomy i," 61–78, and "Learning Anatomy," with an analysis of student notes on the lectures on *methodus anatomica* by Paolo Galeotti and Girolamo Fabrizi d'Acquapendente. In a three-year project at the Institut für Geschichte der Medizin in Würzburg, funded by the *Deutsche Forschungsgemeinschaft*, Fabrizio Bigotti is currently analyzing various sets of students' notes on anatomical teaching in sixteenth-century Padua.

12 For recent studies see Cunningham, *Anatomical Renaissance*; Klestinec, *Theaters of Anatomy*, 67–70; see also the older but still valuable works by Roth, *Andreas*

Vesalius bruxellensis; Sterzi, *Giulio Casseri*; Favaro, *Gabrielle Falloppia*; "Contributi"; "L'insegnamento anatomico."

13 Stolberg, "Learning Anatomy"; "Teaching Anatomy"; cf. Baden-Württembergische Landesbibliothek, Stuttgart, Cod. med. et phys. 4° 4, foll. 469r–513v.

14 Bibliothèque de la Ville de Montpellier, Manuscrits Germain, Ms. 111, "Liber procuratoris."

15 Platter, *Tagebuch*, 240; according to Platter, the old theatre ("alt theatrum anatomicum") was in the "collegij garten in die fierung gebuwen," suggesting that it was a rectangular space, while the new one, in the lower part of the garden, was round like an amphitheatre. Astruc, *Mémoires*, 66, also mentions an "old" anatomical theatre in the college garden.

16 Bibliothèque de la Ville de Montpellier, Manuscrits Germain, Ms. 111, fol. 232r (1530), fol. 233r (1533), fol. 234r, fol. 237r (1534).

17 Platter, *Tagebuch*, 151; Dulieu, "Guillaume Rondelet," 93; Planchon and Planchon, *Rondelet et ses disciples*, 15.

18 Platter, *Tagebuch*, 208, 258–9.

19 Ibid., 207–8.

20 Ibid., 187.

21 Ibid., 209–11, 212, 235.

22 French, *Dissection and Vivisection*, 1.

23 Stolberg, "Teaching Anatomy"; "Learning Anatomy."

24 Platter, *Tagebuch*, 151.

25 Ibid., 207–8.

26 Universitätsbibliothek Erlangen, Ms. 1150, foll. 93r–94r, *Ratio progrediendi in studio medico* by Hieronymus Besler.

27 Siraisi, "Segni evidenti"; Stolberg, "Post-Mortems."

28 Münster, "Ferrara e Bologna," 527–8.

29 See, however, Meier Reeds, *Botany*, and, especially on the links between humanism and botany, Ogilvie, *Science of Describing*.

30 Garbari, Tomasi, and Tosi, *Il giardino dei semplici*; Garbari and Bedini, "Architetture, spazi, tempi e piante."

31 Minelli, *The Botanical Garden of Padua*.

32 Martins, *Le jardin des plantes*; Rioux, *Le jardin des plantes*.

33 Planchon and Planchon, *Rondelet et ses disciples*, 15; Dulieu, "Guillaume Rondelet," 106.

34 Planchon and Planchon, *Rondelet et ses disciples*, 16–18; Lewis, "Clusius in Montpellier."

35 Österreichische Nationalbibliothek, Vienna, Ms. 11210, foll. 115r–120v, "Herbae quas didici in horto Paduano."

36 Strobelberger, *Laureationum medicarum*, 18.

37 E.g. Platter, *Tagebuch*, 174–5, 219.

38 Planchon and Planchon, *Rondelet et ses disciples. Appendice*, 32.

39 Österreichische Nationalbibliothek, Vienna, Ms. 11210, fol. 119v.

40 Ibid., foll. 140r–141r.

41 Universitätsbibliothek Erlangen, Ms. 1150, foll. 93r–94r, *Ratio progrediendi in studio medico* by Hieronymus Besler.

42 Platter, *Tagebuch*, 147, 149, 157.

43 Baden-Württembergische Landesbibliothek, Stuttgart, Cod. med. et phys. 4° 10, foll. 185r–216v, student notes by Konrad Zinn on Felix Platter's lectures on fevers, cit. fol. 214v, "Monspessuli meo tempore sic parabant."

44 Strobelberger, *Laureationum medicarum*, 18.

45 Bylebyl, "School of Padua," 339.

46 See the chronological list in Astruc, *Mémoires*, 225–302.

47 Overview in Bertolaso, "Richerche d'archivio," 7–37; on Mercuriale, in particular, see also Siraisi, "Medicina Practica," 287–305; Calabritto, "*Medicina Practica*."

48 Münster, "Anfänge"; Montesanto, *Dell'origine della clinica medica*; Orsolato, "Sulla prima fondazione"; according to Guarino, "Profilo storico," 79, bedside teaching in the hospital was practised even earlier in Bologna.

49 Cf. da Monte, *Consultationum medicarum*, coll. 455–61, coll. 628–31, coll. 867–9, col. 885, coll. 900–7, coll. 938–43, coll. 956–69 (based on student notes); see also Stolberg, "Bedside Teaching."

50 Da Monte, *Consultationum medicarum*, col. 938.

51 Österreichische Nationalbibliothek, Vienna, Ms. 11238, fol. 120v.

52 See e.g. Maclean, "Trois facultés."

53 Österreichische Nationalbibliothek, Vienna, Cod. 11238, foll. 89v–90v and fol. 110r and Cod. 11226, fol. 175v.

54 Ibid., Cod. 11238, fol. 128v.

55 E.g. ibid., fol. 70r, "Tercia observatio de hydrope ex retentis menstruis"; on the rise of the genre see, in particular, Pomata, "Sharing Cases."

56 See the title of Padoani, *Processus*; Biblioteca Ariostea, Ferrara, Ms Antonelli 531, *Curationes Antonij Musae Brasavoli*, a collection of student notes on a series of individual patients.

57 See Stolberg, "Bedside Teaching," for a more detailed account.

58 Universitätsbibliothek Erlangen, Ms 911, 1–2, 11, 14. On the paramount importance of uroscopy for medical practice at the time, see Stolberg, *Uroscopy*.

59 Universitätsbibliothek Erlangen, Ms 911, 36: "Inspiciebamus excrementa."

60 Österreichische Nationalbibliothek, Vienna, Cod. 11238, fol. 125r.

61 Ibid., fol. 127v.

62 E.g. according to Porter, "The Rise of Physical Examination," a physician who routinely laid hands upon his patients would have been seen as eccentric or indeed offensive.

63 Österreichische Nationalbibliothek, Vienna, Cod. 11238, fol. 89r, foll. 98v–99r, fol. 123v, fol. 129r, fol. 130v.

64 Ibid., fol. 125v.

65 See, e.g., Universitätsbibliothek Erlangen, Ms. 910, with notes on various *collegia*.

66 Da Monte, *Consultationum medicarum*; Trincavella, *Consilia medica*.

67 Brockliss, *French Higher Education*, 395.

68 Platter, *Tagebuch*, 149, "pater."

69 Dulieu, "Guillaume Rondelet," 90; *La médecine à Montpellier*, vol. 2, 71.

70 Strobelberger, *Laureationum medicarum*, 18.

71 Astruc, *Mémoires*, 84–7.

72 Germain, *Les anciennes thèses*, 14–17.

73 Ibid., 18–20.

74 Biblioteca Marciana, Venice, Cod. lat. VII 66 (=9684).

75 Bylebyl, "School of Padua"; Nutton, "The Rise of Medical Humanism."

76 Based on the *Liber lectionum et clavium* and later sources Germain, "La médecine arabe," offers a survey of the authoritative texts, on which the professors in Montpellier taught in the course of the sixteenth century.

77 E.g. Wellcome Library, London, Western Manuscripts, Ms. 602, medical notes of an unidentified student on Bernardino Paterno's lectures, in Padua, on the Hippocratic *Prognostics* and *Aphorisms*.

78 E.g. Universitätsbibliothek Erlangen, Ms. 1002, student notes by Georg Marius on Guillaume Rondelet's lecture on *practica* in 1552.

79 Germain, "La médecine arabe."

80 Wellcome Library, London, Western Manuscripts, Ms. 602; Staatsbibliothek Berlin, Ms. lat. quart. 137, lecture notes by Franz Hildesheim in Padua, 1578–1580.

81 Baden-Württembergische Landesbibliothek, Stuttgart, Cod. med. 4° 4, foll. 255r–280v.

82 Österreichische Nationalbibliothek, Vienna, Cod. 11226, foll. 2r–82r, here fol. 50r: "Proponatur casus. Sit aliquis …"

83 Baden-Württembergische Landesbibliothek, Stuttgart, Cod. med. et phys. 4° 4, foll. 102v–254v.

84 Green, *Making Women's Medicine Masculine*; King, *Midwifery, Obstetrics and the Rise of Gynaecology*.

85 See e.g. University Library Wrocław, M 1473, *De morbis muliebribus lectiones extraordinariae D. Hieronymi Capivaccij*, Padua 1569; Baden-Württembergische Landesbibliothek, Stuttgart, Cod. med. 4° 4, foll. 283r–326v, student notes

by Konrad Zinn on the "scholis privatis et extraordinarijs" on the topic of "de morbis muliebribus" by Alessandro Massaria, in 1593; ibid., foll. 331r–391r, (incomplete) *Tractatus de morbis muliebribus, scholis privatis dictatus a …* *Hercule Saxonia* (1593); Universitätsbibliothek Erlangen, Ms. 981, foll. 1v–27v, student notes by Hieronymus Besler on Massaria's lecture on "De morbis mulierum" in 1591.

86 Forschungsbibliothek Gotha, Chart B 499, foll. 194v–223r, "Curationes … quaedam morborum mulieres infestantium."

87 Österreichische Nationalbibliothek, Vienna, Ms. 11226, foll. 123r–140v, (incomplete) student notes by Georg Handsch on a lecture "De morbo gallico" by Antonio Fracanzano in Padua in 1552; see also Wellcome Library, London, Western Manuscripts, Ms. 602, with a section on "De modo curandi morbum gallicum."

88 Österreichische Nationalbibliothek, Vienna, Ms.11210, foll. 3r–30v, 191v–208v.

89 Baden-Württembergische Landesbibliothek, Stuttgart, Cod. med. et phys. 4° 4, foll. 425r–454r, student notes by Konrad Zinn on Girolamo Fabrizi's lectures on surgery; for an edition and translation of this text see Sambale, *Chirurgischer Unterricht*.

90 Strobelberger, *Laureationum medicarum*, 18. On surgical training in the seventeenth and eighteenth century see Donato, "Surgeons' Training and Hospital Life," ch. 5 in this volume.

91 Strobelberger, *Laureationum medicarum*.

92 Astruc, *Mémoires*, 65–6; Dulieu, *La médecine à Montpellier*, vol. 2, 17.

93 Bertolaso, "I 'terzi luoghi.'"

94 Maclean, *Logic, Signs and Nature in the Renaissance*, 30.

95 Wightman, "Quid sit Methodus?" 360–76; Schmitt, "Aristotle among the Physicians," 1–15, 271–9 (notes).

96 Universitätsbibliothek Erlangen, Ms. 912, student notes by Hieronymus Besler on Capivaccio's lectures on the *methodus medendi* (with a discussion of the meaning of "method") and on the lectures by Emilio Campilongo and Albertino Bottoni on the *methodus consultandi* as well as on Campilongo's lecture on the *methodus semiotica*.

97 Forschungsbibliothek Gotha, Chart. A 629, foll. 221r–240v, student notes by Johann Mattenberg on a lecture on *methodus anatomica* by Fabrizi d'Acquapendente.

98 Da Monte, *Consultationum medicarum*, offers ample evidence for this approach.

99 As Nancy Siraisi put it succinctly: "il più rilevante cambiamento che si può notare nel XV secolo è un'attenzione sempre più seria verso la *practica* da parte dei medici dotti" (Siriasi, "Il Canone di Avicenna," 17).

BIBLIOGRAPHY

Astruc, Jean. *Mémoires pour servir à l'histoire de la faculté de médecine de Montpellier*. Edited by Anne-Charles Lorry. Paris: P.G. Cavelier, 1768.

Basset, Corrine. *Histoire de la faculté de médecine de Valence (1452–1793)*. Thesis. Lyon, France: Université Claude Bernard-Lyon I, 1989.

Berlan, Hélène. *Faire sa médecine au XVIIIe siècle. Recrutement et devenir professionel des étudiants montpéllerains (1707–1789)*. Montpellier, France: Presses Universitaires de la Méditerrannée, 2013.

Bertolaso, Bartolo. "I 'terzi luoghi' nello studio padovano." *Acta Medicae Historiae Patavina* 6 (1958–59): 1–15.

– "Richerche d'archivio su alcuni aspetti dell'insegnamento medico presso la Università di Padova nel cinque- e seicento." *Acta Medicae Historiae Patavina* 6 (1958–59): 17–37.

Brockliss, Laurence W.B. *French Higher Education in the Seventeenth and Eighteenth Centuries: A Cultural History.* Oxford, UK: Clarendon Press, 1987.

Brugi, Biagio. *Gli scolari dello studio di Padova nel Cinquecento. Discorso inaugurale.* Padua, Italy: Bandi, 1903.

Bylebyl, Jerome J. "The School of Padua: Humanistic Medicine in the Sixteenth Century." In *Health, Medicine and Mortality in the Sixteenth Century*, edited by Charles Webster, 335–70. Cambridge: Cambridge University Press, 1979.

Calabritto, Monica. "*Medicina Practica, Consilia* and the Illnesses of the Head in Girolamo Mercuriale and Giulio Cesare Claudini. Similarities and Differences of the Sexes." *Medicina e storia* 11 (2006): 63–83.

Cunningham, Andrew. *The Anatomical Renaissance. The Resurrection of the Anatomical Projects of the Ancients.* Aldershot, UK: Scholar Press, 1997.

Donato, Maria Pia. "Surgeons' Training and Hospital Life in Seventeenth- and Eighteenth-Century Rome." In *Transforming Medical Education: Historical Case Studies of Teaching, Learning, and Belonging in Medicine*, edited by Delia Gavrus and Susan Lamb, 136–60. Montreal, QC, and Kingston, ON: McGill-Queen's University Press, 2022.

Dulieu, Louis. "Guillaume Rondelet." *Clio Medica* 1 (1966): 89–111.

– *La médecine à Montpellier, vol. 2. La Renaissance.* Avignon, France: Presses Universelles, 1979.

– *La médecine à Montpellier, vol. 3. L'époque classique.* Avignon, France: Presses Universelles, 1983.

Ecoiffier, F. *Recherches historiques sur la faculté de médecine d'Avignon (1303–1790).* Montpellier, France: Imprimerie Centrale du Midi, 1877.

Facciolati, Giacomo. *Fasti gymnasii patavini ... collecti ab anno MDXVII quo restitutae scholae sunt ad MDCCLVI.* Padua, Italy: Apud Joannem Manfrè, 1757.

Favaro, Giuseppe. "Contributi alla biografia di Girolamo Fabrici d'Acquapendente." *Memorie e documenti per la storia della Università di Padova* 14 (1922): 241–348.

– *Gabrielle Falloppia modenese (MDXXII–MDLXII). Studio biografico.* Modena, Italy: Tipografia Editrice Immacolata Concezione, 1928.

– "L'insegnamento anatomico di Girolamo Fabrici d'Acquapendente." In *Girolamo Fabrici l'Acquapendente*, edited by Rosario Scipio, 69–93. Viterbo, Italy: Agnesotti, 1978.

French, Roger. *Dissection and Vivisection in the European Renaissance.* Aldershot, UK: Ashgate, 1999.

Garbari, Fabio, and Gianni Bedini. "Architetture, spazi, tempi e piante nell'orto botanico di Pisa. Un'evoluzione simpatrica." In *Nuovi paesaggi. Storia e rinnovamento del giardino botanico in Italia*, edited by Antonio Piva and Pierfranco Galliani, 115–24. Venice, Italy: Marsilio, 2002.

Garbari, Fabio, Lucia Tongiorgi Tomasi, and Alessandro Tosi. *Il giardino dei semplici. L'orto botanico di Pisa dal XVI al XX secolo.* Pisa, Italy: Pacini Editore, 1991.

Germain, Alexandre Charles. *L'école de médecine de Montpellier. Ses origines, sa constitution, son enseignement. Étude historique d'après les documents originaux.* Montpellier, France: J. Martel ainé, 1880.

– *Les anciennes thèses de l'école de médecine de Montpellier. Collation des grades et concours professoraux.* Montpellier, France: Boehm, 1886.

– "Les pèlerins de la science à Montpellier." *Bulletin de la Société Languedocienne de Géographie* (1878): 161–81.

– *Matricule de l'université de médicine de Montpellier (1503–1599).* Edited by Gouron Marcel. Geneva, Switzerland: Droz, 1957.

Green, Monica. *Making Women's Medicine Masculine: The Rise of Male Authority in Pre-Modern Gynecology.* Oxford, UK: Oxford University Press, 2008.

Guarino, Mauro. "Profilo storico degli ospedali di Bologna e Ferrara." In *Le arti della salute. Il patrimonio culturale e scientifico della sanità pubblica in Emilia-Romagna*, edited by Graziano Campanini, Mauro Guarino, and G. Lippi, 77–93. Milan, Italy: Skira, 2005.

King, Helen. *Midwifery, Obstetrics and the Rise of Gynaecology: The Uses of a Sixteenth-Century Compendium.* Aldershot, UK: Ashgate, 2007.

Klestinec, Cynthia. "Medical Education in Padua. Students, Faculty and Facilities." In *Centres of Medical Excellence? Medical Travel and Education in Europe, 1500–1789*, edited by Ole Peter Grell, Andrew Cunningham, and Jon Arrizabalaga, 192–220. Farnham, UK: Ashgate, 2010.

– *Theaters of Anatomy. Students, Teachers, and Traditions of Dissection in Renaissance Venice.* Baltimore, MD: Johns Hopkins University Press, 2011.

Lewis, Gillian. "Clusius in Montpellier, 1551–1554: A Humanist Education Completed?" In *Carolus Clusius: Towards a Cultural History of a Renaissance Naturalist*, edited by Florike Egmond, 65–98. Amsterdam: Koninklijke Nederlandse Akademie van Wetenschappen, 2007.

Maclean, Ian. *Logic, Signs and Nature in the Renaissance. The Case of Learned Medicine.* Cambridge: Cambridge University Press, 2002.

– "Trois facultés de médecine au XVIe siècle: Padoue, Bâle, Montpellier." In *Les échanges entre les universités européennes à la Renaissance,* edited by Madeleine Fragonard and Michel Bideau, 349–58. Geneva, Switzerland: Droz, 2004.

Martins, Ch. *Le jardin des plantes de Montpellier. Essai historique et descriptif, accompagné de neuf planches.* Montpellier, Paris, and Strasbourg, France: Boehm V. Masson and Treuttel, 1854.

Minelli, Alessandro, ed. *The Botanical Garden of Padua / L'orto botanico di Padova, 1545–1995.* Venice, Italy: Marsilio, 1995.

da Monte, Giovanni Battista. *Consultationum medicarum opus absolutissimum.* Edited by Johannes Crato. Basel, Switzerland: per Henricum Petri et Petrum Pernam, 1565.

Münster, Ladislao. "Die Anfänge eines klinischen Unterrichts an der Universität Padua im 16. Jahrhundert." *Medizinische Monatsschrift* 23 (1969): 171–4.

– "Ferrara e Bologna sotto i rapporti delle loro scuole medico-naturalistiche nell'epoca umanistico rinascimentale." In *Atti del XXI Congresso Nazionale di Storia della Medicina (Perugia 11–12 Settembre 1963),* 517–66. Rome: E. Cossidente, 1966.

Nadal, Joseph Cyprien. *Histoire de l'Université de Valence et des autres établissements de cette ville depuis leur fondation jusqu'à nos jours suivie de nombreuses pièces justificatives.* Valence, France: E. Marc Aurel, 1861.

Nauck, E.Th. "Die Zahl der Medizinstudenten deutscher Hochschulen im 14.-18. Jahrhundert." *Sudhoffs Archiv* 38 (1954): 175–86.

Nutton, Vivian. "The Rise of Medical Humanism: Ferrara 1464–1555." *Renaissance Studies* 11 (1997): 2–19.

O'Malley, C.D. "Medical Education during the Renaissance." In *History of Medical Education,* edited by Vivian Nutton, 89–102. Berkeley, CA: University of California Press, 1970.

Ogilvie, Brian W. *The Science of Describing. Natural History in Renaissance Europe.* Chicago, IL, and London: University of Chicago Press, 2006.

Ongaro, Giuseppe. "La medicina nello studio di Padova e nel Veneto." In *Storia della cultura veneta. Dal primo Quattrocento al Consilio di Trento,* vol. 3, 75–134. Vicenza, Italy: Neri Pozza Editore, 1981.

Orsolato, Giuseppe. "Sulla prima fondazione di una clinica in Padova e sul monumento a G. B. Da Monte nella casa che fu del Professore G. A. Giacomini," *Rivista periodica dei lavori della Reale Accademia di Scienze, Lettere ed Arti in Padova* 23 (1872–73): 127–52.

Padoani, Elideo. *Processus, curationes et consilia in curandis in particularibus morbis quae prosperos habuerunt eventus, a ... D. Helidaeo Padoano de Forolivio, professore et archipractico bononiense celeberrimo … medicinae candidatis in praxi eum sequentibus communicata.* Edited by Johannes Wittich. Leipzig, Germany: Sumtibus Nicolai Nerlichii, 1607.

Planchon, Jules-Émile, and Gustave Planchon. *Rondelet et ses disciples ou la botanique de Montpellier au XVIe siècle.* Montpellier, France: Boehm & Fils, 1866.

– *Rondelet et ses disciples ou la botanique à Montpellier au XVIme siècle. Appendice.* Montpellier, France: Boehm & Fils, 1866.

Platter, Felix. *Tagebuch (Lebensbeschreibung) 1536–1567.* Edited by Valentin Lötscher. Basel, Switzerland: Schwabe & Co., 1976.

Pomata, Gianna. "Sharing Cases: The *Observationes* in Early Modern Medicine." *Early Science and Medicine* 15 (2010): 193–236.

Porter, Roy. "The Rise of Physical Examination." In *Medicine and the Five Senses,* edited by W.F. Bynum and Roy Porter, 179–97. Cambridge: Cambridge University Press, 2004.

Primrose, James. "Academia monspeliensis." In *Jacques Primerose. Historien de l'école de médecine de Montpellier,* edited by Alexandre Charles Germain, 9–16. Montpellier, France: Jean Martel ainé, 1883.

Reeds, Karen Meier. *Botany in Medieval and Renaissance Universities.* New York and London: Garland, 1991.

Rioux, Jean-Antoine, ed. *Le jardin des plantes de Montpellier. Quatre siècles d'histoire.* Graulhet, France: Editions Odyssée, 1994.

Roth, Moritz. *Andreas Vesalius bruxellensis.* Berlin: Reimer, 1892.

Sambale, Janine. *Chirurgischer Unterricht in Padua im 16. Jahrhundert. Kommentierte Edition und Übersetzung der studentischen Aufzeichnungen von Konrad Zinn.* Med. diss. Würzburg, Germany: University of Würzburg, 2018.

Schlegelmilch, Sabine. "Promoting a Good Physician: Letters of Application to German Town Authorities (1500–1700)." In *Civic Medicine: Physician, Polity and Pen in Early Modern Europe,* edited by Andrew Mendelsohn, Annemarie Kinzelbach, and Ruth Schilling, 88–109. Abingdon, UK: Routledge, 2019.

Schmitt, Charles B. "Aristotle among the Physicians." In *The Medical Renaissance of the Sixteenth Century,* edited by Andrew Wear, Roger French, and Iain Lonie, 1–15 and 271–9. Cambridge: Cambridge University Press, 1985.

Siraisi, Nancy G. *Avicenna in Renaissance Italy. The Canon and Medical Teaching in Italian Universities after 1500.* Princeton, NJ: Princeton University Press, 1987.

– "Medicina Practica. Girolamo Mercuriale as Teacher and Textbook Author." In *Scholarly Knowledge. Textbooks in Early Modern Europe,* edited by Emidio Campi, Simone De Angelis, Anja-Silvia Goeing, and Anthony T. Grafton, 287–305. Geneva, Switzerland: Droz, 2008.

– "Segni evidenti, teoria e testimonianza nelle narrazioni di autopsie del Rinascimento." *Quaderni storici* 36 (2001): 719–44.

Sterzi, Giuseppe. *Giulio Casseri. Anatomico e chirurgo (1552c.–1616).* Venice, Italy: Istituto Veneto di Arti Grafiche, 1909.

Stolberg, Michael. "Bedside Teaching and the Acquisition of Practical Skills in Mid-Sixteenth-Century Padua." *Journal of the History of Medicine and Allied Sciences* 69 (2014): 633–61.

– "Learning Anatomy in Late Sixteenth-Century Padua." *History of Science* 56 (2018): 381–402.

– "Teaching Anatomy in Post-Vesalian Padua. An Analysis of Student Notes." *Journal of Medieval and Early Modern Studies* 48 (2018): 61–78.

– *Uroscopy in Early Modern Europe.* Farnham, UK: Ashgate, 2015.

Strobelberger, Johann Stefan. *Laureationum medicarum apud exteros promeritarum adversum obtrectatores breves vindiciae, in honorem scholae medicae monspeliensis propositae.* Nürnberg, Germany: Typis Abrahami Wagenmanni, 1628.

Tomasini, Giacomo F. *Gymnasium patavinum … libris V. comprehensum.* Udine, Italy: Nicolai Schiratti, 1654.

Trincavella, Vettore. *Consilia medica.* Basel, Switzerland: Waldkirch, 1587.

Vidor-Borricand, Mireille. *Une université méconnue. L'université d'Orange.* Aix-en-Provence, France: Éditions Borricand, 1977.

Wightman, William P.D. "Quid sit methodus? 'Method' in the Sixteenth Century Medical Teaching and 'Discovery.'" *Journal of the History of Medicine* 19 (1964): 360–76.

5

Surgeons' Training and Hospital Life in Seventeenth- and Eighteenth-Century Rome

Maria Pia Donato

Around 1665, Filippo Paoli, a young apprentice surgeon and caregiver (*giovane di corsia*) in a hospital in Rome, very probably Santo Spirito in Saxia, the city's largest and most important, transcribed some lectures he had attended in a neat copy (maybe with the intention of selling it) under the (wrong) Latin title of *Patologia tumorum preter naturam.*[1] As Paoli duly wrote, a tumour, be it a protuberance, bruise, or bubo, was any "swelling of the parts" caused by the flux or congestion of humours.[2] Traditionally, lessons on tumours were the point of entry into the basic notions of Galenic and humoral medicine, as they had been addressed by Galen's *De tumoribus praeter naturam.* From Celsus to Fabrici of Acquapendente through Avicenna and Guy of Chauliac, tumours were an essential part of the surgical curriculum.

To date, we know practically nothing about Filippo, except that he was one of the many flocking to Rome from the whole Peninsula in order to gain a licence in surgery. Rome was at the time one of the largest Italian cities, at once the centre of the Catholic world and the capital of the Papal State, in Central Italy, and it boasted robust medical infrastructures, including several renowned hospitals where surgical training was imparted. Filippo's notebook and many other similar manuscripts documenting surgical training and practice in seventeenth- and eighteenth-century Italy, which still await in-depth consideration in libraries and archives today, raise several questions about the education, social status, and professional mobility of surgery practitioners. Furthermore, they raise questions on how new philosophical notions were incorporated into medicine and changed – or failed to change – surgical treatments. Although the interplay between natural philosophy and medicine over the centuries is to a great extent obvious (and the object of a vast body of scholarship), the academic distinction between history of science and history of medicine has left such questions in shadow when it comes to surgery; notebooks can help to shed light on them.[3]

Historians of medicine have long ago pointed to the high status of surgery in early modern Italy and have emphasized the interactions that medicine and surgery maintained both intellectually and socially.[4] Recent studies by Cynthia Klestinec, Domenico Bertoloni Meli, and Paolo Savoia, among others, have delved afresh into the Renaissance tradition of learned surgery.[5] Others, such as Jacalyn Duffin and Alessandro Pastore, have traced the activities of surgeons as experts in the sanitary surveillance of towns and in civil and ecclesiastical tribunals.[6] Last but not least, the social world of barber-surgeons has been the object of ground-breaking studies by Sandra Cavallo and Daniela Bartolini.[7] All these scholars have argued that surgery was a highly mobile activity, both socially and geographically.

Yet, the theoretical and practical instruction of early modern surgeons remains largely unexplored. Whereas medieval surgery has sustained a considerable body of scholarship, the relative paucity of studies on the early modern period, particularly after 1600, is puzzling. Available studies are often celebratory in intent or draw heavily upon modern notions of professionalization and clinical education. Contrary to France and England, which have elicited a wider scholarly interest, not much is known about the curriculum, teaching staff, facilities, learning aids, handbooks, or the actual evolution of courses over time. The greatest authors have their place in (more or less Whiggish) histories of surgery, whose origin dates back to the Enlightenment, while common practitioners such as the ones discussed in this chapter remain largely unknown.[8]

The aim of this chapter is to investigate surgeons' training in hospitals, primarily in Rome in the second half of the seventeenth to the mid-eighteenth centuries, a period of tremendous change in medical and scientific culture. As part of wider research on hospitals as sites of knowledge, the narrative begins with description of the institutional background followed by discussion of the style and content of lecture courses for surgical apprentices, drawing upon hospitals' archival records, printed material, and students' notebooks. As I have indicated, these sources enable historians to gain insight into the actual evolution of surgical courses as well as the philosophical and medical ideas that were transmitted. It is argued that under the veil of continuities, changes did, in fact, take place. The slow reform of surgical education began in the late seventeenth century and paralleled the enhancement of practical training for physicians in the context of hospitals. This was the result of the aforementioned Italian tradition of (relative) proximity of medicine and surgery and the long-standing centrality of hospitals in the urban organization of health care, which provided favorable conditions for enhanced training but also arguably hindered in-depth transformations in surgical training.

THE INSTITUTIONAL SETTING:
BECOMING A SURGEON IN EARLY MODERN ROME

In seventeenth-century Rome, like everywhere in Europe, the practice of surgery was a complex reality involving men (and some women) of very different skills, activities, social standing, and legal status. Surgeons encompassed a
broad spectrum, ranging from a vast majority of humble village practitioners
who earned their living by barbering, bloodletting, and simple manual procedures to a few surgeons in large cities whose fame and earnings rivalled those
of physicians and/or who were themselves university-trained physicians.[9]
Although in everyday life, distinctions tended to blur, especially in smaller
towns and the countryside, their education varied too.

Surgical qualification could indeed be acquired in a number of ways.
Although sixteenth-century codification had enhanced the stratification of
the healing arts and helped physicians assert their authority over surgery and
pharmacy, in Italy, learned or "rational" as opposed to "empirical" surgery
was mostly regarded as an integral part of medicine.[10] Hence, the Roman
College of Physicians, chartered in 1471, delivered university grades in medicine and surgery as well as philosophy and medicine. Tellingly, by the 1640s,
a doctorate in surgery cost the same as one in medicine: ten golden *scudi*.
University-trained surgeons accessed the medical corporative organization
and, from 1673 onwards, had to enrol in the College of Physicians' *matricola*
to be allowed to practise and prescribe remedies.[11]

The College of Physicians was also responsible for examining and licensing
surgeons *in gravibus*, who were a step below doctors. In truth, we know very
little about this group of practitioners and their background. Sparse evidence
suggests that they were Latinate and had some academic and practical training, possibly through a formal apprenticeship with a senior practitioner or
hospital training: the apprenticeship-based training was in fact not an alternative to academic instruction. At any rate, letters of recommendation by senior
surgeons were necessary for them to stand for examination. Further down
in the professional hierarchy, the Protomedicus (the first physician, who was
also the head of the college) delivered certificates for surgery *in levibus*, which
was theoretically limited to minor external operations, arteriotomy, venesection, scarification, and the application of plasters and ointments; licences were
temporary or perpetual, and a proof of practice was required.[12] As was typical in early modern Europe, the level of knowledge and experience required
was proportional to the size of the city where the prospective surgeon would
later practise, at the discretion of the Protomedicus and his fellow examiners.
The professional status of any practitioner could anyway evolve over time, as
could his qualification.

The Protomedicus also supervised the concession of licences to barbers, who had their own guild, chartered in 1470. After serving as apprentices and aids for a variable number of years and before taking the Protomedicus's examination, aspiring master barbers had to pass their guild's, which consisted of "knowing all the veins of the human body, how to let blood from said veins, apply leeches and cups, do ligatures, cauterisations and apply egg white [on wounds] and set bones fractures" and any other practical question at the masters' discretion.[13]

It should be noted that learned surgeons had no autonomous organization, neither guild nor college, which was at once an indication of their prestige and a hindrance to the emergence of a strong professional identity. They unsuccessfully attempted to form their own college on multiple occasions. In 1534, an agreement was signed between physicians and surgeons that allowed the latter to be represented on the examining board. Elisa Andretta has argued that this settlement contributed to the permanent appointment of a university lecturer who, besides anatomy, had to teach surgery for four months. Attendance at the annual public anatomical demonstration, for which the College of Physicians had been officially responsible since 1531, was made compulsory for both surgeons and barbers.[14] The agreement, however, was short-lived and by the end of the sixteenth century, the presence of surgeons had disappeared from official texts.[15] Moreover, university lectures and demonstrations in anatomy and surgery were customarily held by physicians and in Latin despite pleas from students for proper surgical teaching.[16] Thus, it is not surprising that few surgeons or barbers actually attended university dissections, as medical authorities complained.[17]

In other words, the corporative structure of surgical practice in Rome followed a common Italian pattern. With a few exceptions, notably Venice and Turin,[18] and contrary to many European countries (except Spain), learned surgeons were affiliated with medical colleges in a subordinate position. However prestigious, this arrangement basically meant that while instruction of lower practitioners was neglected to the benefit of learned surgeons, few actually followed a proper academic surgical curriculum. As Michael McVaugh has noted about fourteenth-century practitioners, learned surgeons who had finally gained access to universities found a medical career more rewarding than a surgical one, at least in big cities.[19] The former did not hinder practising (the noblest part of) surgery, while the latter could be economically precarious because learned surgeons were not supposed to keep a shop like humble artisans and make a living through barbering and hairdressing. Still, in Rome like in many other Italian and European cities, one way of obtaining surgical training was to serve in a hospital. Depending on the number of years an apprentice served, their role in the internal hierarchy, the courses they attended, and the examinations they took, they could obtain the position of "low" or "high" surgeon and could eventually apply for academic grades.

Hospital training seems to have been highly appreciated, such that candidates tried to obtain a place therein by soliciting the favour of the hospital's staff and ecclesiastical patrons, according to one seventeenth-century chronicler.[20] Hospitals enabled young provincials without family networks – which were crucial to the transmission of the trade[21] – to gain some qualification. Unlike private apprentices, hospital trainees did not pay for their education and lodging other than by their work; the senior ones even earned a small wage. Furthermore, hospitals received hundreds of patients, offering opportunities for observing serious conditions. The great French surgeon Ambroise Paré recalled in his *Memories* that at the Hôtel-Dieu in Paris, where he served as an apprentice in the 1530s, he could "see and learn any possible alteration and disease of the human body because of the great variety of patients that lay in it ordinarily and also learn anything about anatomy on an infinite number of corpses."[22] The same was true of other big hospitals in large cities. At Santo Spirito, for instance, four wards were dedicated to 'fevers' and a fifty-bed ward (the *hospitaletto*) to wounded men.[23]

Last but not least, Roman hospitals enjoyed an international reputation, which was carefully crafted by the papacy for the sake of Catholic propaganda.[24] As Domenico Borgarucci, a priest and canon serving Santo Spirito, emphatically wrote in a report on the hospital's activities in 1623, "the goal of the young laypeople who come to the hospital to serve the sick is to learn surgery and observe how to medicate the wounded, draw blood, apply cups and other similar things pertaining to surgeons because in time, they become proficient, and from this hospital came, and still comes so often, the best surgeons in the world."[25] More prosaically, the medical and surgical staff at Santo Spirito usually tended to the papal court, so the apprentices had expectations of being introduced into high circles. For those who left in search of professional opportunities as small-town surgeons or independent practitioners, a certificate from Santo Spirito was anyway an asset.[26]

Admittedly, being a hospital apprentice was a demanding task and implied living a hard, semi-religious life in the hospital's precinct. Hospitals were *luoghi pii*, sacred spaces and charitable institutions under the guidance and surveillance of ecclesiastical authorities, and certainly not modern secular teaching facilities;[27] apprentice-surgeons were, foremost, servants. At Santo Spirito, for instance, their duties included sweeping the halls, making beds, feeding and cleaning the sick, and undressing the dead (though an undertaker was also employed by the hospital). They also kept patients' records, administered surgical treatments and medicines, and prepared the instruments and bandages.[28] Apprentices progressed from fresheners to experienced and senior, and the internal hierarchy also distinguished those in charge of the halls, night wards (*caporali*), and specific tasks, such as administering bloodletting (*caposanguigna*), clysters, and ointments, or taking care of outpatients (*giovane di medicheria*); a step higher was assistant or deputy surgeon for each of the two head surgeons. Every trainee was supposed to learn from his seniors and instruct those below him in the hierarchy. Likewise, four young medical doctors served a one- to three-year internship as *assistenti* (deputies or assistants) to the senior primary physicians. External, most probably fee-paying, apprentices were also admitted to learn the basic precepts and skills for bloodletting and barbering, hoping to be selected for an internship.[29] Their admittance was certainly allowed at another Roman hospital, Santa Maria della Consolazione, which was devoted to traumas and wounds (knife accidents were famously common in Rome).[30]

As in other cities and hospitals – Santa Maria Nuova in Florence, San Giovanni in Turin, Santa Maria della Morte in Bologna, Hôtel-Dieu in Paris and Lyon, and St Bartholomew's and St Thomas' in London, to name but a few – surgical training at Santo Spirito was fundamentally a matter of observing and acquiring a very gradual hands-on experience.[31] Another canon serving Santo Spirito in the seventeenth century and the hospital's historiographer, Pierre Saulnier, reported that the head surgeons "try [to operate] with their own hands when there is great danger, like for trepanning a skull, removing calculi from the bladder how often occurs, amputating a liber when it is necessary because of the virulence of the gangrene; if the thing is lighter, they allow the apprentices to practise, and indeed they encourage and instruct them. They also have the task of examining the surgical novices in order to promote them to a higher position in the art and [they would do so] not on grounds of seniority if those who would have the right [to an advancement] are not learned or have neglected their study."[32]

Formal lectures and demonstrations were also offered. At Santo Spirito, at least since the 1610s, the apprentices collectively paid a fee to a senior staff member to lecture them.[33] Antonio Bucci, who held the position of *chiururgo primario* (head surgeon) from 1616 to 1620 and was a prominent figure in the Roman medical milieu, was seemingly the first to do so.[34] Some years later, teaching had been codified in a more formal and mandatory way. According to Saulnier, "from the group of physicians, or at any rate, from the doctors in surgery, one is always designated who twice weekly gives a lecture in the internal academy of manual medicine and proposes not only elements and principles [of surgery], but also some – so to speak – of the art's secret tricks."[35] Interest in practical surgery and case stories was consistent with the College of Physicians' requirements: doctoral candidates in surgery had first to argue *puncta* from Hippocrates and Galen and then discuss a fictive case devised by the examining board.[36] A chronicler reports that the lecturer also instructed the apprentice on the secrets of the art of "[operating] on dead bodies."[37] As noted, knowledge of anatomy was a further requirement for would-be surgeons and barber-surgeons since the Renaissance. To be sure, surgical literature invariably recommended the study of the human body, at least for practical purposes, with an emphasis on the skeleton and arterial-venous system.

Historians of medicine are increasingly aware that hospitals were sites for research in anatomy since at least the late fifteenth century, but anatomical demonstrations for instructional purposes also regularly took place in hospitals throughout Europe.[38] In Rome, where there was no autonomous guild of surgeons that could host anatomical demonstrations (as was the case in London, Amsterdam, and Paris), hospitals were an alternative or complementary site to the university. In 1649, Saulnier writes that surgery lecturers "train the youths of the hospital and illustrate the precepts not only through little commentaries, but through the very demonstration of things; hence, every year, sometime in the winter months, in the amphitheatre prepared for the goal, he shows with an oration the structure of the human body to those who listen and look, not only the [hospital] pupils, but also to externs desirous of science."[39]

Sparse evidence suggests that, besides the "private" dissections (that is, for training in-house apprentice surgeons), Santo Spirito hosted "public" dissections that were open to both surgical and medical resident staff and to an external audience at least since the early seventeenth century. The best trainees were involved in the procedure. In 1617, for instance, an assistant physician, Giovanni Maria Castellani, demonstrated the arterial and venous system; on that occasion, he published an *in folio* anatomical sheet in Latin under the title *Phylactrion plebotomiae et arteriotomiae*, which presumably helped him obtain the chair in anatomy at La Sapienza in 1619 and the post of *medico primario* at the hospital. Notably, his publication was (re)translated two years later into Italian for the sake of non-Latinate provincial surgeons and barber-surgeons.[40] Half a century later, the teaching of anatomy for surgeons had been unquestionably consolidated. In 1672, Bernardino Genga (1636?–1696?), a practitioner from Mondolfo in the Marches who had climbed the ladder from surgeon apprentice at Santo Spirito to doctor of medicine and philosophy and head surgeon in that same hospital, presented himself as no less than professor of anatomy and surgery on the title page of his compendium of anatomy for surgeons, *Anatomia chirurgica*.[41] During his life, he published several treatises, including a commentary, *In Hippocratis Aphorismos ad chirurgiam spectantes commentaria*, in Latin and Italian, which was consistent with the academic requirements for graduating in surgery.[42]

THE SLOW PACE OF CHANGE

Although the general framework of hospital care and training that has been described thus far did not change, it was not immutable. Starting in the 1660s and more consistently from the 1680s, the statutes and regulations of Roman hospitals were revised and all made additional requirements for the surgical curriculum. The impulse came from both the medical profession, which was undergoing a process of intellectual adjustment, and the papal curia, eager to revive the exemplarity of Catholic charitable institutions.[43] Measuring the gap between good intentions and the realities of care, the Congregation of the Apostolic Visitation, who periodically inspected churches and charitable institutions on behalf of the pope in his capacity as bishop of Rome, repeatedly recommended improvements for the medical and surgical staff. In 1658, the prelates governing Santo Spirito, "considering that the great fame of the venerable hospital depends on the reputation of those great men in medicine, surgery and apothecary who came out of it," stated that no apprentice would receive the hospital's certificate unless he was examined and found proficient.[44] Because the apostolic visitors had pointed out that apprentices were too young and too often employed in vile errands rather than learning the art, it was decided that candidates for apprenticeship should be at least twenty years of age and Latinate in order to be selected through an open call and then promoted by examination.[45]

At San Giacomo of the Incurable, a hospital originally conceived for those affected by the French Pox, the 1659 statutes do not mention any training for young 'servants' who were only supposed to clean and watch the wards; nonetheless, they were entrusted with administering the prescribed medicaments and attending the physician and surgeon while they examined the sick.[46] Following the apostolic visitation in 1677, it was decreed that the apprentices should not be promoted by seniority alone, but after an evaluation of their skills, and the assistant physician would be appointed through an open selection.[47] At least since the 1680s, lectures on anatomy and physiology as well as anatomical demonstrations were also regularly held in the hospital's premises. In the city's fourth largest hospital, San Salvatore (also known as San Giovanni), the head surgeon was formally entrusted in 1693 with lecturing the apprentices twice a week and performing the anatomies; his salary was raised accordingly.[48]

At Santa Maria della Consolazione, the surgical staff was expanded,[49] and the recruitment and internal hierarchy of the *giovani* was altered. In 1685, the hospital board considered "how necessary it is to do the anatomies in our hospital like it was done in the past" and resolved that the head surgeons would perform them in turn for one month "for the public good and to instruct the youths of the said hospital."[50] The following year, new rules or *Regole per il buon governo dell'archispedale della santissima Consolatione di Roma* were issued, which made theoretical and practical training compulsory. Every day, apprentices were required to follow the lectures and anatomies given by the assistant surgeon as well as "any other study and operation from which they may learn surgery in theory and practice."[51] The assistant surgeon would read and explain the theory and question the students (who were eighteen years or older and able to read, write, and "understand Latin books") and supervise their anatomical exercises, whereas the head surgeon was responsible for the public anatomies.[52] Special ornaments were put up at the hospital on the days of public anatomies to celebrate the noble art of surgery.[53]

The practice of anatomy acquired a greater role in the training of surgeons as well as young graduate physicians-in-training. Hospital anatomical theatres staged public anatomy lessons that seriously rivalled those of the university. At San Giacomo's, for instance, they were publicly performed in the 1680s by Mario Cecchini (?–?). Cecchini, after serving as trainee and deputy surgeon at Santo Spirito, graduated from the university and became chief surgeon at San Giacomo and later a surgeon for the cardinals in conclave and to Pope Innocent XIII. He lectured on contemporary mechanical physiology and chemical medicine and introduced the latest anatomical findings.[54] Sparse evidence also points to reputed hospital surgeons offering private tuition and lectures. It is unclear whether this was practised before (it is likely), but it evidently became more common as pressure was put on both surgeons and physicians to increase their practical knowledge.[55]

PHYSICIANS AND SURGEONS TEACHING SURGEONS

One question still remains: who were the hospital lecturers in surgery, and what did they actually teach besides anatomy?

In actuality, not much is known of seventeenth- and eighteenth-century practitioners. They are hardly quoted in local histories and erudite compilations, although in their lifetime they occupied key positions in the city's medical establishment. Rome had long enjoyed a tradition of medical men who were at once academics, hospital practitioners (*medici primari*), collegiate physicians, and possibly physicians to the pope and his household. Hospitals (especially Santo Spirito, which was a papal charity administered by a *commendatore* appointed by the pope) were springboards for success.[56] Therefore, just like physicians, surgeons could craft excellent careers by cumulating positions in hospitals, the papal court, and, albeit more rarely, the university. Practitioners with a hospital background were commonly appointed on the chair of anatomy and surgery at the city's university, La Sapienza, though in actuality academic expectations gave physicians an advantage over surgeons. It should not be overlooked that hospital surgeons were themselves in fact mostly doctors in surgery and even in philosophy and medicine. Accordingly, they shared the same learned understanding of surgery with physicians, but they arguably possessed greater practical experience and sometimes had even begun as simple apprentices. Several such graduated physicians practising surgery have already been mentioned, including Bucci, Genga, and his former pupil Cecchini (both initially trained at Santo Spirito), but the list could be longer.[57]

As for their content, we know that surgery courses taught in Latin at the university dealt with one main topic per year, namely wounds of the head and tumours, on which Hippocrates and Galen had written. Further topics included a thorough analysis of the structure and functions of bodily organs and sometimes *lue venerea*.[58] Hospital teaching was more comprehensive. Courses had the format of a systematic survey of surgical knowledge and practice, grounded in general philosophical and medical principles. This was the learned approach to surgery that had been formalized by the thirteenth-century Latin masters in their effort to provide surgery with a firm scientific fundament and didactic comprehensiveness on the basis of Greek and Arabic sources. Together with a flurry of new editions of (rediscovered) ancient texts, from Galen to Celsus, this tradition of learning was revived in the Renaissance thanks to the printing press, the expanding market for health and beauty services, and the growth of universities, and was expanded by Humanist authorities such as Guido Guidi, Jean Tagault, and Gabriele Falloppia.[59]

Archival evidence suggests that lecture courses were organized into five parts: tumours, wounds, fractures, ulcers, and dislocations, each with their remedies, a survey of major operations (craniotomy, extraction of a dead foetus, lithotomy, etc.), and a general introduction to *materia chirurugica* or surgical pharmaceutics and hygiene.[60] Already used by Avicenna, such a partition had been codified by Guy de Chauliac in the fourteenth century and was known as the *pentateuch*. In the first decades of the eighteenth century, an introduction to natural philosophy was also taught.[61]

More precisely, the template for seventeenth-century Roman hospitals can be found in some of the most successful handbooks of learned surgery of the time, including Gabriele Falloppia's *De parte medicinae, quae chyrurgia nuncupatur* (1571), Giovanni Andrea della Croce's *Chirurgiae universalis opus absolutum* (1573), and especially Girolamo Fabrizi of Acquapendente's *Opera chirurgica* (1623), which nicely combined clarity, erudition, and empiricism in the best Paduan tradition of academic surgery for surgeons. From these authors, lecturers drew the structure and content of their teaching, as well as the Aristotelian argumentative framework and actual treatment of ailments.

Notably, all these books had been translated into Italian and reprinted several times, making them available to non-Latinate surgeons and lay readers.[62] Authors from Northern Italy, especially those from the Republic of Venice, enjoyed wide circulation thanks to the prestige of the University of Padua and the commercial skills of Venetian printers, but a vast number of old and new texts of varying degrees of intellectual complexity addressed to various categories of practitioners were printed in other Italian cities too.[63] Still, in the hospital notebooks under consideration, these works are referred to in their Latin editions. After all, most lecturers were academically trained doctors who did not refrain from quoting lengthy passages in Latin (sometimes providing the translation).

Furthermore, although courses were taught in Italian in an abridged form, the pedagogical techniques of scholastic medicine that the learned tradition of surgery had incorporated were fully at work. Accordingly, explanations proceeded from general definitions and treatment, to genera and then species of ailments. Diseases were classified according to their causes, following a grid of oppositions typical of scholastic logics: the somatic origin (humoral imbalance or ill conformation), type of lesion (*solutio continuitatis* or affection of the similar parts), and so on through binary oppositions of essential and accidental differences (benign/malignant, simple/complex, etc.).[64] Each disorder is discussed following a set order: definition, etymology typically quoted from Galen (who is systematically quoted first, though modern definitions usually follow), causes, signs, and cure, in a genuinely scholastic tradition. Since the Middle Ages, such a structure enabled the learned surgeon who had already mastered the subject to go directly to treatment, while fresheners could start from the definition and learn the rational foundation for it.[65] Ethical recommendations and professional advice, together with the claim that surgery was an integral part of medicine, were disseminated throughout the courses and sketched the ideal portrait of a rational surgeon who masters anatomy and surgical theory, and follows "theory but not abstract speculation" and acts with "prudence"; as Genga expressed it, "being a good and perfect surgeon (morally speaking) does not consist in taking pride at prescribing many medicines only, but a firm knowledge of the nature of diseases is needed together with that of their phases … and when such knowledge is lacking, the surgeon is more empirical or methodical rather than truly rational, who only acts according to reason and rational experience at once."[66]

Still, there was relative latitude in the way teachers could introduce novelties. Just like their medieval and Renaissance predecessors, seventeenth-century surgeons combined, selected from, and adapted their sources and produced their own solutions. It was not only a matter of secret remedies and new instruments and techniques, nor the teacher's personal experience alone, though obviously lecturers incorporated their own experiences and deployed reasons and arguments to defend the correctness of their own practices and ideas. Quite the contrary, it was in the underlying theories that change occurred. As we shall see, adaptation went as far as undermining the Galenic-humoral medical philosophy that ultimately justified the very structure of traditional surgical learning.

FROM HUMOURS TO CORPUSCLES: LESSONS ON TUMOURS

The lessons on tumours prove interesting in this perspective. They provide yet another example of the way surgeons reworked material from the learned tradition and contemporary medical and philosophical debates to suit their own needs, like new wine poured into old bottles. Because tumours were regarded as the superficial outcome of an internal imbalance, they were one of the most theoretically sophisticated parts of surgery and required familiarity with Galenic and humoral medicine (or any other medical system aimed at replacing it). They were where the distinction between 'internal' medicine and 'external' manipulation was more problematic. Tellingly, tumours were commonly dealt with in medical works, including widespread, authoritative treaties on pathology such as Jean Fernel's *Pathologia* or Daniel Sennert's *Medicina practica*.

The first lecture notebook under consideration here, the *Patologia tumorum*, dates from the mid-seventeenth century and is still fully embedded in the Galenic tradition. It is unclear who the lecturer was, but he certainly follows a strict humorism both in the underpinning philosophy and in the explanation of specific conditions.[67] The first lessons are devoted to a general exposition on tumours as a "congestion of escrementitious humours" and "humoural fluxion," asserting that a tumour is formed either by a faulty quantity or quality of blood, yellow bile, black bile, or phlegm (and/or in some instances water). The lecturer then develops his classification of tumours according to essential and accidental specifications, namely the site, form, size, heat, and painfulness of each.

In actuality, close analysis proves Fabricius to be the main reference for this anonymous Roman lecturer; for instance, the chapter on erysipelas is taken nearly word for word from his *Opera*. Fabricius is invariably quoted together with Galen, Hippocrates, Avicenna, Falloppia, and sometimes Celsus, Fernel, Ingrassia, and Sennert. The notions of putrefaction and corruption pervade the text; if the peccant humour is corrupted, the tumour is malignant and the prognosis negative.[68] Occult qualities, a cornerstone of Renaissance Galenism, are used to explain several ailments, such as gangrene.[69] In contrast, the circulation of the blood is introduced once in passing in relation to the phlegmon (a blood tumour), but either the teacher or, more probably, the student is unfamiliar with it and misspells *Harvey* in *Haraclio*.[70] The idea of fermentation, very popular in mid-seventeenth-century European medicine, is also briefly introduced, with black bile being defined as a "fermentative and very bitter humour."[71]

Each type of tumour has a treatment. A good surgeon makes a diagnosis through physical examination of the affected part and sound reasoning and chooses the appropriate remedy for each ailment. The universal cure is, of course, bloodletting, necessary to draw back and adduct overabundant humours. Then, specific topical and/or internal medicines are added. The lecturer avoids any remark for or against chemical medicine but does not refrain from recommending strong chemical medicines, which were very popular among Roman patients at the time. Sometimes he introduces his personal experience explicitly, and while dealing with pestilential buboes, recalls how "we observed in Rome during the plague in the year 1656, that all who were bled died."[72]

If necessary, a qualified surgeon must prescribe oral remedies. Tumours are stated to be the outcome of internal imbalances, and laxatives and corroborants are suggested to help restore the patient's optimal balance. The borders between medicine and surgery are thin regarding cures provided the surgical ailment is visible on the body's surface. Nonetheless, prudence must always guide the surgeon's hand. Internal tumours, and especially an ill-fated condition such as cancer, should be left to the *medicus physicus*. Temerity is morally and professionally bad and surgeons should "let the patient who is doomed to die perish because of the disease and not because of surgical operations."[73]

Two decades later, the conciliation between Ancients and Moderns seems to be the main concern of Bernardino Genga in addressing the same topic. In the notebook of an apprentice named Agostino Cencelli on tumours dated 1692, the same definitions, quotations, grids of classification, and underlying philosophical and medical principles of older manuscripts recur.[74] Genga calmly and learnedly explains Galen's teachings and the humoral aetiology of each tumour following the canonical scholastic progression from genera to species according to their pathogenic elements and qualities. Yet, as soon as he introduces the circulation of the blood, the edifice of Galenism begins to shake.[75]

In fact, in the eyes of the conservative innovator Genga, blood circulation and capillary anastomosis might confer a new, truer meaning to the doctrines of the Ancients. Admittedly, "great difficulties" have long arisen against humoral medicine and surgery. How can melancholy, which is deemed to be "very subtle" humours, cause hard, solid swellings, for instance? Galenic doctrines might satisfy the intellect "sufficiently," but upon closer analysis, they appear to imply mysterious natural faculties inherent to the bodily parts, the existence of which modern anatomy "through experience and reasoning" is disproving. In the light of this tenet, Genga introduces his personal theory: all tumours are formed by blood only; in the circulation, however, blood collects other fluids and escrementitious matter and therefore acquires those different properties that the Ancients attributed to humours.[76] Such a conciliatory approach enables him to salvage the classic taxonomy of tumours.

Hence, tumours might be 'pure' (made by blood alone) or 'spurious' (from blood mixed with other fluids). Genga, however, does not make any thorough explanation of these other fluids. This is why his vision of tumours ultimately does not depart much from the Galenic tradition, apart from disdainful remarks on the "vulgar humourism" of empirics. Indeed, Genga also resorts to modern ideas, especially Willis's and Sylvius's blood fermentation, and speaks of "a mass of putrefied and corrupted particles," but he does not engage in developing any corpuscular interpretation of the bodily fluids and solid parts and prefers to remain on the safe middle ground of eclecticism.[77]

Blood and corpuscles become the key elements in a later notebook of lectures on tumours, titled *Trattato de tumori preternaturali prodotti dal sangue*.[78] The lecturer, Domenico Cecchini (?–1758?), came from a family of learned surgeons, being the son of Mario Cecchini, whom we have already encountered. He graduated in Rome, and at the time the notebook was copied (1732), he was head surgeon and lecturer at San Salvatore and Santo Spirito as well as papal surgeon.

Cecchini heralds modern tenets: he means to disprove the scholastics ("our doctors," he ironically calls them), whom generations of "medicks" followed "like sheep." Thanks to the discoveries and progress made by anatomists "in our blessed century," the time has come to relinquish faculties and other obscurities and embrace a fully circulatory explanation of tumours. Cecchini argues that "the knowledge of so many anatomical facts discovered in our age, and the mechanical way of philosophising" enable the surgeon to "more easily describe and with greater ease explain the causes and essence of the ailments and therefore, acknowledge how much better the doctrine of the moderns suits our intellect."[79] Nonetheless, in dealing with the subject, he also resorts to the conventions of scholastic medicine because he believes the classic method proceeding from the Greek and Latin definition and etymology of signs, causes, and treatment of each ailment is still a valuable guide to surgical knowledge, for lack of a better one. Notably, though, as a further indictment of modernity, Cecchini quotes Galen and Hippocrates abundantly along with Sennert, Descartes, Willis, Sylvius, and Malpighi, but hardly ever any medieval or Renaissance author. Accordingly, Cecchini uses the canonical definition of tumours as swellings resulting from either the plethora or the cacochimia, which are regarded, respectively, as faulty blood circulation or some "unevenness and separation of humours in the blood mass due to which, [the blood mass] is made viscid and fatty"; eventually, fatty or acid particles of an "alien and different nature" than the healthy blood's "globular particles" make it unfit for circulation and fermentation.[80]

In Cecchini's view, a corpuscular understanding of the bodily parts complements the circulation of the blood and both cohere into a proper circulatory pathology combining mechanical and chemical notions. The body is an aggregate of glands and fibres through which fluids, especially the blood, made of different kinds of particles circulate and filter out; their unhealthy composition and movement is responsible for any pathology, including surgical ones. Hence, for instance, pestilential buboes are caused by acids "apt to prick and peel the globules and globular round bodies; these, made flat, compressed or any other form less fit for movement, cause the blood to loose its own movement, not only circulatory but also fermentative," and eventually obstruct viscera, "which, according to Malpighi, are made of innumerable glands."[81]

Of course, by the 1730s when Cecchini taught, such circulatory pathology was hardly a novelty; over more than half a century, it had gradually established itself as the new medical commonplace and a flexible framework for reframing older notions and therapies. Chemical-mechanical medicine does indeed provide the rationale for venesection, frugal lifestyle, and the traditional surgical pharmacopoeia as well as chemical remedies, which Cecchini warmly recommends in a large number of pathologies, though always with "the highest caution and solid reasons."[82]

Emphasis on blood does, however, eventually alter the traditional presentation of tumours. Cecchini concludes his course with a section on aneurysms.[83] An extremely serious and common condition at the intersection of surgery and medicine, aneurysms had already attracted the interest of reputed authors, including the great Roman anatomist and physician Giovanni Maria Lancisi.

Later in the eighteenth century, Cecchini's student, assistant, and successor as papal surgeon, Piedmontese-born Carlo Guattani (1709–73), continued along his master's line in both his teaching and his publications, cautiously modernizing surgical doctrines on tumours.[84] His lectures matter-of-factly posit circulatory pathology and adopt a less heavily scholasticized approach to the subject, and nonetheless remain in the learned tradition.

CONCLUSIONS

In 1751, after he had financed the building of a new wing for Santo Spirito (the *braccio nuovo*), the reformist Pope Benedict XIV promoted a revision of the hospital's statutes in order to define the obligations of each staff member more precisely and introduce new ones.[85] The theoretical and practical instruction for apprentice surgeons that had been consolidated over two centuries was more precisely codified and made compulsory. All had to attend the "school"

in surgical theory and practice twice a week, "write down the treaties in surgery that their masters read and resolve those cases that he will ask them,"
attend private and public anatomies, study in the library daily, and, according
to their seniority, help officials with anatomical preparations, while acquiring
manual dexterity operating on dead and living patients.

In 1758, at the suggestion of chief surgeon Carlo Guattani, the lecture
courses were reframed into *Istituzioni* (basically, surgical theory), anatomy,
practical anatomy, surgical cases, and operations.[86] Guattani, who had spent
some years studying and practising in France, took inspiration from similar
developments at the recently founded Académie Royale de Chirurgie in Paris
in order to instil new life into the old Roman style of instructing young practitioners in hospitals.[87] In contrast, attempts at forming an autonomous College
of Surgeons failed yet again.[88]

Historians generally agree that late-eighteenth-century surgery featured
an increasing emphasis on operations and that teaching accordingly shifted
towards the practical part of surgery, rather than the philosophical side that
had been so important in the medieval and early modern template. This is
certainly true, though it is also true that the history of modern surgery has
largely neglected the study of the medical notions underpinning such a shift.
A second look at students' notebooks and manuscript lectures notes can shed
new light on this point.

Based on far underexploited sources such as lectures on tumours delivered
in Roman hospitals in the period roughly 1650–1750, I have argued that,
within an older scholastic framework, new philosophical notions informed
surgical teaching, while greater emphasis was globally put on the theoretical
and practical education of prospect surgeons and innovations to enhance it
were cautiously introduced. Corpuscularism was blended into humoralism,
and humoralism into circulatory pathology.

However, the Roman case examined in this chapter also shows that the
overall resilience of the traditional intellectual paradigm and the institutional
settings impacted surgical education nonetheless. Notwithstanding innovations in the curriculum and in medical theories, the institutional and social
setting of hospitals did not change radically in papal Rome. At the middle of
the eighteenth century, however, the contours of surgery in Europe were rapidly changing and expanding. Hospital teaching was then becoming a thriving
industry in Paris and London, with all types of courses offered to a rising
number of students. In those countries, opportunities for acquiring surgical
training of different kinds were multiplying and the market for medical and
surgical education continued to grow at a pace the Roman, and more generally the Italian, learned tradition of surgical education and practice, however
venerable, would struggle to follow.

NOTES

1   MS London, Wellcome Library 3819. I would like to thank the editors and the anonymous readers for their comments; my gratitude also goes to the Wellcome Library and staff, which over the years have been an invaluable asset to my research. Translations are mine unless stated otherwise.

2   Ibid., fol. 5.

3   On this point, see Siraisi, "Medicine."

4   Palmer, "Physicians and Surgeons"; Park, *Doctors and Medicine.*

5   Klestinec and Bertoloni Meli, eds., *Renaissance Surgery*; Savoia, *Cosmesi e chirurgia.*

6   Duffin, *Medical Miracles*; Pastore, *Il medico in tribunale.*

7   Cavallo, *Artisans of the Body*; Bartolini, "On the Borders."

8   Lawrence, "Democratic, Divine and Heroic."

9   Pelling, "Occupational Diversity;" Rabier, "Medicalizing the Surgical Trade."

10   The distinction between rational and empirical surgery is explicitly posited in official regulations, e.g. in Mantua, see Carra, Fornari, and Zanca, *Gli statuti.*

11   *Bullarium Collegii Medicorum* Urbis; MS Archivio di Stato di Roma (hereafter ASR), *Università di Roma*, b. 23; *Statuta Collegii DD. Almae Urbis Medicorum.* See further Braconi, "Materiali d'archivio."

12   Cavallo, *Artistans*; Bartolini, "On the Borders." The apprenticeship of surgeons has been thoroughly investigated for England by Lane, "The Role of Apprenticeship," and Chamberland, "From Apprentice to Master."

13   Quoted from the Barbers Company's statutes of 1641, ch. XXVII, reproduced in Calabrini, Marta, and Ricci, *I barbieri di Roma.*

14   Andretta, "Universo dei medici."

15   A "university of surgeons" is still mentioned in *Confirmatio privilegiorum Collegii Medicorum Urbis* of 1562 (a printed copy now in ASR, Biblioteca, *Statuti*, 837/3), but disappears from subsequent papal documents and College of Physicians' statutes.

16   MS ASR, *Università di Roma*, b. 69, fols. 1–2. For an overview of university chairs and their respective lecturers, see Conte, *I maestri della Sapienza.*

17   MS ASR, Università di Roma, b. 61, Lorenzo Garzonio, *Discorso dell'inconvenienti che nascono nella medicina*, 1619.

18   Palmer, "Physicians"; Cavallo, *Artisans*; on the 1721 reform of surgical education in Turin, see Carpanetto, *Scienza e arte del guarire*, 198–209.

19   McVaugh, *The Rational Surgery*, 254.

20   Alveri, *Roma*, 2:256.

21   On this point, see Cavallo, *Artisans.*

22   Quoted in Malgaigne, *Œuvres complètes d'Ambroise Paré*, 1:10.

23 Domenico Borgarucci, "Relazione del modo che si tiene da religiosi di
    Santo Spirito in Sassia di Roma nel governo dell'archiospedale apostolico
    di santo Spirito, e dell'ordine che si osserva nella cura degl'infirmi, et esposti"
    (1623), in Grégoire, "'Servizio dell'anima,'" 235. Borgarucci's report, celebra-
    tory and apologetic in purpose, is nonetheless one of the earliest systematic
    reports on the hospital's internal organization. See further De Angelis, *L'Ospedale
    di Santo Spirito.*

24 Piccialuti, *La carità come metodo.*

25 Borgarucci, "Relazione," 258.

26 Cavallo, *Artisans,* 235.

27 Periodically, ecclesiastical authorities reiterated the prohibition to admit any
    woman in the hospital's precinct; see *Notificazione sopra diversi oggetti,* 14.

28 Saulnier, *De capite sacri,* 148.

29 Borgarucci, "Relazione," 238, names them *forestieri* in opposition to resident
    staff.

30 Antonella Pampalone, *Le botteghe dei barbieri a Roma alla fine del Seicento* (http://
    www.enbach.eu/it/content/le-botteghe-dei-barbieri-roma-alla-fine-del-
    seicento, accessed 31 July 2018), note 22. More in general, see Pericoli,
    L'Ospedale di S. Maria della Consolazione.

31 The Hôtel-Dieu in Paris had an apprentice surgeon *gagnant-maîtrise* who was the
    rough equivalent of Santo Spirito's deputy surgeon. In London, apprentices and
    young surgical and medical students made their arrangements with individual
    practitioners, not the hospital; see Waddington, *Medical Education,* 17–25. On
    Turin, see Cavallo, *Artisans,* 146. On Florence, see Ciuti, "Il medico e
    l'ospedale," and Mannacio, "Teoria e pratica della chirurgia." On Bologna, see
    Savoia, "Skills, Knowledge and Status." The power of ecclesiastical authorities
    in hospital life was obviously greater in papal Rome than elsewhere.

32 Saulnier, *De capite,* 147.

33 Borgarucci, "Relazione," 258.

34 Savio, "Ricerche su medici e chirurghi," 164; Conforti and De Renzi,
    "Sapere anatomico," 443.

35 Saulnier, *De capite,* 143.

36 *Statuta* 1676, 55; see Andretta, "Universo," for earlier requirements.
    Candidates in philosophy and medicine had, in addition, to engage in a
    disputatio with the examiners and college.

37 Alveri, *Roma,* 257.

38 In several towns, it was actually there, and not on the university's premises,
    that the theatres for dissections were built; see Martinez Vidal and Pardo
    Tomas, "Anatomical Theatres," and Diana, "Anatomy between Public and
    Private."

39   Saulnier, *De capite*, 143.

40   Conforti and De Renzi, "Sapere anatomico," 437–41. For a late-seventeenth-century example of anatomical preparations by assistant surgeons at Santo Spirito, see De Angelis, *Accademia Lancisiana*, 15.

41   Genga, *Anatomia chirurgica*, reprinted several times.

42   Genga, *In Hippocratis Aphorismos.*

43   Donato, "La medicina a Roma" and *Sudden Death.*

44   MS ASR, *Santo Spirito*, b. 138, fol. 22–3.

45   The decree was later reprinted in *Notificazione*, 38, 65. Dominici, "Il governo dell'ospedale," discusses the improvements ensuing the apostolic visitation in 1677.

46   *Statuti del venerabile archiospidale di San Giacomo*; Vanti, *S. Giacomo*; Arrizabalaga, Henderson, and French, *The Great Pox.*

47   MS Archivio Segreto Vaticano, *Miscellanea Armadio* VII 59, 3, fol. 17–19.

48   MS Archivio Segreto Vaticano, *Congregazione della Visita Apostolica*, Acta vol. 13, fol. 35.

49   MS ASR, *Ospedale Consolazione*, Congregazioni reg. 11, 1668–80 (non-numbered folios).

50   MS ASR, *Ospedale Consolazione*, Congregazioni reg. 12, 13 December 1696.

51   *Regole per il buon governo.*

52   Ibid., fol. 28–9, 34, 50–8.

53   Posterla, *Esatissima descrizione.*

54   Cecchini, *Elenchus lectionum et ostentiunum.*

55   Guglielmo Riva's anatomical "academy" is mentioned in the prologue to *Statuta* 1676, and Piazza, *Eusevologio romano*, book XII, xxiii–xxvi. See further Savio, "Ricerche sull'anatomico Guglielmo Riva."

56   De Renzi, "A Fountain for the Thirsty."

57   It is noteworthy that the sons of those surgeons such as Genga and Cecchini, who had successfully climbed the professional ladder, practised either surgery or medicine but had invariably secured a doctorate in philosophy and medicine, as did Domenico Cecchini, whose activities are discussed *infra*.

58   Conte, *I maestri*, to be read synoptically with Marini, *Degli Archiatri pontifici*, and Savio, "Ricerche."

59   Nutton, "Humanist Surgery." See a non-exhaustive list of printed editions of medieval authors in surgery in Tabanelli, *Tecniche e strumenti.*

60   This is what can be gathered from the surviving lecture notebooks, namely from MSS London, Wellcome Library 3816-8 and 2494-6.

61   MS London, Wellcome Library 992, *Filosofia in cui si tratta della cartesaa, atomistica e peripatetica tradotta in volgare ad uso mechanico*, "studied and copied" at Santo Spirito by Gaetano Asdrubali, dated 1726; MS Rome, Biblioteca Nazionale

Vittorio Emanuele II, Varia 360, Domenico Cecchini, *Quale sistema di filosofia naturale sia più convenevole alla chiurgia e medicina.*

62   Klestinec, "Translating Learned Surgery." Klestinec convincingly argues that translating and editing were part of the professional identity of learned surgeons, and that vernacular translations were not only meant to meet the demands of non-Latinate practitioners, but to configure relations with other occupational groups and define surgeons' place in urban society.

63   On the Venetian printing industry and book trade, see now Nuovo, *The Book Trade.*

64   Maclean, *Logic, Signs and Nature.*

65   McVaugh, *Rational Surgery*, 46.

66   MS London, Wellcome Library 2496, [Bernardino Genga], *Trattato della farmacia chirurgica*, fol. 4.

67   MS London, Wellcome Library 3819. The lecturer might be Giuseppe Balestra or Bernardino Gentiluzzi, who were head surgeons at Santo Spirito from 1657 to 1661 and from 1661 to 1678, respectively: Savio, "Ricerche," 166. The reader seems to have witnessed the plague outbreak of 1656–57 in person; see MS London, Wellcome Library 3819, fol. 30. Giuseppe Balestra published a book on the plague, *Gli accidenti più gravi.*

68   Wear, *Knowledge and Practice.*

69   MS London, Wellcome Library 3819, fol. 137r.

70   Ibid., fol. 30.

71   Ibid., fol. 11.

72   Ibid., fol. 130.

73   Ibid., fol. 218.

74   MS London, Wellcome Library 2494, [Bernardino Genga], *Delli tumori preternaturali*, copied by Agostino Cencelli in 1692.

75   Ibid., fol. 43–4: "Such a doctrine and way of the generation of tumours cannot be conceded at all, and the reason is because, given the circulation of the blood ... and the blood moving in a way contrary to what Galen says, it necessarily ensues that this doctrine of Galen's is not to be believed, but because it is not enough for a sound teaching to exclude a doctrine as false if one does not bring another one with good reasons ... we will say that the way in which the blood makes a fluxion is the flowing, namely that the said blood goes from major arteries through the minor ones, from minor ones to the smallest ones and capillaries, and from these to the spaces and porosities of the flesh, but if for any cause there happens to be either in these porosities or in the veins, both capillaries and minor ones and major and big ones, an obstruction or obstacle to the regression and circulation of the blood, the said blood ... comes to amass, and staying there in too much quantity, and not well regulated by nature, it comes to be the morbific cause of the tumour."

76   Ibid., fol. 46–7.

77   Ibid., fol. 561–84. It should be added, however, that in addressing surgical
     pharmacy, Genga draws upon corpuscular chemical and mechanical
     explanations much more consistently and recurrently; see MS London,
     Wellcome Library 2496, *Trattato della farmacia chirurgica.*

78   MS London, Wellcome Library 1536, *Trattato de tumori preternaturali prodotti dal
     sangue dettati nel ven. archi. del SS. Salvatore dal sig. Domenico Cecchini dottore in filosofia
     e medicina e chirurgo di Clemente XII e primario in detto ospedale, trascritto da Andrea
     Fresoni.*

79   Ibid, fol. 4–5.

80   Ibid, fol. 41–2.

81   Ibid, fol. 327

82   Ibid, fol. 72.

83   Ibid, fol. 425.

84   MS London, Wellcome Library 2648, [Carlo Guattani], *Trattato generale e parti-
     colare de tumori e delle ulcere; colla giunta di varie operationi chirurgiche*; Carlo Guattani,
     Historiae duae aneurysmatum, and *De externis aneurysmatibus.* On Guattani, see the
     entry by Antonello Pizzaleo in *Dizionario Biografico degli Italiani.*

85   *Regole da osservarsi.*

86   *Notificazione,* 194–6.

87   Gelfand, *Professionalising Modern Medicine.*

88   MS ASR, *Università di Roma,* b. 67 (1765).

BIBLIOGRAPHY

Alveri, Gasparo. *Roma in ogni stato.* Rome: Mascardi, 1664.

Andretta, Elisa. "Universo dei medici e mondo dei chirurghi nella Roma cinquec-
     entesca." *Medicina e Storia* 17–18 (2009): 65–97.

Arrizabalaga, Jon, John Henderson, and Roger French. *The Great Pox: The French
     Disease in Renaissance Europe.* New Haven, CT, and London: Yale University
     Press, 1997.

Balestra, Giuseppe. *Gli accidenti più gravi del mal contagioso osservati nel lazzaretto all'isola,
     con la specialità de medicamenti profittevoli esperimentati per lo spatio di sette mesi.* Rome:
     Moneta, 1657.

Bartolini, Donatella. "On the Borders: Surgeons and Their Activities in the Venetian
     State (1540–1640)." *Medical History* 59 (2015): 83–100.

Braconi, Lucia Alma. "Materiali d'archivio per la storia del Collegio medico romano
     nel Seicento e nel Settecento." *Annali di Storia delle Università Italiane* 4 (2000):
     27–38.

Bullarium Collegii Medicorum Urbis ... in unum volumen provide congestum. Rome: Reverenda
     Camera Apostolica, 1650.

Calabrini, Adriano, Mario Marta, and Sergio Ricci. *I barbieri di Roma. Collegio dei barbieri e parrucchieri di Roma cinque secoli e mezzo di attivita, 1443–1870.* Rome: [no imprint], 1985.

Carpanetto, Dino. *Scienza e arte del guarire. Cultura, formazione universitaria e professioni mediche a Torino nel Settecento.* Turin, Italy: Deputazione subalpina di storia patria, 1998.

Carra, Gilberto, Luciano Fornari, and Attilio Zanca. *Gli statuti del Collegio dei medici di Mantova dal 1313 al 1559.* Mantua, Italy: Sonnetti, 2004.

Cavallo, Sandra. *Artisans of the Body in Early Modern Italy. Identities, Families and Masculinities.* Manchester, UK: Manchester University Press, 2007.

Cecchini, Mario. *Elenchus lectionum et ostentiunum quibus ... humani corporis systema anatomicum ostendetur in theatro anatomico Archixenodochij S. Iacobi Incurabilium. Ob inopiam cadaverum, quibus caret praedictum Archixenodochium non successivis, ut assolent anatomici, sed tribus tantum diebus in hebdomata erunt praedictae ostensiones, diebus adnotatis hora vigesima secunda, & media.* Rome: Hercoli, 1683–88.

Chamberland, Celeste. "From Apprentice to Master: Social Disciplining and Surgical Education in Early Modern London, 1570–1640." *History of Education Quarterly* 53 (2013): 21–44.

Ciuti, Francesco. "Il medico e l'ospedale. Il nosocomio di Santa Maria Nuova e le professioni sanitarie a Firenze in età moderna." *Medicina e Storia* 11 (2011): 63–88.

Conforti, Maria, and Silvia De Renzi. "Sapere anatomico negli ospedali romani: formazione dei chirurghi e pratiche sperimentali (1620–1720)." In *Rome et la science entre Renaissance et Lumières*, edited by Antonella Romano, 433–72. Rome: École française de Rome, 2008.

Conte, Emanuele. *I maestri della Sapienza di Roma dal 1514 al 1787. Studi e Fonti per la storia dell'Università di Roma.* Rome: Istituto Storico per il Medio Evo, 1991.

De Angelis, Pietro. *Accademia Lancisiana e Società Lancisiana nel 3. centenario della nascita di Giovanni Maria Lancisi 1654-1954.* Rome: arte grafica, 1965.

– *L'Ospedale di Santo Spirito in Saxia.* Rome: Nuova tecnica grafica, 1962.

De Renzi, Silvia. "A Fountain for the Thirsty and a Bank for the Pope: Charity, Conflicts, and Medical Careers at the Hospital of Santo Spirito in Seventeenth-Century Rome." In *Health Care and the Poor Relief in Counter-Reformation Europe (1620–1720)*, edited by Andrew Cunningham and Jon Arrizabalaga, 102–31. London: Routledge, 1999.

Diana, Esther. "Anatomy between Public and Private in 14th–16th Century Europe: Social Contexts, Scenarios and Personages." In *Anatomy and Surgery from Antiquity to the Renaissance*, edited by Hélène Perdicoyianni Paléologu, 329–74. Amsterdam: Adolf M. Hakkert, 2016.

Dominici, Silvia. "Il governo dell'ospedale di Santo Spirito e dei suoi annessi nel secolo XVII. Coninuità e riforme." In *L'antico ospedale di Santo Spirito. Dall'istituzione papale alla sanità del terzo millennio*, edited by Luigi Cardilli, 239–51. Rome: il Veltro, 2001–02.

Donato, Maria Pia. "La medicina a Roma tra Sei e Settecento. Una proposta di interpretazione." *Roma moderna e contemporanea* 13 (2005): 99–114.

– *Sudden Death: Medicine and Religion in Eighteenth-Century Rome.* Farnham, UK: Ashgate, 2014.

Duffin, Jacalyn. *Medical Miracles: Doctors, Saints, and Healing in the Modern World.* Oxford, UK: Oxford University Press, 2009.

Gelfand, Toby. *Professionalising Modern Medicine: Paris Surgeons and Medical Science and Institutions in the Eighteenth Century.* Westport, CT: Greenwood Press, 1980.

Genga, Bernardino. *Anatomia chirurgica, cioè historia anatomia dell'ossa e muscoli del corpo humano, con la descrition de' vasi più riguardevoli che scorrono per le parti esterne, e un breve trattato sul moto, che chiamano circulation del sangue.* Rome: Tinassi, 1672.

– *Hippocratis Aphorismos ad chirurgiam spectantes commentaria.* Rome: Stamperia Camerale, 1694.

Grégoire, Réginald. "'Servizio dell'anima quanto del corpo' nell'Ospedale del Santo Spirito (1623)." *Ricerche per la storia religiosa di Roma* 3 (1979): 221–54.

Guattani, Carlo. *De externis aneurysmatibus manu chirurgica methodice pertractandis cum nonnullis circa aneurysmata interna ... opus.* Rome: Pagliarini, 1772.

– *Historiae duae aneurysmatum, quorum alterum in brachio per chirurgicam operationem sanatum in femore alterum paucos intra dies lethale fuit, animadversionibus, et figuris illustratae.* Rome: Pallade, 1745.

Klestinec, Cynthia. "Translating Learned Surgery." *The Journal of the History of Medicine and Allied Sciences* 72 (2017): 34–50.

Klestinec, Cynthia, and Domenico Bertoloni Meli, eds. "Renaissance Surgery: Between Learning and Craft." Special issue of the *Journal of the History of Medicine and Allied Sciences* 72, no. 1 (2016): 1–5.

Lane, Joan. "The Role of Apprenticeship in Eighteenth-Century Medical Education in England." In *William Hunter and the Eighteenth-Century Medical World*, edited by William F. Bynum and Roy Porter, 57–103. Cambridge: Cambridge University Press, 1985.

Lawrence, Christopher. "Democratic, Divine and Heroic: The History and Historiography of Surgery." In *Medical Theory, Surgical Practice. Studies in the History of Surgery*, edited by Christopher Lawrence, 1–47. London: Routledge, 1992.

Maclean, Ian. *Logic, Signs and Nature in the Renaissance: The Case of Learned Medicine.* Cambridge: Cambridge University Press, 2002.

Malgaigne, Joseph-François. *Œuvres complètes d'Ambroise Paré, revues et collationnées sur toutes les éditions antérieurs.* Paris: Baillière, 1840–41.

Mannacio, Anna Teresa. "Teoria e pratica della chirurgia nella Scuola dello «Spedale» fiorentino di Santa Maria Nuova tra XVII e XVIII secolo." *Atti e Memorie dell'Accademia di scienze e lettere La Colombaria* 54 (2003): 189–206.

Marini, Gaetano. *Degli Archiatri pontifici*. Rome: Pagliarini, 1784.

Martinez Vidal, Alvarez, and José Pardo Tomas. "Anatomical Theatres and the Teaching of Anatomy in Early Modern Spain." *Medical History* 49 (2005): 251–80.

McVaugh, Michael. *The Rational Surgery of the Middle Ages*. Florence, Italy: SISMEL- Edizioni del Galluzzo, 2006.

Notificazione sopra diversi oggetti concernenti l'osservanza regolare de' canonici dell'ordine di S. Spirito. Rome: Puccinelli, 1816.

Nuovo, Angela. *The Book Trade in Renaissance Italy*. Leiden, Netherlands: Brill, 2015.

Nutton, Vivian. "Humanist Surgery." In *The Medical Renaissance of the Sixteenth Century*, edited by Andrew Wear, Roger K. French, and Ian M. Lonie, 75–99. Cambridge: Cambridge University Press, 1985.

Palmer, Richard. "Physicians and Surgeons in Sixteenth-Century Venice." *Medical History* 23 (1979): 451–60.

Park, Katharine. *Doctors and Medicine in Early Renaissance Florence*. Princeton, NJ: Princeton University Press, 1985.

Pastore, Alessandro. *Il medico in tribunale. La perizia medica nella procedura penale di antico regime (sec. XVI–XVIII)*. Bellinzona, Switzerland: Casagrande, 1998.

Pelling, Margaret. "Occupational Diversity: Barber-Surgeons and the Trades of Norwich, 1550–1640." *Bulletin for the History of Medicine* 56 (1982): 484–511.

Pericoli, Pietro. *L'Ospedale di S. Maria della Consolazione di Roma dalle sue origini ai giorni nostril*. Imola, Italy: Galeati, 1879.

Piazza, Bartolomeo. *Eusevologio romano*. Rome: Hercoli, 1698.

Piccialuti, Maura. *La carità come metodo di governo. Istituzioni caritative a Roma dal pontificato di Innocenzo XII a quello di Benedetto XIV*. Turin, Italy: Giappichelli, 1991.

Pizzaleo Antonello. "Guattani, Carlo." In *Dizionario Biografico degli Italiani*, vol. 60. Rome: Istituto dell'Enciclopedia Italiana, 2003.

Posterla, Francesco. *Esatissima descrizione dell'istoria rappresentante la dimostrazione anatomica nel ven archiospedale della Consolatione di Roma*. Rome: Corbelletti, 1710.

Rabier, Christelle. "Medicalizing the Surgical Trade, 1650–1820: Workers, Knowledge, Markets and Politics." In *The Palgrave Handbook of the History of Surgery*, edited by Thomas Schlick, 71–94. London: Palgrave MacMillan, 2018.

Regole da osservarsi nel sacro, ed apostolico Archiospedale di Santo Spirito. Rome: Pagliarini, 1751.

Regole per il buon governo dell'archispedale della santissima Consolatione di Roma rinovate l'anno MDCLXXXVI. Rome: Corbelletti, 1686.

Saulnier, Pierre. *De capite sacri Ordinis Sancti Spiritus dissertatio*. Lyons, France: Barbier, 1649.

Savio, Pietro. "Ricerche su medici e chirurgi dell'Ospedale di Santo Spirito nel XVI–XVII secolo." *Archivio della Società Romana di Storia Patria* 25 (1971): 145–67.

– "Ricerche sull'anatomico Guglielmo Riva." *Bolletino storico-bibliografico subalpino* 66 (1968): 229–67.

Savoia, Paolo. *Cosmesi e chirurgia. Bellezza, dolore e medicina nell'Italia moderna*. Milan, Italy: Editrice Bibliografica, 2017.

– "Skills, Knowledge and Status: The Career of an Early Modern Italian Surgeon." *Bulletin for the History of Medicine* 93 (2019): 27–54.

Siraisi, Nancy G. "Medicine, 1450–1620, and the History of Science." *Isis* 103 (2012): 491–514.

Statuta Collegii DD. Almae Urbis Medicorum, ex antiquis Romanorum Pontificum Bullis congesta et hactenus per Sedem Apostolicam recognita et innovatae. Rome: Reverenda Camera Apostolica, 1676.

Statuti del venerabile archiospidale di San Giacomo in Augusta nominato dell'Incurabili di Roma. Rome: Reverenda Camera Apostolica, 1659.

Tabanelli, Mario. *Tecniche e strumenti chirurgici del XIII e XIV secolo*. Florence, Italy: Olschki, 1973.

Vanti, Mario. *S. Giacomo degli incurabili di Roma nel Cinquecento. Dalle compagnie del divino amore a s. Camillo de Lellis*. Rome: Pustet, 1938.

Waddington, Keir. *Medical Education at St Bartholomew's Hospital 1123–1995*. Oxford, UK: Boydell Press, 2003.

Wear, Andrew. *Knowledge and Practice in English Medicine, 1550–1680*. Cambridge: Cambridge University Press, 2000.

PART TWO

Social (In)Justice:
Racism, Inequities,
(De)Colonization

6

The "Indian Predicament": Medical Education and the Nation in India, 1880–1956

Anna Ruddock and Pratik Chakrabarti

There is a general consensus among historians that health care in colonial India was largely, if not exclusively, enclavist in nature and that it originated with a concern for the number of British troops who sickened and died in the encounter with unfamiliar climates and pathogens.[1] The slow shift to a concern with the health of the Indian population was largely provoked by epidemics of cholera and plague in the late nineteenth and early twentieth centuries.[2] On the whole, the colonial approach to public health in India was insubstantial and ineffectual, and reflected the administration's reluctance to intervene, for reasons usually cited as either political or economic, but which were more likely an amalgam of the two.[3] The history of medical education in India, too, is one of political economy, and of contested forms of knowledge and power. Medical education both engendered and was burdened by the political and economic ambitions of India as an emergent nation. In this chapter, we trace the expansion of Western medical training in India through the colonial period and its entanglement with the growing nationalist movement. Then we enter the early decades of independent India to look at the establishment of the All India Institute of Medical Sciences (AIIMS) as an example of the tension in an approach to medical education that placed cutting-edge science at the rhetorical heart of post-colonial development, while expecting an urban-trained elite to respond to the needs of a predominantly rural and impoverished population without infrastructure or incentive. That tension endures today.

THE INDIAN MEDICAL SERVICE AND COLONIAL MEDICAL EDUCATION

The Indian Medical Service (IMS) originated with the "surgeons" placed on East India Company ships – a service organized by the company's own surgeon-general as early as 1614. By the 1670s, these surgeons were recruited specifically to serve the company's civil employees in India, and by the time recruitment began for its standing army in 1749, it recorded thirty "medical men" in its Indian employ. Between the newly established Medical Services of Calcutta, Bombay, and Madras, the numbers of medical employees grew significantly from 1763 onwards: by 1823, there were 630 commissioned officers in the medical departments of the three presidencies.[4]

Various medical colleges in India taught Western medicine,[5] including the Madras Medical College (1835), Grant Medical College, Bombay (1845), and Lahore Medical College (1860). More followed in the early twentieth century, including Lady Hardinge Medical College for Women in Delhi (1916), and others in Patna, Lucknow, Bombay, and Vizagapatnam.[6] Before 1860, other than at these colleges, medical education in India generally took the form of apprenticeships, as it did in Britain. Between 1860 and 1914, however, the IMS determined and controlled the hierarchy of medical education. Medical *schools*, which offered short courses for employment in auxiliary medical services, were subordinated to medical *colleges*, where courses led to university qualifications that allowed a student to take the IMS exam, and whose degrees (from 1892) were recognized in the Colonial List of the British General Medical Council (GMC) in London.

There were some pre-existing medical institutions in the early nineteenth century, which provided more hybrid instruction. The Native Medical Institution had been established in Calcutta in 1822. Students were taught European medical texts translated into Indian languages and they took classes in the Indigenous medical systems of Unani and Ayurveda. Dissection was carried out only on animal bodies, a fact that would prove central to the closure of the institution.[7] This arrangement referenced a political atmosphere in which the parallel existence and occasional syncretism of Western and Indian knowledge systems was tolerated by the colonial administration, and expressly promoted by the era's "Orientalists." An attitudinal shift was expressed in both the report on medical education requested by the Governor of Bengal, William Bentinck, in 1833, and Thomas Macaulay's "Minute on Indian Education" in 1835, which argued for the promotion of Western science and literature through exclusively English-medium curricula.[8]

The Native Medical Institution was replaced by the Medical College in 1835. The first institution in India to teach Western medicine solely in English, its mission was to teach "the principles and practice of the medical science in strict accordance with the mode adopted in Europe."[9] In an effort to stress the parity between Indian and British institutions, the Indian colleges periodically raised their entrance requirements, creating a new market for the medical schools among candidates who did not qualify for college entrance.[10]

The bureaucratic consolidation of Western medicine's supremacy over Indigenous practice stretched into the twentieth century: by the 1920s, medical education "was caught between conflicting pressures of nationalism and a swiftly changing, increasingly scientized European medicine."[11] The Medical Registration Acts and Medical Degrees Act passed between 1912 and 1919 had excluded practitioners trained in Indigenous medicine from claiming the title of "doctor." However, the 1919 Montagu-Chelmsford reforms allowed Indian nationalist politicians to implement policies despite the opposition of British medical advisors, and the Indian National Congress (INC) began to pass resolutions in support of Indigenous medicine. The two positions were never fully reconciled within the party[12]: self-proclaimed modernizers such as Jawaharlal Nehru supported the expansion of Western medicine, while the new regional legislative councils supported Indigenous medicine on nationalist and economic grounds.[13]

The GMC made it clear that Indian medical degrees would only receive international recognition if there was a clear distinction between practitioners trained in Western medicine and those who had studied Indigenous systems. Initial support within the All India Medical Association (1928, later renamed the Indian Medical Association) for the inclusion of Indigenous practitioners was withdrawn, and a separate register for Indigenous doctors was established in Bombay Presidency in 1938.[14]

The numbers of medical colleges, schools, and students grew hesitantly during the nineteenth century, although figures for those who passed the final exams belie the broader impact of medical education. For example, of 2,511 students enrolled at medical colleges in 1916–17, only 512 sat the final exams, and of them 329 passed.[15] However, there were plentiful opportunities for students who left the colleges without a formal qualification to enter private practice, or to take up appointments in one of India's many princely states not directly governed by the British, given the absence of a regulated medical market.[16] This was a somewhat paradoxical outcome for the colonial government from a functional perspective, but the nineteenth-century drive to disseminate the scientific bounty of the Enlightenment among colonized populations was not always separable from the economic motivations of colonialism. An explanation of British policies towards nineteenth-century medical education in India confirms this:

The object [of medical education] was not merely to secure a constant supply of subordinate medical officers for the Government service but also to raise the standard of medical knowledge and encourage the practice of medicine and surgery on established scientific principles.

> That private practitioners possessing the necessary qualifications
> should be able to compete successfully with public medical charities is a
> satisfactory result.[17]

Objections became apparent, however, when Indian doctors threatened the private practice of IMS members. In response, the IMS determinedly prevented Indians from attaining prestigious positions as attending doctors and teachers at major hospitals, as we discuss in the following section.

The grip of the IMS tightened in the early twentieth century, as the GMC began to scrutinize Indian medical education more closely. In 1930, the GMC withdrew recognition of Indian degrees until an Indian medical council was established. As Jeffery puts it, "the rhetoric was that Indian graduates who wished to practise in Britain should meet British standards, but the implications were to affect the patterns of medical education in and for India thereafter."[18]

When the Medical Council of India was established in 1933, the medical schools were excluded from its terms, triggering an effort to dismantle India's "two-tier" system of medical education. Where possible, schools were to be upgraded to colleges, and otherwise closed. The policy received wide support: school-educated doctors hoped to receive the benefits of college graduates; British members of the IMS hoped it would end London's concerns about Indian standards of education; and nationalists were uncomfortable with the notion that medical schools implied second-class care and prompted international mistrust of Indian qualifications. By 1938, the decision was taken to close the medical schools altogether.

THE GRAVE MORAL QUESTION

One of the primary features of medical education in early-twentieth-century India was the tussle between Indian and British doctors and medical students for gaining access to IMS recruitment, and by extension to prestigious positions at prominent medical colleges. Until the 1850s, employment as a doctor did not demand any official qualification. Before 1800 only 6 per cent of doctors had attended a medical school, and at least half had no qualification of any kind. By 1860, however, a growing number of IMS recruits had gained a diploma from the Royal College of Surgeons (RCS) in London or from the Scottish Royal College of Physicians (RCP).[19] Competitive examinations for entry to the IMS were first held in 1855 and were theoretically open to Indians, but the location of the examination centres in London ensured that in practice only 55 Indians had entered by 1913, forming 5 per cent of the Service. By 1921, this had only risen to 6.25 per cent.[20] Some of these early recruits resigned from the service within a short period, citing discrimination by British officers; this criticism would become more audible during the 1920s and 1930s.[21] The pre-eminence of the IMS within the Indian medical education system needs to be seen within wider developments in British imperial medicine from the mid-nineteenth century. Douglas M. Haynes has shown that the GMC, formed in 1858, sought to create a homogenized British medical culture across its empire, by privileging white, male British graduates, through its control of the medical register well into the twentieth century.[22] Indian graduates were fighting this regime of privilege.

While the Indian medical colleges had produced Indian doctors, opportunities for clinical practice and teaching were limited by the dominance of IMS members. In response, Indian doctors formed their own organizations such as the Bombay Medical Union (BMU) in 1883 and the Calcutta Medical Club in 1906. The activities of the groups were mainly directed towards "enhancing the status and dignity of the Indian medical profession."[23] At a time of rising nationalism in the early twentieth century, the BMU in partnership with the nationalist INC challenged the monopoly of the IMS.[24] They demanded greater inclusion of Indian doctors in the IMS cadre and more opportunities for Indian medical graduates outside the IMS in government medical colleges. The BMU wrote to the Royal Commission on the Public Services in India under the chairmanship of Lord Islington (1913), demanding that the IMS examinations be held simultaneously in Britain and India, arguing that the supposedly "open" biennial IMS examinations in London were to all intents and purposes "shut" to the majority of Indians.[25] The letter asserted, "It is high time now that the noxious overgrowth of this service [IMS] were cut off and the numerous civil posts thus liberated from it were thrown open to the indigenous talent of proved merit and ability."[26]

The British Medical Association (BMA) sent its own memorandum to the same commission warning against the Indianization of the IMS. According to the BMA, the "educated Indians who have been trained in our colleges" posed a "grave moral question" for "the future welfare of India in general and the standard of medical education in particular":

The Government of India and the millions it rules will obviously be the first losers, and in this loss its European and Indian subjects will share alike. More gradually, but with equal certainty, the standard of education will fall, thereby inflicting lasting injury on the health of the people. Last, but not the least, comes a grave moral question; India wants our best, in all departments of service. Those who know the Indian most intimately, and who admire most intelligently his many excellent qualities as a professional man, cannot blind themselves to the fact that his standards are still far from being those of his British brother.[27]

The commission made some concessions. It recommended that recruitment to senior posts should be made in both England and India. However, it rejected the main demand to hold competitive exams simultaneously in England and India.[28]

The career of Dr Jivraj N. Mehta (1887–1978), an influential member of the BMU, provides an insight into the history of this conflict over medical knowledge and professional power between Indian and British doctors. Mehta received his first medical degree from the Grant Medical College in Bombay in 1908 and passed his MD examinations in London at the London Hospital Medical College in 1914. He returned to India in 1915, and participated in the nationalist movement and the establishment of one of the most important pre-Independence medical colleges, the Seth Gordhandas Sunderdas Medical College (GS). After Independence, he became minister of finance, prohibition and industries, and later chief minister of the newly formed Gujarat state, as well as Indian High Commissioner to the United Kingdom.[29]

While in London between 1909 and 1915 as a medical student, Mehta became the president of the Indian Students Association. The Association looked after the immediate interests of Indian students studying in England and campaigned for greater inclusion of Indian students in various imperial services, including the IMS. Under Mehta's leadership, the Association sent a statement to the newly established Royal Commission on Public Services in India to explain that while the commission was intended to review educational institutions in India, the situation of Indian students in Britain was "getting worse." The statement complained that the educational institutions in Britain from which most of the imperial public services recruited were "slowly but steadily closing their doors against Indians." The association claimed that London medical colleges were restricting the admission of Indian students, who, as British subjects, should have had equal access to those institutions.[30] It suggested that these colleges should be banned from sending their graduates to sit for the IMS exams. It also alleged that the Indian Students Department, which was formed in 1909 by the British government to ostensibly look after Indian students studying in Britain, was being used to whitewash the real grievances of the Indian students: "we are practically insulted by the existence of the Indian Students' Department, which embodies the official belief that we are either a set of undesirables or incapables."[31] The association also asked that the standards of teaching at Indian medical colleges be improved. It held that despite the curriculum being equal to its British equivalent, poor teaching placed Indian students at a disadvantage when competing with British students in the IMS exams.[32]

Mehta returned to India in 1915 and soon became involved in setting the agenda for nationalist medical education. In a post–World War I context of strained human and financial resources, the government of India actively supported the establishment of private medical institutions. This was also when several colleges of Indigenous medicine, such as the Ayurvedic and Unani Tibbia College in Delhi (1921), were established. The Belgachhia Medical College (later renamed RG Kar Medical College) was established in Calcutta in 1916.[33] Also in 1916, Seth Gordhandas, a Bombay entrepreneur, established an endowment fund for the establishment of a new hospital and medical teaching institution in the city. Until then the Grant Medical College had been the only teaching institution serving the growing metropolis. In this context of increased pressure on medical institutions, the King Edward Memorial hospital (KEM) and GS were established in 1926. The people of Bombay contributed to the fund, and the local government provided the site of an old government house, where the new hospital was built.[34] The GS was located in Parel, a populous and industrial part of the city away from the other medical centres (which were further south), where it served mostly mill workers and their families. It worked closely with the Wadia Maternity Hospital, which was established around the same time, and provided facilities for training in midwifery.

Mehta became the first dean of the KEM and GS in 1926 and defined its principles of medical education in accordance with the Indian nationalist agenda. One of these was that "no member of the staff of this college shall be in Government Service."[35] It was one of the first Indian medical colleges to be almost exclusively staffed by qualified Indian doctors outside government service – and implicitly outside the IMS. The GS and KEM, similar to the Hackett Medical College for Women (HMCW) in China, were much more than just institutions of medical education. As the HMCW became a source of Chinese emancipation (as elaborated in chapter 12 in this volume), these two institutions in Bombay represented the wider ambitions of an emergent nation and its search for autonomy.

In the inter-war period, the Rockefeller Foundation of New York began to play an increasingly active role in funding medical research, education, and facilities in various parts of Asia.[36] Between 1926 and 1927, Dr William S. Carter, a doctor and director of medical education at the Foundation, conducted a thorough evaluation of India's medical colleges, including the GS. Carter was impressed with the new medical college. He recorded that it had "splendid buildings and equipment with excellent laboratory and clinical facilities for teaching, and a staff of able Indians who had good preparation for the positions they hold." The number of students admitted each year was limited to 60, the laboratory could accommodate at least 80, and the hospital had 300 beds. Carter found this to be in "striking contrast with the overcrowding which existed in the Grant Medical College."[37]

He also noted tensions and antagonism between the GS and government-funded medical institutions.[38] British doctors and IMS officers referred to the GS as "an anti-government and political movement" and a legacy of the Non-Cooperation Movement of 1919–20 led by the Indian National Congress against imperial rule. During his visit, Carter met Mehta to discuss these complaints. Mehta insisted that the GS was not an "anti-government" institution, but practised what he described as "natural selection" in order to counteract conditions that privileged government medical officers. He explained that officers of the IMS held all the teaching positions in institutions such as the Grant Medical College, from which he had graduated. These appointments were often not decided according to curriculum requirements but based on the availability of medical officers. Therefore, an officer who taught botany at one time could teach surgery at another. There were also frequent changes in the teaching faculty, as the officers were called up for military service. For Mehta, the practice of excluding government medical officers was a means of creating a stable, dedicated, and specialized teaching faculty for medicine, along with providing opportunities to Indians who had trained in medicine and not joined the government service.[39] On other occasions, Mehta complained about the disparities in salaries of professors and assistant professors and the hierarchical nature of medical colleges. "This has been the bane of the whole educational and medical policy of the British Government," he said.[40]

Mehta's efforts remained anomalous in the wider landscape of medical education in India in the inter-war period. Even as the administration of local health policy and bureaucracy was increasingly devolved to the provinces, the colonial government retained central supervision of the IMS, rather than allowing nationalist politicians further autonomy. This arrangement entrenched the deep suspicion of the IMS among the nationalists and likely informed the decision to abolish it in 1947 and distribute power over medical civil servants to local governments.[41]

THE INDIAN JOHNS HOPKINS

The Health Survey and Development Committee was appointed in October 1943 and was subsequently known as the Bhore Committee after its chairman, Sir Joseph Bhore, a senior civil servant. It was partly an effort to assuage the Indian elite through a demonstration of concern for national welfare in the wake of the recently launched Quit India movement, but it also presaged a broader post-war shift in the West from laissez-faire to greater state interventionism.[42] Its task was twofold: to conduct a "broad survey of the present position in regard to health conditions and health organisation in British India," and to provide "recommendations for future developments."[43]

The four-volume Bhore Report presented in 1946 was implicitly critical of the colonial neglect of Indian public health and of the defeatist attitude of the civil service in the face of a task of such magnitude. The report promoted the dovetailing of preventive and curative care, with recommendations encompassing medical care, education, and administration. Although not without dispute, the report endorsed the policy that saw the closure or upgrading of medical schools.[44] While a minority of members argued for the rapid expansion of all levels of medical education, the report ultimately recommended that India should focus its limited resources on "the highly trained type of physician whom we have termed the 'basic doctor.'"[45]

In 1943, the year of the Bhore Committee's appointment, the colonial government invited Professor A.V. Hill, secretary of the Royal Society in London, and a deputation[46] to visit India and "advise it on the future of scientific research in the context of development."[47] Their report focused on education:

> For the most effective way of producing a change in all this would be to set out deliberately to create teachers and research workers of a new kind, people who would devote their lives to the single object of advancing in India the art, science and practice of medicine. For this purpose a great All-India Medical Centre should be established, an "Indian Johns Hopkins" staffed in all departments by the ablest people available anywhere, employed full-time and adequately paid. The students of the All-India Medical Centre should be highly selected ones, preferably with good degrees in arts or science as a start: and since a large proportion of the most desirable students cannot meet the financial cost of a long training in medicine, all who require help should be given it in the form of scholarships or bursaries ... The intention of the All-India Medical Centre would be to produce the future leaders of Indian medicine and public health, the teachers and research workers.[48]

During the visit, Hill had detailed discussions with members of the Bhore Committee about an institute that would reflect this need for greater integration, the plan for which was briefly known as "Prof. Hill's scheme."[49] Two years later, the Bhore Report included the recommendation that an All-India Medical Institute be established:

> The objects of the Institute should be 1) to bring together in one place educational facilities of the very highest order for the training of all the more important types of health personnel and to emphasize the close interrelation which exists between the different branches of professional education in the field of health; 2) to promote research of the highest type ... ; 3) to co-ordinate training and research; 4) to provide

postgraduate training of an advanced character in an atmosphere which will foster the true scientific outlook and a spirit of initiative; 5) to inspire all persons who undergo training, undergraduate or postgraduate, with the high ideals of the profession to which they belong and 6) to promote in them a community outlook and a high degree of culture, in order that they may become active apostles of the progressive spirit in whatever field they may be called upon to serve.[50]

The ideal of engaging medical education with research, which was behind the suggestions for the All-India Medical Institute, had a wider resonance in the 1940s. A medical mission, chaired by the director general of the IMS, J.B. Hance, and comprising prominent British and Indian doctors and scientists such as C.G. Pandit and W.R. Aykroyd, reported to the Bhore committee in 1944.[51] Among the main problems they highlighted was that in India medical research was distanced from medical education:

The unanimous testimony of the members of the Advisory Committee on Medical Research, of the witnesses examined by them, and of the members of the various groups which have recently toured India, has been that, broadly speaking, medical research receives little or no attention in the Medical Colleges of India.[52]

The main problem was the lack of funding and research staff: "In brief, the absence of research in Medical Colleges in India may be attributed to men and money."[53] The report recommended the nationwide integration of medical research, training, and hospitals.[54] A.V. Hill made a similar point in his report:

The process, therefore, of setting up separate institutes in India for medical research has probably gone far enough: and some advantage would now result from bringing existing research institutes, where practicable, into closer contact with the medical colleges and higher medical education.[55]

Following the submission of Hill's report in 1945, Pandit, a London-trained virologist who was director of the King Institute of Preventive Medicine and Research in Madras, was deputed to accompany Hance on a research trip to the UK, US, and Canada "to study and report on the modern trends in medical education and research." The trip placed particular emphasis on Johns Hopkins University, which was Hill's suggested model for an All India Medical Centre.[56] The terms of reference included the following:

Enquiries should be directed primarily towards securing information which would be of value in the preparations of plans for the organisation of a medical training and research centre, the purpose of which will be to train men, who will eventually be leaders of the medical profession, especially teachers and research workers. *It should be borne in mind that the primary object of such an institution will not be advancement of scientific knowledge, but the training of students.*[57]

In Britain, the Goodenough Committee, which was established to enquire into the changes required in medical education in Britain, released its report in 1944, recommending "the reorganization of medical education and research," particularly for a comprehensive National Health Service.[58] The wartime deputation under Hance and Pandit stated in its own report that "throughout the English speaking world a great renaissance in health provision and education is in formulation and the end of hostilities will see a burst of progress in matter [*sic*] of health unprecedented in history."[59] This reformist enthusiasm permeated discussions during the consultation period, particularly at the University of Oxford, which was developing its own plans for an undergraduate medical school that would adopt innovative teaching arrangements.[60]

Following consultations with the medical faculty of Liverpool University, Professor R.A. Morlan sent a letter to the committee urging that the specificities of India be given as much consideration as international models in establishing the new institute. India, he said, promised new scope for preventive medicine and research, all of which could be part of its new medical training:

In both teaching and research, it could be held that relevance to India should decide priorities. I do not mean simply utility but relevance in [a] wider sense ... The whole problem of geography in relation to disease affords an instance of a long term programme of research to which individuals could contribute and the institute could act as the unifying agency and building up its own peculiar prestige, team spirit and continuity ... One would think that medical anthropology could be cultivated in India as nowhere else. Similarly the problem of "putting over" preventive medicine affects all the world but India affords a unique laboratory for research in the borderland between education and medicine. I hope this makes clear what I mean by relevance as a strategic aim. The Institute should be *itself*, an Indian [*sic*], not a transplanted Johns Hopkins or Mount Vernon.[61]

This fed into the work of the Bhore Committee, whose own report in 1946 led to the establishment of a committee tasked with implementing the All India Medical Institute project. According to Pandit, the plan was shelved for some time due to financial constraints; the upgrading of certain departments in existing medical colleges was agreed as an interim measure, "where suitable leadership was available."[62] Nevertheless, the newly independent Indian government recorded its intention to establish the recommended institution in its first five-year plan (1951–56), and the project was revived by the allocation of a $1.25 million grant by the Government of New Zealand under the auspices of the Colombo Plan.[63] The foundation stone of the All India Institute of Medical Sciences (AIIMS) was laid by New Zealand's minister of industries and commerce in 1952, and the Institute opened in 1956.[64]

JAWAHARLAL NEHRU AND THE SCIENCE OF DEVELOPMENT

The AIIMS foundation stone embodies the intention to place science and technology at the service of post-colonial national development. AIIMS was initially conceived in a report commissioned by the colonial administration. That it was finally built and inaugurated under the auspices of an independent Indian government, with international funding, suggested less an epistemic break in scientific discourse than an opportunity to build on the legacy of Jivraj Mehta and others through a potent narrative that blended the challenges facing the new nation with the promise of scientific remedy. Referring to India's first prime minister, Jawaharlal Nehru, Jahnavi Phalkey describes this developmental discourse as "Nehruvian optimism."[65]

David Arnold suggests that Nehru's understanding of science was not only technical, but also "philosophical and literary," which informed his determination to confirm "the centrality of science in the autobiography of the Indian nation."[66] Science was to serve national interests and inform the redressal of social ills, including disease and poverty. AIIMS represented this intention, and also stood as a symbol of the new government's determined march towards a transnational standard of modernity as represented by science.[67] Despite Pandit's stated ambition for AIIMS to be an "Indian institute established in India, for the training of Indian workers by Indians," the institute carried a wider mandate. When A.L. Mudaliar, chair of the AIIMS planning committee, spoke at the first meeting of the Central Council of Health in 1953, he argued that undergraduate education at AIIMS should be "along the most modern lines that are accepted in international circles":

> It is very important for us to realise that we must look to international standards … When it comes to a question of helping in the cure of the sick and the general welfare of the community you cannot afford to forget international standards or lower your standards below the international level. If you do that, you will be the worse for it.[68]

The preoccupation with Western standards of science and their application to national imperatives was expressed most explicitly through Health Minister Rajkumari Amrit Kaur's speech when she presented the All India Institute of Medical Sciences Bill to Parliament on 18 February 1956. The speech highlights all that was intended to be unique about AIIMS, but also contains insurmountable contradictions of purpose that have had consequences for medical practice within and outside the institute. Towards the beginning of the speech, Kaur asserts:

> Medical education must, above all, take into account the special needs of the country from the point of view of affording health protection to the people ... the continued prevalence of various forms of preventable causes of sickness and suffering necessitates special emphases, if I may so put it, on the preventive aspect of medical care. Further, the extent to which [a doctor] develops a community outlook and a desire to serve the people. Medical education, moreover, is receiving considerable attention in all the progressive countries of the world. I have had the privilege recently to see what is being done in the USA, in the USSR, in Scandinavia and even in the UK to bring it more and more into consonance with present day needs and to promote an increasing realization of the object of equipping the future doctor to give of his best to the community. India cannot afford to keep apart from this broad and steady programme of development that is taking place in other parts of the world.[69]

Shortly afterwards, Kaur notes the initial role of the institute:

> [We are] going to start with a medical training centre which will provide undergraduate study to only a very limited few. *The major emphasis will be on post-graduate study and specialization,* because one reason for our inability to fulfil the desire of so many States today to have medical colleges is the lack of personnel.[70]

In a converse arrangement to that at the GS in Bombay decades earlier, the speech goes on to note the special measure of prohibiting private practice by AIIMS doctors and compensating them with higher salaries to ensure their exclusive focus on the Institute, and the importance of a residential campus to ensure a personal *guru-shishya*, or teacher-student, relationship, in the spirit of one Indian tradition of education. Students were to be given "ample opportunities to participate in both urban and rural health work," and the curriculum was to encourage "a community outlook and also promote powers of initiative and observation and of drawing conclusions from them." The Institute would be "given the powers and functions of a University because it will probably make revolutionary changes, as I hope, in curriculum as well as in modes of teaching," and would "enjoy a large measure of autonomy in order that it may fulfil the objectives." While the government would provide the primary funding for the maintenance of the Institute, Kaur hoped that "philanthropy also will come to the aid, as it so often does, of such institutions because, after all, serving the cause of sick and suffering humanity is always something that appeals to those who would like to give."

In the conclusion of her speech, she stressed that the future of the institute lay in the hands of its members:

I believe it will be their devotion to duty, their desire to promote their work and the spirit of altruism that will actuate [*sic*] them to subordinate personal considerations, as I believe the noble profession of medicine should do, to the fulfilment of the objectives to be achieved that will eventually create and maintain the atmosphere which is necessary for an Institute like this. I therefore do hope that in presenting this Bill for acceptance by Parliament today, the legal structure that is created may facilitate the medical education in the Institute and that, through the influence it exerts, the standards of different forms of professional training in the field of health throughout the country will be raised.[71]

The ambition articulated for the new institution was formidable.[72] AIIMS was intended to transform the nature of medical education and practice in the nation, while deliberately catering to a small number of students to ensure a unique pedagogical experience. Students were to develop a community outlook, to possess a commitment to national service in both rural and urban settings, to develop (in an echo of the Bhore Report) a preventive orientation, and to emulate Western "progress" while responding to Indian needs, while the greater purpose was to focus on post-graduate specialization and the training of teachers. In 1973's *Medicine and Society*, Henry Miller described this as the "Indian predicament":

[T]he Indian predicament is characteristic and understandable. Unless the government trains a medical *corps d'elite* it will be unable to undertake the practical research into preventive medicine that is central to the Indian situation. Furthermore, it will demoralize the medical profession to whom involvement in high technology is a matter of national pride, even if it is not always so easy to justify on utilitarian grounds.[73]

There was an infectious energy in the national ambitions articulated through AIIMS, and also an almost poignant recognition of the scale of the challenge expected to be met by an institution without sufficient supporting primary and secondary infrastructure to protect its mandate, or to ensure that the students it produced were willing and able to establish careers at home rather than leaving the country, as so many of them did.

By 1956, the first year of AIIMS, "technology" was taking precedence over "science" as a key trope in Nehru's speeches. He spoke often about the need to think about the demands of the national planning process "in technological terms."[74] Great energy went into the establishment of the Indian Institutes of Technology in the 1950s, a set of institutions that, in a broader sense than AIIMS, were expected to produce graduates who would shape the future of the country. Arnold suggests that "medicine and public health never stood quite so high in Nehru's esteem" as more explicitly technological pursuits.[75] In the speeches that Arnold cites, however, what is striking is less a lack of esteem for medicine and public health than Nehru's grappling with two separate but related challenges: first, that technology did not offer and could not be considered a magic bullet for public health; and second, how to reconcile a principle of quality over quantity in medical education with the glaring need for a huge number of trained health care professionals. These tensions have always been, and remain, intrinsic to AIIMS.

Despite Nehru's commitment to technology as a tool of national development, in the 1950s he was well aware of the pitfalls of adhering to high technology alone as a public health solution and he foresaw the detrimental consequences of a singular focus on individualized, curative, and largely urban medicine. However, it is also clear, in his address to the silver jubilee celebrations of the Medical Council of India in 1959, that while he was unhappy about the lack of progress in providing comprehensive health care beyond the cities, he did not consider this the sole responsibility of central government:

Now, in spite of 25 years of the All India Medical Council, India is still very poor in the quality of its doctors. In reality and in effect there are vast areas of India where there is practically no medical help available … I do not quite know if you have given thought to this matter. It should be the function of the Medical Council to make suggestions or lay down some rules and regulations even, that it should be incumbent on every new practitioner before he can even practise anywhere to spend a couple of years in a village or in some rural area … It would be a good thing if the Medical Council itself went into this question and laid down some kind of a rule or regulation rather than for Government and Parliament to come in and do something of the kind.[76]

Whether or not it was the lingering influence of the Bhore Report, or a result of Nehru's own observations, or both, he maintained his conviction that social and preventive medicine should take priority, even as he watched the opposite trend become entrenched:

> The actual day-to-day work of a doctor should become more and more preventive than actual treatment, although the latter is of importance. We put up big hospitals and that is inevitable. You must have some big hospitals where there is a concentration of work, but one cannot put up these big hospitals all over India, or even smaller hospitals but rather on a large scale. We should evolve some way of giving medical services to the villagers, because I am constantly thinking as to how to deal with them.[77]

While the prime minister clearly had strong convictions about health and medicine, he did not afford them his direct oversight – unlike the Department of Atomic Energy, for example, of which he retained personal control.[78] This greater distance might partly explain the rather abstract language of hope germane to Nehru's speeches about health and medical policy:

> I should like you to think of these problems which are really vital problems for us, in a sense more vital than the individual big problems of big hospitals and all that you have to deal with. Ultimately, I hope that there would be free medical services for anyone who requires it in India, and high standards of public health.[79]

Five years later, at the second convocation of AIIMS in 1964, Nehru articulated similar preoccupations, with quantity versus quality, technologized curative medicine versus preventive public health care, urban versus rural practice, and here he also dwelt on his concern that India's tradition of Indigenous medicine and learning should not be forgotten. In comparison with the rousing call to arms Nehru delivered to the graduates of IIT Kharagpur in 1951, however, his 1964 address was notably sober, almost weary, as he confronted the divergent challenges that the country still faced in its effort to improve the health of its people. He noted with approval the study of preventive and social medicine at AIIMS and stated that he considered it "particularly important in the modern age."[80] The subject should be, Nehru said, "the dominant function of the Institute and the people who go out of this Institute, because social medicine prevents those things happening which require treatment later on. I hope enough attention will be paid to the social aspects of medicine."[81]

This challenge echoes the parliamentary speech of Amrit Kaur in 1956, wherein the AIIMS mandate was to be at once an exclusive centre of cutting-edge research and technology, and an incubator of doctors who would take social and preventive medicine to the rest of India. "It is comforting," Nehru went on, "to find that your Institute has not so much cared for quantity as for quality. It is essential that we should have higher standards at the top as these will determined the quality of work below to a large extent."[82] Having discussed the need for rural doctors, he then admitted the overwhelming scale of the challenge and his own uncertainty about the remedy:

One thing that troubles me is that in spite of such fine institutes as this one, yet there are vast areas in this country … where the benefits of modern medicine do not reach and sometimes we are rather overwhelmed by the problem. So many people are wanted there – qualified physicians, surgeons and properly equipped institutions – and we have so few. It is obvious that, however good an institute like this may be, that is essential of course; one can only be satisfied if it reaches down to the villages and if thousands, hundreds of thousands of villages feel the impact of it. I do not know how we are going to train the people in such large numbers to go there; and I will suggest to you, those who are trained, have received the benefit of training at these special institutes, should always bear in mind the need of the people of India who live in the villages. Because they are in numbers as well as otherwise the real people of India and unless we know them, we do not function properly. And then how to deal with such vast numbers and how long it will take enough people to go there, is a difficult matter. Whether it is conceivable to have institutes at these villages, some kind of assistance to serve the community, bring up the real cases to experts or how to deal with it, I do not know. But something has to be done to bring modern medicine to the great majority of our people in the country.[83]

There is a retrospective poignancy to these words of an increasingly frail statesman, who once regularly noted the robustness of his health and the rarity with which he consulted doctors, but who could not offer answers to the questions of illness and death that afflicted so much of the population, beyond vaguely articulated hopes. Within two months of his address at AIIMS, Nehru died at the age of seventy-four.

CONCLUSION

Medical education in India was entangled within the broader struggle for civil rights in the colonial period, and then within post-colonial visions of development, health, economic prosperity and industrialization. The Western medical education established by the colonial regime was an elitist and systemically racist endeavour, which Indian politicians and physicians challenged from the early twentieth century. Indian doctors had a combined political and professional motivation for contesting colonial medical institutions, and their demands centred on the greater inclusion of Indians in medical college teaching positions. The Seth Gordhandas Sunderdas Medical College in Bombay was established both to train Indian doctors and to challenge colonial institutions of privilege by employing Indians who were not part of the Indian Medical Service.

Subsequently, in the post-colonial period, AIIMS carried the mandate of the new nation. Modelled on Johns Hopkins, it was to become the premiere medical institution of India, combining the finest research and medical facilities with high-quality training of new generations of Indian doctors. It was also intended to bring social medicine to the nation, to address its wider health challenges. Tasked with this complex mission, AIIMS was caught between the scientific and technological emphases of development and the larger challenges of poverty, population, malnutrition, sanitation, and inadequate medical infrastructure in most of the newly independent country. In this respect, AIIMS became emblematic of the history of medical education in India more broadly: representing the enduring tension between economic growth, social welfare, and the politics of medical professionals – many of whom emigrated upon graduation from AIIMS. Viewed in a contemporary light, while the fight for India's independence was won, the extent to which its approach to medical education has ever served the most pressing needs of its citizens remains a pertinent question.

NOTES

1   Arnold, *Colonizing the Body*; Harrison, *Public Health in British India*; Jeffery, *The Politics of Health in India*; Bhattacharya, *Contagion and Enclaves*.
2   India's mortality rate swelled from 41.3 per 1000 in the 1880s to 48.6 per 1000 in 1911–21; Arnold, *Colonizing the Body*, 200.
3   Amrith, *Decolonizing International Health*.
4   Jeffery, *The Politics of Health in India*, 60–1.
5   We use the description "Western medicine," rather than the more contemporary "biomedicine," in adherence to the terminology used during the period in

question. The term became more contested after 1947. India's first prime minister, Jawaharlal Nehru, preferred "modern medicine" as a means of signifying scientific knowledge that developed as a result of efforts in both the "West" and the "East"; Nehru, *Speeches*, 550. Of course, the longer history of medicine and healing in India begins with the region's earliest populations; Bala, *Medicine and Medical Policies in India.*

6   Jeffery, "Recognizing India's Doctors," 302–3.

7   See Bala, *Medicine and Medical Policies*, 27, for more on the historical politics of dissection that belie the colonial assumption that Indian Indigenous practitioners were averse to the practice by definition.

8   Bala, *Medicine and Medical Policies*, 72–4; Kumar, *Political Agenda of Education*, 52–4.

9   Crawford, *A History of the Indian Medical Service*, vol. 2, 436, cited in Jeffery, *The Politics of Health in India*, 78. Vernacular education was reintroduced at certain institutions (although not the teaching of Indigenous medicine), but was steadily transferred from the major medical colleges to peripheral schools in order to ensure good favour with the medical authorities in Britain: Kumar, *Political Agenda of Education*, 133–6.

10   Reliable data on the precise demographics of medical students is scarce, but we know that there was a broad dominance of high-caste Hindus (although fewer Brahmins than in other sectors of higher education; see Bala, *Medicine and Medical Policies in India*, 30, on the historical association of medicine with impure practice unbefitting Brahmins), and that Christians (initially European and later Eurasian or Anglo-Indian) were disproportionately represented, along with Parsis in Bombay. Muslims only began to be proportionately represented as a consequence of the introduction of reserved seats in the 1920s and 1930; Jeffery, *The Politics of Health in India*, 84.

11   Jeffery, *The Politics of Health in India*, 76.

12   Jeffery, "Doctors and Congress."

13   In later years Nehru seemed more concerned to recognise the achievements of India's own medical traditions, and he suggested in his convocation address to AIIMS graduates in 1964 that the Institute work to "bridge the gap" between the two traditions. Singh, *Jawaharlal Nehru on Science and Society*, 264–6.

14   Jeffery, *The Politics of Health in India*, 53–5.

15   Ibid.

16   Phadke, "Regulation of Doctors."

17   Bengal Administration Report, 1885, 306–7, cited in Jeffery, *The Politics of Health in India*, 83.

18   Jeffery, *The Politics of Health in India*, 33.

19   Harrison, *Public Health in British India*, 20–1.

20   Jeffery, "Recognizing India's Doctors," 311. Following the introduction of a

minimum quota for Indian recruits in 1919, the figure grew to 37 per cent by 1938. Jeffery attributes this rise more to a shortage of British applicants, given improved employment prospects for doctors in Britain, and to a perceived threat to senior positions inherent in the 1919 reforms, than to a willingness to cede more control to Indian medical officers.

21   Jeffery, *The Politics of Health in India*, 64.

22   Haynes, *Fit to Practice*.

23   Quoted in Ramanna, *Western Medicine and Public Health*, 3.

24   Ibid., 217–21.

25   *Representation of the Bombay Medical Union*, 1.

26   Ibid, 3–4.

27   "Memorandum on the Present Position and Future Prospects of the Indian Medical Service, 1913/14, Medical Appeal Board: Constitution of, Appointment, etc.," British Medical Association, India Office Records, Africa and Pacific Collections, British Library, London, IOR/L/S&G/8/305, 1.

28   *Royal Commission on the Public Services in India*, 19–30.

29   For a more detailed account of Mehta's conflict with British colonial medical officials between 1920 and 1940, see Chakrabarti, "Signs of the Times."

30   Scottish training programs were seen as more open to Indian students than their counterparts in London. A significant number of Indian doctors were trained in Edinburgh. Jeffery, *The Politics of Health in India*.

31   "The Status of Indian Students in the United Kingdom, being an Authoritative Statement of their objection to the Existence of an Indian Students' Department and of their grievances at Various Educational Institutions. Adopted at a representative Meeting of Indian Students held in London at Caxton Hall, Westminster on Friday the 8th of May, 1914." Printed by Red Lion Press, London, Printed Material, S. No. 2, 1914, Jivraj Mehta Papers, Manuscript Section, Nehru Memorial Museum and Library, New Delhi, India, 1.

32   Ibid., 1–23.

33   Chakrabarti et al., "R.G. Kar Medical College."

34   Ramanna, *Health Care in Bombay Presidency*, 91.

35   W.S. Carter, "Seth Gorhandas Sunderdas Medical College," vol. XVIII, 1927, 464, Box 10, WS Carter Diaries, The Rockefeller Archive Centre (RAC), New York, 33.

36   Farley, *To Cast Out Disease*; Kavadi, *The Rockefeller Foundation*.

37   Carter, "Seth Gorhandas Sunderdas Medical College," 32, 39.

38   Ibid., 32.

39   Ibid., 33–5.

40   Letter from Mehta, KEM Hospital, Parel, to Mr. Richard B. Gregg, 14 February 1929, Correspondences, File no. 140, Jivraj Mehta Papers,

Manuscript Section, Nehru Memorial Museum and Library, New Delhi, India, 593.

41 Chakrabarti, *Bacteriology in British India*, 84.

42 This was exemplified in Britain by the Beveridge Report of 1942, which presaged the creation of the National Health Service.

43 Government of India, *Health Survey and Development Committee*, vol. 1, 1.

44 Jeffery, *The Politics of Health in India*, 243.

45 Government of India, *Health Survey and Development Committee*, vol. IV, 60.

46 Key figures included Henry Sigerist, the communist historian of medicine at Johns Hopkins University; Janet Vaughan, principal of Somerville College, Oxford, who ran the first blood bank in London during the Blitz and was one of the first people to explore the association between illness and poverty; and John Ryle, the Oxford pioneer of social medicine. Murthy et al., "International Advisors," 76.

47 Madan, *Doctors and Society*, 30.

48 Hill, *A Report to the Government of India*, 17.

49 Pandit, *My World of Preventive Medicine*, 147.

50 Government of India, *Health Survey and Development Committee*, vol. IV, 70.

51 "Medical mission to the Health Survey and Development Committee, India, 1944," C/139/H.2, Manuscripts and Archives, Wellcome Library, London.

52 Ibid., 29.

53 Ibid., 40.

54 Ibid., 41–3.

55 Hill, *A Report to the Government of India*, 20.

56 Pandit, *My World of Preventive Medicine*, 147.

57 Ibid., 157, emphasis added.

58 "The Training of Doctors."

59 Pandit, *My World of Preventive Medicine*, 158.

60 These were particularly promoted by Professor J.A. Ryle, head of the Department of Preventive and Social Medicine, and a pioneer in the field. He described to the committee his method of teaching beyond lectures, including interactive seminars at which patients were present. "The idea that the disease is a social and economic problem is inculcated," he told the visitors. Pandit, *My World of Preventive Medicine*, 161.

61 Ibid., original emphasis.

62 Ibid., 165.

63 International assistance also came from the United States Technical Collaboration Mission in 1960 for construction of the main hospital, and from the Rockefeller Foundation for the purchase of medical equipment and library resources; Madan, *Doctors and Society*, 36. Nehru acknowledged this assistance in his convocation address in 1964.

64 Reflecting the abiding concern to establish an institution not only pre-eminent within India but on par with similar colleges in the West, K.C.K.E. Raja, secretary of the All India Medical Institute Committee, set off in 1952 on another research mission to the US, UK, Canada, Sweden, and Switzerland, "to familiarize himself with the working of medical educational and research institutions in these countries and to establish the necessary contacts for the possible recruitment of overseas staff"; Madan, *Doctors and Society*, 33.

65 Phalkey, "Introduction," 331.

66 Arnold, "Nehruvian Science," 364.

67 Prakash, *Another Reason*, 201–26.

68 Cited in Jeffery, *Politics of Health*, 244–5.

69 Government of India, "All India Institute of Medical Sciences Bill," 263.

70 Ibid., emphasis added.

71 Ibid., 264.

72 The AIIMS Act retains a provision in Article 14 to "provide for the teaching of humanities in the undergraduate courses." This inclusion might have been encouraged by the advocates of comprehensive social medicine teaching, but there is no evidence to suggest such courses ever took place at AIIMS. Also see Madan, *Doctors and Society*, 82–3.

73 Miller, *Medicine and Society*, 81.

74 Arnold, "Nehruvian Science," 366.

75 Ibid.

76 Singh, *Jawaharlal Nehru on Science and Society*, 193.

77 Ibid., 194.

78 Arnold, "Nehruvian Science," 367.

79 Singh, *Jawaharlal Nehru on Science and Society*, 195.

80 Ibid., 265.

81 Ibid.

82 Ibid.

83 Ibid.

BIBLIOGRAPHY

Amrith, Sunil S. *Decolonizing International Health: India and Southeast Asia, 1930–65.* Basingstoke, UK: Palgrave Macmillan, 2006.

Arnold, David. *Colonizing the Body: State Medicine and Epidemic Disease in Nineteenth Century India.* Berkeley, CA: University of California Press, 1993.

– "Nehruvian Science and Postcolonial India." *Isis* 104, no. 2 (2013): 360–70.

Bala, Poonam. *Medicine and Medical Policies in India: Social and Historical Perspectives.* Lanham, MD: Lexington Books, 2007.

Bhattacharya, Nandini. *Contagion and Enclaves: Tropical Medicine in Colonial India.* Liverpool, UK: Liverpool University Press, 2012.

Chakrabarti, Dilip Kumar, Ramanuj Mukherjee, Samik Kumar Bandyopadhyay, Sasank Nath, and Saibal Kumar Mukherjee. "R.G. Kar Medical College, Kolkata – A Premiere Institute of India." *Indian Journal of Surgery* 73, no. 5 (2011): 390–3.

Chakrabarti, Pratik. *Bacteriology in British India: Laboratory Medicine and the Tropics.* Rochester, NY: University of Rochester Press, 2012.

– "Signs of the Times: Medicine and Nationhood in British India." *Osiris* 24, no. 1 (2009): 188–211.

Crawford, D.G. *A History of the Indian Medical Service 1600–1913.* 2 vols. London: W. Thacker, 1914.

Farley, John. *To Cast Out Disease: A History of the International Health Division of the Rockefeller Foundation (1913–1951).* New York: Oxford University Press, 2004.

Government of India. "All India Institute of Medical Sciences Bill." In *Lok Sabha Debates*: 263–4. New Delhi: Lok Sabha Secretariat, 1956.

– *Health Survey and Development Committee*, vols. I–V. Calcutta, India: Government of India Press 1946.

Harrison, Mark. *Public Health in British India: Anglo-Indian Preventive Medicine 1859–1914.* Cambridge: Cambridge University Press, 1994.

Haynes, Douglas M. *Fit to Practice: Empire, Race, Gender, and the Making of British Medicine, 1850–1980.* New York: University of Rochester Press, 2017.

Hill, A.V. *A Report to the Government of India on Scientific Research in India.* London: The Royal Society, 1944.

Jeffery, Roger. "Doctors and Congress: The Role of Medical Men and Medical Politics in Indian Nationalism." In *The Political Economy of Indian Independence and the Indian National Congress, 1885–1985*, edited by Mike Shepperdson and Colin Simmons, 160–73. Aldershot, UK: Avebury, 1988.

– *The Politics of Health in India.* Berkeley, CA: University of California Press, 1988.

– "Recognizing India's Doctors: The Institutionalization of Medical Dependency, 1918–39." *Modern Asian Studies* 13, no. 2 (1979): 301–26.

Kavadi, Shirish N. *The Rockefeller Foundation and Public Health in Colonial India, 1916–1945; A Narrative History.* Pune/Mumbai, India: Foundation for Research in Community Health, 1999.

Kumar, Krishna. *Political Agenda of Education: A Study of Colonialist and Nationalist Ideas.* New Delhi: Sage, 2005.

Madan, T.N., ed. *Doctors and Society: Three Asian Case Studies: India, Malaysia, Sri Lanka.* Ghaziabad, India: Vikas, 1980.

Miller, Henry George. *Medicine and Society.* London: Oxford University Press, 1973.

Murthy, Pratima, Alok Sarin, and Sanjeev Jain. "International Advisers to the Bhore Committee: Perceptions and Visions for Healthcare." *Economic and Political Weekly* 48, no. 10 (2013): 71–7.

Pandit, C.G. *My World of Preventive Medicine*. New Delhi: Leipzig Press, 1982.

Phadke, Anant. "Regulation of Doctors and Private Hospitals in India." *Economic and Political Weekly* 41, no. 6 (2016): 46–55.

Phalkey, Jahnavi. "Introduction." *Isis* 104, no. 2 (2013): 330–6.

Prakash, Gyan. *Another Reason: Science and the Imagination of Modern India*. Princeton, NJ: Princeton University Press, 1999.

Ramanna, Mridula. *Health Care in Bombay Presidency, 1896–1930*. New Delhi: Primus Books, 2012.

– *Western Medicine and Public Health in Colonial Bombay, 1845–1895*. Delhi: Orient Longman, 2002.

Representation of the Bombay Medical Union to the Royal Commission on the Public Services in India, Bombay. Bombay, India: Bombay Medical Union, 1913.

Royal Commission on the Public Services in India. Report of the Commissioners, vol. I. London: His Majesty's Stationary Office, 1917.

Singh, Baldev, ed. *Jawaharlal Nehru on Science and Society: A Collection of His Writings and Speeches*. New Delhi: Nehru Memorial Museum and Library, 1988.

"The Training of Doctors: Report by The Goodenough Committee." *The British Medical Journal* 2, no. 4359 (1944): 121–3.

7

Unequal Global, Racialized Universal, and Colonized Local: Producing Autochthonous Medical Personnel in Cameroon under French Colonial Rule

Jean Baptiste Nzogue

The advent and spread of modern medicine in Africa required considerable human resources. All the European colonial powers encountered many difficulties in their efforts to attract health personnel in general, and medical doctors in particular, to their colonial possessions in Africa. Some reasons for these difficulties were the reluctance of many European doctors to serve in Africa where they could not have the same comfort as in their home countries, the fear of tropical diseases that were serious threats to their lives, low salaries compared to the risks, and the conditions imposed by colonial authorities, such as celibacy. Even in territories such as the Anglo-Egyptian Sudan where British doctors seemed to like the "African adventure," the local government, as in other European colonial empires, limited their recruitment because they found them very costly.[1] The First World War worsened the problem of the availability of European technical staffs. To circumvent the difficulty of recruiting European doctors in the colonies, all colonial powers created categories of Autochthonous[2] "medical assistants" that were unknown in Europe and employed exclusively outside of the European countries.

Due to racial considerations these local staff were, in almost all cases, trained to be inferior to the European doctors; and even when they had completed equal training, they were still either segregated from or considered inferior to the less-experienced European doctor. Studies by Liesbeth Hesselink and Hannah-Louise Clark have discussed this racialization of medical education in the colonial context, be it in Africa or in Asia. Anne Digby and Karin A. Shapiro highlight practices of segregation,[3] while Heather Bell and Vanessa Noble address the inferiority imposed on Africans in the medical professions.[4] One can affirm, with Clark, that the category of medical assistant specifically had spread throughout the French empire as a way of seeking to transform society while preserving racial hierarchy and sparing colonial budgets from the burden of European doctors' salaries.[5] Arguably, a form of colonial hierarchy persisted in medical education despite the independence of African countries and has been transposed to the current post-colonial context in which African medical doctors – trained in Africa – must undergo years of further training to practise in developed countries. Understanding the status of medical assistants is not therefore simply a historical problem, but an issue that continues to reverberate in the present, namely in the perception that developed countries have of medical education in Africa.

In the case of Cameroon under French rule, colonial officials first trained medical assistants locally (1924–44) and only later established training for "African" doctors in Dakar, Senegal (1944–53). It seems that Cameroonians were required to travel to Dakar for advanced medical training because French colonial policy aimed to limit the number of expensive modern structures in Africa. Thus, for the whole French colonial empire in Africa south of the Sahara, except Madagascar, the Dakar Medical School was the only place where "African" doctors were trained, despite the fact that Cameroon was a mandate territory under the League of Nations, and later a trusteeship territory under the United Nations (UN). This special status of Cameroon meant that the territory should be ruled not as part of the French colonial empire, but as an autonomous territory, and was against the League of Nations' philosophy, according to which the mandate was a transitional status leading to self-determination. Although education in Cameroon is not tabula rasa – there is an Autochthonous tradition of education[6] and also remnants of the German era which shaped the uptake of French colonial initiatives[7] – the production of local medical personnel has greatly depended on literacy, and this has led to a model of medical training punctuated by the evolution of school education according to French colonial expectations and standards. Whether as medical assistants or "African" doctors, Cameroonians were trained in "tropical pathologies" only. In other words, the medical education provided to Cameroonians was shaped to treat only the diseases that were known in the African context, and not to understand medicine as a universal science. This is significant because within the framework of the "civilizing mission," European medical thought at the time presented modern medicine as a universal art intended to replace the other forms of Autochthonous medicine that were practised in the colonies.

This chapter analyzes the content of French colonial medical education experienced by Cameroonians who were trained locally for the Medical Service, and later in Dakar, until the late 1940s when they started travelling to France to complete their training as medical doctors. These shifts in medical education were driven by top-down policy that involved all French

Sub-Saharan colonies and mandate territories, except Madagascar. Although the main focus of the chapter is the evolution of colonial medical education in the Cameroonian context, it regularly compares the case of Cameroon to other local experiences across French and other European colonial empires. Pursuing a comparative approach across empires allows me to show the degree to which colonial officials borrowed and adapted policies from other colonial states. This is an empirical study – focused only on French Cameroon and not on British Cameroons – that would have liked to give more room to the archives for a better knowledge of the social history of medical education in Cameroon under French rule. Yet very few files at the Yaounde National Archives provide useful information on the subject. This problem of access to quality information constitutes the main challenge faced by scholars working on colonial and post-colonial history in French-speaking Africa in general and in Cameroon in particular. Very few records relating to these periods have been processed. Nevertheless, through the close study of the existing literature and some archives, I show that medical education in Cameroon evolved in a general context of producing local medical assistants in the African colonies. Unlike previous studies, which have insisted on the role and the place of medical assistants in health action, I especially analyze the (gradual) medical education that was given to these auxiliaries for the practice of colonial medicine.

MEDICAL ASSISTANTS TRAINED ON THE JOB

In a context where many Europeans thought that a "modern" medical education was beyond the capabilities of Africans, colonial rulers chose to train in Africa varieties of local medical personnel destined to assist European doctors. Among these were the medical assistants, who were neither doctors nor nurses but could "assume some of the attributes of a physician."[8] In the case of Cameroon, French and British officials, who officially replaced German authorities in 1922 in line with the League of Nations' mandate, had to start all over due to language barriers and the dispersion of former German-trained Autochthonous health personnel. The unavailability of European doctors in this post-war context (in short supply even in Europe), combined with their reluctance to serve in Africa, made it very difficult for French colonial officials at the beginning of their medical work in Cameroon. In 1921, for example, of the six medical doctors who were expected in Cameroon, only two had arrived.[9] The French therefore needed local personnel with proven intellectual and technical abilities to fill the gap created by insufficient numbers of European medical doctors; to assist the latter in the practice of medicine and surgery; and to coordinate hospital and other medical or health facilities.

To raise these personnel, in 1924 the local government started training medical assistants as an elite professional body made up of staff trained on the job.[10] In French West Africa a comparable professional body of medical assistants trained on the job had been in existence since 7 January 1906.[11] It is important to note that, had the French succeeded in recruiting enough coordinating medical personnel from Europe, they would not have trained and employed medical assistants in these early days of their rule in Cameroon because they took a negative view of the intellectual abilities of the Autochthonous population. This was a general perception, nourished by racial considerations and superiority complexes, that most European intellectuals and colonialists had about Sub-Saharan Africans.[12] They thought that the Africans, who did not undergo formal schooling according to European principles and standards before the advent of colonization, could not have the same intellectual constitution as the Europeans. The French doctors had these prejudices towards the Muslims in Algeria with regard to medical education.[13] Therefore, the employment of a medical assistant in the early 1920s was much more a colonial constraint than an aim to associate the Autochthonous with the medical professions. And it could easily be understood that this position presented many challenges for those who were called in, because assisting the doctor in a hospital, or running a medical station or a mobile medical unit, required proven technical skills and a minimum of managerial qualifications with regard to the expectations of their colonial bosses. This policy of training local personnel as an emergency measure concerned all the colonial trades, and it is not surprising that French officials complained much about their first local auxiliaries because they did not find in them all the desired assets.

Another element that indicates that the employment of medical assistants was for the local elites' sake, at this early stage of French rule in Cameroon, is its selective character. In 1924, the year in which this professional body was organized and when the territory had 146 local nurses, only four of those nurses were accepted as medical assistants.[14] These were Manfred Edanga, Paul Oscho, Bernard Oyage, and Charles Kaledje.[15] However, in the context of the early 1920s, this tiny recruitment should be attributed not only to Autochthonous intellectual limitations but also to budgetary restrictions that made it impossible to recruit in large numbers. In Cameroon's particular context, these budgetary restrictions were not due to the 1921 international economic crisis since, according to the figures produced by the French colonial officials, Cameroon regained economic prosperity in 1923 and it was in that very year that the Territory had its first autonomous budget. The surplus revenues were above 6 million francs in 1923, 9 million in 1925, and 17 million in 1926.[16] Although colonial documents provide information on general health budgets, they do not give details such as funds budgeted for medical education. Until 1946, when France decided to sponsor socio-economic development of its African colonies and territories, the health and medical services in Cameroon were fully funded by the local budget that consisted of local resources. In the French colonial philosophy, it was clearly established that each territory must provide for its own development and contribute to the metropolitan economy.[17] This profit-based colonial philosophy seems to have been a leitmotiv for all the European powers; for example, Bell highlights the fact that British "conquest and administration were accomplished with few resources" in the Anglo-Egyptian Sudan.[18]

In the minds of French officials, medical assistants that would be trained on the job would have to be recruited from among the most senior male nurses, who would need to hold the certificate of Upper Primary School and be proposed by the Director of the Health Service. As well, the proposed nurses would have to become medical assistants by competition. But this was just an ideal at this stage of French rule in Cameroon. Earlier, with the creation of the League of Nations in 1919, the French local government decided to organize a regular professional body of local nurses, a move that was supposed to put an end to the recruitment of nursing volunteers, who had been employed since 1916[19] and who did not know how to write, read, or speak French.[20] The opening of the Upper Primary School in Yaounde in the early 1920s, at the French colonial headquarters in Cameroon, was supposed to provide the Medical Service with learned Autochthonous personnel who could assist European medical doctors. Thenceforth, local nurses required a minimum general school instruction and a minimum of six years' nursing experience to qualify and be recruited as medical assistants.[21]

However, when the professional body of local medical assistants was organized in 1924, the territory had not yet produced its first graduates. As a transitional arrangement, French colonial officials had to start, in the meantime, with the best former nursing volunteers who had been confirmed as nurses in 1919. Instead of proceeding by competition, officials made direct appointments. Manfred Edanga, Paul Oscho, Bernard Oyage, and Charles Kaledje were appointed medical assistants from among the most qualified nurses due to their professional conscience and knowledge. The testimony from Dr Gustave Martin, the first director of the French Health Service in Cameroon, on these Autochthonous early health personnel is very striking: "They are very intelligent; often even quite devoted ... They are superior in terms of work output to our nurse skirmishers, mainly those coming from Congo. Many are excellent servants. The Health Service would therefore have every interest in increasing the number."[22] The first competition for the recruitment of medical assistants was organized in July 1929, once French Cameroon had started producing graduates from the Upper Primary School.[23] The oral and written examination focused on nine specific topics: role of the medical assistant; anatomy and physiology; minor surgery; hygiene; medicine; etiology and prophylaxis; administration; organization and functioning of health facilities in Cameroon; pharmacy.[24]

By studying the qualities that were required of a local medical assistant and the subjects on which applicants were assessed, we can better understand the assumptions and ideological values that guided the French colonial administration in its approach to Autochthonous medical education in Cameroon. The questions on the role of the health assistant, for example, dealt with the following detailed topics: the medical assistant in a health facility; the medical assistant and his substitute when needed; relationship between the medical assistant and the doctor and between the medical assistant and the sick; moral qualities that a good medical assistant must possess; assiduity, zeal, punctuality in the service, correction, and politeness towards all; patience, gentleness, and devotion to the sick; the responsibility of the medical assistant in the general execution of the services in a health facility; the initiatives that a medical assistant could take as well as those he should not; the medical assistant in a dispensary without a doctor; and limitations on actions in the treatment of patients. All these details clearly show that the medical assistants were destined for management positions in health facilities, either as assistants to the European doctor or as managers of health facilities where it had not been possible to assign a doctor. The limitation on the action of medical assistants in the treatment of patients is explained by the insufficiency of the training that was given to them on the job. It is understandable that the colonial administration wanted to specify their attributions so that they did not view themselves as qualified at the level of a doctor.

There is a second line of evidence that shows that medical assistants were superior in value to nurses trained on the job: the position they occupied in preventive disease control and in the treatment of patients. First, they were initiated in the etiology and prophylaxis of cosmopolitan diseases: smallpox and vaccines, chickenpox, pneumococcal diseases, tetanus, tuberculosis, tumours, skin diseases, diseases of nutrition, diseases of the respiratory system, diseases of the circulatory system, diseases of the genito-urinary system, diseases of the nervous system, and diseases of the sense organs. Second, medical assistants were specially trained to manage diseases specific to the tropical environment, also called "exotic" diseases by the Europeans, such as amoebic and bacillary dysentery, leprosy, yaws, ulcers, mycetoma, hookworm, or flea-ticks.

While medical assistant trainees learned certain skills and procedures, they were not taught the scientific or clinical rationale behind them. In Cameroon, as in Algeria, trainees were kept at arm's length from clinical instruction and demonstration, and, as a result, their practical knowledge was limited to what they were told and shown how to do. They were taught the task with the expectation that they would then be able to perform it mechanically, efficiently, and effectively. Even in countries such as Algeria, where youth literacy was more developed than in Cameroon, medical assistant curricula did not include scientific knowledge about diseases such as smallpox until the late 1920s, even though they routinely administered smallpox vaccinations. Discrimination against Muslim medical assistant students also meant they had far fewer opportunities for hands-on or bedside demonstrations on real patients during their training.[25] They were regularly criticized by senior doctors for having knowledge that was too abstract and for lacking clinical experience.[26] It is reasonable to speculate that colonial authorities did not expect incoming Autochthonous students to have a broad base of science education, as did European medical students. Nor were medical assistants trained to be "practitioners" of medicine; rather, their role was to become an effective means of delivering medical treatments and information.

Three entrance examinations were organized in Cameroon between 1930 and 1932. Two candidates were admitted in 1930, one in 1931, and one in 1932.[27] Even French colonial statistics show that after 1924 they never recruited more than three medical assistants trained on the job per year, and never more than eleven for the whole country.[28] In line with their status of "auxiliary," and as elsewhere in the French empire, the pedagogical method privileged visual learning. "Students were first to be exposed to the most 'eye-catching' services at the hospital."[29] They were expected to recognize the different "local" diseases and to learn how to prevent them.

For these medical assistants trained on the job, the intended scope of their role may have been narrow with regard to active medical treatment, but it was very broad in terms of hygiene and prophylaxis within local communities. They were trained mainly for the fight against sleeping sickness and smallpox, which, due to their epidemic and deadly character, were the priority for French colonial officials in the 1920s. Medical assistants were often in charge, or second-in-charge to European doctors, of mobile medical units and were responsible for sensitizing local populations to the dangers of infectious diseases and the poor hygiene that could cause them. Their role in this mobile medicine was of great importance since they had greater audience and impact within local communities than white doctors, who were often military men against whom the Autochthonous inhabitants held many grudges due to their brutal methods. In this line – since their periodic visits were the only opportunities that rural communities had to receive medical attention from the colonizers – the local government entrusted medical assistants with the responsibility for overthrowing the prejudices local populations had about European medicine. In hospitals, these local medical elites trained on the job were the closest auxiliaries to European doctors, and they exercised their managerial role in dispensaries and in medical stations.

Even with the requirement of a general level of education, taught-on-the-job medical assistants still had several shortcomings related to their lack of theoretical training. It is true that their practical training in hospitals and extensive experience as nurses made them very valuable, and some were as skillful as the European doctors, whose many years of medical education were both practical and theoretical. The low numbers of medical assistants who were recruited per year, moreover – only one or two annually, despite the territory's desperate need for more medical personnel – shows that French colonial officials found it risky to multiply this category of auxiliaries imposed by the colonial context. This professional body trained on the job, therefore, was an intermediary step towards the creation of a school for the training of local medical personnel in Cameroon, as was the case in French West Africa where a medical school had been organized in Dakar in 1918 for the training of African auxiliary doctors.

CERTIFIED LOCAL MEDICAL ASSISTANTS

Recruitment of medical assistants trained on the job ended in 1932 with the creation of the School of "Certified Local Medical Assistants" at Ayos, a suburb of Yaounde. In common with medics trained on the job, this new category of medical personnel was organized to provide the Medical Service with well-equipped Autochthonous medics who could assist European doctors in the practice of medicine and in running medical facilities in Cameroon. The initial category of local medical assistants, those trained on the job, seemed to have been organized mainly for the fight against sleeping sickness, especially through mobile medical units run by medical assistants. Due to shortages of European doctors, they were posted instead to hospitals and dispensaries, either to assist European doctors or to run dispensaries and medical stations. With the decline of sleeping sickness and the gradual increase of youth literacy, they no longer fit the vision that the French colonial authorities had for the fight against tropical diseases in Africa in general, and in Cameroon in particular. These medical personnel from the on-the job training model had to be phased out as they retired.

The professional body of certified local medical assistants fitted more, at this stage, the ideal pursued by French colonial officials to have in Cameroon local auxiliaries with both practical and theoretical medical training, as was the case in places such as West Africa and Algeria. As such, the recruitment of local medical personnel took a decisive turn in 1932 with the organization of the School of Medical Assistants.[30] If in 1924 the French colonial officials had selected the best nurses trained on the job to become medical assistants, in 1932 they began to prepare candidates from the Yaounde Upper Primary School before sending them to attend vocational training at Ayos. It was the same policy in French West Africa.[31] To increase numbers of certified medical assistants, the local government created a medical option at the Upper Primary School in order to attract more graduates to the medical sector. But its pupils were not prepared for studies in basic sciences that accorded with European standards of general education, where recruitment to medical schools required preliminary knowledge on specific subjects. It is to emphasize this comparatively low standard, in contrast with programs in schools for Europeans, that Clark states that in Algeria, "[d]uring study for the [Certificat d'Etudes Primaires], pupils were given no textbook instructions in physics, chemistry, or natural history, nor formally introduced to these subjects by means of experimental or physical apparatus."[32] This educational policy, based on narrow colonial objectives, was common throughout the French colonial empire in Africa, where not only was the Upper Primary School very selective, but getting the Certificat d'Etudes Primaires (CEP) required for medical education "was an exceptional achievement that remained rare until 1945."[33] Moreover, graduates from this local elite school were solicited by other sectors of the French colonial civil service, where they could get better wages. Thus, only very few of them chose the medical profession.

Students who chose the medical option were admitted without competition to the School of Local Medical Assistants – after they graduated from the Upper Primary School – and they started their vocational training as trainee nurses. Successful candidates were trained for three years. This training consisted of theoretical courses, practical exercises, and hospital internships. During the first year, students competed in the nursing rank service. The program focused on anatomy and physiology, medical semeiology, and first-year nursing courses. Candidates who were admitted to the second year served as rank-grade nursing staff. Students were trained on notions of internal pathology and diagnosis, external pathology and surgical semeiology, and obstetrics, as well as taking second-year nursing courses. The third year, finally, prepared them more for the fight against tropical diseases; it concerned the hygiene of the individual, the hygiene of the pregnant woman and the child, the prophylaxis of contagious diseases, and the elements of therapeutics.[34] It can thus be seen that medical assistants were trained to play a leading and supervising role in the field. Those trained on the job were also admitted to the school to complete their training. The training of Cameroonian medical assistant students in basic obstetrics – which was emphatically not the case in Muslim countries such as Algeria – shows that, even though the colonial model of medical assistant was picked up and transferred from place to place, some concessions were made to what colonial officials supposed to be local cultural norms.

During the school year, students were subject to monthly assessments and they underwent a final examination before a jury.[35] This exam covered subjects taught during the year; it included written, oral, and practical tests. The former local medical assistants from on-the-job training who were admitted to the school had to pass, like the other candidates, the tests relating to the nursing course. The first year consisted mainly of a level test, and those who were judged unfit for the medical profession were simply dismissed at the end of this probationary year. As for the second year, successful candidates were admitted to the courses of the higher class and were appointed fourth-class nurses. Finally, for the third year, successful medical assistant students were ranked in order of merit, based on the total points obtained in various exams – all the passing exam scores and marks obtained during the school years. This classification was submitted by the Examination Committee to the Commissioner of the French Republic, who made the appointments to the rank of medical assistant within the limits of places determined by the Public Health Budget. Appointments were not automatic for everyone who completed the training of medical assistant; priority was given to the most deserving.

From the foregoing, it appears that the admission of the Autochthonous to the School of Medical Assistants offered them two employment alternatives: nurse or medical assistant. The French colonial authorities, at this stage of colonization and of youth literacy, were looking for the most skillful among young Cameroonians to train and to employ as medical assistants. Such an approach in a colonial context shows that even though the French colonial authorities needed medical assistants, they were committed to employing only the most successful of those who were trained. Another interesting point in this approach is the classification according to skills. The most talented were appointed medical assistants, and, due to budget restrictions, only somewhat-less-talented graduates were appointed nurses of a higher rank who would be first in line to be promoted to medical assistants in case of vacancy. The students' performances were therefore very decisive for their professional futures. French colonial officials published on 16 June 1934, in the *Journal Officiel* of French Cameroon, the list of medical assistant students who, after their second year of study at Ayos, were admitted to the third year; it also published the list of trainee nurses, first-year medical assistant students, who were admitted to the second year. What is striking here is the number of students who were admitted in the third and second years. They were very few: only five for the third year (Eyidi Bebey Marcel, André Ndondo, Wilson Manfred, Avele Williams, Ze Charles) and six for the second year (Nseme Pensy, Kouo Moundi, Ngando Jacques, Monayong Daniel, Essombe Joseph, Esso Jacques).

Most of these trainees, if not all, were from the coastal, central, and southern regions of French Cameroon, where the European colonial system of education had been well-established since the German Protectorate. Some of them, such as Eyidi Bebey, later became medical doctors who owned private clinics, and who contested the colonial order when the Autochthonous were given social and political rights at the end of the Second World War and were jailed for their political engagement.

From 1932 to 1938, four cohorts of medical assistants were trained at Ayos.[36] From the testimony of the French colonial physicians, who seldom appreciated the Autochthonous, the training of medical assistants at Ayos succeeded perfectly. Medical assistants served as excellent auxiliaries to European doctors and were often valued by the European population in Cameroon.[37] The physician-director of the Ayos Medical Training Center vocalized his pride in them enough to inspire the famed French novelist, Martin du Gard, to recount: "Who were these collaborators? Certified medical assistants, graduates from the Ayos Medical School, I was told. Not doctors, but they aren't nurses either. A professional conscience equal to that of European doctors ... Most, after their third year of study in Ayos, do what doctors in the French countryside did fifty years ago: emergency surgery, ligatures, fractures of the femur, strangulated hernias."[38] Professor Mülhens from the Tropical Institute of Hambourg visited the School of Ayos in 1938 and paid homage to medical assistant trainees after observing their skills. He concluded that many European medical students were not as skillful as these "Negroes."[39]

Compared to those who were formally trained on the job, certified medical assistants had a broader place in the colonial medical system. Although curricula always emphasized so-called "tropical" diseases, medical assistants were mainly trained for medical purposes. This choice is understandable with regards to the context of the early 1930s: smallpox had disappeared thanks to vaccination; sleeping sickness was under control and no longer demanded the deployment of mobile medical units. It was now time to train medical assistants to treat the numerous other endemic diseases that affected local populations. The pedagogical method continued to privilege visual learning. For this new category of medical assistants, not only did they learn how to recognize and prevent "tropical" diseases, they were mainly taught how to treat them. Yet, due to racial considerations, the aim of this medical education was not to produce a medical assistant who understood the principles of "modern" medicine, but to cultivate a skillful local "practitioner" who could apply what he was taught at Ayos. These medical assistants, often positioned at the head of medical centres when they were not assisting European doctors in divisional or "regional" hospitals, realized their shortcomings and managed themselves to enhance their medical knowledge. Clark states that, in Algeria, some medical assistants "borrowed medical textbooks from their supervisors or took out a subscription to French scientific journals to develop their medical knowledge."[40] However, in 1944 near the end of the Second World War, France decided to require increased formal qualifications from local medical personnel in the territory. It repealed the cadre of certified medical assistants due to the advent of another, more competitive type of practitioner who was more closely linked with the European doctor, and whose career prospects allowed him to become a medical doctor: these were the "African" doctors.

A NEW CATEGORY: "AFRICAN" DOCTOR

With the advent of a new international order at the end of the Second World War, one of the main purposes of the newly created United Nations (UN) was to accelerate the process of self-determination for colonized people. This required the "Africanization" of colonial personnel even in those areas where Africans were not recognized as having the same skills as Europeans, since colonial powers were asked to grant independence to their colonies and territories under their rule.

In the field of medicine, colonial officials created another variety of medical assistant before they started producing doctors according to European standards. The new category created at the end of the war to assist European doctors bore the designate title "African" doctor – that is to say, doctors trained for Africa and able to practise only in Africa. France had already organized medical education in the French Indies (1882), in Madagascar (1896), and in Indochina (1902). In each case, only strictly local diplomas were awarded. Once more, the logic of "races" prevailed in the advent of this professional body, despite a new international context requiring more and more the right of colonized people to self-determination. If in Asia, namely in Indochina, French officials finally created in 1939 a common cadre of medical doctors in which the Indochinese had the same status as the Europeans,[41] in postwar Africa they were still applying the philosophy of the "civilizing mission," which envisaged the progress, step by step, of Black Africans. Medical education and the practice of "modern" medicine had been one of the main fields where expressions of marginalization in colonial societies were seen most visibly. In South Africa, though the country had had its independence since the early twentieth century, not only were Black citizens not officially given the right to undergo full medical training until the early 1940s when a "reformist climate" appeared,[42] but those who forced their way into medicine by training themselves abroad could not practise in places where there was a white doctor; nor could they treat white patients.[43] This was a general stance that Europeans had in colonies: other races were inferior and white patients could only be treated by white doctors. This racialization is clearly apparent in works such as those of Bell, Clark, Hesselink, and Monnais-Rousselot that we have already quoted in this study.

The title "doctor" was new only for Cameroon and Togo (former German protectorates), which had been placed under the mandate of the League of Nations and whose administration was entrusted to France and Great Britain. To provide its colonies in Africa south of the Sahara with more qualified medical assistants, France had created the African School of Medicine in Dakar, Senegal, on 1 November 1918 at the close of World War I.[44] From that date, French officials began to train "auxiliary doctors" for their African colonies. The advent of this category of local medical personnel – auxiliary doctors – put an end to the training of "medical helps" in French West Africa.[45] Students were admitted to the Dakar school after they had completed their upper primary education, and the duration of the medical training was three years. One could wonder why French colonial officials did not give the title of "auxiliary doctors" to the certified medical assistants they trained for Cameroon when both categories were trained for three years and the trainees were admitted to medical schools with the CEP. This delay in Cameroon's context could be explained by the difficulty of getting enough candidates from the Upper Primary School due to its selective character, and to the fact that its products also had to serve in numerous other areas of the colonial civil service. This situation of the scarcity of "learned" youths for medical education was not specific to Cameroon, as highlighted by Clark for Algeria, although Algerian schools required fees whereas Cameroon public education, up to the Upper Primary School, was free of charge.[46] As a result, insufficient supplies of graduates might have led to the perpetuation of recruitment among the most experienced and skillful nurses with an elementary-level education. With regard to medical education, it was therefore necessary to wait for Cameroon to produce enough graduates who possessed the required educational level. The title "African" doctor could be justified by the extension in 1944 of the training of local "doctors" to all nationals of African countries that were under France's rule, and by the fact that the duration of the training was extended from three to four years.

The decision in 1944 to send Cameroonians to the Dakar Medical School led to the closure of the Ayos School of Medical Assistants,[47] and, as a transitional measure, recruitment started from among medical assistants who were already in the field and those already in training at Ayos. Medical assistants already out of school needed at least three years of professional experience to qualify. As for those who were still in school, the French colonial authorities took into account their current level of training. First-year students were allowed to enter the second year of medical studies. Those in the second year at Ayos were admitted to the third year of the medical school program; the medical assistant students who were at the end of their training had direct access to the fourth year of the Dakar School of Medicine and Pharmacy. This concordance did not proceed randomly; in the case of both schools, for students who entered at the level of the Upper Primary School the program was practically the same, except in the fourth year at Dakar, in which courses corresponded much more to the profile of "doctors."[48] In short, apart from dissection and general science courses, which constituted the added value of the training in Dakar before 1944, the medical assistant students from Ayos had undergone in three years all the training that was given to the auxiliary doctors of Dakar during their three years of medical studies. The fourth year that completed the training of "African" doctor students in Dakar included subjects such as operative medicine (surgery?), surgical (post-operative?) syndromes, medical syndromes, bacteriology, otorhinolaryngology specialties, ophthalmology, dermatovenereology, administration, deontology (professionalism? ethics?), and so on.

Medical education in French colonies was given by general practitioners practising the same "tropical" medicine that learners were called to practise. It was the same lecturer of general medicine who did the theoretical courses who received the trainees in his hospital. The pathologies observed at the hospital corresponded to those students would meet every day in the field.[49] The very first Cameroonian "African" doctor students admitted to the fourth year at the Dakar School of Medicine and Pharmacy in 1944 were three in number: Etienne Bilounga, Manassé Belinga Beke, and Mathieu Tagny.[50] When they departed for Dakar, they had just graduated from the School of Medical Assistants at Ayos. With regard to practical training, the first Cameroonian trainees had been supervised at the Dakar Central Hospital from April to July 1945. At the end of the three months of practical training, the trainees underwent a test on the following subjects: clinical examination of a hospital patient; clinical examination of a dispensary patient; medical pathology and therapy; epidemiology and hygiene; and bacteriology.

By 1953 – the year that the Dakar School of Medicine and Pharmacy closed – all Cameroonian medical assistants, even those from on-the-job training, were already in Dakar to be trained as "African" doctors. The Dakar School was replaced by the Institute of Advanced Studies of Dakar, which opened on 6 April 1950 and was affiliated with the Universities of Paris and Bordeaux. By attaching colonial medical education to Paris and Bordeaux, the French colonial officials were at last awarding recognition to "African" doctors within a more "universal" form of French medicine. However, compared to the British, the French delayed this recognition for much longer. After all, Great Britain found it very useful to produce local practitioners in countries such as the Anglo-Egyptian Sudan in the 1920s. Bell highlights that "British doctors in Sudan believed in the universalism of scientific and medical discourse: by following appropriate standards of behaviour and by mastering the correct techniques, Sudanese … too could become practitioners of Western medicine."[51] In the field, "African" doctors were running sub-divisional hospitals or medical centres, and they assisted European doctors in the major hospitals. They supervised consultations, care, and surgical operations. Unlike auxiliary doctors, who were prohibited from performing autopsies and major surgical operations, "African" doctors were authorized to undertake these procedures under the supervision of European doctors.[52] Some of them were assigned to the Mobile Hygiene and Prophylaxis Department, where they sometimes ran prophylaxis areas.

However, the advent of the professional category of "African" doctors in a context of decolonization, according to which Africans should have the same rights as Europeans in the colonies, aroused the anger of European doctors who did not want to admit that Africans could claim equality with them. In French Cameroon, in 1946, the physician-director of the Health Service, Lieutenant-Colonel Beaudiment, expressed his disagreement to the metropolitan colonial authorities in Paris, who had decided to harmonize Europeans' and Africans' positions and salaries: "Should a doctor-lieutenant therefore consider as an equal a first-class African doctor and as his superior a fourth-class principal? … Can we set up a system for subordinates to have higher pay than their chiefs? Or should we admit that because of this superiority of pay African doctors are taking precedence over European doctors?"[53] This reaction, which surely reflected the views of many European doctors in Cameroon, sufficiently shows that the posture of Europeans in the colonies was that the Autochthonous should never expect equality with their colonizers. It goes without saying that even in their decision to harmonize European and African colonial cadres, colonial authorities in Cameroon were merely yielding to international pressure, which had become more and more pressing.

This new context of "equality" in the colonies was undoubtedly to affect the appreciation that European physicians had for the professional value of their African collaborators. Dr Beaudiment, in one of the reports to his hierarchy, described "African" doctors as pretentious, and noted their recurring errors in the diagnosis of diseases. Such testimonies about the Autochthonous medical elite were rare before the advent of the new "equality" ethos. One can see, through this, manifestations of conflicts in the relationship between the medical authorities and the "African" doctors. Joseph-Joël Timba, an "African" doctor interviewed by Wang Sonne, affirms that his hierarchal head, Dr Gallaud, had never criticized him directly during their years of collaboration. Timba discovered after Gallaud's departure, however, secret letters that Gallaud had written to the director of the Health Service in which he made the following accusations: "Timba is lazy and incompetent, difficult to manage and imbued with his quality as African doctor. He always retorts: *Listen! I too am a doctor.*"[54] It is difficult to determine the root of the problem solely from such reports and testimonies. However, the performance of Cameroonian "African" doctor students in Dakar, and the training prospects that followed, can illuminate more about their professional value.

The qualifications of these Cameroonians trained in Dakar can be appreciated through the time frame during which Cameroon had "African" doctors; by the ranking of many of them at the end of their medical studies; and through the prospects open to them to become medical doctors in their own right, on par with Europeans. Between 1944 and 1947, in three years, Cameroon trained 52 "African" doctors[55] in Dakar, an average of 17 per year. And, before the Dakar school closed its doors, they reached the number of 64 out of 582 "African" doctors trained for all the French colonies and territories in Black Africa.[56] The levels of excellence achieved by Cameroonian students encouraged French colonial authorities to increasingly adopt a policy of replacing European physicians with qualified Africans. To achieve this aim, they began to send to France, from the late 1940s, the best laureates of Dakar to pursue further medical studies with a view to obtaining a university medical degree (MD). A metropolitan decree of 18 August 1949 set the conditions for granting scholarships to African doctors. These scholarships for higher education, at the expense of local budgets, were of two kinds. Their number was fixed each year by the French minister of overseas.[57] The first type of scholarship was reserved for the best laureates graduating from the Dakar School, according to their rank at the end of training. As for the second type, it corresponded to scholarships for which the "African" doctors who were already in service could compete. Fifty-nine "African" doctors were still in service in Cameroon in 1956, and five of them, after being admitted to assert their right in retirement, were practising their art as private doctors.[58] In addition to their impressive number in a short period of time, several Cameroonian "African" doctor students were at the top of their class at the end of their medical studies in Dakar.

In 1949, three Cameroonian "African" doctors were pursuing their medical studies in France,[59] and in 1951, they were already practising in Cameroon as medical doctors. The French colonial authorities rather expressed their satisfaction at having in the territory these new local medical elite who had graduated from the Paris Faculty of Medicine.[60] In 1952, two other grant holders from the Dakar School were pursuing their medical studies in France. At home in Cameroon, four "African" doctors who had just graduated were preparing their Baccalaureates in order to benefit from the scholarships obtained due to their high ranking at the end of their training in Dakar.[61] In 1956, four other Cameroonian grant holders from Dakar went on to study medicine in France.[62] One can therefore conclude that "African" doctors had proven their skills in a colonial context, in which the intellectual and technical abilities of Africans were not readily recognized by their European bosses in the colonies.[63] The central power in Paris, aware of the stakes related to these local medical elite in the process of Africanizing human resources, capitalized on the potential of the "African" doctors, to the point of recognizing them as full medical doctors qualified to ensure the succession of European technical staff.

CONCLUSION

Analyzing the methods of training and curricula, and comparing local experiences of medical education, improves our knowledge of how colonial rulers perceived so-called "tropical medicine." Cultivating local medical personnel in Cameroon depended mostly on youth literacy and on perceptions held by Europeans about Africans and their capacity to profitably act as medical professionals. The medical assistants recruited beginning in 1924 to be trained on the job were able to reach this position because they had proved themselves to be the most talented of the local nurses. The lack of theoretical training for these early medical assistants shows that they were employed because of colonial constraints on French officials early in their mandate in Cameroon. They could only work under orders since they did not have a wide knowledge of modern medicine in terms of their years of training and practical knowledge. The certified medical assistants from the School of Ayos had the advantage of both theoretical and practical training, but they were also shaped for colonial constraints and limited to working only in Africa. Due to racial considerations, they were not trained to understand modern medicine as universal, but rather to fit specific French needs to reduce the incidence of tropical diseases. With a multitude of such diseases to treat and prevent, the training of auxiliaries did not lead them to acquire diversified clinical skills, nor to become specialists during a period in which medical specialization proliferated. Although the training of medical assistants improved during this period, the curricula show that their medical education remained basic and typically colonial.

The elite of local medical staff were later on trained in Dakar for all French possessions in Black Africa except Madagascar. It is at this level that one can easily understand that the training given to the medical assistants was significantly influenced by French perceptions of Africans and their intellectual abilities. The category and title "African doctor" make clear that these personnel were trained to be in all respects inferior to European doctors. This discrimination considerably slowed the spread of modern medicine in Cameroon

under French rule – even as colonial officials continually complained about
shortages of European doctors. This low standard of medical education
can also be explained by the non-transfer to the colonies of the technologies
available in Europe. Medical education in France for "African doctors" from
Cameroon did not begin until the late 1940s. There was therefore no colonial
project – as there was in other African colonies and territories – of full medical
training (theoretical and practical) of Cameroonians.

This study makes it possible to understand that medical education in
Cameroon under French rule was not part of a global program to implement modern medicine in the colonies. This training was justified by colonial
necessities that led French officials to create categories of medical assistants
(akin to "auxiliaries" in other colonial contexts) that could help them achieve
their objectives with regard to the preservation of the territory's human capital. The non-transfer of technologies and knowledge, and curricula specially
adapted for Africa, show medical education at a discount. Medicine, in other
words, was not "universal" when it came to African practitioners. This colonial situation has been transposed to the post-colonial state, as is the case in
most African countries. In order to practise in developed countries, medical
doctors trained in Cameroon are still obliged to follow complementary courses
for years.

NOTES

1   Bell, *Frontiers of Medicine*.
2   I use the terms "Autochthonous" and "Autochthone" throughout this chapter
    in preference to terminology such as "indigenous" and "native," since both of
    the latter terms were used pejoratively in the colonial period and can still do
    harm in the present. Where I have translated verbatim from colonial records,
    the original language of French colonial officials appears in quotation marks.
3   Digby, "Early Black Doctors in South Africa"; Shapiro, "Doctors or Medical
    Aids."
4   Bell, *Frontiers of Medicine in the Anglo-Egyptian Sudan*; Monnais-Rousselot,
    "Paradoxes d'une médicalisation coloniale"; Noble, "A Medical Education
    with a Difference."
5   Clark, "Administering Vaccination," 36.
6   Ware, *The Walking Qur'an*.
7   Martin, *L'existence au Cameroun*.
8   Rosinski and Spencer, "The Training and Duties."
9   Rapport Annuel à la Société des Nations (SDN), 1921, 34.
10 *Journal Officiel des Territoires du Cameroun*, 4 June 1924.
11 Ndao and Nzogue, "Acteurs et structures."

12   Sarraut, *Grandeur et servitude coloniale*, 168–9.

13   Clark, "Doctoring the Bled," 82.

14   Rapport Annuel à la SDN, 1924, 38.

15   *Journal Officiel des Territoires du Cameroun*, 1924, 446.

16   Rapport Annuel à la SDN, 1925, 44.

17   Colombani, *Mémoires coloniales*, 13; Monnais-Rousselot, "Paradoxes d'une médicalisation," 36.

18   Bell, *Frontiers of Medicine*, 4.

19   *Journal Officiel des Territoires du Cameroun*, 1919, 3–6.

20   This language barrier was the cause of many burrs in the work of local nurses. Internal correspondences between French medical and administrative officials in Cameroon are full of complaints to this effect.

21   *Journal Officiel des Territoires du Cameroun*, 1929, 483–4.

22   Martin, *L'existence au Cameroun*, 485.

23   The Certificate of Upper Primary School was the highest level of education that the Autochthonous could have in French Cameroon until the end of World War II, when secondary education was organized in the territory.

24   *Journal Officiel des Territoires du Cameroun*, 1929, 483–4.

25   Clark, "Administering Vaccination," 39.

26   Ibid., 82.

27   Sonnè, "Les auxiliaires autochtones," 172–3.

28   Archives Nationales de Yaoundé (ANY), Service de santé, Rapport Annuel, Année 1938.

29   Clark, "Doctoring the Bled," 72.

30   *Journal Officiel des Territoires du Cameroun*, 1932, 747–53.

31   *Bulletin de la Société de Pathologie Exotique*, 1920, 625.

32   Clark, "Doctoring the Bled," 64.

33   Ibid.

34   *Journal Officiel des Territoires du Cameroun*, 1932, 747.

35   The jury was made up of the director of the Health Service or his representative, the chief medical official of the School of Medical Assistants, and two medical doctors appointed by the director of the Health Service (*Journal Officiel*, 1932, 716).

36   ANY, 2AC 11707, Service de santé, Rapport Annuel, Année 1938.

37   Ibid.

38   Du Gard, *L'appel du Cameroun*, 71–2.

39   Mveng, *Histoire du Cameroun*, 151–2.

40   Clark, "Administering Vaccination," 39.

41   Monnais-Rousselot, "Paradoxes d'une médicalisation," 39.

42   Noble, "A Medical Education with a Difference," 555–6.

43   Digby, "Early Black Doctors," 429–33.

44   Sankalé, *Médecins et action sanitaire en Afrique Noire*, 39.
45   Ndao and Nzogue, "Acteurs et structures de santé," 130.
46   Clark, "Administering Vaccination," 39.
47   *Journal Officiel de l'Afrique Occidentale Française*, 1944; 815–17.
48   Sonnè, "Les auxiliaires autochtones," 238–9.
49   Ndao and Nzogue, "Acteurs et structures de santé," 132–3.
50   Sonnè, "Les auxiliaires autochtones," 236–7.
51   Bell, *Frontiers of Medicine*, 40.
52   *Bulletin de la Société de Pathologie Exotique*, 625.
53   ANY VT 39/239, Renseignements confidentiels … Lettre du Médecin-
      Lieutenant-Colonel Beaudiment, 4 November 1946.
54   Sonnè, "Les auxiliaires autochtones," 249–50.
55   Rapport Annuel à l'Organisation des Nations Unies (ONU), 1947, 107.
56   *Afrique Documents*, 1960, 89.
57   Rapport Annuel à l'ONU, 1949, 363–5.
58   Rapport Annuel à l'ONU, 1956, 213.
59   Rapport Annuel à l'ONU, 1949, 156.
60   Rapport Annuel à l'ONU, 1951, 221.
61   Rapport Annuel à l'ONU, 1952, 226.
62   Rapport Annuel à l'ONU, 1956, 213.
63   ANY, VT 39/239, Renseignements confidentiels … Lettre du Haut-
      Commissaire de la République Française au Ministre de la France d'Outre-
      mer, 28 January 1947.

BIBLIOGRAPHY

Bell, Heather. *Frontiers of Medicine in the Anglo-Egyptian Sudan, 1899–1940*. Oxford
    Scholarship Online, 2011. doi: 10.1093/acprof:
    oso/9780198207498.001.0001.
Clark, Hannah-Louise. "Administering Vaccination in Interwar Algeria. Medical
    Auxiliaries, Smallpox, and the Colonial State in the Communes mixtes." *French
    Politics, Cultures and Society* 34, no. 2 (2016): 32–56.
– "Doctoring the Bled: Medical Auxiliaries and the Administration of Rural Life in
    Colonial Algeria, 1904–1954." PhD diss. Princeton, NJ: Princeton University,
    2014.
Colombani, Olivier. Mémoires coloniales. *La fin de l'Empire français d'Afrique vue par les
    administrateurs coloniaux*. Paris: La Découverte, 1991.
Digby, Anne. "Early Black Doctors in South Africa." *The Journal of African History* 46,
    no. 3 (2005): 427–54.
Du Gard, Martin. *L'appel du Cameroun*. Paris: Flammarion, 1939.

Hesselink, Liesbeth. *Healers on the Colonial Market. Native Doctors and Midwives in the Dutch East Indies.* Leiden, Netherlands: KITLV Press, 2011.

Martin, Gustave. *L'existence au Cameroun. Etudes sociales, études médicales, études d'hygiène et de prophylaxie.* Paris: Emile Larose, 1921.

Monnais-Rousselot, Laurence. "Paradoxes d'une médicalisation coloniale. La professionnalisation du 'médecin indochinois' au XXe siècle." *Actes de la recherche en sciences sociales,* no. 143 (2002/03): 36–43.

Mveng, Engelbert. *Histoire du Cameroun.* Yaoundé: CEPER, 1985.

Ndao, Mor, and Jean Baptiste Nzogue. "Acteurs et structures de santé dans la prise en charge de la tuberculose au Cameroun et au Sénégal colonial." In *Sida et tuberculose: La double peine? Institutions, personnels et sociétés face à la coinfection au Cameroun et au Sénégal,* edited by Laurent Vidal and Christopher Kuaban, 109–40. Louvain-La-Neuve, Belgium: Academia Bruylant, 2010.

Noble, Vanessa. "A Medical Education with a Difference: A History of the Training of Black Student Doctors in Social, Preventive and Community-Oriented Primary Health Care at the University of Natal Medical School, 1940s–1960s." *South African Historical Journal* 61, no. 3 (2009): 550–74.

Rosinski, Edwin, and Frederick J. Spencer. "The Training and Duties of the Medical Auxiliary known as the Assistant Medical Officer." *American Journal of Public Health* 57, no. 9 (September 1967): 663.

Shapiro, Karin A. "Doctors or Medical Aids – the Debate over the Training of Black Medical Personnel for the Rural Black Population in South Africa in the 1920s and 1930s." *Journal of Southern African Studies* 13, no. 2 (1987): 234–55.

Sankalé, Marc. *Médecins et action sanitaire en Afrique Noire.* Paris: Présence Africaine, 1969.

Sarraut, Albert. *Grandeur et servitude coloniale.* Paris: Editions du Sagittaire, 1931.

Ware, Rudolph, III. *The Walking Qur'an: Islamic Education, Embodied Knowledge and History in West Africa.* Chapel Hill, NC: University of North Carolina Press, 2014.

8

An Undesirable Past: Free Medical Schools and the First Doctors of the Mexican Revolution, 1910–45

Jethro Hernández Berrones

A closed book does not make you wise, nor does a diploma make you a master.

Mexican proverb

In September of 1932, Mexico City's Beneficencia Pública (Welfare Office) hired Alfredo Zendejas to lead one of its public dispensaries. Fernando Oca-ranza joined this Office's Executive Board the same month. With a long academic trajectory as faculty member of the Military Medical School and as faculty member, secretary, and dean of Escuela Nacional de Medicina (ENM; National School of Medicine) of the Universidad Nacional de Mex-ico (currently UNAM; National Autonomous University of Mexico) in the 1920s, Ocaranza prided himself of having met most practitioners of med-icine. For this reason, he questioned Zendejas's educational and professional background. Zendejas had studied at the Military Medical School and grad-uated from the Free School of Homeopathy of Mexico. He had practised in public medical institutions after he completed his academic preparation. Yet, Ocaranza pointed to Zendejas's degree as proof of his unsuitability for the position. At the hospital of the free school, faculty "teach surgery with tires, assuming the rubber coating resembles the skin and the hollow part, the body's cavities," Ocaranza said to the board. He argued that while Zendejas's diploma – "finely printed and with the regulatory seal of the Department of Public Health" – allowed him to practise medicine legally, the medical com-munity would question the office's decision to hire a person who lacked the training – and implicitly the academic lineage – required by the position. The board agreed to remove Zendejas from the dispensary.[1]

The tension between free schools and the ENM after the outbreak of the Mexican Revolution (1910) resulted from a shift in the model of health provi-sion implemented by post-revolutionary governments. If nineteenth-century liberalism regarded medicine as an individual and private concern, where individuals were responsible for educating themselves on and providing themselves with medicine, twentieth-century social medicine considered health a responsibility of nation-states. Post-revolutionary governments in Mexico embarked on an ambitious program to bring medicine to all Mexicans and raise healthy citizens. These programs included legislative reforms, administrative reorganization, new and renovated medical infrastructure such as schools and hospitals, and public health works and campaigns. Yet the programs opened up opportunities for medical practitioners who supported either of the models. ENM graduates signed up for social medicine because it allowed them to extend further their already important presence in medical institutions supported and controlled by the government, allowing them to implement a type of medicine they believed would improve the health and lifespan of Mexicans. Founders of free schools sided with liberal medicine. Regarding public medical schools as elitist, reactionary, conservative, and restrictive, they organized an alternative model of free − private − schools, financially, ideologically, and pedagogically independent from government regulation.[2] These liberal doctors believed that free medical schools trained working-class and poor Mexicans who were more likely to return and provide.medical services to their communities, where few − if any − ENM graduates practised.

The *título* or diploma turned into the symbol of the tensions between supporters of private and government-regulated medical education. A legal document, a proof of someone's medical expertise, a symbol of professional identity, and an opportunity for economic revenue, the diploma became in the 1920s and 30s an element of social control. The idea of a medical *título* dates back to the colonial period, when the Spanish monarchy established the Protomedicato, an institution that regulated medical curricula, imposed requirements to study medicine at the university, and granted authorization to practise medicine. In a piece of parchment, the *título* embodied the holder's knowledge, skills, socio-economic status, and sometimes even ethnic and religious background. After independence (1822), liberals fought to create institutions and legislation to end colonial privileges, though physicians sought to retain some control over their education and practice. In the second half of the nineteenth century, the tension between freedom of education and labour conflicted with physicians' authoritative claims over bodies, disease, hygiene, and sanitation.[3] The Constitution of 1857 aimed to undermine corporations' control over education and occupational elitism by granting Mexicans the freedom of education and occupation. Yet medical institutions such as the School of Medicine − predecessor of the ENM − unified surgery and medicine, previously taught separately at the university, and gained control over its own curriculum. The Superior Sanitary Board − an office that evolved from the Protomedicato and preceded the post-revolutionary Departamento de Salubridad Pública (DSP; Department of Public Health) – kept a registry of professional medical degrees. *Títulos* lost their legal value in the Constitution, but their cultural value increased, turning into symbols of professional identity and expertise widely used by physicians and sanitary authorities, and acknowledged by many upper- and middle-class Mexicans. During the Porfiriato (1886–1910), medical and sanitary institutions gained power, yet the revolution of 1910 did not mitigate the tension between professional liberalism and state control. The Constitution of 1917 retained the educational and labour liberalism of the 1857 mandate, but it granted the DSP national oversight on matters of hygiene, sanitation, and control of epidemic disease. This office established special educational requirements to register medical degrees, limiting medical activities for unregistered practitioners and imposing fines on offenders. Staffed by ENM graduates, the DSP became an office that used medical diplomas for professional control, targeting, as the introductory vignette shows, free schools.

Historians have examined how state institutions, politicians, and international health agents catalyzed the transformation of Mexican medicine from a liberal to a social model.[4] Social medicine promoted the intervention of the state in disseminating hygienic values, providing medical staff and services, and preventing and controlling epidemic disease. These were goals oriented particularly towards rural and working-class populations. Historians have also studied the challenges state officers faced in the formation and regulation of a new type of health professional and the implementation of state programs to socialize medicine.[5] Free medical schools, however, have received much less scholarly attention. Faculty, students, and graduates from free schools defended the freedom of medical education and professional practice. Furthermore, they promoted homeopathy, an approach to medicine disregarded by the medical community associated with the ENM, but that homeopaths believed was suitable for underserved Mexicans. Consequently, free school supporters represented a threat to the project of social medicine as imagined by ENM graduates. Yet free schools trained doctors who offered medical services to underserved Mexicans decades before education authorities implemented programs to bring students at state medical schools to experience the social realities in rural communities. These free schools thrived for three decades until sanitary and educative authorities discovered, targeted, and eliminated them.

Borrowing methodologies from the social history of medicine and the history of public health, I place free schools, their founders, their graduates, their knowledges, and their practices at the centre of historical analysis and in dialogue with state efforts to modernize health interventions.[6] I give voice to the subaltern voices of these schools' faculty and students through a wide array of sources including diplomas, lawsuits, school reports, inspection reports, applications, examinations, transcripts, clinical reports, and correspondence. Amplifying the voices of these social actors is an issue of social justice. It is particularly important because post-revolutionary sanitary and education agencies intentionally tried to erase their professional history. In this chapter, I examine free medical schools and the concerted effort of sanitary and educational authorities to regulate them and their graduates. My analysis demonstrates that free schools occupied an ambivalent position in the revolutionary project for social medicine, a position that was the outcome of negotiations between popular initiatives and state projects. Free schools provided modern medical education to the working class and the poor while they also challenged the state model of medical education and practice from 1910 to 1940. Contradictorily, state surveillance forced free-school graduates to operate in the margins of state oversight and unintentionally pushed them to continue offering health services to workers and peasants, fulfilling the goal of the revolution to socialize the medical profession.

THE TWENTIETH-CENTURY CONTEXT

In 1910, professional medicine was an urban phenomenon only partially and locally regulated. Post-revolutionary governments sought to regulate medical training and practice at the national level through UNAM and the DSP. The National University was an office created in 1910 to organize different professional schools, including the ENM. This school became the model to which new medical schools in the states aspired during the Porfiriato and after the revolution. Graduates from the ENM and other medical schools, including free schools, received a diploma that certified their academic training. In 1920, the DSP required the registration of diplomas of health practitioners all over the nation.[7] Registration was required to perform certain professional functions, and there were fines and penalties for offenders. Yet, university authorities decided to align with the 1917 Constitution and refused to sanction the diplomas that authorized an individual to engage in a professional practice. The Secretaría de Educación Pública (SEP; Ministry of Public Education) emerged as an independent institution in 1924 to regulate elementary education, but in the 1930s, it became responsible for certifying free schools and their diplomas. Medical staff at the DSP first and later at the SEP used the ENM academic model to assess medical training at free schools. In turn, legal staff used the medical staff's judgment, ruling sanitary codes, and federal and local legislation to establish the "official" status of medical schools and their graduates. However, free schools challenged these institutions' regulatory efforts since legislation was different from state to state and since it changed in the span of thirty years. Therefore, despite thorough documentary research, DSP and SEP authorities found it hard to substantiate legally their claims to erase the institutions that they regarded as an undesirable past.

BEGINNINGS

Free schools emerged in the reformist context of the revolution. Disappointed with Porfirian (1876–1910) schemes of training, some academically trained homeopaths opened schools independent from government regulation and funding. Historians suggest that the first free schools were the Free School of Law and the Free School of Homeopathy of Mexico (ELHM).[8] Established in 1914 in Mexico City, these schools brought together a solid group of professionals that resisted professional reforms in the 1920s and 1930s. Still functioning today, they are relics of the first efforts to create an alternative model of professional schools after the armed struggle. They were, however, neither the first ones nor the only ones.

There were at least ten free schools offering programs in medicine, nursing, and midwifery in Mexico after 1910. They resulted from the individual efforts of doctors committed to providing medical training to students who could not afford or whose working schedules did not allow them to attend public medical schools.[9] Some schools had sponsors; others had industrious and financially stable founders. Founders' efforts were not selfless, however. Having a school gave them the means to rent the facilities where they lived, taught, and practised. As schools recruited more students, they became more financially viable, graduated more students, and were more visible to government authorities. Financial hardships resulted in conflicts among faculty, between faculty and school administrations, and between these and government authorities. Administrators, for instance, generally invited faculty who wanted to teach without remuneration. Faculty were disappointed, however, when their altruism did not pay social or professional dividends. Consequently, there was a high turnover of faculty. Students attended these schools for their low cost or their suitable schedules. Symbols in diplomas suggest founders hoped to create a model of medical training that addressed working-class needs. This sensibility made some schools susceptible to receiving political support from workers' organizations. Most schools had a connection with homeopathy, a therapeutic system that gathered a group of doctors critical of contemporary changes in medical institutions.[10]

These schools had diverse genealogies, institutional trajectories, curricular organization, and impact on the student population. Juan Ollivier founded the Free School of Medicine of Puebla (ELMP) in 1910.[11] The schools' original homeopathic denomination changed after interim president Venustiano Carranza decreed the school's "official" status in 1915, arguing curricular parity with the ENM.[12] A high-school diploma was not required and the program lasted five years.[13] The school continued issuing diplomas until the 1930s and graduated at least 56 students. Alfredo Ortega founded the Free Homeopathic Institute of Mexico (ILHM) in 1914. He was a 1904 graduate from the National School of Homeopathic Medicine (ENMH), a strong advocate for homeopathy, and director of the dispensary at the National Homeopathic Hospital.[14] The school merged with the ENMH in 1945.[15] It graduated about 84 students from 1920 to 1936.[16] J. Rodríguez Toriello founded the Institute of Medical Sciences in 1922, later renamed the Free Mexican University (ULM). This institution offered programs in medicine, dentistry, nursing, and midwifery. The medical program lasted five years. The school charged $10 monthly and had 200 students in the early 1930s.

New free schools in the provinces followed the model of those in the capital.[17] In 1925, Onésimo Gómez, a 1916 graduate from the ELHM, began negotiations to establish a free school in Guadalajara.[18] ELHM founder Higinio Pérez was his sponsor. Pérez provided cash as well as books and homeopathic globules for selling. He also gave academic advice, moral support, and even legal recommendations. Leadership conflicts and economic hardships delayed the school's continuous work until 1930. Of the 35 students who enrolled in 1925 and 1926, only 13 graduated in 1929, suggesting the school had a program of four years. From 1930 to 1937, the school had an average enrollment of 21 students per year. By 1938, the school had graduated 37 students.

Free schools also had programs for midwifery and nursing in the 1920s. A detailed analysis of these is beyond the scope of this chapter. I use their information, however, to illuminate the organization of free medical schools, their student population, and their graduates' practice. The ELHM began a midwifery program in the 1920s.[19] In 1920, Arturo Palmero opened the Free School of Obstetrics and Nursing of Mexico (ELOE), which operated until 1934.[20] In 1924, Isaac Torres founded the Free School of Obstetrics (ELO) in honor of Juan N. Arriaga, an important homeopath during the Porfiriato (1886–1910).[21] Founders claimed they offered the same programs as UNAM, but followed the business model of free schools. Students in Palmero's school paid $25 pesos for tuition and $100 for their internship. Torres charged $3–4 a month for tuition. Faculty had no salary. About 150 students attended these schools in the 1920s and 1930s.[22]

STUDENTS

In the 1910s, founders of free schools advertised their institutions to working-class students. They argued that such schools provided medical training to young men and women who migrated from the countryside to the cities and had to work to make a living. In the 1920s, they operated alongside state programs aimed at bringing trained medical staff to working-class and rural communities. Free schools justified their special role: to train students from working-class and rural backgrounds who were inclined to return to their own communities to provide medical services, or even to create new free schools in similarly needy communities. In the context of a revolution, propaganda that appealed to industrial workers and peasants' educational, socio-economic, and medical needs resonated ideologically and politically. Circumstantial and direct evidence, moreover, indicates that such discourses mirrored the realities of student demographics at free schools.

The fact that free schools began as student-led efforts suggests that founders' narratives about working-class sensibilities were authentic rather than merely discourses constructed to echo the rhetoric around social programs. For instance, students who could not attend classes at the ENMH requested Higinio Pérez to create study groups in the late evening so they could study medicine after working hours.[23] The ELHM retained such schedules after it was officially established. Similarly, a group of women interested in helping pregnant women in the town of Tacubaya decided to study midwifery and organized the ELO.[24] Many students had a working-class or rural background. Palmero argued that his students came from towns and villages around Mexico City and could not afford the trip or paperwork to get their diplomas after having finished coursework.[25] Some of them worked in Mexico City before enrolling at the ELOE.[26] In an expression of solidarity with students who had financial difficulties, the ELHG's founder refused to charge fees to students – even after local authorities threatened to ban his own private medical practice and leave him without the financial resources to keep the school open. These examples indicate that founders genuinely conceived of their schools as opportunities for the working class.

Most medical students were male and most midwifery and nursing students were female. Only 1 out of 56 graduates of medicine from the ELMP was a woman, and the ILHM in Mexico City had a similar ratio.[27] The female-to-male ratio of medical graduates at the ELHG was somewhat higher (8:76). The ELHM had a similar ratio (36:322) from 1914 to 1950.[28] In midwifery, 2 out of 72 graduates from the ELHM in the same period were male. At the ELOE, 12 out of 82 students were male. There were exceptions to this trend. For instance, only 1 out of 20 graduates from the ULM in nursing was a woman. A proportion of 1 per cent women graduating from medical schools in Mexico in the 1900s was a common trend. The ENM had a ratio of 1:90 in 1911.[29] Women with a degree in medicine from the UNAM in the second half of the 1940s represented 5.2 per cent of the total number of graduates in medicine.[30] The ELHM and ELHG's 10 per cent female graduation proportion was higher than the ENM's, which suggests an initial openness towards professional medical education for women. While the ELHG retained this proportion, the proportion of both woman students and woman graduates at the ELHM decreased from the 1910s to the 1920s, partly because the ELHM opened its midwifery program then. Midwifery programs in free schools offered spaces for women interested in medicine that public schools did not.[31]

Most students were from Mexico City, but many were from towns neighbouring the capital or from other states. 26.8 per cent of the student population at the ELOE had recently migrated from four neighbouring towns and eleven states. More than half of the students (55.4 per cent) at the ELHM were immigrants to Mexico City from three neighbouring towns, twenty-three states, and two countries (Spain and Japan).[32] Given the working-class orientation of free schools, recent immigrants to Mexico City found free schools suitable for their economic, scheduling, and social needs.

Prospective students had varying degrees of academic preparation. In the 1920s, SEP mandated all schools, including free schools, to require evidence (e.g., a diploma) that incoming students had completed elementary education, and, by the 1930s, secondary education. In addition to the SEP's requirements, some free-school administrators created middle- and high-school programs and instituted qualifying exams in order to attract higher numbers of students.[33] With a diploma and professional experience in elementary education, Palmero examined 82 prospective students, of which he considered 25 qualified to begin the ELOE's nursing and midwifery program. In 1930, he implemented a preparatory course. A few ELOE prospective students had completed coursework at the secondary or professional level, and even at other free schools such as the Free University of Veracruz. These students may have held an advantage over other students since Palmero expedited students who showed proficiency in the course content. In rare cases, free schools revalidated all coursework done at similar institutions. This was the case for Arnulfo Durán Jiménez, an ILHM graduate who relocated to Guadalajara in 1924. Dr Rosas, dean of the ELHG, issued a diploma for him, arguing parity of coursework and professional examination procedures between both institutions.[34] The objective of most free-school administrators was to ensure that students could master foundational scientific concepts.

Qualifying exams offer a window into the scientific knowledge students were required to attain in order to enroll in a professional medical program at free schools. These records also show the differences in conceptual depth between middle- and high-school students. The ELOE's qualifying exam for high school required students to define concepts, give examples, and explain applications of concepts in zoology, botany, physics, and chemistry. In 1932, Magdalena Cruz wrote a three-page essay on general notions of cellular, tissue, and general anatomy.[35] She explained the cellular nature of living matter, the parts of different kinds of cells, the possibility of living functions beyond the cellular level, and the levels of organization defined by cellular structures and functions. She defined in a two-page essay two botanical groups, giving some examples and suggesting their uses. In another two-page essay, she explained a chemical reaction to produce hydrogen and drew a diagram to illustrate how to carry out the experiment in the laboratory. In a half-page essay, she provided a physical explanation of the sense of touch. In 1934, Esperanza Cerda González, who had only attended elementary school, was required to elaborate on reptiles, the plant genus *Solanum*, the centre of gravity, and Berthelot's law.[36] She did it succinctly, using only half a page for each answer. The two prospective students had a similar degree of elaboration, showing a command of scientific concepts. However, responses from students who had had some preparatory education were more sophisticated and provided practical applications.[37] Examination answers suggest that prospective students knew scientific concepts that prepared them to study in a professional program, at least in nursing and midwifery, in the late 1920s.

CURRICULUM

Once enrolled in a free medical school, students took two and five years of coursework to complete the program of nursing/midwifery or medicine, respectively. ENM graduates and government authorities knew these schools existed, but they did not have a clear idea of their programs, facilities, and activities.[38] Furthermore, they considered them "manifestations of medical piracy" that endured only in a country of liberties such as Mexico.[39] The DSP learned about some of them in 1920, when many free schools' graduates sent in their diplomas to comply with the medical registry, but the Office of Legal Affairs and Revalidation was interested in the legal status of free-school diplomas rather than the schools' curricula. The UNAM disengaged from any regulatory role of professional education during the 1910s and 20s. The SEP assumed this role in 1929 and discovered what medical education for the working class looked like.

Most free schools had a homeopathic orientation. However, homeopathic did not mean non-medical – as homeopathy's detractors wanted Mexicans to believe. Homeopaths, many of them professional physicians, had pushed for the popularization of medical knowledge and the inclusion of homeopathy in the curriculum of medical schools since their arrival in Mexico in 1853.[40] Faculty at the ENM resisted and homeopaths responded by creating their own school in 1895, the ENMH, with an inclusive curriculum, state support, and the ENM faculty's criticism.[41] Notably, free medical schools provided homeopaths opportunities to extend their curriculum to other schools without state surveillance.

The politics of the revolution and the modification of the ENM's medical curriculum in the 1920s influenced the pedagogical approach of free schools. After 1910, ENM faculty argued over preserving the theoretical approach of the Porfiriato or introducing a practical one. As an ENM and UNAM administrative staff member in the 1910s, 1920s, and 1930s, Fernando Ocaranza pushed for establishing a systematized laboratory and clinical instruction based on the physiology of Claude Bernard.[42] If ENM faculty had resisted this transformation in the 1910s, Ocaranza's leadership as the UNAM's dean helped him transform medical curricula and training methods in the second half of the 1920s. With a physiological and clinical orientation, a new generation of physicians staffed the public health and education offices responsible for inspecting and evaluating free medical schools in the 1920s and 1930s. For this generation, free schools did not meet contemporary standards of modern medical training because they lacked opportunities for bedside clinical instruction and laboratory work. In other words, graduates of free medical schools were not qualified to guarantee the right to health of Mexicans.

In contrast, free-school founders criticized contemporary medical education as encyclopedic, positivistic, and unpractical. They designed programs that made efficient use of time and focused on essential knowledge with practical relevance. Supporters of free schools believed they trained a generation of practitioners with the basic requirements to attend to the health needs of the destitute, the working-class, and the rural population. Accessible, affordable, practical, and with a social orientation, free schools institutionalized the exchange of medical and homeopathic knowledge that already happened domestically in local communities. This exchange began elsewhere perhaps as it did in Mexico City, discussing and using homeopathic and other medical domestic manuals and later adding technical knowledge as required by academic medicine. Nevertheless, it lacked the facilities and orientation that official medical schools required.

Most free schools followed ELHM and ENMH medical programs in the 1910s.[43] These programs focused on anatomy, surgery, physiology, pathology, and therapeutics. There were no special courses in basic sciences such as pharmacy, chemistry, histology, or bacteriology. There was a clinic in surgery and in internal medicine. Some programs also offered a class on obstetrics. While programs dedicated less time to each course compared to the ENM, some had additional courses that the ENM did not.[44] For instance, the ELHM offered philosophy of medicine and hygiene. Coursework took five years. In 1916, 1925, and 1933, ELHM administrators realigned the program with the ENM in response to various regulatory pressures from the DSP and SEP.

The SEP discovered the ILHM's medical program in 1930. It had the same practical and medical focus of the ELHM's first program, but selected courses rather arbitrarily from other homeopathic programs. The institute offered fewer anatomy courses and similar numbers of courses in basic science, pathology, therapeutics, obstetrics, pediatrics, hygiene, and medical humanities (legal medicine, history of medicine). It also introduced a new course on toxicology, a subject that the ELHM and ENMH did not offer. In 1944, the institute extended this program from four to five years.[45]

Despite the curricular update to free schools in the 1920s and 30s, the government's main concern was that students might receive inadequate clinical training. With no access to public hospitals, most free-school teachers and students reported that clinical practice took place in the school's dispensary or with the faculty's own clientele.[46] Palmero's midwifery and nursing students submitted internship reports that confirm these accounts.[47] At "Sanatorio Palmero," students practised taking and recording patients' vital signs, including temperature and blood pressure.[48] They also assisted with childbirths, usually at patients' homes, and occasionally at public hospitals.[49] Their practical skills were exceptional, delivering babies successfully most of the time from normal and difficult pregnancies. Furthermore, they knew and applied obstetrical practices doctors used in the early twentieth century, though they preferred non-surgical procedures.[50] Reports also describe interactions with physicians who graduated from free schools. The interactions suggest that these doctors followed the same procedures that were employed by doctors who had graduated elsewhere. While evidence on the specific training of free-school graduates may not be as thorough as that on midwives, circumstantial evidence suggests that medical students were as knowledgeable in medical matters as their counterparts were in midwifery.

REGULATION

Post-revolutionary governments did not acknowledge the training, skills, or diplomas of doctors who graduated from free schools. Sanitary officers in the 1920s and SEP staff in the 1930s questioned free schools as they discovered the high number of practitioners the schools produced: at least 544 health providers (497 doctors, 35 nurses, and 12 midwives) by the mid-1930s.[51] Doctors represented 16 per cent of those registered with the DSP in 1929.[52]

Diploma in hand, free-school graduates felt entitled to practise in the profession they had studied for years. In the search for a healthy nation and a manageable medical profession, however, DSP and SEP authorities contravened the professional liberties granted in the Constitution and used the ENM's academic model to deny them professional citizenship.

The DSP systematically denied the registration of free-school diplomas throughout the 1920s. In 1920, sanitary authorities began to register diplomas from "official" schools – those authorized by local governments – or practitioners who passed special examinations. Sanitary codes imposed restrictions on unregistered practitioners.[53] During the 1920s, the DSP kept most free-school diplomas out of the registry, even when their holders won lawsuits against the Department.[54] Ignoring the constitutionally legal status and technical level of free schools, sanitary authorities based their policy on presumptions about them. Supported by courts, DSP staff exerted a sanitary dictatorship, blocking free-school graduates' access to the medical registry.[55]

Free-school doctors found alternative ways to ratify their professional credentials. Many requested public authorities to endorse the signatures on their diplomas.[56] Endorsed diplomas may have convinced employers of a diploma's "official" status. Some state governments registered these diplomas in spite of federal sanitary policies.[57] Their holders, though, had to register in every single state where they practised, even when the Constitution required all states to acknowledge particular acts by local governments. As more local states began to align with federal sanitary regulation, free-school graduates found it more difficult to register their diplomas. Changing legislation and the animosity of local medical and public health officials limited free-school doctors' opportunities to register their diplomas in local boards. Ignacio Vázquez Gómez, a 1927 ULM graduate who had fulfilled Morelos's established requirements to obtain a medical diploma, barely made it to the scheduled examination proposed by the local Sanitary Board on very short notice.[58] The abrupt procedure suggests the board either doubted the candidate's preparation or wanted him to miss the examination. During this decade, free-school doctors used various means to legalize their diplomas locally, but this did not have the national registry's acceptance they needed.

In the 1930s, the DSP continued exerting its influence when the SEP became responsible for certifications. The secretary began to revalidate free-school diplomas and certify some free-school programs.[59] The department registered these diplomas, but the political and legal instability in the early 1930s that allowed the registration of 170 ELHM diplomas made the department reconsider SEP policies. The DSP stopped registering diplomas from free schools and convinced the SEP to reframe certification guidelines, a shift that negatively affected free schools with pending applications.[60] Affected graduates sued the department. This time the DSP officers carried out detailed investigations to find out the "official" status of a school at the time it issued diplomas in order to justify in court DSP denials of registration.[61] In the most iconic of these lawsuits, the DSP discovered President Carranza had actually legalized the ELMP in 1915, but that a local professional regulation had made this legalization inapplicable by 1919.[62] Courts selectively allowed the registration of some but not all graduates from free schools in the early 1930s based on these types of investigations.[63] DSP officers specifically blocked the registration of students who had graduated in the 1910s and 1920s, consistently framing free schools as having been unable to legally issue medical diplomas during these decades.

The SEP adopted DSP policies in the 1930s, assuming the surveillance of free schools and their diplomas. As ENM graduates working at the SEP's Department of Psycho-Pedagogy and Hygiene (DPPH) confronted their ideals of medical training with the realities of free schools, they decided to incorporate the DSP's discriminatory policies, disqualifying free schools as institutions unfit to provide a practical and scientific medical education. They did it by establishing procedures to revalidate diplomas. Petitioners had to demonstrate they had studied and passed examinations in a program similar to the ENM's and had approved a professional exam.[64] Instead, the DPPH used free schools' lack of documentation to deny revalidations in the 1930s, as in the case of Faustino Fernández Mayor, an ELMP graduate.[65] Medical inspectors found he had studied for five years, when the ENM program required students to study for six; the university had only partially revalidated his high-school studies when he enrolled in the school; and he had obtained school certificates from "official" middle and high schools fifteen years after he obtained his medical diploma. The candidate's sequence of studies was irregular and the fulfillment of enrolling requirements questionable, yet the commission recommended not revalidating the diploma because he did not provide evidence of the school's enrollment requirements, academic program, and syllabi.

Certification of schools was the SEP's second gatekeeping strategy; it substituted degree revalidation and gave SEP authorities insight into free schools.[66] For certification, the SEP required free schools to provide detailed documentation of their academic programs, enrollment requirements, facilities, proficiency of faculty members, and plans to sustain "academic efficiency and efficacy."[67] After certifying the ELHM and ELOE in 1930 and 1931, the SEP went through staff and policy changes that subverted the willingness to certify free schools.[68] DPPH medical staff began to scrutinize schools' documentation very closely – including each course's syllabus, students' current and previous academic records, and student and faculty members' attendance records. They also paid close attention to facilities – enough and adequate rooms for clinical practices and equipped laboratories for practical instruction in the sciences. DPPH inspectors found free schools lacking. They denied certification to the ILHM in 1931 because its documentation did not include a list of faculty members.[69] They did the same to the ELO, because both documentation and facilities were lacking and therefore they believed the school could not provide "good professional instruction" that cultivated "good social and moral principles for the practice of medicine."[70]

SEP authorities also became suspicious of free schools' long-term success and implemented in-situ inspections to verify the accuracy of school reports. For instance, after the ELOE had submitted reports and stopped SEP attempts to cancel its certification, DPPH staff subjected the ELOE to inspections.[71] Inspectors depicted the ELOE as radically different from its portrayal in Palmero's reports. If Palmero praised its efficient and practical program, inspectors characterized it as abbreviated, narrow, and superficial. Inspectors dismissed student practical training as domestic, unsupervised, irregular, and anti-pedagogical (not teaching them hygienic procedures and not exposing them to difficult deliveries). To them, the school had "dark classrooms with low ceilings," containing old-fashioned models "unsuitable for teaching the practice of obstetrics" and outdated laboratory instruments.[72] Despite the SEP's close surveillance, the school remained open until 1938, when Palmero died.[73] Other schools were less successful. SEP inspections of the ULM revealed that the director did not follow SEP recommendations, allowing the enrollment of students rejected from the UNAM and issuing them diplomas when he saw fit. Inspectors also considered the school's program "rudimentary."[74] The SEP never incorporated this school. The SEP's inspections came later to the provinces, though they had the same aim and effect. Six years after the ELHG requested certification in 1931, inspectors reported that "a medical school could not exist with [such] facilities" and that it needed to have an amphitheatre with cadavers, well-equipped laboratories for every single course on basic sciences, and a hospital for clinical practices, as well as detailed programs for each course.[75] Inspectors framed their evaluation based on the scientific and medical culture of the university, with the aim of discrediting medical training at free schools and shutting them down.

CAREERS

The outcome of registration denials, revalidation procedures, certification requests, and inspection reports by DSP and DPPH medical officers resulted in a culture of distrust towards free schools. The idea of poor practical training created a climate of uncertainty about them. How prevalent was this perception among the public and how did it affect employment of free-school graduates?

Mexican society was ambivalent about free schools. Some Mexicans expressed a lack of confidence, and others showed complete trust. The governments of Puebla and the State of Mexico denied legal status to free-school diplomas in the 1930s.[76] Graduates with degrees from both official and free schools preferred to use the former for the DSP registry.[77] ELOE graduates revalidated their diplomas when legally they did not need to do it.[78] The SEP secretary in 1931 justified the ELOE's certification by the need for midwives with "at least some deficient scientific training" to help with the deliveries of poor Mexican women, who usually sought the services of "completely ignorant *comadronas*." For state officers, if free schools served a social function, they did it at the expense of medical quality. Parents were concerned free schools deceived their children, promising them an official diploma.[79]

Many graduates, however, were confident about their training and their credentials. In multiple lawsuits and correspondence, they proved their conviction about their proficient training and their diplomas' legal status.[80] They accused governments of imposing a "state medicine" without recognizing the characteristics of free schools and the legal and material conditions schools faced.[81] They cited the ENMH as an example of a state-funded school that, in the early 1930s, did not have the laboratory facilities state authorities demanded – and yet the DSP had registered its diplomas.[82]

In spite of people's ambivalence on the medical quality of free schools, patients used free-school doctors' services, predominantly in urban working-class neighbourhoods and rural areas. Graduates primarily offered private services. ELOE midwives' and nurses' reports mention ELHM and ILHM graduates as bedside doctors in the early 1930s.[83] Some of them had consulting offices in Mexico City.[84] ILHM graduates practised in Durango.[85] ELHP graduates practised in several states such as Durango (where they founded a professional society), Chihuahua, Baja California, San Luis Potosí, Sinaloa, Colima, and Puebla.[86] Others changed locations and positions several times.[87] ULM graduates worked in Guerrero, Durango, Morelos, Chihuahua, and Tamaulipas.[88] A few held important positions at state institutions; for instance, Antonio Herrera practised in the Secretariat of the Navy and the Army and directed the General Hospital of Guerrero and Texcoco.[89]

Free-school graduates argued that their practice favoured *campesinos* and the proletariat. If some of them practised in Mexico City and state capitals, many offered their services in small towns and villages. Patients of Alfonso Bonilla, Ángel Crespo Delgado, and Salvador Dosamantes lived in Tacubaya, a town neighbouring Mexico City, on the road to Lecumberri prison east of Mexico City – a poor neighbourhood – and in a working-class neighbourhood located northwest of Mexico City. These physicians' and patients' geographic distribution suggests the working-class and rural contexts where medical consultations happened. Privately employed, these doctors did not generally serve elites or even middle-class urban patients. They fulfilled the mandate of social medicine after the revolution, though in a private manner and on the margins of state control.

CONCLUSIONS

Free medical schools were a model of medical training in tension with the post-revolutionary project of social medicine in Mexico. The liberal model in the late nineteenth century was based on a free market of health providers and consumers. In this model, academically trained doctors usually remained in cities where they had attended medical school and where the middle class and elites could afford their services. The Federal District, where Mexico City is located, had 526 doctors in 1900.[90] In 1895, the density of doctors was 276.74 per 1,000km², and the doctor-to-patient ratio 9.9 per 10,000.[91] Government officers after the revolution sought to change this trend. For them, Mexicans' access to health was a right with social and economic benefits for the nation. Therefore, not only did the state have a responsibility, but a gain in providing it. One approach state agents took was the "socialization" of medical students after the revolution in order to shift the liberal culture of professional medicine. Sanitary officers, for instance, created the National School of Public Health in 1922 to train a new generation of health providers with a holistic view of disease and medicine that considered not only the biomedical, but also the social, cultural, and economic aspect of disease and health.[92] This, however, was not enough to satisfy the health needs of Mexicans. Using the 1930 census, Dr Esther Chapa exposed the fact that 2,359 out of 4,520 doctors practised in Mexico City; 1,542 in major cities; and 628 in smaller towns.[93] She calculated that 11.5 million Mexicans living in 84,000 communities out of a total 16.5 million inhabitants did not have any form of medical care. Originally resisting change, the ENM implemented a social service in 1936, a program where medical students who had completed coursework at a government-funded medical school spent a year in rural towns before they took the professional examination and earned their diplomas.[94] Authorities ignored free schools and their graduates in their sanitary and educational projects to build a healthier nation after the revolution.

Free medical schools were a hybrid and transitional model aligned with the revolutionary ideal of socialized medicine, but also in conflict with emerging and consolidating state institutions of public health and education. Their curricula integrated contemporary medical science with homeopathy. While free schools aligned with the social orientation of the revolutionary state, they defended their independence from state regulations, surveillance, and subsidy.

Government officers knew that free-school graduates provided medical services to patients and in places ENM graduates would not venture, but these
officers also lamented the poor quality of free schools' facilities and programs.
Free schools offered medical training and services to non-elites in the 1910s
and 1920s. When sanitary and education institutions created and consolidated programs to bring doctors with a "scientific" and social understanding
of health and medicine to the countryside, they discovered free schools and
treated them as an epidemic outbreak. They located the germ of free medical
education, designed a sanitary campaign against their diplomas, and eliminated free schools by the mid-1940s. Free schools were inclusive of diverse
medical perspectives, innovative in the efficient and pragmatic use of resources
to deliver good practical training, and attentive to the needs of Mexicans.
Their model, however, lasted only a couple of decades until the state assumed
this role.

Sanitary policies against free schools were unintendedly self-serving. By
aiming to get rid of free schools, these policies brought free-school graduates
to underserved Mexicans. The medical registry forced free-school doctors to
practise on the margins of state surveillance. The rural countryside and urban
working-class neighbourhoods were spaces where these doctors could practise
without exposing themselves to the growing number of sanitary officers in
the country. This implied that practitioners with actual academic training did
bring health services to the population the revolutionary state aimed to serve.

Sanitary policies were also ambivalent. By not recognizing free-school
graduates' credentials, the state rendered these practitioners invisible when
it required knowing their number and distribution to plan the provision of
health services accordingly. Sanitary officers, therefore, did not plan the distribution of health care providers in the nation based on the actual number of
practitioners on the ground. Officers needed to consider free-school graduates
in their calculations in order to have a more accurate picture of the provision
of medicine in Mexico after the revolution. They did not. In *not* doing so, they
ignored a past for the sake of the construction of a new and healthier nation.
Medical and public health authorities prescribed the remedy for a new nation,
eliminating the past of liberal professional training and practice in order to
forge the future of a socialized medical profession.

The ELHM, however, endured, becoming a symbol of the limits of state
authority in controlling doctors and a constant reminder of the relevance of
free schools in the construction of the Mexican medical profession after the
Mexican Revolution. Free schools emerged in 1910 and formed the first doctors of the revolution: doctors who challenged the status quo of medical education. Doctors who created new schools to train working-class, itinerant, and
foreign students in medicine. Doctors oriented towards fulfilling the medical

needs of middle-class, working-class, poor, and destitute Mexicans. Doctors who exposed and fought against the despotism of sanitary legislation and policy. Doctors whose lives broaden our historical understanding of the complexities of the revolutionary ideal of providing health to all Mexicans.

NOTES

1   Archivo Histórico de la Secretaría de Salud (AHSS), Beneficencia Pública (BP), Dirección, Actas de Sesión, 9, 9, 22 September 1932 and 27 October 1932.

2   Free medical schools in Mexico resemble the model of proprietary schools in the United States to a certain extent. Free medical schools were associated with homeopathy, as many proprietary schools were to a wide variety of medical systems in the nineteenth-century US. The push to organize the medical community into what sociologists have called the medical profession came from a subgroup of this community in both countries. However, the historiography suggests that the regulatory process in the United States depended very significantly on the internal reorganization of the medical community, while in Mexico state institutions mediated this process in substantial ways. A comparative study lies beyond the scope of this chapter. For an overview of medical systems and their role in medical education in the United States see Gevitz, *Other Healers*.

3   Hernández Sáenz, *Carving a Niche*; Carrillo, "Profesiones sanitarias y lucha de poderes."

4   Birn, *Marriage of Convenience*; Sowell, *Medicine on the Periphery*; Agostoni, *Médicos, campañas y vacunas*.

5   Gudiño-Cejudo, Magaña-Valladares, and Hernández Ávila, "La Escuela de Salud Pública de México"; Agostoni, "Médicos rurales y medicina social"; Soto Laveaga, "Bringing the Revolution to Medical Schools."

6   Birn and Necochea López, "Footprints on the Future"; Diego Armus, "Disease in the Historiography of Modern Latin America."

7   Pruneda, "Por el Departamento de Salubridad Pública."

8   Garciadiego, *Los orígenes de la Escuela Libre de Derecho*; Francois Flores, *Escuela Libre de Homeopatía*.

9   Correspondence between Onésimo Gómez and Higinio Pérez, Fernando Darío Francois Flores's private archives (OG); Francois Flores, *Escuela Libre de Homeopatía*.

10 Carrillo, "¿Indivisibilidad o bifuración de la ciencia?"; Francois Flores, *Historia de la homeopatía en México*; Francois Flores, *Escuela Libre de Homeopatía*.

11 Also known as the Free School of Homeopathy of Puebla. See AHSS, Secretaría de Salubridad y Asistencia (SSA), Dirección General de Asuntos Jurídicos (DGAJ), Registro de Títulos de Médicos Homeópatas (RTMH); AHSS,

SSA, DGAJ, Títulos, 2, 11; Tesis aislada 2ª sala, *Semanario Judicial de la Federación y su Gaceta*, Quinta Época (SJFG), t. XXVII, 4 November 1929, p. 1502; SJFG, t. XXXIII, 22 October 1931, p. 1501; SJFG, t. XXXIV, 11 April 1932, p. 2156; SJFG, t. XXXV, 10 June 1932, p. 911; SJFG, t. LXX, 10 June 1937, p. 4667; SJFG, t. XXVIII, 16 January 1930, p. 249. SJ, 45, 17.

12   Dr Leonides Andreu Almazán certified Carranza's legal recognition on 5 January 1931: Archivo General de la Nación (AGN), Abelardo L. Rodríguez (ALR), 011/13.

13   AGN, Secretaría de Educación Pública (SEP), Departamento de Psicopedagogía e Higiene (DPPH), 35489.

14   He published two articles in the journal *La homeopatía* XIII, 2 (1907) and XVI, 2 (1912). Nombramientos, AHSS, BP, Hospitales, Hospital Nacional Homeopático (HNH), 1, 22, 9 October 1914. Correspondence between President Pascual Ortiz Rubio and F. Corsá and J.O. Montenegro, ALR, 582/2, 3 October 1932.

15   AGN, SEP, Departamento Jurídico y de Revalidación (DJR), 31724, 32-3-1-1 and s/n.

16   Títulos, 1, 36; 1, 49; 1, 49; 2, 1; 2, 2; 2, 24; 2, 48; 3, 9; 3, 17-21; DJR, 31726, 17-2-7-19.

17   Gutiérrez López, "Lucha por el control de la educación superior."

18   OG.

19   "Registro general de médicos y parteras recibidos de la ELHM," Archivo histórico de la Escuela Libre de Homeopatía de México (AELHM).

20   Arturo Palmero 1934 annual report, DJR, 31737, 17-1-10-41.

21   Correspondence, Isaac Torres, DJR, s/n, s/n, 17 September 1931.

22   Arturo Palmero, annual reports, 1933, 1934, 1935, DJR, 31737, 17-1-10-41; 31737, 17-1-10-41; and 31737, 17-1-10-41.

23   Moheno, "En defensa de los homeópatas," 75–6. Francois Flores, *Escuela Libre de Homeopatía*, 71–81.

24   See note 21.

25   See note 22.

26   DJR, 31726, 17-2-7-6 and 17-2-6-70.

27   2 women out of 84 graduates at the ILHM.

28   Transcripts, AHELHM.

29   Castañeda López and Rodríguez de Romo, "Mujeres médico graduadas."

30   Penyak, "Obstetrics and the Emergence of Women."

31   SEP statistics for 1945–49 show that 12 out of 223 women had a university degree in obstetrics, midwifery, or gynecology, and 9 were ELHM graduates in midwifery: Penyak, "Obstetrics and the Emergence of Women," 77.

32 "Registro general de médicos y parteras recibidos de la ELHM" and historias
    académicas de médicos, AELHM.

33 Francois-Flores, *Escuela Libre de Homeopatía,* 73; Moheno, "En defensa de los
    homeópatas," 77; Pérez, *Programas y métodos de enseñanza;* transcripts, AELHM;
    ILHM programs, DJR, 31737, 17-1-10-41, 20 February 1933; 1933 and
    1934 annual reports in note 22; ILHM programs, DJR, 31724, 32-3-1-1 and
    s/n.

34 Títulos, 1, 51.

35 DJR, 31726, 17-2-6-192.

36 DJR, 31726, 17-2-6-184.

37 Paz Patiño, DJR, 31726, 17-2-6-196; Esperanza Cerda González, DJR,
    31726, 17-2-6-184.

38 "Dictamen que presenta la comisión."

39 Pous Cházaro, "Juicio crítico."

40 Hernandez Berrones, "Homeopathy 'for Mexicans.'"

41 Quevedo y Zubieta, "La Homeopatía oficial ó la bifurcación de la ciencia."

42 Ocaranza, *Historia de la medicina en México,* 208–10.

43 Transcripts, AELHM; Pérez, *Programas y métodos de enseñanza.*

44 Herrera Moreno, "La Escuela de Medicina de México"; Ocaranza, *Historia de
    la medicina en México.*

45 ILHM programs, see note 15.

46 Union of Professionals of the Free Mexican University, letter, DJR, 31878,
    17-2-8-182. See also AHSS, Salubridad Pública (SP), Servicio Jurídico (SJ),
    29, 14.

47 DJR, 31726 and 31729.

48 DJR, 31726, 17-2-6-194 and 195.

49 DJR, 31729, 17-2 6-82; 17-2-6-63; and 31726, 17-2 6-185.

50 Carrillo, "Nacimiento y muerte de una profesion."

51 Figures are certainly larger. Records only show information for a few years,
    and most schools functioned for more than a decade.

52 "Lista de los médicos cirujanos," 1929, AHSS, SP, Ejercicio de la Medicina
    (EM), 10, 20.

53 The 1894 Sanitary Code restrictions included advertising services, working at
    government institutions, and issuing death certificates. The 1926 and 1934
    Sanitary Code's new restrictions included leading private clinics and hospitals,
    prescribing heroic drugs, or heading dispensaries. Pruneda, "Por el
    Departamento de Salubridad Pública"; AHSS, SP, Secretaría, 11, 1, pp. 33–5;
    "Un dique al ejercicio de la medicina por charlatanes," *El Universal,* 2
    September 1934, reprinted in "Los Charlatanes y el Nuevo Código
    Sanitario," *Acción Médica* V (January 1935): 7.

54   Moheno, "En defensa de los homeópatas," 34–65; EM, 4, 14; Archivo
      Histórico de la Universidad Nacional Autónoma de México (AHUNAM),
      Universidad Nacional (UN), Rectoría, 29, 381; AHUNAM, UN, Rectoría,
      Asuntos Generales, Dirección General de Incorporación y Revalidación de
      Estudios, cajas 63–4, exp. 597.

55   Aréchiga, "Educación, propaganda o 'dictadura sanitaria.'"

56   Including public notaries, local governments, public health offices, the
      Subsecretary of the Interior, and the Subsecretary of Foreign Relations.
      Títulos, 1, 26; 1, 36; 2, 11; and 1, 36.

57   Ismael Rendón from the ELMP registered his diploma in Veracruz (1924),
      Mexico City (1925), Morelos (1925), Tamaulipas (1927), and back in Puebla
      (1929); Antonio Mendoza y Calderón from the ILHM, in Colima (1933) and
      Querétaro (1933); Pedro M. Cobos from the ILHM, in Morelos (1926). DJR,
      31726, 17-2-7-19; Títulos, 1, 48.

58   DPPH, 35557, 17-9-8-187.

59   DJR, 31831, 17-2-7-116.

60   Particularly the ILHM, ALR, 582/2.

61   ULM's case, SJ, 28, 3. ILHM's case, DJR, 31726, 17-2-7-19.

62   Unsuccessful ELMP graduates' lawsuits are in note 12. See also SJ, 38, 12, and
      EM, 12, 22; Tesis aislada 2ª sala, SJFG, t. XXXIII, 18 November 1931, p.
      3145; SJFG, 21 October 1931, p. 1501; SJ, 41, 12 and 45, 17; SJFG, t. LIII,
      29 July 1937, p. 1162; SJFG, t. LXXIII, 21 August 1942, p. 4407; SJFG, t.
      LXXXI, 24 August 1944, p. 4207; SJFG, t. LXXXI, 24 August 1944, p.
      4172. Only Rafael Chávez de Alba was registered.

63   2 out of 14 ELMP graduates, 33 ILHM graduates, and 1 ELHG graduate.

64   Títulos, 1, 36, and DJR, 31831, 17-2-7-116.

65   Report, DPPH, 35489.

66   Revalidations could still happen if students were examined on every single
      course of "official" medical programs. To my knowledge no student
      revalidated a medical diploma this way. Opinion of SEP's Legal Office, DPPH,
      35557, 17-9-8-187.

67   "Decreto por el cual se reglamenta el funcionamiento de las escuelas libres."

68   "Decreto por el cual se concede a la Escuela Libre de Homeopatía"; "Decreto
      por el cual se concede a la Escuela Libre de Obstetricia y Enfermería de
      México."

69   Correspondence, ALR, 582/2.

70   See note 21.

71   DJR, 31737, 17-1-10-41; Tesis aislada 2ª sala, SJFG, t. XXXVII, 12 January
      1933, p. 88; Tesis aislada 2ª sala, Quinta Época, t. I, Const., P.R; SCJN,
      12 January 1933, p. 724; ELOE's 1933, 1934, and 1935 annual plans are in

note 22; AGN, SEP, Dirección de Enseñanza Técnica (DET), 34911, 15-4-10-224.

72 Inspection report, DPPH, 35543, 17-14-1-272.

73 Memo, DJR, 31737, 17-1-10-41.

74 Lawsuit, DJR, 31831, 17-2-7-123.

75 Correspondence, DET, 34911, 15-4-10-219.

76 Court rule, EM, 12, 22; letter, SJ, 26, 8.

77 Letter, EM, 13, 5, p. 88.

78 DJR, s/n, 13-9-3-150; Tesis aislada 2ª sala, SJFG, t. XL, 17 February 1934, p. 1565.

79 DJR, 31944, 17-3-6-86.

80 Lawsuits of ELMP see notes 11 and 65. Lawsuits from ILHM graduates in Tesis aislada 2ª sala, SJFG, t. LXXI, 27 January 1942, p. 1424; SJFG, 3 February 1942, p. 7231; SJFG, t. LXXIII, 20 July 1942, p. 1631; SJFG, Informe 1946, 20 July 1942, p. 80; SJFG, Informe 1942, 11 February 1946, p. 63; SJFG, t. LVII, Tercera Parte, 7 March 1962, 91. Lawsuits from ULM graduates are in DJR, 31831, 17-2-7-116; correspondence, DJR, 31878, 17-2-8-182; DJR, 31831, 17-2-7-123; SJ, 29, 14; correspondence, SJ 29, 14.

81 Correspondence, EM, 13, 12, p. 2-7.

82 Correspondence, DJR, 31878, 17-2-8-182. Also, SJ, 29, 14.

83 DJR, 31729, 17-2-6-82, 17-2-6-91; DJR, 31726, 17-2-7-7.

84 AHSS agents' reports, SJ, 41, 21; 45, 15; and 45, 18.

85 Telegram, DPPH, 35511, 17-14-5-150.

86 Letters, EM, 13, 5, p. 64-5, and EM, 13, 14, p. 11-2; SJ, 38, 12 and EM 12, 22; EM, 13, 5, p. 41; EM 13, 12, p. 20; EM 13, 12, p. 24; and AGN, Pascual Ortiz Rubio, 1932, 24/1959.

87 Títulos 1, 26.

88 DET, 34913, 15-4-10-69; Tesis aislada 2ª sala, SJFG, t. LXXIX, 23 February 1944, p. 3904; DPPH, 35557, 17-9-8-187; Tesis aislada 2ª sala, SJFG, t. XLVI, 9 November 1935, p. 3248; SJFG, LXXI, 28 January 1942, p. 1485.

89 Lawsuit, SJ, 38, 12, p. 3-6.

90 González Navarro, *Estadísticas sociales del Porfiriato, 1877–1910*, cited in Arce Gurza et al., *Historia de las profesiones en México*. Anexo 10.

91 González Navarro, *Estadísticas.* Anexo 9.

92 Gudiño-Cejudo, Magaña-Valladares, and Hernández Ávila, "La Escuela de Salud Pública de México."

93 Esther Chapa, "Faltan médicos en México," 1.

94 Agostoni, "Médicos rurales y medicina social," 776–86; Soto Laveaga, "Bringing the Revolution to Medical Schools."

BIBLIOGRAPHY

Agostoni, Claudia. *Médicos, campañas y vacunas. La viruela y la cultura de su prevención en México, 1870–1952.* Mexico: UNAM, Instituto de Investigaciones Históricas, Instituto de Investigaciones Doctor José María Luis Mora, 2016.

– "Médicos rurales y medicina social en el México posrevolucionario (1920–1940)." *Historia Mexicana* 63, no. 2 (2013): 745–801.

Arce Gurza, Francis, Mílada Bazant, Anne Staples, Dorothy Tanck de Estrada, and Josefina Zoraida Vázquez. *Historia de las profesiones en México.* Edited by Lilia Cárdenas Treviño. Mexico: El Colegio de México, 1982.

Aréchiga, Ernesto. "Educación, propaganda o 'dictadura sanitaria.' Estrategias discursivas de higiene y salubridad públicas en le México posrevolucionario, 1917–1945." *Estudios de historia moderna y contemporánea de México*, no. 33 (2007): 57–88.

Armus, Diego. "Disease in the Historiography of Modern Latin America." In *Disease in the History of Modern Latin America: From Malaria to AIDS*, edited by Diego Armus, 1–24. Durham, NC: Duke University Press, 2003.

Birn, Anne-Emanuelle. *Marriage of Convenience: Rockefeller International Health and Revolutionary Mexico.* Rochester Studies in Medical History. Rochester, NY: University of Rochester Press, 2006.

Birn, Anne-Emanuelle, and Raúl Necochea López. "Footprints on the Future: Looking Forward to the History of Health and Medicine in Latin America in the Twenty-First Century." *Hispanic American Historical Review* 91, no. 3 (2011): 503–27.

Carrillo, Ana María. "¿Indivisibilidad o bifuración de la ciencia?: La institucionalización de la homeopatía en México." In *Continuidades y rupturas. Una historia tensa de la ciencia en México*, edited by Francisco Javier Dosil Mancilla and Gerardo Sánchez Díaz, 277–310. Morelia, Mexico: UMSNH, Instituto de Investigaciones Históricas, UNAM, Facultad de Ciencias, 2010.

– "Nacimiento y muerte de una profesión. Las parteras tituladas en México." *Dynamis* 19 (1999): 167–90.

– "Profesiones sanitarias y lucha de poderes en el México del siglo XIX." *Asclepio* 50, no. 2 (1998): 149–68.

Castañeda López, Gabriela, and Ana Cecilia Rodríguez de Romo. "Mujeres médico graduadas en la Escuela Nacional de Medicina de México durante el Porfiriato (1876–1910)." *Revista Inclusiones* 2, no. 1 (2015): 88–121.

Chapa, Esther. "Faltan médicos en México." *Acción médica*, no. 15–16 (1935): 1.

"Decreto por el cual se reglamenta el funcionamiento de las escuelas libres." *Diario Oficial*, LVII, 18 (23 November 1929), http://www.dof.gob.mx/index. php?year=1929&month=11&day=23.

"Decreto por el cual se concede a la Escuela Libre de Homeopatía, el reconocimiento y los privilegios a que se refiere la Ley Reglamentaria de Escuelas

Libres." *Diario Oficial*, LVIII, 24 (29 January 1930), http://www.dof.gob.mx/index.php?year=1930&month=01&day=29.

"Decreto por el cual se concede a la Escuela Libre de Obstetricia y Enfermería de México, el reconocimiento y los privilegios a que se refiere la Ley Reglamentaria de Escuelas Libres." *Diario Oficial*, LXV, 20 (24 March 1931), http://www.dof.gob.mx/index.php?year=1931&month=3&day=24.

"Dictamen que presenta la comisión designada por la Academia Nacional de Medicina para juzgar los trabajos presentados al concurso anual. Primer Tema: 'Estado Actual de la Medicina en la República.'" *Gaceta médica de México* 57 (1926): 51-7.

Francois Flores, Fernando Darío. *La Escuela Libre de Homeopatía*. Mexico: Biblioteca de Homeopatía de México, A.C., 2004.

– *Historia de la homeopatía en México*. Mexico: Biblioteca de Homeopatía de México, A.C., 2007.

Garciadiego, Javier. *Los orígenes de la Escuela Libre de Derecho. El Derecho y sus Maestros.* Mexico: UNAM, Facultad de Derecho, 2006.

Gevitz, Norman. *Other Healers: Unorthodox Medicine in America*. Baltimore, MD: Johns Hopkins University Press, 1988.

Gudiño-Cejudo, María Rosa, Laura Magaña-Valladares, and Mauricio Hernández Ávila. "La Escuela de Salud Pública de México: su fundación y primera época, 1922-1945." *Salud pública de México* 55, no. 1 (2013): 81-91.

Gutiérrez López, Miguel Ángel. "La lucha por el control de la educación superior. La Universidad Michoacana contra las escuelas libres, 1921-1938." *Historia Mexicana* 59, no. 2 (2009): 669-709.

Hernandez Berrones, Jethro. "Homeopathy 'for Mexicans': Medical Popularisation, Commercial Endeavours, and Patients' Choice in the Mexican Medical Marketplace, 1853-1872." *Medical History* 61, no. 4 (October 2017): 568-89.

Hernández Sáenz, Luz María. *Carving a Niche: The Medical Profession in Mexico, 1800-1870*. Montreal, QC: McGill-Queen's University Press, 2018.

Herrera Moreno, Enrique. "La Escuela de Medicina de México." *Memorias y revista de la Academia Nacional de Ciencias Antonio Alzate* 43 (1925): 369-445.

"Los Charlatanes y el Nuevo Código Sanitario." *Acción Médica* V (January 1935): 7.

Moheno, Querido. "En defensa de los homeópatas." Mexico: 1924.

Ocaranza, Fernando. *Historia de la medicina en México*. Mexico: CONACULTA, 1995.

– *Historia de la medicina en México*. Mexico: Laboratorios Midy, 1934.

Penyak, Lee M. "Obstetrics and the Emergence of Women in Mexico's Medical Establishment." *The Americas* 60, no. 1 (2003): 59-85.

Pérez, Higinio G. *Programas y métodos de enseñanza de la Escuela Libre de Homeopatía y preparatoria anexa*. Mexico: J.L. Muñoz, 1925.

Pous Cházaro, Esteban. "Juicio crítico acerca del estado actual de la enseñanza de la medicina en la república. *Amicus Plato: sed magis amica veritas.*" *Gaceta médica de México* 57 (1926): 58–66.

Pruneda, Alfonso. "Por el Departamento de Salubridad Pública. Importante para los que ejercen la medicina, la cirujía, la farmacia, la obstetricia, la odontología, la medicina veterinaria y la homeopatía, en el Distrito Federal." *Asociación Médica Mexicana. Boletín de Propaganda* I, no. 2 (1920): 58–9.

Quevedo y Zubieta. "La Homeopatía oficial ó la bifurcación de la ciencia." *La medicina científica* VIII, no. 22 (1895): 346–7.

Soto Laveaga, Gabriela. "Bringing the Revolution to Medical Schools: Social Service and a Rural Health Emphasis in 1930s Mexico." *Mexican Studies / Estudios Mexicanos* 29, no. 2 (2013): 397–427.

Sowell, David. *Medicine on the Periphery: Public Health in the Yucatan, Mexico, 1870–1960.* Lanham, MD: Lexington Books, 2015.

Tesis aislada 2a sala, *Semanario Judicial de la Federación y su Gaceta*, Quinta Época, t. XXVII, 4 November 1929, p. 1502.

– t. XXVIII, 16 January 1930, p. 249.

– t. XXXIII, 21 October 1931, p. 1501.

– t. XXXIII, 22 October 1931, p. 1501.

– t. XXXIII, 18 November 1931, p. 3145.

– t. XXXIV, 11 April 1932, p. 2156.

– t. XXXV, 10 June 1932, p. 911.

– t. XXXVII, 12 January 1933, p. 88.

– t. XL, 17 February 1934, p. 1565.

– t. XLVI, 9 November 1935, p. 3248.

– t. LXX, 10 June 1937, p. 4667.

– t. LIII, 29 July 1937, p. 1162.

– t. LXXI, 27 January 1942, p. 1424.

– t. LXXI, 28 January 1942, p. 1485.

– t. LXXI, 3 February 1942, p. 7231.

– t. LXXIII, 20 July 1942, p. 1631.

– t. LXXIII, 21 August 1942, p. 4407.

– t. LXXXI, 24 August 1944, p. 4207.

– t. LXXXI, 24 August 1944, p. 4172.

– t. LXXIX, 23 February 1944, p. 3904.

– Informe 1942, 11 February 1946, p. 63.

– Informe 1946, 20 July 1942, p. 80.

Tesis aislada 2ª sala, *Semanario Judicial de la Federación y su Gaceta*, Quinta Época, t. I, Const., P.R. SCJN, 12 January 1933, p. 724.

Tesis aislada 2ª sala, *Semanario Judicial de la Federación y su Gaceta*, t. LVII, Tercera Parte, 7 March 1962, p. 91.

9

From Objectified Body to Silent Teacher: Decolonizing the Anatomical Body in Taiwan's Modern Medical Education

Harry Yi-Jui Wu

Professor Bor-shen Hsieh (1942–2018) of National Taiwan University, one of the most respected personalities in modern Taiwanese medical education, died in 2018. Before he slipped into a coma, he pledged to donate his body for educational purposes. This was not the first such pledge in Taiwan, but the ability for an individual to make such a pledge – and for a medical institution to accept such a donation – took decades of work. The development of modern medicine resulted in a shortage of cadavers for anatomy education, and thus medical schools had to strategically source bodies. Professor Hsieh's action catalyzed the call for selfless and dedicated followers in the enterprise of medical education. This episode encompassed multiple layers of significance in the history of the use of human bodies in modern medical education. It also attested to how bodies were decolonized from being subjects of imperial knowledge production during the colonial era to becoming essential living elements in contemporary medical education at the beginning of the new millennium. Over a century ago, cadavers were objects under the anatomical knife of colonial medicine; today they are respected as "silent mentors" in modern anatomical classes. This chapter provides a context-based ethical analysis of life education for medical teachers and shows how contemporary medical knowledge has advanced from an unjust past.

The human bodies used in anatomical research and education in pre– and post–World War II Taiwan have shifted from being considered a "subordinate race" to being treated as respected individuals. This transformation was shaped by the various social, cultural, and political factors involved in the shifts Taiwan underwent from a colonial territory to a post-colonial country and from an authoritarian to a liberal, altruistic society. Cadavers used to be unnamed bodies belonging to races considered subordinate in the context of colonial science. They then became objects in the discourse of post-war authoritarian state-building. Finally, they became respected and dignified persons in a democratized society. However, the *bona fide* decolonization of human bodies in Taiwan's anatomical education did not occur until the late 1990s, half a century after the end of World War II.

ANATOMY AS THE FOUNDATION OF MODERN MEDICAL EDUCATION

In many East Asian countries, including Taiwan, where medicine was introduced via colonialism, anatomy is an essential component of modern medical education. A majority of physicians in Taiwan once claimed that knowledge of gross anatomy was perceived to be what made medical students unique.[1] Modern medicine was introduced in Taiwan toward the end of the nineteenth century under Japanese rule. Developed along biological principles according to Gotō Shinpei, the first head of civilian affairs in the colony, modern medicine was used as part of the efforts of the Japanese colonial government to modernize the country and thereby legitimize its governance.[2] The continuing development of modern medicine during the post–World War II period ensured Taiwan's status as a modern state. Despite several rounds of pedagogical reformation, gross anatomy has remained an indispensable part of formal medical curricula since the beginning of medical education in Taiwan.

Medical historians have long studied the differences between how bodies have been observed, perceived, and explained in the Eastern and Western worlds. For example, Shigehisa Kuriyama explains how sensory experiences in ancient Chinese culture shaped the ways in which human bodies were viewed, and he compares these findings with those from ancient Greece.[3] Che-Chia Chang systematically examines, from intellectual as well as linguistic perspectives, how anatomical terms were translated and created in modern China.[4] In addition, from the perspective of the management of bodies, historians have argued that anatomy is not only an instrument used by modern scientists to gain deep knowledge of the human body, but it also represents an invasion by the colonial or state power of ownership and autonomy of citizens' bodies.[5]

Recent studies look at the disciplinary power over bodies in East Asia. David Luesink makes the Foucauldian argument that anatomical knowledge in Republican China was based on the practice of dissection in the military, medical schools, and hospitals.[6] More specifically, taking forensic medicine as a lens, Daniel Asen documents the growth of anatomical practice and pathological research at Peking Union Medical College, despite public opposition.[7] From a transnational perspective, James Poskett shows that certain anatomical knowledge, based at the time on physiological anthropology, was introduced to China in the early twentieth century via the circulation of books and translations through inter-imperial connections.[8] However, few studies have touched upon what the bodies utilized in anatomy meant in medical education throughout East Asia's complex history. In addition to being the source of anatomical knowledge, cadavers were human beings before they were procured and used as pedagogical instruments.

ANATOMY AS AN OFFSHOOT OF PHYSIOLOGICAL ANTHROPOLOGY

Medical education was one of the most important infrastructures developed in Taiwan under Japanese colonial rule. Using Germany's *Staatsmedizin* as a model, the colonial government used modern medicine as a bio-governance tool to transform Taiwan from what they regarded as a reservoir of diseases into a modern state.[9] In contrast to the majority of European colonizers, the colonial government in Taiwan established a medical school offering university-level education to prospective physicians soon after it took power. In 1897 Yamaguchi Hidetaka (1866–1916) established a school to train native physicians, becoming the superintendent of Taiwan Hospital, the colony's first modern hospital. Two years later, a second colonial state-sponsored medical school was established by the Office of the Taiwan Governor-General, with Yamaguchi as its first director. In 1936, this medical school was incorporated into the newly established Taihoku Imperial University, the precursor of the present-day National Taiwan University. University-trained physicians offered colonial medical services and became the force driving the sustainable development of modern medicine in Taiwan.

Along with the development of modern medicine in Taiwan, anatomical education was closely associated with the highly racialized physiological anthropology that was first advanced by European colonial empires in the nineteenth century. Michael Shiyung Liu describes the colonial medical system in Taiwan as being hybrid in nature. Regarding the staffing of medical services, university-trained doctors were favoured rather than discriminated against by those trained in Japan.[10] Toward the end of World War II, under the policy of assimilation, university-trained Taiwanese doctors had equal status with those of Japanese descent. Thus, modern medicine effectively transformed colonized subjects into modern citizens under the power of the Japanese Empire. However, the medical theories developed in colonial Taiwan were greatly influenced by then-popular racial thinking.[11]

During the process of knowledge-making in the Japanese empire, native bodies became the subject under the "gaze" of physiological anthropologists. This tradition can be best exemplified by the construction of an Ainu "race"

in Hokkaido since the mid-nineteenth century.[12] Similar scientific activities
were extended to Japan's colony in the south. At the beginning of modern
medical education in Taiwan, the delivery of anatomical knowledge depended
on limited translated sources; most textbooks were translated from German.
One of the most important anatomists at this time was Mori Oto (1890–
1967), the son of army surgeon general officer Mori Ōgai (1862–1922), who
was considered a leading writer and medical statistician in Meiji Japan.[13] In
anatomy textbooks, human bodies were simply detailed atlases that were conceived as purely scientific objects. Upon the establishment of the Office of the
Taiwan Governor-General Medical School, medical education consisted of
a one-year preparatory program and four years of undergraduate training.
The preparatory program included basic science, languages, humanities, and
ethics. Undergraduate training consisted of basic and clinical medicine. The
anatomical sciences, including gross anatomy and histology, were the most
important of these basic sciences.[14] Few teachers were formally trained anatomists due to a shortage of teaching faculty. The first generation of medical
students in colonial Taiwan recollected that anatomy teachers either recited
what was written in their books or drew a detailed diagram of the body on the
blackboard for students to copy and memorize.[15] Given the shortage of qualified anatomists, anatomy teachers were assisted by clinicians or other basic
scientists until the end of World War I.[16]

In the Euro-American world, Samuel George Morton's *Crania Americana*
and similar works gained popularity in the mid-nineteenth century, unlike
early-twentieth-century East Asia, where scientific racism first entered the
region and predominantly accompanied the existing intellectual foundation
in Japanese science.[17] The concept of race was first introduced to Japan by
the American zoologist Edward S. Morse (1838–1925) in the 1870s via his
teaching of anthropological and biological methods. Morse also introduced
Darwinian evolutionary theory by promoting Darwin's translated works. By
the mid-1880s, intellectuals in Japan were already actively discussing the
"Japanese race" and other racial groups. Racial thinking also influenced physicians who adopted the concept of "inferior races" in the Japanese Empire,
a concept they applied to the Ainu in Hokkaido, the Chinese and Indigenous
peoples in Taiwan, and the people who inhabited the Ryukyu Islands.[18]

In Taiwan, research on anatomical sciences in the early twentieth century
furthered the interests of Japanese cultural anthropologists. Ethnographers
conducting fieldwork in Taiwan documented the lifestyles, religious rituals, and folklore of the various Indigenous peoples, but they also collected
information on their skin colour, hair distribution, and limb proportions.[19]
According to anthropologists, these physical characteristics determined the
biological constitution of races, embodying different levels of acculturation.

For example, in 1908, Mori Ushinosuke (1877–1926) published his preliminary physical anthropological observation on the Atayal community, who were then considered the most "primitive" and "uncivilized" Indigenous group in Taiwan.[20] Anthropologists also documented various types of diseases, either physical or psychological, that supposedly afflicted only the particular race observed. Even before the Japanese occupation, Dutch military medical officers had already taken the basic body measurements of Indigenous populations in Taiwan. The earliest systematic physiological anthropology surveys were initiated by Torii Ryūzō (1870–1953), who came to Taiwan from Japan. By comparing body characteristics among his research subjects, Ryūzō concluded that the Indigenous Taiwanese populations had migrated to the area via the Philippines, Polynesia, and the Malaysian peninsula.[21]

From the mid-1920s to the advent of World War II, researchers based either in Japan or at the Governor-General Medical School published articles on the measurement of skulls, spines, teeth, and palm prints. Relying on the scarce teaching materials translated from German, these researchers produced a considerable number of studies, which were published in medical journals in Japan and Taiwan. The most crucial of these studies was *Lehrbuch der Anthropologie* by Swiss anthropologist Rudolf Martin (1864–1925), who managed to standardize anthropological methods and techniques through anthropometric photography.[22] Martin was famous at the time for his pioneering works in cranial measurement, and his textbook was circulated as one of the most important sources of its kind in Japan's colonies. In a laboratory in Taiwan, researchers used the seeds of true indigo, a plant widely grown in the tropics in Asia, to replace the sand or millet seeds widely used in Europe to measure the cranial volume of a skull.[23] To obtain human skulls and other body parts, these anthropologists reached out to collections held at Tokyo University and in other small and private laboratories. An additional few cadavers were obtained from Japan's early battles against Taiwanese Indigenous communities. One famous collection included four skulls of members of the Paiwan tribe, killed when the Japanese military attacked Botans in southern Taiwan one year before colonization in 1895, as well as remains of the Atayal people who died in the famous conflict of 1930.[24] Other sources included bodies found in the woods or disinterred without permission and stolen from Indigenous communities' graves.[25]

At Taihoku Imperial University, Takeo Kanaseki (1897–1983) consolidated the relationship between physiological anthropology and anatomy. With the resources provided by the university, he systematically developed research methods with an established research team. The team developed systematic surveys for somatometry and osteometry. The researchers studied the Indigenous and Chinese people in Taiwan and extended their observations

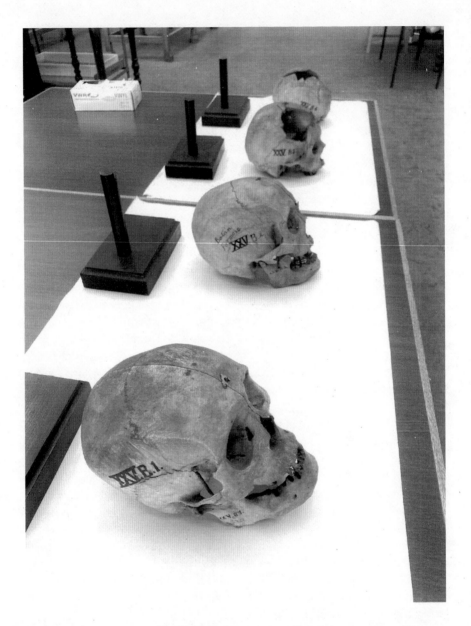

Figure 9.1 | Four skulls of members of the Paiwan tribe, killed when the Japanese military attacked Botans in southern Taiwan in 1894. The skulls were first obtained by the American physician Stuart Eldridge, who worked in Japan, and later the Scottish zoologist John Anderson, before they became part of English anatomist Sir William Turner's collection at the University of Edinburgh. (Photograph by author, © University of Edinburgh, Anatomical Museum Collection)

and measurements of bodies to Indigenous and Chinese populations in various other coastal areas in Southeast China. In the 1940s, following Japan's *nanshin-ron* policy to include Southeast Asia and the Pacific Islands in the empire's sphere of military interest, the team also studied the physical anthropology of populations on Hainan Island.[26] The two leading anatomists, Mori Oto and Takeo Kanaseki, remained in Taiwan until the 1950s, as Japanese scholars were gradually repatriated to Japan after the war.

CONTINUING THE FOCUS OF THE COLONIAL GAZE
ON TAIWANESE BODIES AFTER WORLD WAR II

Following Japan's defeat in World War II, Taihoku Imperial University became National Taiwan University in 1945. The defeat of the armed forces of the Republic of China forced its government to relocate to Taiwan in 1949, allowing the Communist Party of China to establish a new state in the mainland. The Chinese Nationalist Government took over the infrastructure on the island left behind by Japan in a speedy handover that included all levels of educational institutions. Under this framework, all university departments were restaffed in accordance with the new nation-state's higher education policy. However, at National Taiwan University, for example, six academic schools were renamed and restructured but the teaching and research programs remained largely unchanged.[27]

According to Daniel Asen, prewar physical anthropology had a great impact on the rebirth of dermatoglyphics.[28] Highly racialized science under colonial rule was reincarnated as a new form of national knowledge. Due to the shortage of teaching staff and the scarcity of teaching resources, academics at the Department of Anatomy of the reinstituted National Taiwan University continued their research and teaching by relying on theories and practices developed during the Japanese colonial era. Their research was still heavily painted with racialized colours. In post–World War II Taiwan, many teachers of anatomy were systematically trained physical anthropologists who had conducted island-wide fieldwork documenting the body measurements of various Indigenous communities under the supervision of Takeo and Mori. Unlike the Japanese anatomists, however, these scholars no longer translated textbooks or developed innovative research methods. Instead, having adopted the theories they had learned, these scholars began to use devices that were precisely designed for their fieldwork. Relying on the textbooks used during the Japanese period, which described practical anthropometrical methods, research teams spent days to weeks in various Indigenous communities that had not yet been surveyed.[29]

Given the travel policy constraints instituted during the beginning of the Cold War, researchers no longer conducted surveys outside Taiwan. Using the

remaining body samples and the method of observation and measurement
in somatometry, these researchers compared different Indigenous Formosan
groups to one another and Indigenous to Chinese people.[30] Notably, not being
able to conduct fieldwork in mainland China, researchers recruited soldiers
who had been relocated to Taiwan with the Chinese Nationalist Government
and measured photos of their palms. To researchers, labelling different
Chinese groups could still denote racial meanings. However, it is difficult to
say whether their observations implied a belief in the existence of any racial
hierarchy made specifically for the purpose of colonization. Such categoriza-
tion efforts may have merely reflected how traditionally Chinese communities
classified themselves as "subnations" according to geographical origins, languages, and customs.[31]

SOURCES OF CADAVERS FOR ANATOMY AND THE STATE'S GOVERNANCE OVER HUMAN BODIES

From pre- to post-war Taiwan, the methods used to obtain cadavers for medical education represent the transformation in how human bodies were perceived and treated by different authorities. Although decolonization never
actually occurred with regard to knowledge production, the social status of
cadavers used in gross anatomy shifted from the perspective of citizenship and
the legal system. Japanese colonial rule gradually brought about the regulation
of cadavers for anatomical purposes in Taiwan. From the very beginning of
Japanese colonization, the dead bodies of sick prisoners or of executed death
row inmates not claimed by their families could be handed over to the medical
school for anatomical research or education.[32] However, such regulations did
not meet the demand from the medical school, which resorted to publishing
in newspapers public requests for unclaimed cadavers from the judicial sector.[33] The tradition of donating bodies for anatomy was unpopular until the
establishment of Taiwan Zenshukai (台湾全終会), a charitable society.[34] The
society was established in 1908 by the director of the Taihoku Inari Shinshia
as a token of thanks to the head of the medical school at the time, Horiuchi
Tsugio (1873–1955). Medical schools would hold ceremonies to commem-
orate those "comrades" who donated bodies for anatomical education. The
Zenshukai played an important role by sending representatives annually to
participate in these ceremonies. The Zenshukai hoped that these ceremonies
would persuade people to donate their bodies for anatomical education after
their passing. However, bodies remained far more available for pathological
investigation than for anatomical education.[35] One of the main reasons for
this is thought to be the Chinese cultural belief that human bodies should be
preserved intact.[36]

In the immediate post-war period, following the political unrest before the actual government relocation took place, martial law was imposed on the island. For almost four decades, the bodies of unidentified individuals and prisoners had been the main source for anatomical education. However, martial law shifted this colonial power over dead bodies to the newly established state. There are several explanations for the shift of authority over human bodies. One could take the Foucauldian view that the bodies of people who were deemed by the racist science of the time to be from "inferior races" were subjected to the medical gaze; however, the racial boundary between those who observed the bodies and the bodies under the anatomist's knife was no longer clear. Julia Kristeva's concept of abjection, which emphasizes the materiality of human bodies, might be useful to illustrate the use of the corpse by the newly established Chinese authority in Taiwan. Bodies dissected were of those individuals considered disturbing or threatening to the system and order.[37] However, this phenomenon can also be explained from the perspective of legal history.

Historian Chin-Lin Huang has noted that during the reform of the legal system of modern China toward the end of the nineteenth century, the shift from ancient Chinese ethical codes to an emphasis on rights was not extended to the ownership of bodies and body parts,[38] which explains the Chinese state's authority over dead bodies. In December 1948, the Ordinance of Anatomy on Cadavers was legislated under the new Regime of the Republic of China. The ordinance was then adopted in Taiwan after the government relocated from Nanjing to Taipei. According to the ordinance, the bodies of people who died in public institutions, whether in a prison or a hospital, could be handed over to medical schools if the individual's family failed to claim the body within one month. In Taiwan, the time immediately following the 228 Incident, a massacre followed by an anti-government uprising in 1947, was known as the "White Terror." The White Terror period saw severe suppression, murder, and frequent imprisonment of political dissidents who were perceived to be a threat to the government's one-party rule. This period provided the National Defense Medical Center with a relatively rich source of dead bodies for anatomical education due to the number of prisoners executed at the time.[39] During my own medical student days, my neurological anatomy professor described how cadavers were sourced: while receiving training at National Defense Medical College as a boarding student, he had to collect the bodies of political prisoners who had been executed in groups, their bodies riddled with scattergun bullets.

Medical schools that had less access to dead bodies followed the tradition of the Japanese colonial period and held annual rituals at local temples and sanatoriums to express gratitude to the families who provided dead bodies for anatomical education, in the hope that the number of such donations would increase.[40] However, these efforts had a limited effect. Furthermore, during the first two decades after World War II, funeral directors took control of almost all cadavers, and a market emerged in which unknown cadavers became tradable commodities, with prices surging toward the end of the 1960s. In 1972, a centre for cadaver distribution was established in response to this pernicious practice. However, the situation did not improve until the Ordinance of Anatomy on Cadavers was revised in 1984.

This revision was a watershed moment in history. First, it elevated the status of cadavers to that of human persons. Second, it shifted authority over dead bodies from the state to medical professionals. In the new law, the term *dati* (gross body) replaced the Chinese expression *shiti* (cadaver), which was originally perceived as morbid and objectivized. The new law also decreed that the dead bodies of prisoners or death row inmates could not be used without the permission of their family members. In hospitals as well as in medical schools, families were given the right to decide whether the body could be dissected for pathological examination. Regarding the required information about the dead body, in addition to name, gender, age, profession, and the documentation of fingerprints, the dates of birth and death, national identity card number, and address while still alive were also required. Nevertheless, during the process of legislation, legal experts and medical professionals clashed over how long a time should be permitted to elapse between death and the embalming of the body. To protect the legal status of the dead, legal experts suggested lengthening the period for the family to claim the body as long as no morbid changes had yet occurred. The "civil rights" of the dead bodies were at the centre of this debate. Medical professionals, however, insisted on a period of six hours to meet medical interests, including organ transplantation and pathological investigation.[41] After this legislation came into effect, medical schools became the centres for gathering and distributing cadavers.

CADAVERS REGAIN HUMAN PERSON STATUS
IN CONTEMPORARY MEDICAL EDUCATION

The 1990s witnessed a milestone in anatomy education: dead bodies were finally deemed to have the status of a human person. The "Silent Mentor" Campaign, initiated by Tzu Chi, a Buddhist medical college and renowned religious charity group, was critical to this transition. The work emerged alongside the rise of engaged Buddhism, which is best exemplified by Tzu Chi. Such social organizations proliferated in the late 1980s with other service- and advocacy-oriented initiatives. After martial law was lifted in 1987, Taiwanese society changed drastically; middle-class populations began to ask for de facto democracy and to pursue liberal lifestyles, creating a third sector of society in addition to the government in transition and to budding enterprises.[42] Through the charisma of the group's founder and the organization's humanitarian works, including medical missions and disaster relief, Tzu Chi's impact was recognized in Taiwan and internationally.[43] According to the organization's own publication, Tzu Chi's medical college received its first pledge of body donation in 1995, the year after its medical school was founded. The donor, Ms Hui-min Lin (林蕙敏), died one month after she pledged to contribute her body for medical education purposes. Before her body was used for educational dissection, a ceremony was held to commence the Silent Mentor Campaign. The most prominent characteristic of Tzu Chi's campaign was that it directly addressed and involved the bereaved family, relying on their consent to and engagement with the process of donation throughout the whole course of anatomy teaching and learning activities.[44]

A typical silent mentor program involved a complex ritual consisting of seven steps associated with the receipt, treatment, and commemoration of the donated body. The anatomy class was led by a surgeon-turned-anatomist and was described as a simulated surgical procedure rather than as a dissection of the dead body. Before the class began, students had to meet the members of the donor's family and familiarize themselves with the donor's life and medical history. A Buddhist-style commemoration ceremony was held on campus before the class began. After the ceremony, the students were encouraged to review the life lived by the deceased person. In the anatomy laboratory, each screen displayed a portrait and the name of the body donor, the silent mentor. After one semester, students had to stitch up each body, dress it in white fabric, place it in a coffin, and accompany the individual's family members on the journey to the crematorium. Another ceremony followed immediately, where students dedicated various forms of gratitude to their silent mentors, who were now placed in glass urns.

Tzu Chi's Silent Mentor Campaign was influential in two ways. First, it led to many bodies being pledged and donated for educational purposes – so many that the number of pledged bodies exceeded the usage capacity of the organization's teaching hospitals.[45] Second, it prompted other medical schools in Taiwan and elsewhere in Asia, including Malaysia and Hong Kong, to follow.[46] It also had a significant impact on medical education: a study shows that the program helped medical students cultivate a humanistic approach to patients. A three-year survey of medical students found that they became more positive every time they dealt with a new body and with the individual's family being present at the "bedside" of the anatomical table. The students treated the cadaver as a teacher or friend rather than as a teaching and learning tool, and they thought such treatment was appropriate. The students also felt that the requirement to suture the body after dissection and the opportunity to learn about the life stories of their silent mentors helped them nurture compassion toward future patients.[47] When the program was introduced in other medical schools, the religious aspects may have been altered or removed based on the nature of the school. A recent documentary produced in Taiwan followed the entire process of an anatomy course, featuring the family of a body donor who had died from breast cancer and a group of medical students from the Catholic Fujen University, and it focused on what the process meant to all participants before, during, and after the dissection.[48] The documentary was well-received at various international film festivals, as well as at hospitals and medical schools, many of which are non-religious institutions.

In post-millennium Taiwan, most medical schools have implemented a silent mentor program, with the ritualistic procedures and religious elements varying across institutions. This extensive process can be attributed to the initiatives promoting the teaching of medical humanities in curriculum reform at medical schools. As a part of these reforms, medical schools began to emphasize the importance of education in humanities. A large number of teachers educated in the United States returned to Taiwan during this time. The silent mentor program was a perfect vehicle to spread this new pedagogical spirit. However, this pedagogy was criticized for conflicting with conventional medical education, which emphasized the anonymity of cadavers and required detached concern in anatomical training.[49] A study conducted among students who participated in an anatomy course following the silent mentor practice at a secular medical school showed that medical students experienced conflict about perceiving the cadaver as both a learning tool and a human being.[50] The students swung between seeing their silent mentors as neutral materials and as living persons, which generated an intense sense of helplessness.[51]

CONCLUSION

The transformation of human bodies used in anatomy education in Taiwan enables historians of medicine to rethink how anatomy research was transformed from physiological anthropology to functional anatomy, and how bodies under the anatomists' knives were decolonized across contexts. In a two-phase process, the bodies were liberated first from subordination to Japanese racial science, then from the Chinese Nationalist Government's sovereignty, and finally from the dominance of the medical profession.

During the era of research under Japanese colonial rule, bodies of either Indigenous or Chinese origin scrutinized by modern medicine were considered inferior in terms of racial status. The bodies were observed and measured, becoming useful tools in the development of modern medicine in the Japanese

Empire. After World War II, however, bodies were not fully emancipated from the colonial gaze. The pedagogy and practice of anatomy education informed by pre-war physiological anthropology were continued under the auspices of a new authoritarian state. Physical anthropology gradually faded from history, partially because this generation of anatomists exited the stage due to old age. The new pedagogy focused strongly on functional anatomy.

The process of sourcing human bodies for anatomy education was not profoundly transformed until the last two decades of the twentieth century. Cadavers used during Japanese colonial times were sourced in unjust ways, being the bodies of executed prisoners or combatants killed in inter-ethnic battles and not claimed by their families. After World War II, the Chinese Nationalist government exerted dominance over the dead and continued using the bodies of prisoners who died in custody and the bodies of unclaimed and unidentified individuals. This was due in part to the nature of the government as a settler/colonizer, which was little different from that of the Japanese colonizers. The state retained control of the final decision regarding the disposal of citizens' bodies.

The 1980s marked an actual turning point at which the social and legal identity and meaning of human bodies in medical education were revised. First, toward the end of martial law in the 1980s, the voices of civil society were increasingly recognized. Numerous medical professionals were elected to parliament, and their efforts shifted the power of gathering and distributing cadavers from the government to hospitals. These medical professionals also enabled families to decide whether the bodies of their loved ones could be dissected for either legal or medical purposes. However, conflicts also arose between the "civil rights" of the dead and the medical interest in dead bodies. Second, in the 1990s, the Silent Mentor Campaign initiated by the Buddhist organization Tzu Chi prompted pledges of body donation from across the island. Cadavers used in medical education now became human persons with names, life histories, personalities, and memories, and anatomy laboratories became surgical theatres for simulated procedures. Medical students were thus trained to act with humility and cultivate an additional capacity to reflect on their roles. The newly fathomed rituals in the program also became important elements shaping medical students' professional identity.

Recently, challenges have inevitably emerged regarding the conflict between scientists' prompt decision-making and humanists' hesitation. In this latest phase I described, even though cadavers are non-living things, they have gradually been given several rights equivalent to those accorded to living citizens. From anatomy materials to human persons with civil identities, cadavers' multiple roles have been altered by political transformations, the rise and fall of physical anthropology, the development of modern medicine, and social changes. In Taiwan, the history of anatomy education and the ways in which bodies have been used epitomize changes in society regarding the transformation of ethnic relationships and the formation of civil society. The ever-changing bond between medical students and cadavers also poses a challenge in medical education, implying the shifting identity of future medical doctors from solely scientific physicians to emotive and contemplative humanists.

NOTES

1   Chang, "Knowledge Transfer and Practice," 75–128.

2   Liu, *Prescribing Colonization.*

3   Kuriyama, *The Expressiveness of the Body.*

4   Chang, "*Yü Huai Wei Chih,*" 21–52.

5   Chen, "Anatomy and Punishment," 105–59; Tai, "Circus, Anatomy, Museums."

6   Luesink, "Anatomy and the Reconfiguration of Life and Death," 1009–34.

7   Asen, *Death in Beijing.*

8   Poskett, *Materials of the Mind.*

9   Liu, *Prescribing Colonization.*

10   Ibid.

11   For example, the discourse of tropical neurasthenia is a major subject in psychiatry studies. In the process of identifying diseases, the Japanese colonizers attempted to claim that the composition of their bodies was superior. See Wu and Teng, "Tropics, Neurasthenia, and Japanese Colonizers."

12   Roellinghoff, "Osteo-hermeneutics," 295–310.

13   For Mori Oto's accounts on anatomy, for example, see Mori, *Learning on the Anatomical Table.*

14   Chang, "Knowledge Transfer and Practice."

15   Han, *Memories at 60,* 48–9.

16   For example, Professor of Pathology Tanaka Sukekichi (田中祐吉) had to lecture on anatomy in addition to his own discipline in 1902. In the 1910s, the famous parasitologist Yokokawa Sadamu (横川定) lectured on anatomy at the Office of the Governor-General Medical School. In 1919, resources for medical research and education were improved following the end of World War I, and the anatomical sciences were consolidated in Taiwan. Lecturers were sent abroad for further anatomical graduate studies, and professionally trained lecturers began to enter the scene. For example, Tsusaki Takamichi (津崎孝道), a former assistant at the anatomical laboratory of Keio University in Tokyo, came to Taipei to teach anatomy. In 1919, the first anatomy specialist, Adachi Tsumaji (安達島次), was appointed to a professorship at the

Governor-General Medical School in anatomical science. See Tsai and Lu, "Pioneers of Anatomical Sciences in Taiwan."

17 For the case of China, see Poskett, *Materials of the Mind*, "Epilogue."

18 Terazawa, "Racializing Bodies."

19 Chen, *Ino Kanori*.

20 Mori, "Physique of Northern Aboriginal Taiwanese."

21 Tsai and Lu, "Physical Anthropology in Taiwan."

22 Morris-Reich, "Anthropology, Standardization and Measurement."

23 Tsai and Lu, "Physical Anthropology in Taiwan."

24 The four Paiwan skulls were first collected by the University of Tokyo and studied by American anatomist Stuart Eldridge. They were then eventually given to William Turner, a Scottish physician. Currently, the four skulls are still stored at Edinburgh University. See Eldridge, "Notes on the Crania," and Turner, "A Contribution to the Craniology."

25 For further research see Imai, "Research on the Morphology of Lacrimal Glands," Maruyama, "The Anatomy of Oral Cavity Base in Formosan Indigenous and Formosan Chinese."

26 See, for example, Asai and Sakai, "Das Hautleistensystem," 91–111.

27 Ou, "The Japanese Teachers That Were Kept."

28 See Asen, "'Dermatoglyphics' and Race."

29 Martin, *Lehrbuch der Anthropologie*.

30 For example, see Yu and Chang, "Physical Anthropology of the Thao"; Chang and Liao, "Palmar Dermatoglyphics in the Atayal"; Yu, "An Anthropometric Study of the Shukuoluan-Ami"; Yu, "An Anthropometric Study of the Taroko Atayal."

31 See Lo, *Introduction to Hakka Studies*.

32 See Ordinance No. 350, implemented by the Governor's Office in December 1899.

33 Chang, "Knowledge Transfer and Practice."

34 See Oda, *50 Years of Medicine in Taiwan*.

35 Ibid.

36 Similarly, public resistance to bodies being dissected arose when Peking Union Medical College was developing its anatomical science. See Asen, *Death in Beijing*.

37 Kristeva, *Powers of Horror*.

38 Huang, *History, Body, Nation-State*.

39 See Shen and Lin, "Interviews with Mr. Ts'ai Yang-Te," 470; Huang and Sung, *Gardener of the Apricot Forest*, 140.

40 Tu, *Memoir of Dr Tu Tsung-Ming*, 146.

41 Cadaver Dissection Ordinance (1st Rev), Legislative Yuan Secretariat, 1983. Legal Case no. 72, *Gazette of Legislative Yuan*, Republic of China.

42   For further details on democratization, see Ho and Hsiao, "Civil Society and Democracy-Making"; for further details on Tzu Chi, see Yao, *Taiwan's Tzu Chi*.

43   Huang, *Charisma and Compassion*.

44   Douglas-Jones, "Silent Mentors." In the following paragraphs, I use "silent mentors" to denote the same practices; some other documents use the phrase "silent teachers" instead.

45   Chen, "The Making of a Tzu Chi Surgeon."

46   Chen, Chang, et al., "Letters to Silent Teachers."

47   Lai et al., "An Experience in the Integration of Humanities and Medical Science."

48   Chen, *The Silent Teacher*.

49   See Douglas-Jones, "Silent Mentors."

50   Tseng and Lin, "'Detached Concern' of Medical Students."

51   Lin, "The Conception of Life and Body," 71–103.

BIBLIOGRAPHY

Asai, Masawo [淺井政雄], and Mituru Sakai [酒井堅]. "Das Hautleistensystem der Vola an Chinesen auf der Insel Hainan" [海南島支那人ノ生體人類學的研究]. *Taiwan Igakkai Zassi* 40, no. 12 (1941): 94–111.

Asen, Daniel. *Death in Beijing: Murder and Forensic Science in Republican China*. Cambridge: Cambridge University Press, 2016.

– "'Dermatoglyphics' and Race after the Second World War: The View from East Asia." In *Global Transformations in the Life Sciences, 1945–1980*, edited by Patrick Manning and Mat Savelli, 61–77. Pittsburgh, PA: University of Pittsburgh Press, 2018.

Chang, Che-Chia. "*Yü Huai Wei Chih*: Creation of Chinese Anatomical Terms under Linguistic Constraints." In *The Construction of New Knowledge in Modern China*, edited by P'ei-Te Sha and Che-Chia Chang, 21–52. Taipei: Academia Sinica, 2013.

Chang, Ping-Lung, and Shu-Yen Liao. "Palmar Dermatoglyphics in the Atayal in Tung-Shih District, Taiwan." *Bulletin of the Department of Archaeology and Anthropology* 12 (1958): 20–35.

Chang, Shu-Ching [張淑卿]. "Knowledge Transfer and Practice: The Case of Anatomy in Taiwanese Medical Schools, 1900–1980." *Taiwanese Journal for Science, Technology and Medicine* 20 (April 2015): 75–128.

Chen, Guo-Ming, Chien Chang, and Tong Yu. "Letters to Silent Teachers in Tzu Chi Medical School: A Spiritual Interaction." *Death Studies* 35 (2011): 441–54.

Chen, Maso [陳志漢]. *The Silent Teacher* [那個靜默的陽光午後]. DVD. Taipei: Activator Licensing, 2017.

Chen, Mei-Yi. "The Making of a Tzu Chi Surgeon." Translated by Yau-Yang Tang. Hualien City, Taiwan: Buddhist Compassion Relief Tzu Chi Foundation, 25 January 2008.

Chen, Wei-Chi. *Ino Kanori and the Emergence of Historical Ethnography in Taiwan.* Taipei: National Taiwan University Press, 2014.

Chen, Yueh-Yüan. "Anatomy and Punishment: Exploring the Relationship between French Anatomical Pedagogy and Human Anatomy from the Sixteenth to Eighteenth Century." *New History* 22, no. 1 (March 2011): 105–59.

Douglas-Jones, Rachel. "'Silent Mentors': Donation, Education, and Bodies in Taiwan." *Medicine Anthropology Theory* 4, no. 4 (October 2017): 69–98.

Eldridge, Stuart. "Notes on the Crania of the Botans of Formosa." *Transactions of the Asiatic Society of Japan* 5 (1877): 158–69.

Han, Shi-Quan [韓石泉]. *Memories at 60: The Autobiography of Dr. Han Shi-Quen* [六十回憶：韓石泉醫師自傳]. Edited by Han Liang-Chün [韓良俊]. Taipei: Wang Ch'un Feng Culture/Publishing [望春風文化], 2009.

Ho, Ming-sho, and Michael Hsin-huang Hsiao. "Civil Society and Democracy-Making in Taiwan: Reexamining Its Link." In *East Asia's New Democracies: Deepening, Reversal, and Non-liberal Alternatives,* edited by Yin-wah Chu and Siu-lun Wong, 43–64. London: Routledge, 2010.

Huang, Hsiao-K'eng, and Chü-Ch'in Sung. *Gardener of the Apricot Forest: Memoir of Huang Hsiao-K'eng.* Taipei: Passion Fruit, 2008.

Huang, Jin-Lin. *History, Body, Nation-State: The Formation of Human Body in Contemporary China.* Taipei: Linking Publishing, 2001.

Huang, Julia C. *Charisma and Compassion: Cheng Yen and the Buddhist Tzu Chi Movement.* Cambridge, MA: Harvard University Press, 2009.

Imai, Shōan [今井倭武]. "Research on the Morphology of Lacrimal Glands." *Taiwan Igakkai Zassi* 30, no. 2 (1931): 311–25.

Kristeva, Julia. *Powers of Horror: An Essay on Abjection.* New York: Columbia University Press, 1980.

Kuriyama, Shigehisa. *The Expressiveness of the Body and the Divergence of Greek and Chinese Medicine.* New York: Zone Books, 2002.

Lai, Chi-Wan, et al. "An Experience in the Integration of Humanities and Medical Science in a Gross Anatomy Curriculum." *Medical Education* 6, no. 2 (2002): 166–72.

Lin, T'ien-Yu. *A Record of Recurring Dreams in the Ivory Tower.* Taipei: Biographical Literature, 1975.

Lin, Ya-Ping. "The Conception of Life and Body in Modern Medicine: Reflections on Medical Students' Encounters with Cadavers in Gross Anatomy." *Journal of Life Education* 9, no. 1 (2017): 71–103.

Liu, Michael Shi-Yung. 2009. *Prescribing Colonization: The Role of Medical Practices and Policies in Japan-Ruled Taiwan, 1895–1945*. Ann Arbor, MI: Association for Asian Studies, 2009.

Lo, Hsiang-lin. *Introduction to Hakka Studies*. Shanghai, China: Shanghai Literature and Art Publishing House, 1933.

Luesink, David. "Anatomy and the Reconfiguration of Life and Death in Republican China." *The Journal of Asian Studies* 76, no. 4 (2017): 1009–34.

Martin, Rudolf. *Lehrbuch der Anthropologie*, 2nd ed. Jena, Germany: Verlag von Gustav Fischer, 1928.

Maruyama, Yoshiro [丸山芳郎]. "The Anatomy of Oral Cavity Base in Formosan Indigenous and Formosan Chinese." *Taiwan Igakkai Zassi* 36, no. 8 (1937): 1–37.

Mori, Oto [森於菟]. *Leaning on the Autopsy Table* [解剖臺に凭りて]. Tokyo: Showa Bookstore, 1934.

Mori, Ushinosuke. "Physique of the Northern Aboriginal Taiwanese from an Anthropological Perspective" [森丑之助人類學上より見たる北蕃の體質]. *Taiwan Times* (1910): 20–1.

Morris-Reich, Amos. "Anthropology, Standardization and Measurement: Rudolf Martin and Anthropometric Photography." *British Journal for the History of Science* 46, no. 3 (2013): 487–516.

Oda, Oshirou. *50 Years of Medicine in Taiwan*. Taipei: Avanguard Publishing, 2009.

Ou, Su-Ying [歐素瑛]. "The Japanese Teachers Who Were Kept for Employment in National Taiwan University 1945–1949" [戰後初期臺灣大學留用的日籍師資, 1945–1949]. *Bulletin of Academia Historica* [國史館學術集刊], no. 6 (2005): 145–92.

Poskett, James. *Materials of the Mind: Phrenology, Race, and the Global History of Science, 1815–1920*. Chicago, IL: University of Chicago Press, 2019.

Roellinghoff, Michael. "Osteo-hermeneutics: Ainu Racialization, De-indigenization, and Bone Theft in Japanese Hokkaido." *Settler Colonial Studies* 10, no. 3 (2020): 295–310.

Shen, Huai-Yü, and Lin Tung-Ching. "Interviews with Mr. Ts'ai Yang-Te." In *30th Anniversary of Taichung Veterans General Hospital: A Review of Oral History*, vol. 1, 467–507. Taipei: Institute of Modern History, Academia Sinica, 2012.

Tai, Li-Chuan. "Circus, Anatomy, Museums – The Hottentot Venus in the French Empire." In *Empire and Modern Medicine*, edited by Li Shang-Ren, 177–212. Taipei: Liking Publishing, 2008.

Terazawa, Yuki. "Racializing Bodies through Science in Meiji Japan: The Rise of Race-Based Research in Gynecology." In *Building a Modern Japan: Science, Technology, and Medicine in the Meiji Era and Beyond*, edited by Morris Low, 83–102. London: Palgrave Macmillan, 2005.

Tsai, Hsi-Kuiy, and Kuo-Shyan Lu. "Physical Anthropology in Taiwan: Retrospect and Results." *Journal of the Formosan Medical Association* 7, no. 1 (2003): 85–9.

– "Pioneers of Anatomical Sciences in Taiwan." *Jing-Fu Bulletin* 29, no. 8 (2012): 2–9.

Tseng, Wei-Ting, and Ya-Ping Lin. "'Detached Concern' of Medical Students in a Cadaver Dissection Course: A Phenomenological Study." *Anatomical Sciences Education* 9, no. 3 (2016): 265–71.

Tu, Tsung-Ming [杜聰明]. *Memoir of Dr Tu Tsung-Ming* [回憶錄——台灣首位醫學博士杜聰明(上)]. Taipei: Long-Wen, 2001.

Turner, William. "A Contribution to the Craniology of the Natives of Borneo, the Malays, the Natives of Formosa, and the Tibetans." *Transactions of the Royal Society of Edinburgh* 45, no. 3 (1907): 781–818.

Wu, Yu-Chuan, and Hui-Wen Teng. "Tropics, Neurasthenia, and Japanese Colonizers: The Psychiatric Discourses in Late Colonial Taiwan." *Taiwan, a Radical Quarterly in Social Studies*, no. 54 (2004): 61–103.

Yang, Lien-Sheng [楊蓮生]. *The Inside Story of Sixty Years of Medical History: Dr. Yang Lien-Sheng's Autobiography* [診療秘話六十年]. Taipei: Yüan Ch'i Chai, 2008.

Yao, Yu-Shuang. *Taiwan's Tzu Chi as Engaged Buddhism: Origins, Organization, Appeal and Social Impact*. Leiden, Netherlands: Brill, 2012.

Yu, Chin-Chuan. "An Anthropometric Study of the Shukuoluan-Ami in Eastern Formosa." *Bulletin of the Department of Archaeology and Anthropology* 19–20 (1962): 11–22.

– "An Anthropometric Study of the Taroko Atayal in Eastern Formosa." *Bulletin of the Department of Archaeology and Anthropology* 21, no. 22 (1963): 22–31.

Yu, Chin-Chuan, and Chang Ts'ong-Ming. "Physical Anthropology of the Thao." *Bulletin of the Department of Archaeology and Anthropology*, no. 9–10 (1956): 125–36.

The Making of the World's Only Medical School Mandatory Placement in Indigenous Communities: Northern Ontario School of Medicine (NOSM)

Geoffrey L. Hudson and Marion Maar

In this chapter we will introduce our unique medical school placement in the context of medical and health professional education. The main focus will be on the history of program development, from early considerations to the commitment to create a mandatory Indigenous community placement (2003–04). In addition, we will examine the development, implementation, and review of the placement pilot in 2005, the first full iteration with the (initial) charter class of 2005–06 at the end of that academic year, and subsequent developments.

The Northern Ontario School of Medicine (NOSM) is the first new Canadian medical school since McMaster (Hamilton, Ontario) in the late 1960s. It was created by the Ontario provincial government to serve the interests of northern Ontario, which includes remote, rural, and urban hubs over an area roughly half the size of Europe. It has been argued that it is "the first medical school to be established with an explicit social accountability mandate as defined by the World Health Organization."[1] The school currently serves as the Faculty of Medicine for Lakehead University in Thunder Bay and Laurentian University in Sudbury, and now has over seventy teaching sites across the north. As the Faculty of Medicine for two universities, it currently reports academically via its academic council to a joint senate committee for NOSM established by the two university senates. This joint senate committee then submits identical papers for approval to each senate. As of the time of writing, NOSM is to shortly become a stand-alone University, academically independent of Lakehead and Laurentian. For non-academic purposes, it is (and will continue to be) a non-profit corporation with a board, and thus, for example, it hires its own faculty and staff.[2]

IMMERSION CURRICULUM JUST PRIOR TO THE PILOT
AND FIRST ITERATION OF THE PROGRAM

The intent behind creating an immersion curriculum is for health care students to reach a level of understanding of culture and its relationship to health from a patient perspective. Different terms have been used for this understanding. In medical education, the concept of 'cultural competence' is useful, as it can be assessed to some degree. It is the mastery of knowledge, a set of measurable skills, attitudes, and behaviours in which practitioners begin to become aware of their own culture and biases as they prepare to provide quality care to diverse populations.[3] This understanding, when embodied by the student, enables effective work in cross-cultural situations but does not address the inherent power imbalance between the recipient of the care and the health care provider.[4] Cultural safety does incorporate this, focuses on the "social, structural and power inequities that underpin health inequalities/ disparities," and is experienced by both service-users and practitioners.[5] However, it is a difficult concept to assess in education because 'culturally safe' can, by definition, only be evaluated from the patient perspective.[6] Understanding historical power imbalances is particularly important when working with Indigenous peoples in order to understand how colonial policies such as dispossession of lands and lifestyles, forced assimilation, marginalization, and racism are the determinants of health that have led to, and still reinforce today, ill health among Indigenous people.

At the time of the development of the placement module (known in the school as Module 106), there were few cultural immersion curricula worldwide in health provider education. A segment on "Culture in Medicine" in the journal *Academic Medicine* in 2001 showed that immersive cultural experiences were limited in medical curricula, and when present at all were mostly at a pilot stage of development, providing short-term experiential opportunities such as "Increasing Cultural Competency in Native Hawaiian Physicians."[7] Cultural immersion in Indigenous communities had not been applied on a *mandatory* basis to an entire cohort of medical students or other health professionals from any ethnic backgrounds, and the school is, to the best of our knowledge, still unique in that aspect, in requiring successful completion by *all* students for their degree. In the United States, Kavanagh described an innovative six-week nursing field school that provided immersion learning experiences in High Plains Oglala Lakota tribal areas.[8] In New Zealand, a one-week cultural immersion in Māori communities of third-year medical students in groups of eight to fifteen was supported by critical reflection on biases related to culture and ethnicity. Outcomes included positive student evaluations, and it helped to address the problem of unconscious inherent racism.[9] The authors saw immersion as a promising approach to "consciousness raising to counter the insidious effects of non-conscious inherited racism."[10]

The cultural immersion program at the end of the first year exists along with a range of other Indigenous health curriculum components, delivered as core curriculum at other times in the Undergraduate Medical Education (UME) program (with summative assessment). As the immersion placement was developed, Indigenous health curriculum components were also created in the required courses and integrated into small and large group sessions as well as structured clinical skills development. Indigenous knowledge was, as a significant part of that process, integrated into student learning. As Jacklin, Strasser, and Peltier outline, overall the curriculum came to include a variety of topics concerning Indigenous people in Canada and worldwide: culture and history, health services, culture and medicine, disease trends, patient care, health research. In addition, the curriculum explicitly deals with the role of future physicians and physicians in relationship development.[11]

PEDAGOGICAL BACKGROUND TO IMMERSION

The immersive approach to learning is rooted in ethnographic research in anthropology, where researchers use a methodology called 'participant observation' to learn about other cultures by participating in their everyday life. The objective of that practice is to better understand the worldviews, language, and structure of the culture "by doing." Insights that one might have while practising participant observation are captured, and analysis is supported, by ethnographic writing. Ethnographic writing in the form of a self-reflexive field journal provides a forum for documentation and interrogation of a wide range of topics, including one's own unconscious biases, that can be discovered and critically re-examined at various points in the curriculum, and how past experiences and emotions colour perceptions and attitudes about other cultures. The writing thus helps to expose one's own tacit culture, interrogate assumptions, validate questions, and expose the epistemology of subconscious conclusion. It allows a critical examination of power relationships and inequities; it also helps to navigate the discomfort of cognitive dissonance that may occur in cultural encounters and lead to transformation of self, understanding, and interpretation.[12] "The ethnographer's personal experiences, especially those of participation and empathy[,] are recognized as central to the research process."[13]

When applied to medical education, it allows learners to deepen their understanding of socio-cultural worldviews and perspectives as they observe lived experiences of health care by Indigenous people. They are encouraged to learn in a continuing manner. Supported by critical reflection, they build on previous personal insights to transform their understanding of Indigenous health. The immersive curriculum has the potential to spiral on a personalized level, offering students different learning depending on their own preparedness and at different times in their lives.

INDIGENOUS PERSPECTIVES ON IMMERSION

In a literature review, Battiste explains that "[t]he first principle of Aboriginal learning is a preference for experiential knowledge. Indigenous pedagogy values a person's ability to learn independently by observing, listening, and participating with a minimum of intervention or instruction." [14] Congruent with this Indigenous pedagogy, as will be discussed, during engagement sessions prior to the start of the school, Indigenous communities voiced their preference for having medical students attend immersive learning in their communities during their first year. [15]

REACHING THE GOALS OF IMMERSION LEARNING

The role of cultural immersion in health-provider learning is to observe firsthand, to understand what is meaningful to people, and to expose one's own unconscious preconceptions. A recent review of the literature showed that cultural immersion experiences that offer a broad array of learning opportunities affect learning in several positive ways: students acquire new knowledge and skills, experience emotional growth, improve their cultural awareness in interactions with patients, and develop an improved outlook when considering the importance of culture. [16]

Indigenous cultural immersion programs for health care providers are geared towards improving cultural sensitivity, cultural competence, or cultural safety related to Indigenous health by encouraging self-reflection on attitudes and biases, and provide opportunities to work with Indigenous peoples and patients in a supervised setting. [17]

SOCIAL ACCOUNTABILITY AND INDIGENOUS NORTHERN ONTARIO

In 2000, Lakehead University president Dr Fred Gilbert approached the Nishnawbe Aski Nation (NAN), a political territorial organization representing forty-nine First Nations communities within northern Ontario with an estimated affiliated population of 45,000 people, and asked it to help with a proposal to create a new medical school in northern Ontario. NAN leaders agreed on several conditions, one of which was involvement in curriculum development. [18]

Subsequently this included several opportunities for Indigenous persons and representatives to participate in curriculum workshops. In May 2003, a consultative workshop included the following recommendation: "it was not enough to have the students read about Aboriginal people but instead they needed to live with them. Thus the curriculum should include a placement into Aboriginal communities for all students." This recommendation also built on recommendations made at a community curriculum workshop held in January 2003, at which it was suggested that the school have a community-based curriculum that "will provide students with a unique mix of learning opportunities in a diverse range of sites including aboriginal and francophone communities."[19]

As well as responding to the articulated needs of Indigenous and Northern communities, the school was also influenced by medical educational developments towards social accountability. In 1995 Boelen and Heck argued that there was a societal requirement for medical school accountability to society, and especially to the local communities within which schools are situated, including increasing student sensitivity to underserved communities in order to improve community health status. The World Health Organization (WHO) defined social accountability as "the obligation of medical schools to direct education, research and service activities towards addressing the priority health concerns of the community," with the priorities "to be identified jointly by governments, health care organizations, health professionals and the public."[20] Health Canada responded by adapting this definition and advocated for medical schools to respond in deed. The school picked up on these valuable suggestions, which contributed to the decision of the Accredited MD Program Group in July 2003 to include an Aboriginal placement for students in first year.

The founding dean, Roger Strasser, has spoken subsequently about the resistance that came from a number of northern physicians to the Indigenous communities' request for an Indigenous placement. Strasser commented in an interview in 2014 that "it was interesting and quite challenging to persuade people who thought they knew[,] that this was actually a good idea and in particular the physicians who service remote First Nations[,] especially in the Sioux Lookout zone. Those physicians said 'oh no you know it's not a good idea to have medical students living in these communities' … It's a variation on the theme that only doctors should teach medical students[;] and of course those doctors visit those communities but don't live in those communities."[21]

To operationalize the decision to create the placement, in July 2003 the school placed an ad looking for people to contribute to curriculum development in northern and rural health. A variety of individuals responded, starting their work within weeks. One participant, Kristen Jacklin, has said that the group concurred with the decision to create a placement in northern Indigenous communities, wanting to send them to the communities to experience life with Indigenous peoples.[22]

In 2003–04 the school's five Undergraduate Medical Education (UME) course committees were struck, with one being "Northern and Rural Health." The initial course description stated that students "will examine and treat peoples of diverse ethnic origins including Francophone and Aboriginal Peoples … As you learn and work in Northern Ontario, you have the opportunity to experience activities such as fishing, camping, hiking, and canoeing in a setting of exquisite northern wilderness."[23] Richard Denton, the chair of the Northern and Rural Health Theme Course Committee, wrote in an email to the committee members on 8 July 2004: "I think our Theme is a bit different from the others, in that Northern and Rural Health is something that needs to be *experienced* … at the end of year one, on a reserve."[24]

The importance of Indigenous people having a crucial role in educating the students was highlighted in an email from the interim director of Aboriginal Affairs to the Northern and Rural Health Course Committee on 20 July 2004: "Aboriginal resource people can provide the teachings and perspective to students [when] written materials don't necessarily do the job … This would be especially crucial in the areas of teaching of historical influences in the lives of Aboriginal peoples from an Aboriginal perspective and how Aboriginal peoples are working on healing initiatives and preserving their languages, culture and customs today."[25]

The goals and nature of the Indigenous community placement went through several phases of development. Initially, in early 2004, all placements were seen through a clinically focused educational lens. In a document dated 5 February 2004 titled "Draft of DLS Clinical Clerkship Definitions" there is a summary table of anticipated types of learning clerkship. The Aboriginal Clerkship, to take place in year one with the related community health resources, was to include: "nursing stations (volume of at least 10–12 patients per day) or physicians who service for extended period of time; may have a small hospital … or a contiguous community with a physician who services Reserves and/or Settlements."[26] In an email from Dean Strasser to those in the school, titled "Dean's Desk," Strasser discusses a meeting of the school's board representatives with Ontario officials from the ministries of Health and Higher Education as well as from hospitals and post-graduate residencies in which "there was recognition of the [school's] … model of medical education including Community Based Medical Education involving a range of clinical settings including long term facilities, rehabilitation services, mental health services, family practice clinics, community hospitals and nursing stations in remote communities." An instructional designer from the school noted beside the email: "description of model for clinical experiences."[27]

So too the school produced a communication in June 2004 titled "Update to faculty and staff from the Distributed Clinical Learning Sites Unit," which purported to answer the question "What are Distributed Learning Sites?" The answer in part was "compulsory … clinical clerkships … throughout each of the four years of our curriculum … [to] expose our students to Aboriginal, Franco-Ontarian, rural and urban settings." The "Update" stated further that "this will allow them to build their diagnostic and examination skills with respect to the particular clinical context in which they will find themselves after graduation. The learning sites will be supported by high quality internet in order to provide a reliable virtual learning environment for students, linking them back to educators and resources at the School's two main campuses. Clinical educators within the community will also have full access to faculty development resources and full support from the Medical School's faculty and staff."[28]

The goal of a *clinically* focused placement in Indigenous communities would not be met, and instead a different focus slowly emerged over time. This was not for want of trying, however. An obvious problem with a clinical focus was that First Nations communities are medically underserved. For example, the remote fly-in communities were only visited by a physician monthly. The Northern and Rural Health Course Committee Minutes of 5 October 2004 mention that "it was suggested to have students work with allied health professionals during their 6 week placement."[29] The UME coordinator responsible for recruiting sites for students in the communities, Martha Mussico, reported at a Course Chairs' Retreat on 12 and 13 October 2004 that she had engaged with thirty-five communities who were interested, with ten memoranda of intent signed. There were nursing stations and health providers but only two physicians. The plan was to have preceptors in each community, "someone who works in health care" such as community health nurses, as well as a "local champion."[30]

The notebooks of an instructional designer, Holly Rupert, also reveal other decisions were being made and potential difficulties of immersion considered: students would be sent in pairs; small group learning in real time over vast distances would be challenging; it would need to be "computer mediated."[31]

By January 2005 Martha Mussico suggested at a meeting of the Committee responsible for the pre-clerkship years – Phase One – that they expand the definition of "'Aboriginal Communities' to include those other than in remote and rural areas. They can also include those [near] urban areas. Examples would be Fort William, Ontario (located in the West) near Thunder Bay and Nipissing, Ontario (located in the East) near North Bay." Mussico argued that then "students will have the chance to experience *different [Indigenous] cultures*" (our emphasis).[32] And it was mentioned that this definitional change and new direction was supported by the interim director of Indigenous Affairs, Orpah McKenzie. It would additionally allow for "at least 6–10 new placements."[33]

INDIGENOUS COMMUNITY PLACEMENT PILOT

It was decided in early 2005 that it would be wise to pilot the Indigenous community placement that year prior to the school taking on its charter students in September. The month of June was selected. Communities that had already signed up to take the charter class students were picked to take on the pilot based on factors such as the degree of readiness, an appropriate geographical distribution of communities, whether they had accommodations for the pilot students, and the state of their IT infrastructure. Those tasked to prepare the running of the pilot included the first author as pilot coordinator; two faculty administrators, including Dr Sarah Newbery; crucially, Aboriginal (now Indigenous) Affairs staff; and Student (now Learner) Affairs. Fifteen medical and nursing students were selected from medical and nursing schools in southern Ontario, Manitoba, and (for nursing) Lakehead University in Thunder Bay. Eight Aboriginal communities and agencies accepted the call in total – Kingfisher First Nation, Deer Lake First Nation, Muskrat Dam First Nation, Kenora's Waasegiizhig Nanaandawe'iyewigamig Health Access Centre, Pic River First Nation, Constance Lake First Nation, Wikwemikong Unceded Indian Reserve (now Wiikwemkoong Unceded Territory), and Moose Cree First Nation. The faculty involved in putting together the pilot read the relevant literature mentioned above, and especially drew from the more extensive pioneering experience of nursing schools globally.[34] At the time the emphasis was still on cultural competency, with very little on cultural safety. Soon enough that would change. Holly Rupert, the instructional designer on the pilot and subsequent module, commented in an interview that "[d]uring the time of developing" the pilot and module "we were thinking very much about ... if students could just understand this population, then they could be more competent in delivering the care to this population. That was the rationale and I think that was the ... momentum behind all of our curriculum decisions. So, we were not thinking about ... cultural safety ... My perception is that what I described as cultural competence is what nosm was presenting and thinking and applying."[35]

For the pilot coordinator, looking through old correspondence with colleagues, the following contemporary reflections of the experience of the pilot are revealing: "spent last six weeks planning for and coordinating a pilot in which medical students spent two weeks in Aboriginal communities across Northern Ontario. [During the] last fascinating week [I was] in Sudbury coordinating the orientation week for the pilot in which students are now in Aboriginal communities across northern Ontario. The Aboriginal teachings were incredibly interesting and sometimes very, very powerful (e.g. residential schools: history and effect). Wow." Hudson described the experience as "extremely hectic. I did my best to be appropriately charming, intense and bossy, behind the scenes and it all went well, with much chopping and changing. Our School is not yet in operational mode and so staff needed to be given clear ... instructions and encouragement to get practical things done as and when needed, even if technically it wasn't their job. With the students out in the communities there are many logistical challenges we're dealing with now." During the end of the second week of students in community, the pilot coordinator was invited to visit Deer Lake First Nation, a fly-in community of "900 people in far northwestern Ontario (where the Manitoba border turns right). From there T[hunder]-Bay is the deep-south. And Toronto, what is that?" There were two students there and the pilot coordinator "was invited along for a fish fry which took 3 hours to prepare and cook the food from scratch (with freshly caught fish arriving all the time): fish, home fries, elder prepared bannock, onions." The pilot coordinator remarked that he found it "interesting [the] way even male teenagers respected the old[er] female elders who ordered them about at will." "One woman [was] very proud [that] the men do [the] cooking at [the] fish fry; fairly unusual among northern rezs." His correspondence reveals his own culture shock: there were "many little kids: throwing rocks at me and everyone, trying to run out on the runway at the airport, riding around in boxes in the back of pickup trucks, carrying puppies around, smiling all the time." Other notes highlight the unfamiliar poverty and lack of infrastructure that confronts students and faculty from the south: the "bathroom at the airport was an outhouse perched precariously over a ditch. It swayed, the hole covered by a rough piece of wood. Sign over the entrance: 'Deer Lake Toilet: Coed.'" The "students did really well over the last two weeks, playing baseball, fishing, working well with the nurses," among other placement activities.[36] Since it was a relatively short visit, discussion of the cultural learning experience awaited the students' return from Deer Lake the following week.

The pilot coordinator had some reflections on the student experience after the final week which he shared, based on his conversations with students and on their evaluations of the pilot and other materials. Overall, he found that a majority thought the pilot community placement was a positive experience, especially in terms of cultural education. An impressive range of cultural teaching and learning took place, with an acknowledgment by students of the difference between first impressions (and southern stereotypes) and the reality that students began to learn about in the communities. Some examples include community resourcefulness, strength and resilience, the significant extent of physical activity, health of community life and strong social ties, impact of the residential school system, a less materialistic way of life, inadequate federal government funding vs. community needs, and the expanded scope of practice of nursing in remote communities. The students had begun to learn about talking to patients with cultural awareness and respect, the nature of community life, and what respect for the land means to Indigenous peoples. Students also took time to identify community health needs (e.g. resources, delayed emergency care, preventative programs, sports facilities). Those students who communicated with northern physicians were very much encouraged to learn about the diversity and scope of practice in the north. Two medical students told the pilot coordinator that the pilot was such a positive experience that it had made them decide to engage in further clinical experiences in northern communities. Students found the orientation helpful, commenting that it should be extended to help students better deal with the culture shock and isolation, as well as the nature of individual communities including the effects of poverty, as well as mental and substance abuse problems, on health and medicine. Students, while praising many of the community coordinators, were careful to recommend that all community coordinators be trained well in advance, and that community placement plans be developed in cooperation with NOSM and approved by the school (the latter has never been the school's approach, with the communities trusted with organizing community activities for students as part of the partnership).

The pilot coordinator, in weekly meetings with the students, discovered that the balance between cultural learning and scientific/clinical education was delicate; the pilot taught the school that attention does need to be given to the quantity and timing of assignments, among other things. Too much school-based curriculum was inappropriate, and clinical case report requirements during the pilot had to be dropped, a written reflection exercise was replaced by an oral presentation, and a narrow list of required readings for the final pilot exam was shared with the students to make study manageable.

The pilot coordinator found that the school, in emphasizing the clinical opportunities to the pilot students, set them up for some disappointment. There was never going to be enough clinical time, given that physicians are in most cases not in the communities while students were there, and there is not necessarily the range of patients in the nursing stations in all communities. This experience was to continue the process of a reorientation of the Indigenous community placement from a clinical to a community-cultural focus.[37]

The chair of the pilot steering committee, Dr Sarah Newbery, has reflected since in an interview (2017) that a key reason for the success of the pilot was the Aboriginal Affairs staff, Tom Terry and Cindy Crowe, who worked with the communities: "I think they really did help shape the development of it. If not from the School internal curriculum standpoint, from the community receptivity standpoint. And I think the role that they played was really key in ensuring that communities understood what this could mean for them and the importance of participating and really creating the momentum around the on-the-ground implementation of it."[38]

Newbery had some concerns about the lack of clinical opportunities, and an ad hoc committee meeting was held on 31 August 2005 to talk about the placement and the clinical experience. Topics discussed were the role of the clinical teacher and the distinction between this role and that of community learning facilitator; a list of objectives and clinical settings; and the importance of students spending time with a health care professional "to enhance the students' understanding of culture and impact on health and access to the health care system. No firm plan emerged however, and beside 'next meeting' was 'no meeting is scheduled.'"[39] Subsequently the position of clinical teacher was never heard of again in the context of the Indigenous placement, and although some communities appointed community learning facilitators, not all did so; this was reflected in a decision not to provide funding for community learning facilitators to come to the local community coordinator two-day orientation in early 2006 (although some communities themselves paid for their community learning facilitator to come).

The orientation of the instructional designer is evident in her notebook. She comments in her notes on the UME Committee minutes of 8 August 2005 that "[Module] 106 is *cultural immersion* but [the] 4 w[ee]k exp[erience] has to be supported in other modules before & after" (our emphasis).[40]

In an interview, Newbery commented, "I feel like as a clinician one of the concessions was not making it a clinical experience, and really focusing on the cultural and community experience. That, I feel was a concession to enable the success from an Aboriginal community perspective, but also … people who are wiser than I am, who felt that the importance of really being in the community and having the opportunity to be as immersed in the culture as one can be while one is also pursuing the rest of the curriculum, that there was enough value in that to make that experience worthwhile. So, from my standpoint, the shift of focus felt like a concession from a clinician lens."[41]

The pilot provided lessons for the school, which were discussed in several reports as well as in a symposium. Initially the problems that had arisen in the pilot resulted in some hesitation in the school. In late July at the Phase One committee meeting, a member "questioned if UME was considering either altering or removing the [A]boriginal placement for CBM 106, due to the many concerns noted during the pilot." The decision of the committee was to "continue to move forward with the curriculum content for 106."[42] It was a tentative decision, however; a plan was created to proceed with another pilot for the charter class year if sufficient preparation was untimely. In addition, Holly Rupert wrote in her notebook against comments made in the UME Committee in early August that the question of the significant cost of the placement arose: it was "[f]inancially doable at least for next 3 yrs."[43] In her 2017 interview, Newbery commented, "I remember conversations about the expense, I remember conversations about the challenge of an immersive experience. And the logistical challenges for communities and the optics of overcoming those logistical challenges. So things like how we say to a community that absolutely we'll find housing for these two wealthy, largely white medical students. It's too bad your own community is struggling so much with hous[ing]."[44]

Recommendations from the pilot included increased support for the communities, extra administrative support, improved curriculum delivery, and preparatory curriculum work. A symposium on the pilot placement held on 20 October 2005 included discussion of the student experience in improved cultural awareness and understanding, as well as consideration of how they could advocate for and with the communities for health needs. At the symposium, Katherine Turner, a community representative for Moose Cree First Nation, argued that the experience was positive for the communities in the short and long term, including welcoming the medical school role models for Aboriginal youth in the community, as well as better physicians for Indigenous patients and communities. She also identified the need for the communities to engage in more extensive planning and staffing preparation.[45]

In the pilot, web-based discussion boards proved unworkable because of the lack of reliable internet in some communities. In addition, students were not building on each other's postings. Instead, it was decided that for the charter class the school would employ the telephone for small and large group discussions. Resources would be made available for the students on their laptops in advance of going into the communities so they could be sure to be able to do preparatory readings prior to classes. In addition, the (rather boring!) recordings of lectures were to be replaced by distributed tutorial sessions (suggested by school faculty member Dr Brian Ross, from a University of the Highlands and Islands model) with pre-packaged readings, questions, and a take-up session over the phone.

To improve community preparation for the 2005 charter class, the communities would be approached months in advance and the school would use a site-readiness committee. Each community would hire local community coordinators, who would be provided with a two-day orientation meeting several months before the placement at the two main campuses in Thunder Bay and Sudbury. In the pilot placement symposium, Tom Terry and Cindy Crowe discussed how the communities were being approached for the 2006 placement for the charter class. First, they were contacting the communities "(Health Directors, Leaders, Chiefs …)" with expression of interest documents (community information packages) followed up by visits to the communities. Then letters of interest were signed between the school and the communities. This was followed by the distribution of an "Aboriginal Year 1 Planning Checklist to interested communities" and meetings to work with the communities to complete the placement details. Then, Terry and Crowe explained, the school for its part would evaluate the fit between the communities and the curriculum (and vice versa for the communities), followed by the school working with the community to sign an Affiliation Agreement.[46] From 2006 Sam Senecal joined the Aboriginal Affairs staff as a regional Aboriginal community coordinator. Terry and Crowe, for the pilot, had been based in northwestern Ontario. Sam was based in the east. His good work in 2006 and since has built on the work of Terry and Crowe to improve community engagement with, and preparedness for, the placement. One of the major tasks for the Aboriginal Affairs Unit became the ongoing communication and partnership development with over forty communities. The Unit also took on responding to concerns by communities or students over the placement and conflict resolution.

To improve the curriculum, new sessions were created to improve the students' preparedness to address their own unconscious biases and begin to learn about Indigenous culture and culturally safe care, developed principally by school founding faculty and medical anthropologists, Marion Maar (who had eight years' prior experience working for a Northern Ontario First Nations organization where she supported the evaluation of cultural training for health care providers), Kristen Jacklin, and collaborating, experienced Indigenous health care providers. The first author also assisted as a historian of medicine, as did others. Indigenous health services, policies, history, and resilience would be taught by faculty and Indigenous resource persons. The pilot's self-study project was significantly improved for the charter class curriculum so that students better reflected on and understood what it would take for them to become effective health care providers for Indigenous patients. The students were asked to answer a number of questions including the history of health care in the community, the social determinants of health, barriers to care, their own personal and professional growth, and related subjects. They gave the presentation first in the community at a venue determined by the local community coordinator and then incorporated feedback from community members in a final presentation in their small case-based group once they returned from the placement. There was an opportunity for a question-and-answer session, with the project being double-marked by faculty.

Concerning the curriculum development and the role of the Self-Study Project, the instructional designer, Holly Rupert, who supported faculty, commented, "I worked on every module in the first two years; so that's 11 modules. I helped faculty to write a lot of cases and … in many ways [Module] 106 was the most challenging. And I think that the self-study [project] was brilliant, a really brilliant thing to have included. And I was, I think out of everything in the module, I was happiest as an instructional designer about that because it was an important self-reflection component of the curriculum."[47]

2006, FIRST ITERATION

The first iteration of the placement with the school's charter class in 2006 was much better for (and than) the pilot. All fifty-six students went in pairs to communities across the north for four weeks: remote northern fly-in, rural with road access, and a limited number of urban or near-urban placements. Students submitted three preferred choices for their placement, and most got one of them. They had a much greater range of preparatory sessions. The community got more support from the school, principally through the assistance offered by the Aboriginal Affairs Unit, and the communities learned, shared, and incorporated their own lessons from the pilot. Students reported that the experience was meaningful and impactful.[48] The first author was the module coordinator and made a number of recommendations subsequently which were implemented. These included, on the medical science side, focusing on the endocrine system rather than the relatively lab-intensive musculoskeletal system (implemented after a multi-year phase-in during the 2008–09 academic year). The successful on-campus orientation sessions for the students and local community coordinators were kept. The pre-packaging of the curriculum was maintained, as was the use of teleconferencing for classes.

From the beginning, the communities scheduled clinical and community-cultural opportunities for the students without school interference, and this was to be continued, with conversations with the students about the need to be flexible in dealing with the changes in the community schedule necessitated by changes in community plans and needs. At the module coordinator's suggestion, in future there would be two module coordinators, with the second author coming in for 2007 and thereafter.

After the first iteration with the school's charter class was the next Indigenous workshop in August 2006, "Keeping the Vision – Mii Kwen Daan," which included twenty of the twenty-eight local community coordinators from the placement earlier that year.[49] They shared their experience and came up with ideas about best and improved practice for themselves and the school. These recommendations included a plan to "provide several opportunities for students and local community staff to interact and learn from each other regarding their expectations and other student or community-specific issues to better prepare both parties for successful design and delivery of community and cultural learning/immersion experiences."[50]

DEVELOPMENTS SINCE 2006

Since the first iteration of the placement, the school has added an Indigenous health (as well as culture and health) curriculum to students throughout their first year, which is particularly intense in the two weeks prior to their placement, while they are still on the two main campuses.[51] Although the need for two weeks – rather than one week as in the second-year rural health placements – was questioned by the associate dean UME at a Phase 1 committee meeting on 13 October 2005, this was seen to be needed to better prepare the students. From the second iteration, the community/cultural experiences scheduled by the communities while the students were on placement were increased to 10–12 hours each week, and the clinical experiences were reduced from 10–12 to 6–8 hours. The community/cultural experiences continue to be created by each Indigenous community without being subject to any approval process by the school. The local community coordinators teach each other about best practices when they meet each year in a two-day orientation. The communities make their decisions on the basis of what they know future physicians need to learn in order to be effective physicians who provide culturally safe care for Indigenous people. Students participate in a wide variety of activities and learn about many aspects of community life. This includes observing traditional healing and ceremonies, visits with elders, well baby clinics, sex education in the classroom, band council governance, living off the land (hunting, fishing, harvesting wild rice, etc.), and shadowing the nurses and community health workers, among many other things.

Students in nursing stations or health centres are supervised by nurses and physicians and before they leave for the communities the students participate in an orientation session so that they all have an appropriate understanding of relevant matters such as the scope of appropriate clinical activities. In the light of some experiences in the first iteration of the placement, which posed serious risk management challenges for the school – with students dealing with a gunshot wound and a delivery on the weekend – a decision was made to place students only in those communities in which there were nurses present at all times.

From 2007 to 2019, where possible, the authors have both served as module coordinators, one on each campus. An important aspect of preparing students continues to be a series of mandatory sessions led by the module coordinators and regional Indigenous community coordinators that complement other academic sessions. Practical information is shared, such as how students should demonstrate cultural awareness and practise cultural humility in the communities, the health, social, and political system(s) on reserves, and the treaties in operation in northern Ontario. These sessions have taken place every year, with only one exception when the Learner Affairs Unit, which initially sponsored them under the directorship of Darcia Borg (currently executive director for Dilico Anishinabek Family Care, which provides health services in the northwest), then withdrew them without any notice to UME, resulting in a year with no scheduled preparation sessions for the students. In 2018–19 a new Indigenous full-time faculty member, Lorrilee McGregor (member of Whitefish River First Nation), took the lead in these sessions in her role as a new Module 106 coordinator. Another key aspect of preparing students effectively has been the second author's successful effort (over multiple years) to spiral – weave – the cultural safety and critical reflection curriculum throughout the first year. Placing that enhanced curriculum early and repeatedly throughout the first year allows students time to integrate their learning effectively over six months by initially increasing their intellectual knowledge and then applying cultural safety and critical reflection at their weekly community learning sites, during the Francophone health module, and finally during the immersion experience.

The community engagement with students in advance of the module has also been improved. Students now engage with their local community coordinator months before the placement, during the yearly LCC workshop, and there is ongoing communication prior to the students' arrival. This followed the recommendation from the communities at the "Keeping the Vision – Mii Kwen Daan" gathering in August 2006.[52]

Teleconference guides and instructions for students and faculty have undergone development, and faculty are provided with both written orientation material and, more recently, preparation sessions at module start. Detailed contingency plans exist and are utilized. Students are given instruction on professional conduct and it is assessed by the module coordinators acting on advice from the local community coordinators. The preparation includes faculty advice on such things as postings about the placement, community, and patients on the internet (in the light of some unfortunate inappropriate occurrences during a couple of early iterations of the module). In more recent iterations the first and second authors, as module coordinators, have had a role in ensuring that the student small groups include students from a variety of communities (remote fly-in, rural drive-in, and peri-urban) in each group in order to enable the students to share their diverse experiences. In addition, the module coordinators advise on the appointment of case-based-session small-group facilitators to ensure that they are faculty with the necessary background and experience (given the role of the sessions in dealing with subjects related to Indigenous health, including preparing the students for the self-study project and its self-reflection and professional development components). Students are now required to live in the communities for the entire experience, including weekends, and if absent for any reason for more than three days must construct and be evaluated on an alternative learning plan in order to be deemed to have completed the cultural immersion experience. To enhance the immersion experience, student billeting with community members is always employed if possible. The students very helpfully provide evaluations about the success of the placement for program evaluation purposes. Information about the student evaluations is shared with the local community coordinators at their annual orientation.

A number of faculty, including the two authors, are researching the effectiveness of this cultural immersion experience. Some early results were recently published, drawing on interviews with graduates. The main themes that arose from the interview centred on "the common thread of the value of community-engaged learning." Many of the students interviewed commented on their "greater understanding and empathy with patients from the cultural groups of Northern Ontario": "I think that you gain ... insight from this experience, how culture does play a huge part in daily life and decisions"; "things that we would consider basically standard but are not there in some of these smaller fly-in reserves." The article's conclusion on the interviews was that "the overall evaluation from the respondents was that the cultural immersion experience was worthwhile, had lasting effects on their knowledge and practice, and provided an effective learning environment."[53] So too, an article written by University of Toronto faculty concerning Kenora's Waasegiizhig Nanaandawe'iyewigamig Health Access Centre found a significant difference between trainees from the school and other medical schools. On the basis of interviews, it was discovered that the NOSM learners had a better understanding of relevant matters concerning the rural north, including Indigenous peoples, their communities, and the existing economic and social conditions.[54] Some NOSM learners have been matched with their Indigenous placement communities interested in collaborating in summer health research, which relies on trust and cultural learning established during the immersion as the foundation. This is a positive development, as it increases capacity for social accountability in research.[55]

CONCLUSION

How often does a medical school pilot include a press conference in its schedule for students and faculty? Seldom, if ever. The pilot for this unique placement did. And there were news releases, and a report published in three languages. All of which touted Success! When, afterwards, the vice dean asked the pilot coordinator quietly how successful the pilot actually was, he was told "shambolic, but we learned lots." This gap in perspective reflects the lack of readiness of the school at the time of the pilot and the dramatic learning curve that had to be overcome to achieve the goal of a successful Indigenous immersion placement.

That a press conference was scheduled is perhaps not such a surprise. Indigenous peoples in Canada and across the globe experience health inequities which are to a significant extent due to limited access to culturally safe care. Culture is an important, relevant factor. This was acknowledged locally when the provincial government created an Indigenous health policy in consultation with Indigenous people to emphasize their involvement in planning and designing health care in ways that reflected their perspective.[56] And as discussed early in this chapter, cultural safety, with its origins with the Māori of Aotearoa (New Zealand), has also gained increasing recognition as a vital component of medical education and practice. In this context medical education that focuses on cultural safety via a cultural immersion experience is highly relevant. The skills, knowledge, and attitudes of practitioners will hopefully be improved by living with Indigenous people, learning from them, and incorporating professional self-reflection in the process of medical education.

Recent reviews of the literature that include attention to Indigenous health curricula globally reveal that, except for NOSM, Indigenous health immersion programs have still not been applied on a mandatory basis to an entire medical school cohort as a degree requirement. One article reviewing cultural competency interventions concluded that lectures continue to be "the predominant teaching modality" and medical schools should "expand their teaching to include non-traditional modalities."[57] A review of health sciences cultural safety education explicitly considered a range of "experiential instructional approaches."[58] In several medical schools in North America, Australia, New Zealand, and elsewhere, placement electives are provided for self-selected students. Schools also provide Indigenous health curricula on campus that take the form of lectures, orientations, clinical skills developments, and/or small group sessions/tutorials to a greater or lesser extent. Day and weekend camps also exist, usually on a volunteer basis.[59] In Canada, as elsewhere, the NOSM immersion program has been noticed. This includes being featured in a Canadian Federation of Medical Students position paper entitled "Indigenous Peoples and Health in Canadian Medical Education": "Indigenous health modules should move beyond solely didactic teaching methods and instead use experiential methods that enable students to take part in culturally safe approaches to medicine and [I]ndigenous healing by engaging more directly with [I]ndigenous peoples ... [I]immersive experiences are one manner in which NOSM has been able to overcome ... Western biases and place value on Indigenous knowledge."[60]

Cultural immersion is thus an experiential approach to learning about Indigenous culture that is fairly new, certainly for entire classes rather than just in the form of elective opportunities. Research to provide evidence that will provide the basis to further enhance this approach is needed, and has been ongoing, with early results mentioned above, and with more detailed analysis to be shared in due course. There is the potential to raise consciousness among medical students, reveal tacit inappropriate biases (including racism), and assist students to learn about not only themselves but also other cultures in ways that will, we hope, go a long way to assist them in their preparation for work in culturally diverse settings as future physicians.

One of the charter class students, (now Dr) Kim Varty, came to a relevant conclusion: "cultural immersion provides an opportunity for health professionals to practice their trade in a new setting, with new interactions, and the development of new relationships. All of which affect the individual and have the potential to affect the way they practice ... Medicine is written in textbooks, but lived while talking with and examining a patient, and doing these things while in the context of the patient's Aboriginal, rural or international life. It is seeing life in a different context which takes the science of medicine and allows it to become an art."[61]

There is always, however, the danger of unintended consequences, which the research is attempting to discover, among other things. Indeed, Dean Strasser in his 2014 interview cautioned that "there are certainly students for whom this experience has reinforced their prejudices ... and so that's something that we have to be aware of and [to] continue to guard against ... I think it is actually a small number of students ... [for which] ... their learning outcomes are ... the opposite of what we'd hope for."[62] In this respect, carefully selecting, preparing, and evaluating faculty who themselves are experienced in Indigenous health issues and skilled at guiding students towards cultural humility throughout the placement is an important but still somewhat neglected priority up until this point. The main rationale for the placement was that the cultural immersion experience would enhance our future physicians' ability to care for Indigenous patients, wherever they encountered them. Research and experience will tell (and continue) the tale.

ACKNOWLEDGMENT

The authors are very appreciative of the partnership with, and generosity of, the Indigenous community partners, who have provided about 28–30 placement sites each year since 2006.

NOTES

1   During the history of this placement, common and official usage in Canada has altered from "Aboriginal" to "Indigenous." The authors use "Indigenous" but keep the term "Aboriginal" in contemporary citations, titles, and quotations. All material cited that is not in the bibliography is in the private archive of the first author. Hodge et al., "From Lancelot to Lapland," 131.

2   Aberman and Wright, "Governance and Organization," 131–56.

3   Hart-Wasekeesikaw, "Cultural Competence and Cultural Safety."

4   Kurtz et al., "Social Justice and Health Equity," 13–26.

5   Smye, Josewski, and Kendall, "Cultural Safety: An Overview"; Lee et al., "Health Sciences Cultural Safety Education," 271–85.

6   Ramsden, "Cultural Safety and Nursing Education."

7   Kamaka, "Cultural Immersion in a Cultural Competency Curriculum," 512.

8   Kavanagh, "Summers of No Return," 71–9.

9   Dowell, Crampton, and Parkin, "The First Sunrise," 242–9.

10 Crampton, Dowell, and Parkin, "Combating Effects of Racism," 595–8.

11 Jacklin, Strasser, and Peltier, "From the Community to the Classroom," 143–50.

12 Spradley, *Participant Observation*; Clifford and Marcus, *Writing Culture*.

13 Clifford and Marcus, *Writing Culture*.

14 Battiste, "Indigenous Knowledge and Pedagogy."

15 NOSM, "Report of the NOSM Aboriginal Workshop."

16 Brock et al., "Cultural Immersion in the Education of Healthcare Professionals."

17 Hudson and Maar, "Faculty Analysis of Distributed Medical Education," 2664; Thackrah, Thompson, and Durey, "'Listening to the Silence Quietly,'" 685.

18 J. Morris, letter to F. Gilbert, President Lakehead University, 2 June 2000; Nishnawbe Aski Nation, "Resolution 00/16 re. proposed Northern Medical School," 20 July 2000.

19 NOSM, "A Flying Start: Report of the NOMS Curriculum Workshop – Getting Started in the North, 16–18 January 2003," 5.

20 Boelen and Heck, *Defining and Measuring*, 3.

21 Roger Strasser, interview with Hudson, 23 February 2014.

22 Kristen Jacklin, interview with Hudson, 21 September 2007.

23 NOSM, "Northern and Rural Health (Theme 1) Course Committee Description, 2003–04."

24 Richard Denton, email correspondence, 8 July 2004.

25   Orpah McKenzie, email correspondence, 20 July 2004.

26   NOSM, "Draft of DLS Clinical Clerkship Definitions," 5 February 2004.

27   Holly Rupert, notebooks vol. 1, 20 February 2004.

28   NOSM, "Update to faculty and staff from the Distributed Clinical Learning Sites Unit," June 2004.

29   NOSM, "Minutes of Northern and Rural Health (Theme 1) Course Committee, 5 October 2004."

30   NOSM, "Minutes of Course Chairs' Retreat, 12 and 13 October 2004."

31   Rupert, notebooks vol. 1, p. 17, 14 October 2003.

32   One could quibble with Mussico's terminology as recorded in the minutes: remote usually is interpreted to mean fly-in (or very bad road to get there) when it comes to First Nations in Northern Ontario, and there are rural communities that are not remote but accessible by road (albeit sometimes at considerable distance). So too the communities she cites as urban would usually be considered near an urban area (or peri-urban).

33   NOSM, "Minutes of Phase One Committee, January 2005."

34   Literature that was especially influential at the time with the faculty at the school: Smith, "Concept Analysis: Cultural Competence," 4–10; Jazrozik, "Going Bush," 18; Crandall et al., "Applying Theory," 588–94. Nursing literature included: Armitage and McMaster, "Rural and Remote Mental Health Placements," 75–9; Bernal and Froman, "The Confidence of Community Health Nurses," 201–3; Bernal and Froman, "Influences on the Cultural Self-Efficacy," 24–31; Thomas et al., "An Intensive Cultural Experience in a Rural Area," 126–33; Ryan and Twibell, "Outcomes of a Transcultural Nursing Immersion Experience," 30–9.

35   Rupert, interview with Hudson, 1 November 2017.

36   Hudson, e-mail correspondence, 25 June 2005.

37   NOSM, "Report on the Module 106 Integrated Community Experience."

38   Sarah Newbery, interview with Hudson, 14 August 2017.

39   NOSM, "Minutes of Meeting, Phase 1 – Ad Hoc committee re. Module 106 and the Clinical Experience."

40   Rupert, notebooks vol. III, p. 17, 8 August 2005.

41   Newbery, interview with Hudson.

42   NOSM, Phase One Committee Meeting Minutes, 26 July 2005.

43   Rupert, notebooks vol. III, p. 17, 8 August 2005.

44   Newbery, interview with Hudson.

45   Hudson, Geoffrey, Katherine Turner, Sarah Newbery, Orpah McKenzie, Cindy Crowe, Thomas Terry, Dan Hunt, and Loretta Baratta, "Examination of an Aboriginal Pilot Elective," NOSM Symposium, 20 October 2005, PowerPoint Slides.

46   Ibid.

47   Rupert, interview with Hudson.

48   Hudson and Hunt, "The Northern Ontario School of Medicine and Social Accountability," 163–8.

49   Strasser, interview with Hudson.

50   NOSM, "Keeping the Vision – Mii Kwen Daan"; Strasser, interview with Hudson.

51   Jacklin, Strasser, and Peltier, "From the Community to the Classroom," 143–50.

52   NOSM, "Keeping the Vision – Mii Kwen Daan."

53   Strasser et al., "Community Engagement," e33–e43.

54   Coke et al., "A Northern Perspective on Medical Elective Tourism," E227–E283.

55   Maar, Boesch, and Tobe, "Enhancing Indigenous Health Research Capacity," e21–e32.

56   Ontario Ministry of Health, *New Directions*.

57   Deliz et al., "Cultural Competency Interventions," 568–77.

58   Kurtz et al., "Health Sciences Cultural Safety Education," 271–85.

59   Immersion experience examples: overnight camp, first year students, Bond University Australia: Sargeant, Smith, and Springer, "Enhancing Cultural Awareness Education," 224–30; two-day visit, fourth-year students who volunteer, University of Adelaide and Flinders University: Benson et al., "A Brief Experience for Medical Students in a Remote Aboriginal Community," 752–9; clinical rotation of one month, three third-year students and a resident, University of Alberta: Betkowski, "Med Students Gain Aboriginal Perspective on Health"; two-day Aboriginal cultural orientation as part of a two-week placement in year two, rural area (50% Aboriginal), University of Notre Dame, Australia: Mak and Miflin, "Living and Working with the People of 'the Bush,'" e603–e610; weekend, 24% of first year students randomly selected, University of Hawai'i: Carpenter, Kamaka, and Kaulukukui, "An Innovative Approach," 15–19; weekend, fourth-year students, voluntary, Dunedin School of Medicine, University of Otago, New Zealand: Sopoaga et al., "Training a Medical Workforce," 19.

60   Arkle et al., "Indigenous Peoples and Health in Canadian Medical Education," 1–22, 8. See also Robinson, Savia, and Shanmuganathan, "Approaches to Incorporating Indigenous Health," 57–8; Madjedi and Daya, "Cultural Immersion Placements," 28–9.

61   Varty, "Leaving on a Jet Plane for a House Call," 275–86, 286.

62   Strasser, interview with Hudson.

BIBLIOGRAPHY

Aberman, Arnie, and Dorothy Wright. "Governance and Organization." In *The Making of the Northern Ontario School of Medicine: A Case Study in the History of Medical Education*, edited by Geoffrey Tesson, Geoffrey L. Hudson, Roger Strasser, and Dan Hunt, 131–56. Montreal, QC, and Kingston, ON: McGill-Queen's University Press, 2009.

Arkle, Madeline, Max Deschner, Ryan Giroux, Reed Morrison, Danielle Nelson, Amanda Sauvé, and Kelita Singh. "Indigenous Peoples and Health in Canadian Medical Education Position Paper." *Canadian Federation of Medical Students*. 2015. https://www.cfms.org/files/position-papers/2015_indigenous_people_in_ canadian_med_ed.pdf.

Armitage, Sue, and Rose McMaster. "Rural and Remote Mental Health Placements for Nursing Students." *Australian Journal of Rural Health* 8, no. 3 (June 2000): 175–9.

Battiste, Marie. "Indigenous Knowledge and Pedagogy in First Nations Education: A Literature Review with Recommendations." In "National Working Group on Education and the Minister of Indian Affairs, Indian and Northern Affairs Canada." Apamuwek Institute, 2002. https://www.afn.ca/uploads/files/ education/24._2002_oct_marie_battiste_indigenousknowledgeandpedagogy_ lit_review_for_min_working_group.pdf.

Benson, Jill, Courtney Ryder, Madeleine Gill, and Anna Balabanski. "A Brief Experience for Medical Students in a Remote Aboriginal Community." *Australian Family Physician* 10 (2015): 752–9.

Bernal, Henrietta, and Robin Froman. "Influences on the Cultural Self-Efficacy of Community Health Nurses." *Journal of Transcultural Nursing* 4, no. 2 (Winter 1993): 24–31.

– "The Confidence of Community Health Nurses in Caring for Ethnically Diverse Populations." *The Journal of Nursing Scholarship* 19, no. 4 (December 1987): 201–3.

Betkowski, Bev. "Med Students Gain Aboriginal Perspective on Health." *Folio*, 22 October 2015. https://www.folio.ca/med-students-gain-aboriginal-perspective-on-health/.

Boelen, Charles, and Jeffery E. Heck. *Defining and Measuring the Social Accountability of Medical Schools*. Geneva, Switzerland: World Health Organization, 1995.

Brock, Marty J., Levi B. Fowler, Johnathan G. Freeman, Devan C. Richardson, and Lisa J. Barnes. "Cultural Immersion in the Education of Healthcare Professionals: A Systematic Review." *Journal of Educational Evaluation for Health Professions* 16, no. 4 (2019).

Carpenter, Dee-Ann, Martina Kamaka, and C. Malina Kaulukukui. "An Innovative Approach to Developing a Cultural Competency Curriculum; Efforts at the John A. Burns School of Medicine, Department of Native Hawaiian Health." *Hawai'i Medical Journal* 70, Supplement 2, no. 11 (2011): 15–19.

Clifford, James, and George E. Marcus. *Writing Culture: The Poetics and Politics of Ethnography.* Berkeley, CA: University of California Press, 1986.

Coke, Sarah, Ayelet Kuper, Lisa Richardson, and Anita Cameron. "A Northern Perspective on Medical Elective Tourism: A Qualitative Study." *Canadian Medical Association Journal* 4, no. 2 (2016): E227–E283.

Crampton, Peter, Anthony Dowell, and Chris Parkin. "Combating Effects of Racism through a Cultural Immersion Medical Education Program." *Academic Medicine* 78, no. 6 (June 2003): 595–8.

Crandall, Sonia J., Geeta George, Gail S. Marion, and Steve Davis. "Applying Theory to the Design of Cultural Competency Training for Medical Students: A Case Study." *Academic Medicine* 78, no. 6 (June 2003): 588–94.

Deliz, Juan, Fayola Fears, Kai Jones, Jenny Tobat, Douglas Char, and Will Ross. "Cultural Competency Interventions during Medical School: A Scoping Review and Narrative Synthesis." *Journal of General Internal Medicine* 35, no. 2 (2019): 568–77.

Dowell, Anthony, Peter Crampton, and Chris Parkin. "The First Sunrise: An Experience of Cultural Immersion and Community Health Needs Assessment by Undergraduate Medical Students in New Zealand." *Medical Education* 35, no. 3 (March 2001): 242–9.

Hart-Wasekeesikaw, Fijola. "Cultural Competence and Cultural Safety in First Nations, Inuit and Métis Nursing Education: An Integrated Review of the Literature." Aboriginal Nurses Association of Canada, 2009. https://opus.uleth.ca/bitstream/handle/10133/720/An_Integrated_Review_of_the_Literature.pdf.

Hodge, Heidi, Dean Carson, Peter Berggren, and Roger Strasser. "From Lancelot to Lapland: Implications of Engaged Rural Universities." In *University Partnerships for International Development*, edited by Patrick Blessinger and Barbara Cozza, 123–39. Bingley, UK: Emerald Group, 2017.

Hudson, Geoffrey L., and Dan Hunt. "The Northern Ontario School of Medicine and Social Accountability." In *The Making of the Northern Ontario School of Medicine: A Case Study in the History of Medical Education*, edited by Geoffrey Tesson, Geoffrey L. Hudson, Roger Strasser, and Dan Hunt, 157–82. Montreal, QC, and Kingston, ON: McGill-Queen's University Press, 2009.

Hudson, Geoffrey L., and Marion Maar. "Faculty Analysis of Distributed Medical Education in Northern Canadian Aboriginal Communities." *Rural and Remote Health* 14, no. 4 (2014): 2664.

Jacklin, Kristen, Roger Strasser, and Ian Peltier. "From the Community to the Classroom: The Aboriginal Health Curriculum at the Northern Ontario School of Medicine." *Canadian Journal of Rural Medicine* 19, no. 4 (2014): 143–50.

Jazrozik, Konrad. "Going Bush – Helping Medical Students Learn from Aboriginal People." *The Medical Journal of Australia* 163, no. 11–12 (December 1995): 591–4.

Kamaka, Martina L. "Cultural Immersion in a Cultural Competency Curriculum." *Academic Medicine* 76, no. 5 (May 2001): 512.

Kavanagh, Kathryn. "Summers of No Return: Transforming Care through a Nursing Field School." *The Journal of Nursing Education* 37, no. 2 (1998): 71–9.

Kurtz, Donna, Robert Janke, Jeanette Vinek, Taylor Wells, Pete Hutchinson, and Amber Frost. "Health Sciences Cultural Safety Education in Australia, Canada, New Zealand, and the United States: A Literature Review." *International Journal of Medical Education* 9 (2018): 271–85.

Kurtz, Donna L.M., deSales Turner, Jessie Nyberg, and Diana Moar. "Social Justice and Health Equity: Urban Aboriginal Women's Actions for Health Reform." *International Journal of Health, Wellness, and Society* 3 (2014): 13–26.

Lee, Donna, Marie Kurtz, Robert Janke, Jeanette Vinek, Taylor Wells, Pete Hutchinson, and Amber Froste. "Health Sciences Cultural Safety Education in Australia, Canada, New Zealand, and the United States: A Literature Review." *International Journal of Medical Education* 9 (2018): 271–85.

Maar, Marion, Lisa Boesch, and Sheldon Tobe. "Enhancing Indigenous Health Research Capacity in Northern Ontario through Distributed Community Engaged Medical Education at NOSM: A Qualitative Evaluation of the Community Engagement through Research Pilot Program." *Canadian Medical Education Journal* 9, no. 1 (2018): e21–e32.

Madjedi, Kian, and Rukhsaar Daya. "Cultural Immersion Placements as a Tool for Cultural Safety Education for Medical Students." *University of British Columbia Medical Journal* 7, no. 2 (2016): 28–9.

Mak, Donna, and Barbara Miflin. "Living and Working with the People of 'the Bush': A Foundation for Rural and Remote Clinical Placements in Undergraduate Medical Education." *Medical Teacher* 34, (2012): e603–e610.

NOSM. "Keeping the Vision – Mii Kwen Daan." 2006. https://www.nosm.ca/wp-content/uploads/2018/06/2006-Keeping-The-Vison-Report-English.pdf.

– "Report of the NOMS Aboriginal Workshop 'Follow Your Dreams.'" June 2003. https://www.nosm.ca/wp-content/uploads/2018/06/2003_06_03_FollowYourDreams_en.pdf.

Ontario Ministry of Health. *New Directions: Aboriginal Health Policy for Ontario*. Toronto: Queen's Printer for Ontario, 1994.

Ramsden, Irihapeti Merenia. "Cultural Safety and Nursing Education in Aotearoa and Te Waipounamu." PhD diss. Melbourne: Victoria University of Wellington, 2002. https://www.nzno.org.nz/Portals/0/Files/Documents/Services/Library/2002%20RAMSDEN%20I%20Cultural%20Safety_Full.pdf.

Robinson, Danielle, Chowdhury Ankika Savia, and Purathani Shanmuganathan. "Approaches to Incorporating Indigenous Health into the Canadian Medical School Curriculum." *University of Western Ontario Medical Journal* 86, no. 2 (Fall 2017): 57–8.

Ryan, Marilyn, and Renee S. Twibell. "Outcomes of a Transcultural Nursing Immersion Experience: Confirmation of a Dimensional Matrix." *Journal of Transcultural Nursing* 13, no. 1 (January 2002): 30–9.

Sargeant, Sally, Janie Dade Smith, and Shannon Springer. "Enhancing Cultural Awareness Education for Undergraduate Medical Students: Initial Findings from a Unique Cultural Immersion Activity." *Australian Medical Journal* 9, no. 7 (2016): 224–30.

Smith, L.S. "Concept Analysis: Cultural Competence." *Journal of Cultural Diversity* 5, no. 1 (Spring 1998): 4–10.

Smye, Victoria, Viviane Josewski, and Emma Kendall. "Cultural Safety: An Overview." First Nations, Inuit and Métis Advisory Committee Mental Health Commission of Canada, 2010. http://www.troubleshumeur.ca/documents/Publications/CULTURAL%20SAFETY%20AN%20OVERVIEW%20%28draft%20mar%202010%29.pdf.

Sopoaga, Faafetai, Tony Zaharic, Jesse Kokaua, and Sahra Covello. "Training a Medical Workforce to Meet the Needs of Diverse Minority Communities." BMC *Medical Education* 17, no. 19 (2017): 17–19.

Spradley, James P. *Participant Observation*, reissue edition. Long Grove, IL: Waveland, 2016.

Strasser, Roger, John Hogenbirk, Kristen Jacklin, Marion Maar, Geoffrey L. Hudson, Wayne Warry, Hoi Cheu, et al. "Community Engagement: A Central Feature of NOSM's Socially Accountable Distributed Medical Education." *Canadian Medical Education Journal* 9, no. 1 (2018): e33–e43.

Thackrah, Rosalie D., Sandra C. Thompson, and Angela Durey. "'Listening to the Silence Quietly': Investigating the Value of Cultural Immersion and Remote Experiential Learning in Preparing Midwifery Students for Clinical Practice." *British Medical Council Research Notes* 7, no. 1 (2014).

Thomas, Mary Durand, Sergio A. Olivares, Hyun Jung Kim, and Cheryle Beilke. "An Intensive Cultural Experience in a Rural Area." *Journal of Professional Nursing* 19, no. 3 (May 2003): 126–33.

Varty, Kim. "Leaving on a Jet Plane for a House Call: A Review of the Implementation of Cultural Competency in Medical Education." In *The Proceedings of the 17th Annual History of Medicine Days*, edited by Melanie Stapleton, Jennifer Lewis, and Frank W. Stahnisch, 275–86. Calgary, AB: Faculty of Medicine, University of Calgary, 2008.

PART THREE

Educational Spaces: Architectural, Gendered, Marginal, Digital

Opening Doors for Men:
Women's Medical Education in South China, 1899–1936

Kim Girouard

When Dr Mary Fulton founded the Hackett Medical College for Women (HMCW) in 1899 in Guangzhou, she could have hardly imagined that her new all-female school would eventually become the lifeblood for the development of modern medical education in South China for men and women alike.[1] Guangzhou, also known as Canton, was the capital of the southern Chinese province of Guangdong, and the first place in China where women could formally train in modern medicine.[2] Indeed, at Canton Hospital, the first Western-style hospital to be established in China in 1835, women had been admitted to medical classes beginning in 1879. After a quarrel between two male hospital chiefs twenty years later, however, all the male students withdrew from the program in support of their mentor's resignation. Medical classes ceased indefinitely, leaving the female medical students suddenly without educational prospects in medicine. Fulton's objectives were straightforward when she accepted funds donated by Edward A.K. Hackett to build the HMCW: to resume the training of Canton Hospital's female students. Instigated by determined individuals under the auspices of the Board of Foreign Missions of the Presbyterian Church in the United States of America (PCUSA), which had overseen the foreign and domestic missionary activities of the church since 1837, what began as an unassuming training program for women physicians nevertheless changed the medical landscape of the region.

In China, the first decades of the twentieth century were characterized by an unregulated and eclectic influx of interventions and influences from modern medicine. Consequently, studies examining the development of medical education tend to focus on centralization efforts by the China Medical Board (CMB) founded in 1914 by the Rockefeller Foundation, a private charitable organization based in the United States. In particular, standard historiographies emphasize the contribution of the Peking Union Medical College (PUMC), which was reorganized in 1917 by the CMB as a co-educational

institution modelled after the Johns Hopkins University Medical School in the
United States. This model introduced new standards for medical education
and practice in China that were based on laboratory and clinical methods.[3]
None of these studies, moreover, engage an explicit gendered perspective.
Some historians have analyzed the educational and professional trajectories
of several famous Chinese female doctors, particularly those trained in the
United States, in order to illustrate their importance to the professionalization of nursing and midwifery in China, as well as subsequent increases in
women's professional and political empowerment.[4] No comprehensive work,
however, analyzes the importance of medical training for women in China
beyond this vital sociological significance – that is, to view it as a cornerstone
for modern Chinese medical education itself. To redress this deficit, this chapter examines closely the Hackett Medical College for Women in Guangzhou,
one of three medical schools for women that opened in China at the beginning of the twentieth century, and certainly the most important in terms of
longevity and number of graduates.

A few scholars have explored the history of the HMCW and the women who
created it. Sara W. Tucker and, more recently, Xu Guangqiu both demonstrate how the school transformed the lives of numerous Chinese women
and non-Chinese female missionaries by offering career opportunities and
encouraging them to enter the public sphere.[5] Nonetheless, neither historian
challenges the official but inaccurate version of history propagated by the
American Presbyterian Mission: that the demise of segregated women's medical training in South China was brought about when the Canton Hospital
(the men's institution) absorbed the HMCW founded by Mary Fulton to create
the new Sun Yat-sen Medical College – today the Faculty of Medicine of the
Sun Yat-sen University, the most important medical school in South China.
To the contrary, as this chapter shows, it was Fulton's HMCW that took up the
educational aspirations of the Canton Hospital to form a new co-educational
institution that eventually became the Sun Yat-sen Medical College in 1936.
The historical inaccuracy is institutionalized on the official website of Sun Yat-
sen University, an account that does not mention the HMCW and refers only
to the medical training program of the old Canton Hospital, namely the Bo Ji
Medical School, as the precursor of its prestigious Faculty of Medicine.[6] This
chapter reveals the fundamental but overlooked role played by the HMCW in
the development of modern medical education in South China.

This chapter challenges official narratives by showing how the Hackett
Medical College for Women, not the Canton Hospital, was the foundation for
the new co-ed medical school that emerged in the 1930s. It does so by examining the formative influences of specific personalities and everyday realities for
female medical students and educators in the preceding period. By adapting

to local socio-cultural environments, the HMCW served both the professional expectations and the health needs of Chinese women. The school's leadership also shrewdly negotiated evolving standards of scientific medicine and medical education in order to gain legitimacy in the eyes of emergent local health authorities and simultaneously serve women's educational and health needs. Contrary to the dominant and persistent historical narrative – the view that the Hackett Medical College was closed because it was outdated – I show how the institution became a gateway for the development of modern medical education in South China, not only for women, but also for men.

LOCAL CONTEXTS AND WOMEN'S PROFESSIONAL EXPECTATIONS

When the Hackett Medical College for Women (HMCW) was created in 1899, Mary Fulton, the school's founder, had no trouble recruiting female students. In Guangzhou, especially, the social environment was conducive to the establishment of a women's medical school. In particular, the HMCW responded to two demands. On the one hand, it supported the professional ambitions expressed by local women who both understood the "traditional" role of female healers and embraced ideas about women holding paid jobs outside the domestic confines of the home. On the other hand, the HMCW answered the medical and health needs of local women by providing access to female doctors, both Chinese and missionary, with advanced training in the fields of gynecology, obstetrics, and pediatrics within, importantly, an institutional context that conformed to existing social norms of sex-segregation. In doing so, the school successfully positioned itself as a space in which some women could embody the new educational and professional standards of modern medicine, and in which others could access such physicians and diagnostic technology within an acceptable homosocial setting. It was a strong position that enabled the directors, educators, and students to tackle the challenges ahead.

Modern medicine was first introduced in China in Guangzhou under the auspices of Christian missions. Following the end of the Opium Wars (1840–42; 1856–60), Chinese authorities gave missionaries the right to proselytize throughout China. Modern medicine was often framed as a tool for evangelization, and dispensaries and hospitals of varying degrees of sophistication were set up in conjunction with chapels and churches. Because the port in Guangzhou was the only one opened to foreign trade prior to 1840, and because the city became the anchor and the gateway for Western imperialists in China, this evangelical medicine phenomenon was significant and began even before that turning point. In 1835, the American missionary doctor Peter Parker established there the first Western-style hospital in China, first called the Ophthalmic Hospital and later renamed the Canton Hospital. In 1866, the Canton Hospital – which had provided some informal training to medical assistants – established a more formal training program in medicine for local Chinese men.[7]

As the work of Connie Shemo demonstrates, it was at the request of two Chinese pupils from the True Light Seminary, a boarding school for girls operated by the American Presbyterian Mission, that the head of Canton Hospital, physician John G. Kerr, consented to admit female students to his medical class in 1879.[8] There were no female missionary doctors in this period to inspire young Chinese schoolgirls who were keen to train in medicine. Contrary to long-standing historical narratives conveyed by the Mission, then, it was Chinese women, not missionaries, who instigated the development of formal medical education for women in Guangzhou.[9]

As recent historical interpretations demonstrate, there existed a long tradition of women medical practitioners in China, not only as midwives, but also as healers and literate practitioners educated in the Chinese scholar tradition.[10] These Chinese women left very few formal records of their knowledge and practice. The evidence compiled by Wu Yi-Li suggests, however, that some belonged to reputable medical families, so that women in late imperial China could have acquired medical knowledge and legitimacy by means of family lineage.[11] Some of the first female students to train at the Canton Hospital also undoubtedly fit this narrative. Harriet Noyes, head of the True Light Seminary, for example, indicated in her memoirs that one of the female medical trainees at the Canton Hospital had a father and brother who had also graduated from Kerr's formal medical program.[12] It is reasonable to speculate, therefore, that women medical trainees at Canton Hospital were inspired to join the ancient sorority of female healers and learned practitioners in China, or, more directly, by medical role models within their own families.

For these young women, medical training might have been considered a good way to eventually support themselves or supplement the income of their households. Indeed, in Guangdong province, and especially in the region of the Pearl River Delta where Guangzhou is located, women had more room to manoeuvre within the Confucian social order than elsewhere in China. Notably, it was not unusual for them to contribute to the family economy by working outside the home. Within the peasant class and even among the richest family landowners, as well as in smaller trading communities, sex segregation was less strict. Numerous women were active in the agricultural, manufacturing, and commercial sectors.[13] According to a 1914 report of the Rockefeller Foundation, in South China, "the opportunity to become a doctor, or even something which will allow [women] to assume the title of doctor, and bring back the financial and social rewards, seems to appeal to a considerable number of young women."[14]

From the end of the nineteenth century onward, Chinese women who entered medical education in Guangzhou were not driven solely by a desire to "minister like angels to their suffering sisters," as Christian missions might have hoped, "with the self-denying and benevolent fervour that characterizes the sex."[15] Without dismissing the reasonable idea that Guangzhou's female medical students may have been animated by the altruistic nature of medical work, it is equally reasonable that this was not the only aspect of medicine that motivated them to enter its professional ranks. Rockefeller Foundation Commissioner Simon Flexner implied as much when he acknowledged that local women training in the missionary medical schools of South China "could earn what are almost fabulous sums for those people" (Flexner was referring to Chinese women as "those people").[16] In a regional context in which the female population was more widely involved in economic affairs and public society, it is likely that women viewed the medical profession as a lucrative business opportunity, and therefore as a path to their own economic independence.

By the end of the nineteenth century, female students and "assistants" at the Canton Hospital could already measure the financial prospect of a medical private practice. Just before the opening of the HMCW in 1899, two Chinese women "assistants" on staff at the Canton Hospital amassed $832 for the hospital through their home practices, aided by female medical students. This amount would have represented a monthly revenue of approximately $35 each, had the women earned the income themselves in private practice.[17] These profits were reported by Canton Hospital administrators in American dollars and have not been adjusted. During the same period, by comparison, less-educated Chinese scholars teaching in the area's village schools earned roughly $8 per month, and skilled workers might receive a monthly salary of $9 to $13 in a big city such as Guangzhou.[18] A private medical practice, then – even that of a female physician – appears to have been as lucrative as Flexner suggested.

It is therefore less surprising that at the beginning of the twentieth century the management at Canton Hospital considered itself fortunate to retain the services of the HMCW's graduates, since "any of them could easily establish themselves in a lucrative private practice if they desired it in preference to their self-denying efforts in Hospital service."[19] Indeed, it was common for Chinese women doctors to leave their institutional functions after several years to establish themselves in private practice; many even did so immediately after graduation. It was so common, in fact, that the HMCW had little choice but to train its students accordingly. As mentioned in the report of the school for the academic year 1915–16: "each Senior student spends two weeks with one of the foreign doctors of the city ... to study the practical methods used in an extensive private practice."[20] Not only were the management and teaching staff of the HMCW aware of the appeal of private practice, they also provided their students with tools to embark and succeed on this path.

Although institutional employment opportunities became more numerous, diversified, and financially more attractive over time, the HMCW's graduates continued to favour private practice. In the middle of the 1920s, for example, the management of the school reported that the majority of its graduates, 51%, worked in private practice, compared to 16% in missionary medical work, 7% in Chinese private hospitals, and 6% in governmental or philanthropic institutions; the rest pursued graduate studies (4%), were deceased (4%), or their circumstances were unknown (12%).[21] In the early 1930s, the portrait was practically the same. Of the HMCW's 214 graduates, 109 (51%) were identified as working in the private sector.[22] For the school's teachers, the fact that private practice was still generally more remunerative (not to mention less demanding and restrictive than a hospital position) largely explained this persistent preference.[23]

Despite tenacious efforts by American missionaries to persuade both themselves and their supporters at home that their medico-religious missions had paved the way for women's medical education in South China – specifically by modelling female doctors as intermediaries of their holy mission – much of the historical evidence points in the opposite direction. Not only was women's medical education in the mission's own Canton Hospital instigated by Chinese women themselves, female Chinese physicians continued to serve their own medical interests and professional prospects through the establishment and success of Hackett Medical College for Women.

SOCIAL NORMS OF SEX SEGREGATION

In addition to the educational and financial opportunities it afforded to Chinese women with professional aspirations, the HMCW was all the more germane in this regional context because it met Chinese social conventions of sex segregation. Although women of Guangdong province, and in particular in the Pearl River Delta, had more room to manoeuvre within the Confucian order, they were expected to minimally conform to such social norms. As was the case throughout China, women of Guangzhou preferred to be treated by medical practitioners of their own sex, especially for medical conditions involving their genitalia and reproductive functions. As historians have shown, therapies in late imperial China that involved discussions or examination of female genitals, including assistance during childbirth, were the exclusive domain of women.[24] Consequently, in the eyes of Christian missionaries, there was a need for modern female doctors in South China.

In his annual report of 1880, John Kerr noted that the female students in his medical class at Canton Hospital gave "promise of being very useful ... in cases of diseases peculiar to females."[25] Earlier that year, when a messenger was dispatched to the hospital to fetch a doctor for a woman suffering from "retention of urine," Kerr, who had only male doctors available, instead "sent one of the female medical pupils to relieve her, as it would be more in accordance with Chinese ideas of propriety to have a female attendant in such a case."[26] Recognizing that the women's wards at Canton Hospital could be more effective if female students received more extensive training in obstetrics, gynecology, and reproductive diseases – and further recognizing that male instructors could not effectively provide such training to Chinese women – Kerr finally requested that the Board of Foreign Missions send a female missionary doctor to the Canton Hospital as an instructor.

Dr Mary W. Niles arrived in 1882 and officially commenced her duties in the hospital the following year, after completing her studies in the Cantonese language.[27] A second female physician, Dr Mary Fulton, arrived in 1884. In 1892, Niles was officially assigned to teach lectures in gynecology and obstetrics to all medical students at Canton Hospital, including men. According to archival evidence, however, Canton's male students did not receive any hands-on clinical training in these specialties, which continued to be the case until the school's closure in the early twentieth century. In reality, only Niles's female students continued to perfect their obstetrical and gynecological skills in practical settings.[28] From 1896 onwards – likely to facilitate this expanded program of specialized clinical instruction for women physicians – female students spent some time learning apart from their male counterparts and were "taught separately under the direction of Dr Niles, assisted by U Mi Tak, one of the women graduates."[29] At the end of the nineteenth century, therefore, the male graduates of Canton Hospital had possibly never attended a case of childbirth. Yet their female classmates received comprehensive theoretical and clinical education in gynecology and obstetrics.

If the missionary training programs at Canton Hospital already differed according to the sex of the students, Mary Fulton's determination to open the Hackett Medical College for Women at the turn of the twentieth century signalled the effective division between women's and men's medical education in South China. Educated at the Women's Medical College of Pennsylvania, it was perhaps only natural for Fulton to envision a separate medical school for women in Guangzhou. During her employment as a medical instructor for female pupils at Canton Hospital, moreover, she and her male colleagues repeatedly noted in reports that more suitable accommodations to teach and house female students were needed in order to develop women's clinical training further.[30] In this same period in North America, respected women's medical schools increasingly provided exceptionally advanced training in gynecology and obstetrics, and, in some cases, pediatrics.[31] Fulton and her missionary colleagues applied the same principles at their new medical school for women.[32]

In 1909, the list of theoretical courses taught to female students at the HMCW and to their male counterparts at Canton Hospital were very similar, although the women's curriculum included pediatrics and the men's program did not. At Canton Hospital, male students had two didactic lectures dedicated to obstetrics and one to gynecology, but no curricular time allotted for clinical training in either specialty.[33] At its affiliated hospital, the David Gregg Hospital for Women and Children, HMCW students, by contrast, gained clinical experience in all medical fields, including gynecology, obstetrics, and pediatrics.

The HMCW remained a women's institution committed to training female doctors who were especially proficient in the fields of gynecology, obstetrics, and pediatrics, even when its management passed into the hands of male doctors beginning in 1925, discussed in more detail below. In the early 1930s, Hackett's four-year medical program provided 378 hours of training in gynecology, of which 234 were dedicated to clinical teaching. In addition, 296 hours of instruction were specified for the field of obstetrics, of which 152 were devoted to practical training. By comparison, the medical faculty of National Zhongshan University in Guangzhou (formerly the Gongyi Medical School), which had readmitted women to its program in 1926, offered only 187 hours of combined instruction in those fields during its four years of training. And, while the co-educational institution provided only 136 hours of pediatrics instruction, the HMCW offered 252 hours of teaching in this specialty, of which 180 were dedicated to clinical training.[34]

By providing local women with access to highly capable female doctors who were able to respond to the special health needs of the female population in South China, the HMCW filled a gap that a men's institution could not. By the 1930s, Chinese women were gradually less reluctant to be seen by male doctors, although they still largely preferred to be treated by women physicians, especially for gynecological complaints and obstetrical procedures. From this perspective, the HMCW's mandate to serve the local female population meant that it remained relevant. To pursue it into the twentieth century, however, the school had to adapt to new medical and educational exigencies.

NEGOTIATING EVOLVING STANDARDS OF MEDICAL EDUCATION

The evolving medical landscape of the first decades of the twentieth century was challenging for the HMCW. To endure, it had to maintain up-to-date medical standards and approval from emergent authorities. Successive directors and faculties adapted curricula to new scientific and educational standards established, first, by the Rockefeller Foundation's China Medical Board from the mid-1910s, and, later, during the Nanjing decade (1927–37), by China's Nationalist government (Guomindang).[35] On one hand, they implemented more rigorous entrance requirements and strengthened training programs, without ignoring the social realities of Chinese women's education. On the other, they endorsed co-educational approaches promoted by the scientific medical community and the central government, without abandoning the HMCW's commitment towards women's education and health.

At the end of the nineteenth and beginning of the twentieth century, the country's intelligentsia and ruling authorities were concerned by imperialist incursions into China. Those in power increasingly considered science and medicine as vectors for modernity and as political tools to eventually regain full sovereignty over the nation. The idea of the "Sick Man of Asia" was integral, a well-studied narrative that conveyed the image of a weak and degenerate China, in opposition to the strong and vigorous white civilization.[36] By linking Chinese women's inferior condition to this narrative, Chinese rulers endorsed initiatives proposed by Christian missions to improve the health and material conditions of the female population, regarded as essential to national survival.[37] It was within this political and social context that Guangdong authorities supported Mary Fulton and the Hackett Medical College for Women.

In light of this broader socio-political context, remarks made by Canton's daodai on the occasion of the HMCW's 1908 Commencement resonated as especially significant.[38] The daodai began by stating that he was ashamed that it had taken foreigners so far removed from China to establish the first women's medical school in the region. He subsequently urged the Chinese population and government to support the work of the HMCW because such institutions "will bring vast relief, dissipate prejudice and open the way for other needed reforms that will enable China to take a high place amongst other nations."[39] Indeed, the viceroy of Liangguang (the provinces of Guangdong and Guangxi) also personally attended the ceremony in recognition of the school's efforts and successes, accompanied by a formal guard of 500 soldiers.[40] The previous year, the viceroy had started placing his official seal on all of its diplomas, making Fulton's school the only Western-type medical school recognized by the highest authorities in the province.[41]

Local authorities may have viewed the HMCW as a tool of modernity, yet representatives of the Rockefeller Foundation, who contributed to produce the final report of their commission of inquiry on Medicine in China in 1914, did not. According to details in one of their preliminary reports, the school's entrance requirements were too low, almost nonexistent, except for a "knowledge of Chinese, reading and writing." The report's authors described the training program as outdated and lacking rigor because, they claimed, director Mary Fulton's "ideas of medical work and medical education are those of a generation ago." The report also questioned the quality of the education because some members of the foreign staff "had not been in the hospital for a very long time and practically had no connection with the work." In reality, most of the teaching appears to have been carried out by Fulton herself, who, by that point, did much less clinical and surgical work at the hospital because she was helped by her "Chinese assistants." According to the Rockefeller report, the HMCW's female graduates were "of very little value, except that they know a little obstetrics." In short, it concluded, they were competent midwives.[42] From 1914 onward, powerful philanthropic agencies such as the Rockefeller Foundation that funded (and thus adjudicated) medical schools expected clinical and laboratory training to go hand in hand.

Fulton had obtained the MD in 1884, an era in which the best-trained physicians continued to grapple with the validity of new bacteriological explanations of infectious disease. Described in Mission documents as "one of the most busy women in the world," it is indeed conceivable that she had not kept up with the latest laboratory developments in medicine, especially those emerging outside China.[43] Indeed, she regularly advocated for medical education based on apprenticeship and practical bedside training. She explained her pedagogical perspective in the following terms: "Better to turn out a hundred doctors a year who will intelligently minister to the relief of suffering *now* than to wait twenty years and be able to turn out three or four 'as good as doctors at home.'"[44] But after the publication in 1910 of Abraham Flexner's influential report on medical education in North America, sponsored by the Carnegie Foundation, learning medicine by apprenticeship was ruled unsatisfactory. Not only Rockefeller commissioners, but also the missionary medical community in China, viewed medical training without scientific training as deficient. Indeed, when two young female doctors arrived in Guangzhou in 1913, both were disappointed by what they perceived as the institution's low quality and standards. Martha Hackett was a graduate of Rush Medical College in Chicago and the daughter of the HMCW's founding donor. Not a physician, Harriet Allyn had a PhD in biology from the University of Chicago. Subtle tensions persisted between Fulton and her new, younger medical colleagues.

That Hackett's graduates were merely good midwives was an unfair and inaccurate assessment. All evidence points to the reality that they were not only knowledgeable gynecologists and obstetricians, but also skilled general surgeons. According to the Rockefeller report itself, they performed almost all surgical operations at the hospital. Physician Luo Xiuyun, for example, performed "forty-five consecutive abdominal operations without the loss of a patient."[45] She was also renowned to have performed more than 200 caesarean sections in her career, and to have successfully removed an ovarian tumour weighing 105 pounds.[46] After the reorganization of the HMCW in 1916, Luo Xiuyun was retained as chief surgeon as well as the only instructor of surgery.[47] At a time when obstetrics was not as valued as highly as other emerging medical specialties – in part because of its roots in the female sphere and historical connections with midwifery – Chinese female doctors were routinely perceived as solely and merely gynecological and obstetrical technicians. Both their professional status and clinical performance were often presumptively categorized second-rate.[48]

Doctors Hackett and Allyn were initially sent to the HMCW to assist Fulton, but eventually replaced her and took over operations. When Fulton resigned from her position as director of the HMCW in 1915, she cited her ill health and desire to dedicate herself to translation work. Her resignation resolved latent conflicts between herself and Hackett and Allyn, and left the school in the hands of a new generation of female leadership.

While Hackett and Allyn took issue with the school's inadequate scientific training, they never suggested that the competencies of the school's graduates were limited to obstetrics (nor did their eventual male successors, for that matter). As evidenced by the hours dedicated to this specialty in the training program during their tenure, moreover, they did not try to divert the school from its expertise in the field. Nor did Hackett and Allyn doubt the medical and surgical skills of the Chinese women doctors, since they continued to rely on them to provide clinical care and perform surgeries in the hospital. They remained concerned, however, by the lack of pre-medical education in basic maths and sciences, which were becoming increasingly standard entrance requirements in North American medical schools at the beginning of the twentieth century. Indeed, from the mid-1910s, both medical missionaries and Rockefeller representatives recognized that the main obstacle to the training of female doctors in China was inadequate preliminary education for girls.[49]

The Chinese school system was reorganized by the Qing Dynasty in the early twentieth century, which included and promoted the education of girls. A few years after the advent of the Chinese Republic in 1912, however, it was still difficult to find women candidates who possessed the knowledge needed to enter medical training. The main goal of girls' schools in Guangdong in this period, as elsewhere in the country, was to produce good wives and virtuous mothers, a mandate that accorded with the Confucian principles that still permeated the Chinese society, even in the south.[50] In 1915, Hackett and Allyn observed that the educational aims of missionary schools reflected similar social expectations for girls, and were more focused on domestic arts than on science. Even the True Light Seminary, they reported, the boarding school for girls operated by the American Presbyterian Mission, could not be considered a proper high school, but rather a "grammar school," because apart from simple arithmetic, no other scientific subject was taught to its female pupils.[51]

Appointed president and dean of the HMCW, respectively, Hackett and Allyn had the power to implement changes that brought the quality of its medical training program up to the new Flexnerian standards. This enhanced its credibility in the eyes of the authorities that controlled funding and policy. The new leaders recognized, however, that they risked alienating prospective Chinese students if they did not also adapt the school's policies to local contexts. They did not simply make the entrance requirements more rigorous, however, as did many North American schools, a measure that prevented most students in marginalized groups from entering medicine. To avoid precisely this effect, therefore, Hackett and Allyn instituted a pre-medical year of training for all new students. This enabled the HMCW to continue admitting high numbers of local applicants, while ensuring that those offered a place in the medical training program possessed the essential scientific preparation to pursue medical study.

The measure was applied in 1915 and intended to be temporary in order to allow adequate time for girls' education to develop further in the region. Again in 1922, however, Allyn reported that the HMCW's students had to "come first to pre-medical work in the foundation of science, because it is so difficult to get these in other schools and colleges."[52] While by the early 1920s more girls in Guangdong were attending school, it was mostly in primary education that their numbers increased.[53] In 1923, 468 girls were enrolled in secondary school in the province compared to 8,639 boys.[54]

In 1925, physician J. Allen Hofmann was appointed successor to Hackett and Allyn. Male and American, he was also reluctant to implement entrance requirements that would limit too severely the intake of female Chinese medical students. In 1928, the new Chinese Nationalist authorities requested that all medical schools in China register with the Ministry of Education, and increase their minimum entrance requirements to a recognized senior middle school diploma. Hofmann did not want to comply. Apart from his assumed reluctance to hand over the presidential reins of the HMCW to a Chinese physician, which the new national regulation also required, Hofmann expressed concern about the school's ability to improve its infrastructure in order to meet the registration standards. He also worried, reasonably, that more restrictive entrance requirements would reduce or prevent the successful admission of new local candidates.[55]

The consensus reached by HMCW officials was to proceed gradually with the state registration of the school, and to raise the entrance requirements accordingly little by little. In 1929, consequently, they added a second pre-medical year to the training program in order to "give opportunity for the instructors to train the students very thoroughly in the methods of careful and logical thinking, before they come up to the more important medical courses."[56] The same year, applicants who had not graduated from an accredited senior middle school, yet who had completed twelve years of schooling, were provided with the opportunity to pass an entrance examination that included mathematics and basic sciences.[57] Evidently, this incremental strategy was justified, since the number of enrollees in the pre-medical courses steadily decreased from fourteen to ten students between 1929 and 1930. It fell to only four in 1931, the year that the HMCW finally strictly applied the central government's rules on standardized entrance requirements.[58] In 1932, the two-year premedical course was reduced to one intensive year in order to fully comply with the policies of nationalist authorities, and the HMCW was officially registered and recognized as a "school of medicine of college grade."[59]

From the mid-1910s onward, those who managed the HMCW had been aware that the school needed to adjust its curricula to the increasing standards of medical education in order to legitimize itself in the eyes of the medical and governmental authorities in China. At the end of the 1920s, such changes had become a matter of survival, since schools that refused or failed were, by then, obviously doomed to disappear. As a women's medical college, however, the HMCW also necessarily had to address reduced opportunities for local girls to receive adequate preliminary education. By implementing solutions for this plain reality, the school not only assured itself a ready supply of local female medical students to train, it remained equally steadfast in its commitment to women's medical education, and, by extension, to women's health in the region.

OPENING THE DOORS TO MEN

In order to pursue this joint mandate further, the school's leadership recognized that the Hackett Medical College for Women must eventually face the realities and challenges of teaching and learning modern medicine in an all-female medical school. On the one hand, beginning in the mid-1910s, there had been a constant shortage of women missionary doctors in Guangzhou, as everywhere else in China. The situation was explained in part by declining numbers of female medical graduates in North America, and the impossibility for American missionary women to combine medical practice and marriage.[60] On the other hand, the HMCW gradually disqualified Chinese women doctors from holding chairs and professorships if they lacked post-graduate training outside China. It became practically impossible, therefore, to operate the school and teaching hospital exclusively with female staff and faculty. In parallel, in the rise of the New Culture and May Fourth Movement (1915–21) – which was characterized by an eclectic rejection of Confucianism – Chinese intellectuals and students, male and female, began to advocate generally for co-education, and for equal access to higher learning for women.[61] From the early 1920s, Chinese public universities gradually accepted women, and the Chinese government authorized co-education at all levels of schooling in 1923. The same year, the North China Union Medical College for Women merged with the Medical Faculty of the Shandong Christian University. Only two women's medical colleges established in China remained: the HMCW and the Women's Christian College of Medicine, which had relocated from Suzhou to Shanghai.[62] Meanwhile in the United States, all women's medical schools but one (Woman's Medical College of Pennsylvania) had closed.[63] Consequently, the segregated medical training that the HMCW had proudly and reliably offered suddenly appeared less modern, and, as the American experience demonstrated, less viable.

In Guangzhou, since the closing of the Canton Hospital training program in Guangzhou in 1912, and a failed attempt by Canton Christian College (later Lingnan University) to set up its own medical school for men between 1906 and 1914, the male medical missionary community in the region had continued to develop plans for a "union" medical school for men (that is, a school resulting from the collaboration of several different Christian missions). By the beginning of the 1920s, they viewed the HMCW as a good "adjunct" to their scheme to reinstate strong medical educational programs for men in South China, and they assumed that the HMCW would see a union affiliation as advantageous. The Council on Medical Education of the China Medical Missionary Association (CMMA) had a mandate to promote and guide the development of modern medicine and medical education under Christian auspices throughout the country. In 1923, the council adopted a resolution stipulating that if extensive efforts were not immediately enacted to uplift the HMCW to the standards of the CMMA, the female-only medical training program should be abandoned. Furthermore, it advised against the maintenance of separate medical schools for women in China, and therefore urged the HMCW to affiliate more closely with Canton Hospital and its male doctors. The ultimate goal, the council made clear, should be a single co-educational institution in the near future.

Initially, the directors of both the HMCW and the Canton Hospital had agreed that the women's institution would cooperate as an independent partner in the new scheme of Christian medical education in Guangzhou. After the warning from the CMMA in 1923, however, members of the medical missionary community applied additional pressure. In a letter addressed to the representatives of the Presbyterian Mission, for example, physician Joseph L. Harvey emphasized that, in order for a new Christian union medical school to materialize, the project must be co-educational because, according to Harvey, "other Missions will not join in with Hackett as a strictly women's medical school." The HMCW had two options: "either become a part of the larger medical work," Harvey insisted, "or close."[65]

It took almost a decade to coalesce, but, in 1933, co-education under Christian auspices concretized in Guangzhou. The previous year, an agreement was signed between the Hackett Medical College for Women, Canton Hospital, and Lingnan University (previously Canton Christian College). Alongside its female students, the HMCW welcomed its first male students, who were at this time very few. At the time, men counted for half of newly admitted first-year candidates at the HMCW, more precisely four of eight, and were in total six of fifty students in the school.[66] The 1933 unification was the end of separate medical education for women in South China. It also initiated the administrative incorporation of the HMCW into Lingnan University, even before the historical school's original facilities were shuttered in 1936 when the entire medical faculty moved to the new site of the Sun Yat-sen Medical College, located next to Canton Hospital.

From an administrative perspective – and especially if viewed as a correlate of the American experience of co-educational medical training at the beginning of the twentieth century – it is tempting to conclude that the unification was a defeat for women's medical education in Guangzhou. However, closer examination of everyday realities, decisions, and practices shows that the Hackett Medical College for Women was not shut down or pushed out. On the contrary, it was the HMCW that opened its doors to male students in the 1930s. The men were forced to adapt and prove themselves to the school's well-established medical sisterhood, and to be accepted by their female colleagues and teachers. Physician Jessie MacBean, for instance, affiliated with the Presbyterian Canadian Mission and chair of obstetrics at the HMCW, was not keen to welcome young men into her class. MacBean urged the school's administration to be more selective with regard to which male applicants it admitted because she thought that "women put more of themselves into the work they undertake."[67] New male students also had to adapt themselves to an environment not designed for the accommodation of both sexes. For example, a lack of co-educational infrastructure at the HMCW forced them to reside outside the premises of the school, whereas female medical trainees remained true "residents" according to the American system.

Male medical trainees, moreover, were obliged to follow the HMCW's existing curriculum – designed especially to prepare female physicians to serve the region's female patient population – because the medical training program was already fully registered with the central government before becoming co-educational. Even when the HMCW became Sun Yat-sen Medical College, no compromise was made for male students hoping to decrease or avoid the 306 hours of training in gynecology and obstetrics or the 234 hours dedicated to pediatrics. Like their female classmates, male trainees were required to manage at least five "confinement cases" (childbirths) by themselves before the end of their fifth year of training, including delivery and pre- and post-natal care. During the internship year at Canton Hospital or Hackett Medical Center (formerly the affiliated hospital of the HMCW), all students also had to successfully complete a six-week rotation in the departments of both gynecology and obstetrics.[68] In the late 1920s and the first half of the 1930s, the HMCW's mandate to train women doctors who would serve the female population of the region remained the institution's priority, even if the necessity of a separate women's medical school was soon deemed obsolete.

While the end of the era of separate women's medical education in the United States resulted in a decrease of the proportion of female trainees, the same was not true in China, and especially not in South China. In the 1890s, the percentage of female medical graduates in the United States was as high as 20 per cent. Since the favoured co-educational training programs – that is, those legitimized by adhering to the new Flexnerian standards – tended to impose formal and informal quotas on female entrants, however, this proportion rapidly declined, and between 1929 and 1940 never surpassed four per cent. Indeed, it was not until the mid-to-late 1970s that women returned to the study of medicine in similar proportions to those of the pre-Flexner era.[69] Evidently, co-education did not have the same effect in China, where medical schools did not impose quotas and made more than marginal space for women by the 1930s. According to a study published in the *Chinese Medical Journal* in 1933, roughly 17 per cent of medical students in the country were women that year, and in Guangdong province it was more than 30 per cent.[70] The proportion of the HMCW's female trainees clearly decreased when it became co-educational, but the school's new admissions policy did not lead to a quasi-disappearance of women from its training program. In 1946, for instance, women represented 33 per cent of the students of the Sun Yat-sen Medical College, and two years later that number had risen to 36 per cent.[71] The HMCW had to embrace co-education eventually. The historical record indicates that the transition went more smoothly for its female students than for their male counterparts, and that the outcome did not have the expected devastating effect on women's medical education.

CONCLUSIONS

The Hackett Medical College for Women had little choice but to embrace co-educational medical training and open its doors to male medical students. Unlike in the American context, however, it was not female medical students that were forced to transition and adapt themselves to a curriculum designed for the opposite sex – it was men. These developments, moreover, did not result in a decrease of female medical graduates, as they had in the United States.

The Hackett Medical College for Women was more than an ephemeral missionary endeavour designed to convey the Gospel to the Chinese female population. Not only was it a vector for Chinese women's emancipation, it was instrumental to the development of modern medical education in South China. Indeed, far from having been a ground-breaking progressive initiative by the Mission to produce, according to missionary narratives, "self-denying angels," the medical training that the HMCW provided was, in fact, the product of its particular regional context. First established in Canton Hospital at the request of local schoolgirls at the end of the nineteenth century, it continued to support the practical expectations of ambitious young women who recognized medical training as a means to earn a good living. By offering a training program well suited to the particular health needs of local women and expectant mothers, the HMCW simultaneously respected the realities created by Chinese social norms of sex segregation. The institution was also in tune with the persistent preference of local women for medical attendants of their own sex. As it entered the twentieth century, the HMCW confronted the equally challenging realities of new entrance and curricular standards for medical education, influenced by American developments such as the publication of the Flexner Report and demands from philanthropic agencies in exchange for funding medical education. The HMCW understood how to redefine and, when necessary, reinvent itself on its own terms to meet these new standards while measuring the real capacity of women in the region to adapt and succeed accordingly. In the early 1930s, the school also met state and missionary calls for co-education without compromising female physicians' enviable place in the local medical landscape, and, by extension, without depriving the local female population of access to advanced health care services in gynecology, obstetrics, and pediatrics. By consistently overcoming these challenging realities, the HMCW not only ensured its immediate survival, it was courted by the male medical missionary community in South China as a valuable, indeed essential, affiliate institution for the training of men. It remained an integral institution in the region's ongoing development of medical education.

While Canton Hospital lay educationally dormant for more than twenty-five years, the Hackett Medical College for Women was developing successful curricula, effective teaching, and female graduates – so successful, in fact, that it was eventually asked to open its doors to male students. In light of this analysis, the Hackett Medical College for Women should be recognized for its legitimate place in the history of the formidable Sun Yat-sen Medical College, and in the broader history of modern Chinese medical education. Sun Yat-sen Medical College customarily claims the Canton Hospital as its only ancestor. But, if the Canton Hospital represents its paternity, its maternal line – the Hackett Medical College for Women – played an equally foundational role in its inception and success.

NOTES

1   Born in Ashland, Ohio, in 1854, Mary Hannah Fulton was the second
    woman physician to be appointed to the South China Mission by the Foreign
    Mission Board of the Presbyterian Church in the USA. She graduated from
    the Woman's Medical College of Pennsylvania in 1884, and arrived in South
    China the same year. She died in Pasadena, California, in 1927. See Tucker,
    "A Mission for Change"; Xu, *American Doctors in Canton*, 131–86.
2   The term "modern medicine" is used throughout this chapter to designate a
    set of knowledge and practices about health that emerged in Europe at the
    beginning of the nineteenth century and was subsequently adopted in North
    America and elsewhere in the world. As Tina Phillips Johnson argues, the
    term is particularly suited in the context of modern China, because it captures
    the essence of the Chinese term *xiyi* (literally "Western medicine"). Equally so,
    it conveys an ideal of modernity pursued by local actors in China at the time,
    as well as the scientific component of the discipline. Furthermore, "modern
    medicine" does not imply an inherent Westernness. See Johnson, *Childbirth in
    Republican China*, xxiii.
3   See for instance Bullock, *An American Transplant*. Also Bullock, "A Case Study
    of Transnational Flows"; Yip, *Health and National Reconstruction*, 132–75.
4   Shemo, *The Chinese Medical Ministries*; Johnson, *Childbirth in Republican China*.
5   Tucker, "A Mission for Change," 137–57; Xu, *American Doctors in Canton*,
    131–86.
6   Sun Yat-sen University, "About SYSU: SYSU History," https://www.sysu.edu.
    cn/en/about/about04/667.htm (accessed 28 November 2021).
7   For more on Canton Hospital and the medical training it provided see Xu,
    American Doctors in Canton, 23–130.
8   Born in Duncansville, Ohio, in 1824, John G. Kerr graduated from Jefferson
    Medical College, Philadelphia, in 1847. He was appointed to the South

China Mission by the Foreign Mission Board of the Presbyterian Church in the USA. in 1854 and succeeded Dr Peter Parker as the head of the Canton Ophthalmic Hospital the year after. He was superintendent of the Canton Hospital for almost 45 years before devoting the rest of his life and career to the mentally ill. He died in Guangzhou in 1901. See Fu, "Medical Missionaries in China."

9   Shemo, "'Her Chinese Attended to Almost Everything,'" 324.

10   Leung, "Women Practicing Medicine," 128.

11   Wu, *Reproducing Women*, 19.

12   Noyes, *A Light in the Land of Sinim*, 88. Unfortunately, the name of Kerr's trainee is unknown.

13   Siu and Chan, "Introduction," 4–5.

14   Women's Hospital of the English Presbyterian Mission, Swatow, July 25, 1914, China Medical Board, Record Group 4, Series 1, Box 24, Folder 483, Rockefeller Archive Center, North Tarrytown.

15   *Report of the Medical Missionary Society in China for the Year 1889*, 9.

16   Cited in Shemo, "'Wants Learn Cut, Finish People,'" 65.

17   *Report of the Medical Missionary Society in China for the Year 1899*, 12.

18   Mary H. Fulton, *Inasmuch*, 84–5; Gamble and Meng, *Prices, Wages*, 92.

19   *Annual Report of the Medical Missionary Society in China for the Year 1903*, 13.

20   *Bulletin of The Hackett Medical College for Women, Catalogue 1915–1916*, 8.

21   *Hackett Medical College for Women, Bulletin 1924–1925*, 13.

22   *Annual Report of the Hackett Medical College for Women, Hospital Number 1933*, 13.

23   Annual Report of the South China Mission, 1934, Presbyterian Church in the USA, Board of Foreign Missions, Record Group 82, Box 49, Folder 09, Presbyterian Historical Society, Philadelphia.

24   Furth, "Concepts of Pregnancy," 16; Wu, *Reproducing Women*, 15–18.

25   *Report of the Medical Missionary Society in China for the Year 1880*, 20.

26   Ibid., 17.

27   Born in 1854 in Watertown, Wisconsin, Mary West Niles graduated from the Woman's Medical College of the New York Infirmary for Women and Children in 1882. Appointed to South China Mission by the Foreign Mission Board of the Presbyterian Church in the USA the same year, she became head of the Woman's Department of the Canton Hospital for fifteen years. She later joined the staff of the HMCW and pursued a private medical practice in Guangzhou until 1923, when she decided to dedicate herself entirely to the Mingxin School for the Blind she founded in 1889. She retired in 1928 in Pasadena, California, where she died in 1933. See Xu, *American Doctors in Canton*, 138–40, 204–8.

28   *Report of the Medical Missionary Society in China for the Year 1892*, 41.

29   *Report of the Medical Missionary Society in China for the Year 1896*, 31.

30   *Report of the Medical Missionary Society in China for the Year 1898*, 13, 29.

31   Morantz-Sanchez, *Sympathy and Science*, 64–89.

32   This was the case, for instance, for Dr Mary W. Niles; Dr Ruth C. Bliss, who
     graduated from the Women's Medical College in Pennsylvania in 1892, and
     Dr Eleanor Chestnut, who was stationed at the Lianzhou Presbyterian
     Women's Hospital, received medical degrees from the Women's Medical
     College of Chicago in 1893, and sporadically taught at the HMCW.

33   Swan, "South China Medical College," 307; Fulton, "Hackett Medical
     College," 327; *E.A.K. Hackett Medical College for Women, 1910–1911*.

34   Lee, "Some Statistics on Medical Schools," 1034. *Hackett Medical College for
     Women, Catalogue June 1930*, 25, 33–8.

35   The Nanjing decade refers to a period of relative political stability in China.
     It began in 1927 with the nominal unification of the country by Chiang
     Kai-shek (Jiang Jieshi) and the establishment of its Nationalist government
     (Guomindang) in Nanjing. Marked by a relative acceleration of modernizing
     efforts, it ended with the Japanese invasion in 1937.

36   Historians attribute the construction of this identity to medical iconography
     and attitudes towards specific health problems such as plague, leprosy, sperma-
     torrhea, and infant mortality. See Heinrich, *The Afterlife of Images*; Leung,
     Leprosy in China: A History; Shapiro, "The Puzzle of Spermatorrhea"; Johnson,
     Childbirth in Republican China.

37   Johnson and Wu, "Maternal and Child Health"; Johnson, *Childbirth in
     Republican China*.

38   The daodai was the intendant of Canton. As an official of the Qing Court he
     had administrative control over the city, and was mandated to deal with the
     foreign consuls.

39   Fulton, *Inasmuch*, 98.

40   The viceroy was the highest official of the Qing court in the area. He had
     administrative control over a territory that covers the current provinces of
     Guangdong and Guangxi.

41   Fulton, "Hackett Medical College," 325.

42   Women's Hospital of the Presbyterian Mission and Hackett Medical College
     for Women, F.W.P. & R.S.G., Canton, July 1st, 1914, China Medical Board,
     Record Group 4, Series 1, Box 24, Folder 461, Rockefeller Archive Center,
     North Tarrytown.

43   *The Seventy-Second Annual Report*, 156.

44   Fulton, "Hackett Medical College," 326.

45   Fulton, *Inasmuch*, 83.

46   Xu, *American Doctors in Canton*, 150–1.

47   *Bulletin of The Hackett Medical College for Women, Catalogue 1915–1916*, 3–5.

48   Morantz-Sanchez, *Sympathy and Science*, 63.

49   *Medicine in China*, 37.

50   Hershatter, *Women in China's Long Twentieth Century*, 84.

51   Letter from Dr Martha Hackett and Dr Harriet M. Allyn to Dr Brown, September 1st, 1915, Presbyterian Church in the USA, Board of Foreign Missions, Record Group 82, Box 05, Folder 04, Presbyterian Historical Society, Philadelphia.

52   Allyn, "The Hackett Medical College," 218.

53   Bailey, *Gender and Education in China*, tables 2.1, 4.3.

54   Ibid., table 4.4.

55   Report of the President of Hackett Medical College and Affiliated Institution, 1927–1928; President's Report of Hackett Medical College and Affiliated Institutions, February 1927, Record Group 82, Box 05, Folder 04, Presbyterian Historical Society, Philadelphia.

56   *Hackett Medical College for Women, Catalogue 1928–1929*, 13.

57   Ibid., 12.

58   Report of the President of Hackett Medical College and Affiliated Institutions, November 1931, Presbyterian Church in the USA, Board of Foreign Missions, Record Group 82, Box 05, Folder 04, Presbyterian Historical Society, Philadelphia; *Catalogue of the Hackett Medical College for Women (June 1930)*, 13; *Bulletin of the David Gregg Hospital for Women and Children (April 1929)*, 40.

59   *Annual Report of the Hackett Medical College, Hospital Number 1933*, 4.

60   Love, *Chinese Women in Medicine*; Tucker, "A Mission for Change," 145–6.

61   For more details concerning the debate on the value of co-education during the May Fourth period, see Wang, *Women in the Chinese Enlightenment*, 67–116.

62   Tao, "Medical Education of Chinese Women," 1012–13.

63   Morantz-Sanchez, *Sympathy and Science*, 243–8.

64   Medical Education for Women, March 12, 1923, Presbyterian Church in the USA, Board of Foreign Missions, Record Group 82, Box 05, Folder 04, Presbyterian Historical Society, Philadelphia.

65   Letter from Joseph L. Harvey to Mr Scott, June 20th, 1924, Presbyterian Church in the USA, Board of Foreign Missions, Record Group 82, Box 27, Folder 08, Presbyterian Historical Society, Philadelphia.

66   *Report of the Hackett Medical, Hospital Number January 1, 1933 to June 30, 1934*, 12.

67   Ballantyne, *Dr. Jessie MacBean*, 30.

68   *Lingnan University, Bulletin No. 61*, 138–43.

69   Warsh, *Prescribed Norms*, 201. Statistics for the United States concern students of the graduate class.

70   Tao, "Medical Education of Chinese Women," 1018–19.

71   Lingnan University, A Statistic of Enrolment, Academic Year 1945–1946,
      United Board for Christian Education in Asia, Lingnan University, Record
      Group 11, Box 187, Folder 3311, Yale Divinity School Library, New Haven,
      CT; Y.Y. Huang, Lingnan University Academic Report, First Semester 1948–
      1949, United Board for Christian Education in Asia, Lingnan University,
      Record Group 11, Box 182, Folder 3263, Yale Divinity School Library, New
      Haven, CT.

BIBLIOGRAPHY

Allyn, Harriet M. "The Hackett Medical College: The Healing of His Seamless
    Dress by Chinese Beds of Pain." *The Presbyterian Magazine* (April 1922): 218.
*Annual Report of the Hackett Medical College for Women and Affiliated Institutions, Hospital
    Number 1933*. Canton, China.
Annual Report of the Medical Missionary Society in China for the Year 1903. Canton, China.
Bailey, Paul J. *Gender and Education in China: Gender Discourses and Women's Schooling in the
    Early Twentieth Century*. New York: Routledge, 2007.
Ballantyne, Lereine. *Dr. Jessie MacBean and the Work at Hackett Medial College, Canton,
    China*. Toronto: Women's Missionary Society of the Presbyterian Church in
    Canada, 1918.
*Bulletin of the David Gregg Hospital for Women and Children, Hackett Medical College for
    Women, Turner Training School for Nurses (April 1929)*. Canton, China.
*Bulletin of The Hackett Medical College for Women, The David Gregg Hospital for Women and
    Children, The Turner Training School for Nurses, Catalogue 1915–1916*. Canton, China.
Bullock, Mary Brown. *An American Transplant: The Rockefeller Foundation and Peking Union
    Medical College*. Berkeley, CA: University of California Press, 1980.
– "A Case Study of Transnational Flows of Chinese Medical Professionals: China
    Medical Board and Rockefeller Foundation Fellows." In *Medical Transitions in
    Twentieth Century China*, edited by Bridie Andrews and Mary Brown Bullock, 285–
    96. Bloomington and Indianapolis: Indiana University Press, 2014.
*Catalogue of the Hackett Medical College for Women, Turner Training School for Nurses (June
    1930)*. Canton.
E.A.K. Hackett Medical College for Women, 1910–1911. Canton, China.
Fu, Louis. "Medical Missionaries in China: John Glasgow Kerr (1824–1901) and
    Cutting for Stone." *Journal of Medical Biography* 26, no. 3 (2018): 194–202.
Fulton, Mary H. "Hackett Medical College for Women, Canton." *The China Medical
    Journal* 23, no. 5 (1909): 324–9.
– *Inasmuch, Extracts from Letters, Journals, Papers, etc.* West Medford, MA: The Central
    Committee of the United Study of Foreign Missions, n.d.
Furth, Charlotte. "Concepts of Pregnancy, Childbirth, and Infancy in Ch'ing
    Dynasty China." *Journal of Asian Studies* 46, no. 1 (1987): 7–35.

Gamble, Sydney David, and Meng, T'ien-p'ei. *Prices, Wages, and the Standard of Living in Peking, 1900–1924*. Peking: Peking Express Press, 1926.

Hackett Medical College for Women, Turner Training School for Nurses, David Gregg Hospital for Women and Children, Bulletin 1924–1925. Canton, China.

Hackett Medical College for Women, Turner Training School for Nurses, Catalogue 1928–1929. Canton, China.

Hackett Medical College for Women and Turner Training School for Nurses, Catalogue June 1930. Canton, China.

Heinrich, Larissa N. *The Afterlife of Images: Translating the Pathological Body between China and the West*. Durham, NC, and London: Duke University Press, 2008.

Hershatter, Gail. *Women in China's Long Twentieth Century*. Berkeley, CA, Los Angeles, CA, and London: University of California Press, 2007.

Johnson, Tina Phillips. *Childbirth in Republican China: Delivering Modernity*. Lanham, MD, and Plymouth, MA: Lexington Books, 2011.

Johnson, Tina Phillips, and Wu, Yi-Li. "Maternal and Child Health in Nineteenth- to Twenty-First-Century China." In *Medical Transitions in Twentieth Century China*, edited by Bridie Andrews and Mary Brown Bullock, 51–68. Bloomington and Indianapolis: Indiana University Press, 2014.

Lee, T'ao. "Some Statistics on Medical Schools in China for 1932–1933." *Chinese Medical Journal* 47 (1933): 1029–39.

Leung, Angela Ki Che. *Leprosy in China: A History*. New York: Columbia University Press, 2009.

– "Women Practicing Medicine in Premodern China." In *Chinese Women in the Imperial Past: New Perspectives*, edited by Harriett T. Zurndorfer, 101–34. Leiden, Netherlands: Brill Academic Publishers, 1999.

Lingnan University, Bulletin No. 61, Catalogue of the College of Arts and Sciences, College of Agriculture, College of Engineering, and College of Medicine, With Announcements for the Academic Year 1937–38. Canton, China: June 1937.

Love, Hattie F. *Chinese Women in Medicine*. Soochow, China: Soochow Women's Medical School, 1917.

Medicine in China, by the China Medical Commission of the Rockefeller Foundation. New York: Rockefeller Foundation, 1914.

Morantz-Sanchez, Regina. *Sympathy and Science: Women Physicians in American Medicine*. Chapel Hill, NC: University of North Carolina Press, 2000 [1985].

Noyes, Harriett Newell. *A Light in the Land of Sinim: Forty-Five Years in the True Light Seminary, 1872–1917*. New York: Fleming H. Revell Company, 1919.

Report of the Hackett Medical College and Affiliated Institutions, Hospital Number January 1, 1933 to June 30, 1934. Canton, China.

Report of the Medical Missionary Society in China for the Year 1880. Hong Kong, 1881.

Report of the Medical Missionary Society in China for the Year 1889. Hong Kong, 1890.

Report of the Medical Missionary Society in China for the Year 1892. Hong Kong, 1893.

Report of the Medical Missionary Society in China for the Year 1896. Hong Kong, 1897.

Report of the Medical Missionary Society in China for the Year 1898. Hong Kong, 1899.

Report of the Medical Missionary Society in China for the Year 1899. Hong Kong, 1900.

The Seventy-Second Annual Report of the Board of Foreign Missions of the Presbyterian Church of the United States of America. New York: 1909.

Shapiro, Hugh. "The Puzzle of Spermatorrhea in Republican China." *Positions. East Asian Culture Critique* 6, no. 3 (1998): 551–96.

Shemo, Connie. *The Chinese Medical Ministries of Kang Cheng and Shi Meiyu, 1872–1937: On a Cross-Cultural Frontier of Gender, Race, and Nation*. Bethlehem, pa: Lehigh University Press, 2011.

– "'Her Chinese Attended to Almost Everything': Relationships of Power in the Hackett Medical College for Women, Guangzhou, China, 1901–1915." *Journal of American-East Asian Relations* 24 (2017): 321–46.

– "'Wants Learn Cut, Finish People': American Medical Missionary Education for Chinese Women and Cultural Imperialism in the Missionary Enterprise, 1890s–1920." *The Chinese Historical Review* 20, no. 1 (2013): 54–69.

Siu, Helen F., and Chan, Wing-hoi. "Introduction." In *Merchant's Daughters: Women, Commerce, and Regional Culture in South China*, edited by Helen F. Siu, 1–22. Hong Kong: Hong Kong University Press, 2010.

Swan, John M. "South China Medical College." *Chinese Medical Journal* 23, no. 5 (1909): 303–8.

Tao, S.M. "Medical Education of Chinese Women." *Chinese Medical Journal* 47 (1933): 1010–28.

Tucker, Sara W. "A Mission for Change in China: The Hackett Women's Medical Center of Canton, China, 1900–1930." In *Women's Work for Women: Missionaries and Social Change in Asia*, edited by Leslie A. Flemming, 137–57. Boulder, co: Westview Press, 1989.

Wang, Zheng. *Women in the Chinese Enlightenment: Oral and Textual Histories*. Berkeley, ca: University of California Press, 1999.

Warsh, Cheryl Krasnick. *Prescribed Norms: Women and Health in Canada and the United States since 1800*. Toronto: University of Toronto Press, 2012.

Wu, Yi-Li. *Reproducing Women: Medicine, Metaphor, and Childbirth in Late Imperial China*. Berkeley, ca: University of California Press 2010.

Xu, Guangqiu. *American Doctors in Canton: Modernization in China, 1835–1935*. New Brunswick, nj, and London: Transaction Publishers, 2011.

Yip, Ka-Che. *Health and National Reconstruction in Nationalist China: The Development of Modern Health Services, 1928–1937*. Ann Arbor, mi: Association for Asian Studies, 1995.

Nothing to Write Home About? The Tuberculosis Sanatorium as a Site of Clinical Training in Finland, 1900–60

Heini Hakosalo

In 1910, the newly graduated Suoma Loimaranta (1881–1954) was offered a junior house physician's post at Takaharju Sanatorium for Consumptives. She hesitated, being

> well aware that the work of a sanatorium physician was hardly interesting at that time. The only surgical procedure in use was [artificial] pneumothorax, and even that was very limited because it was a very risky procedure without an X-ray machine, which Takaharju did not have until 1914. There was no specific medication either; not even tuberculin was used any more. Only hygienic-dietetic and symptomatic treatments were carried out.

Loimaranta accepted the offer, only to find her suspicions confirmed. Life in the sanatorium was confined and isolated, especially during the winter, and the work "was monotonous, and somewhat hopeless even, as there was hardly anything I could do as a doctor."[1] By 1960 – that is, by the end of the period discussed in this chapter – the way that tuberculosis was diagnosed and treated had undergone drastic changes. However, as we will see, neither the sanatorium as a site of learning nor the students' "sanatorium experience" had completely lost their specific features.

Although many early-twentieth-century doctors shared Loimaranta's misgivings about sanatoria, these places nevertheless became an important site of clinical training. This chapter asks why. Three factors, I argue, conspired to give sanatoria a prominent role in clinical training. The first was the great demand for tuberculosis physicians, a demand that was driven by government public health policies. The foremost platform of clinical training, Helsinki University Hospital, was unable, and perhaps also unwilling, to meet the demand. Second, a series of internal changes gradually turned the sanatorium into a more hospital-like, and thus more attractive, place of training and work. Third, the development of tuberculosis outpatient services made "sanatorium skills" (clinical skills that a trainee could acquire or perfect in a sanatorium) increasingly useful outside sanatoria as well.

I will start by discussing the place and forms of clinical training in Finnish medical education, move on to consider a sample of "sanatorium skills," and last, address the trainees' sanatorium experience. In tackling structural changes, I mainly rely on administrative documents produced by the medical school, sanatoria, and anti-tuberculosis organizations. In discussing the experiences of clinical trainees, I make use of a variety of published and unpublished autobiographical texts and a selection of contemporary egodocuments (letters and diaries). The greatest bulk of unpublished autobiographical material is an extensive life-writing collection called *Memories of Medical Work*. There is something of a gender imbalance in the more personal part of the material: while there are no women among the authors of the published autobiographies, women and men are represented in roughly equal proportion in the unpublished autobiographical material, and women are overrepresented in the egodocuments used in this chapter.[2]

Secondary sources are both plentiful and scarce. The history of medical education and the history of sanatoria have each been intensively studied but seldom, if ever, in conjunction. In the historiography of medical education, two strands stand out as especially relevant here: studies on teaching hospitals and studies highlighting the student experience.[3] The two strands fruitfully meet in Laura Kelly's *Irish Medical Education and Student Culture, c. 1850–1950*. Kelly contends, and the same holds true for my material, that "it was clinical experience that was viewed as being the most important formative experience, by students and teachers alike."[4] The historiography of medical education in Finland was long restricted to chapters in the commissioned histories of the universities, which tend to focus on administrative and curricular changes, as well as on notable faculty members.[5] The situation has recently been improved, thanks above all to Sari Aalto's solid studies on medical education at the University of Helsinki during the middle decades of the twentieth century. Aalto not only accounts for the major structural changes but also attends to the tacit, extracurricular aspects of medical education. Pieter Dhondt has analyzed early-twentieth-century Finnish medical education within a broader European context, and I have discussed the first generations of Finnish female medical students in a series of papers.[6] This research also adds to important discussions among historians about the role of skill in medicine and medical education.[7]

International historiography of tuberculosis is voluminous. All major studies on the history of tuberculosis include some discussion of sanatoria, and some specifically focus on them.[8] One thing that they widely agree upon is that treatment was not the only, and perhaps not even the primary, function of the twentieth-century tuberculosis sanatorium. The other two prominent functions were isolation and re-education. Sanatoria contained patients with contagious forms of tuberculosis and sought to inculcate hygienic habits into them.[9] However, there are unexplored aspects as well. Thus, existing scholarship has paid very little attention to the fact that some sanatoria became important loci of research, or that many functioned as sites of clinical training. Although the latter functions were admittedly subsidiary, they did increase the number of people with a stake in sanatoria and may thereby go some way towards explaining why these institutions – in Finland at least – so clearly outlived their therapeutic usefulness.

THE PLACE OF CLINICAL TRAINING IN MEDICAL EDUCATION

With the term "clinical training," I refer to any medical work done by undergraduates and post-graduates with the purpose of gaining clinical experience in a hospital or other institution of care under the supervision of a senior member of the profession. The twentieth century witnessed a general tendency away from informal and personalized teaching arrangements towards more regulated and uniform training programs.

In Finland, as in Germany, medical education has been exclusively provided by state-owned universities. This, together with the small size of the population, accounts for the uniformity of Finnish medical education during the period that we are looking into. Between 1828, when the university was transplanted to the new capital, and 1943, when a second medical faculty was founded in Turku, all Finnish doctors were trained at the Medical Faculty of the University of Helsinki (called Imperial Alexander's University until 1917). The faculty was responsible for both theoretical and practical instruction, for examination, and *de facto* also for licensing, as all duly examined graduates were automatically, without further tests or examinations, licensed by the National Board of Health (NBH).[10] This concentration of power in the hands of the faculty sets Finland apart from Britain, where an assortment of different public, private, and professional bodies provided theoretical and practical instruction and were responsible for examining and licensing doctors; from Germany and the Netherlands, where medical graduates took a separate state examination before being licensed; and even from neighbouring Sweden, where students were encouraged to move between the three medical schools.[11]

During the first part of the twentieth century, Finnish medical education had three clearly demarcated parts: the premedical, the preclinical (or theoretical), and the clinical. Premedical studies lasted around two years, consisted of natural sciences, and culminated in the "medico-philosophical examination," the passing of which opened the doors to the Medical Faculty. In 1945, pre-medical studies were replaced by a competitive entrance examination, preceded by a six-week preparatory course. Preclinical studies included courses on anatomy, physiology, medical chemistry, and pharmacology. This phase ended with a major examination and the conferral of the degree of Candidate of Medicine. The step from preclinical to clinical studies emerges as especially important in medical autobiographies.[12] After years of theoretical study, students welcomed the "real work" awaiting them at the university clinics. The clinical-stage student, known as a "candidate" but addressed, somewhat confusingly, as "doctor," presented himself or herself at a clinic in a crisp white coat. The efforts of the newly minted candidates to compensate for their lack of practical experience by putting on professional airs were often met with more or less benevolent mockery by nurses, patients, and elder colleagues. In patient recollections, a fumbling candidate, especially one equipped with a sharp instrument, may also emerge as a fear-inspiring figure.[13]

The mandatory part of clinical studies consisted of lectures, examinations, and above all clinical clerkships. Custers and ten Cate's characterization of clerkships in early-twentieth-century Germany and the Netherlands perfectly applies to Finland, too:

> For a long time, clerkships lacked clear educational objectives and examinations, and they were based on a fixed-time principle: Students "served their time" in a system that was described as "jumping from one clinic to the other." Faculty showed little interest in what happened during clerkships, and students were often mere spectators. Hands-on experience was usually "scut-work": patient intakes or routine laboratory tests.[14]

After three or more years of clinical studies, the student was examined and received a licentiate of medicine, which was, and still is, the basic medical degree in Finland.

During the first part of the century, the average total length of medical studies was over ten years, which was a recurring cause of concern for the faculty.[15] Nevertheless, it was widely agreed that mandatory clinical studies did not sufficiently prepare the student for independent medical work. Students were expected and usually also eager to complement their studies with voluntary clinical practice. The two most common ways of obtaining extra experience were to work as an intern in a secondary care unit or to substitute for a rural medical officer.[16] Internships can be further divided into two categories: an internship at a university clinic was regarded as more official and valuable, and was entered into the personal register of professional merit that was maintained by the National Board of Health. Training periods in other major hospitals, sanatoria, or asylums could also be called internships but were considered less valuable and (unfortunately for us) not registered by the NBH. A compulsory three-month internship at one of the university clinics was integrated into the curriculum in 1945, but students continued to seek clinical experience at other clinics and hospitals, too.[17]

By definition, a licentiate is someone allowed to practise medicine without supervision.[18] However, the profession increasingly placed value on advanced post-graduate training. Such training was for a long time voluntary and unregulated, and graduates sought it from different quarters. Prior to the First World War, Finnish medical graduates had the habit of taking a grand tour of well-known European – usually German or French – clinics. Back home, the best way to gain advanced post-graduate training was to secure a two-to-three-year residency in a major hospital.[19] The majority of these residencies were "voluntary," i.e. unsalaried, especially after specialization became common and made such posts coveted. At the beginning of the century, specialization was a local matter of self-identification and tacit collegial consent. This changed in 1931, when the Finnish Medical Association published a list of full and subsidiary specialties, introduced formal requirements for specialization and established a board to confer specialist status.[20] Initially, the basic requirements were a year in general practice and two years of specialist training at a university clinic or an equivalent hospital or sanatorium. Precisely what "equivalent" meant in this context remained a contentious issue. Other long-term causes of disagreement were remuneration – a system that relied on unsalaried residencies clearly favoured the wealthy – and lack of transparency in the selection of residents.[21]

TUBERCULOSIS SANATORIA AS A TRAINING GROUND

Tuberculosis was a public health priority in Finland from the beginning of the twentieth century until the 1970s, much longer than in most European or the other Nordic countries. Public health interventions started with a vigorous but poorly co-ordinated anti-tuberculosis campaign at the beginning of the century, evolved into a full-blown public tuberculosis service during the post-war years, and ceased only in the mid-1980s, when the service was dissolved and its remaining parts integrated into the general health care system. During its heyday, the tuberculosis service constituted a health care system within the health care system, with its own legislation and its own primary health care institutions (urban and rural tuberculosis dispensaries) and secondary care institutions (sanatoria and tuberculosis hospitals). Both dispensaries and sanatoria were staffed by full-time tuberculosis physicians, and the tuberculosis services came to employ a considerable proportion of the medical work force. In 1955, for instance, 5 per cent of all physicians and 13.2 per cent of all specialists specialized in tuberculosis.[22] Practically all of them would have been working in public health care. Between 1931 and 1944, tuberculosis medicine was the most popular (or at least the most populated) specialty, surpassing even internal medicine and surgery, and it remained among the top five until the 1960s.[23]

Sanatorium practice was an experience shared by all doctors who ended up working in tuberculosis medicine and by many who did not. Sanatoria employed students at a stage when they were not yet allowed to stand in for communal or hospital physicians, and, for many, the sanatorium thus provided their first contact with medical work outside university clinics. Undergraduates attended the sanatoria in the capacity of "summer candidates" and interns. The former was a clinical-stage undergraduate who worked in the sanatorium during a term break. She or he observed and assisted, usually in exchange for accommodation and food. The graduate seeking specialized clinical experience would work as a (voluntary) resident or stand in for a junior house physician. In 1912, the national anti-tuberculosis associations started to offer three-month "sanatorium grants" for graduates who wanted to train in a sanatorium. The attitude of sanatorium chief physicians towards clinical trainees varied. They might complain about the extra work that supervising the trainees entailed,[24] but they were also aware that their often-understaffed institutions needed these inexpensive extra pairs of hands.

George Weisz has discussed the different forces that drove medical specialization in the nineteenth and twentieth centuries. These include academic and scientific developments, the needs of specialist practice, and government-supported public health programs.[25] In the case of Finnish tuberculosis medicine, it was clearly the last factor that mattered the most. It is fitting that, in opening the inaugural meeting of the Finnish Society of Tuberculosis Physicians in 1928, Richard Sievers (1852–1931), the grand old man of tuberculosis medicine, reminded the audience of the "great *social* importance" of their work.[26] In contrast, tuberculosis medicine remained academically weak. It waited for a long time to obtain a chair and a clinic, the hallmarks of a medical discipline. A course on tuberculosis was introduced into the curriculum in 1922, but the part-time lecturer responsible for teaching the course complained that the nine beds designated for tuberculous patients at the university hospital were far too few to enable effective clinical instruction. A chair was established in 1943 and the first chair-holder appointed in 1945. A teaching clinic opened at the new Helsinki City Tuberculosis Hospital in 1929, but sanatoria continued to play an important role in clinical training.[27]

Given the aura of social medicine and the almost non-existent chances of academic advancement, it will not come as a surprise that the status of tuberculosis medicine was relatively low and that women physicians, who faced both overt and covert discrimination in the job market, often opted for it. For many aspiring women doctors, the rapidly expanding field offered the line of least resistance. Women were well represented among both sanatorium and dispensary physicians, and tuberculosis/pulmonary medicine was the single most popular specialty among women doctors until the 1950s. However, female physicians-in-chief remained a rarity in public sanatoria. The only exception is the northernmost sanatorium, located about thirty kilometres south from the Polar Circle. This institution was headed by a woman in 1927–43 and again in 1953–60.[28]

SANATORIUM LESSONS

Although the broad outline of Finnish sanatorium history follows international trends, it also has some distinctive features. For instance, there were no completely private, elite sanatoria in Finland – in an agrarian country with small and not very wealthy middle and upper classes, no major sanatorium could function wholly without public support, and the clear majority were in public ownership. Another idiosyncratic feature pertains to timing. Major public investments in tuberculosis control could start only after the country had gained independence in 1917 and recovered from the short but socially and economically destructive civil war of 1918. Anti-tuberculosis work thus got off to a relatively late start, and tuberculosis would remain a major public health issue longer than in most European and the other Nordic countries.

Finnish sanatorium history can be divided into three phases. *The time of the traditional sanatorium* (1900–25) saw the establishment of three major sanatoria – Takaharju (1903), Nummela (1903), and Halila (1920). In addition, there were four medium-sized institutions with 30–50 beds in each and a host of smaller "cottage sanatoria" with fewer than 30 beds apiece. The large sanatoria played an important role in clinical training, and the medium-size sanatoria welcomed trainees, too. The second period (1925–52) can be called *the time of the folk sanatorium*. In the Finnish context, the term "folk sanatorium" is applied to public sanatoria that emerged as the result of a specific form of financial collaboration between the state and local municipalities. Patients were predominantly, but not exclusively, working-class. The first folk sanatorium was opened in 1925, but the real boom started in 1930, when the state legislated to generously subsidize their construction. This financial incentive, combined with the massive demand, led to the founding of fourteen major sanatoria between 1930 and 1952. The total number of sanatorium beds grew from roughly 600 in 1918 to approximately 4,500 by 1941.[29]

The time of the central sanatorium (1952–70) started with a major legal and administrative realignment that transferred the responsibility for both preventive and curative operations in the public sector. The whole country was now divided into tuberculosis districts, each with a central sanatorium that was owned and run by the local municipalities and co-funded and monitored by the state. No new sanatoria were opened, but many of the old folk sanatoria were enlarged and modernized. Small private sanatoria disappeared, and the role of private organizations in anti-tuberculosis work became marginal. The number of sanatorium beds peaked as late as 1960, after which it went into rapid decline. By the mid-1960s, sanatoria were admitting non-tuberculous patients, too. Ten years later, the age of the tuberculosis sanatorium was over.

Traditional sanatorium care relied almost exclusively on so-called general or hygienic-dietetic treatment, i.e. on a combination of rest and moderate, incremental exercise, fresh air, and wholesome food. This regimen was complemented by various symptomatic or experimental treatments whose curative power had not been established but were used *faute de mieux*. As Suoma Loimaranta implied when she regretted that there was little she could do *as a doctor*, general treatment required managerial rather than specifically medical skills. The trainees who benefited the most from learning the principles of general treatment were those who went on to reproduce the whole set-up elsewhere, i.e. to found or run sanatoria themselves.

The most important individual "sanatorium skill" during the age of the traditional sanatorium was mediate auscultation, or stethoscopy. The sanatorium was neither the first nor the only place where a medical student practised stethoscopy, but the environment did provide an excellent opportunity to hone the skill. The stethoscope is a simple instrument, and the basic technique is easy to learn, but the potential for refinement is almost endless. Eva Piispanen (1877–1950), who trained at Nummela Sanatorium in 1907–08, described her daily routine in a letter to a friend. After the morning ward round, she examined patients with the chief physician in the latter's office. They would sit on opposite sides of the patient with their stethoscopes, and the superior would draw Piispanen's attention to various sounds emanating from the patient's chest.[30] Göta Tingvald (1896–1982) sought specialized clinical experience in Takaharju twenty years later. She still all but equated the practical part of her work with mediate auscultation: "I do have practical work," she wrote to her friends back in Helsinki. "I already know how to recognize clicking, bubbling, rattling etc. rales. And should you come here, we'd find plenty of tuberculosis in each one of you too!"[31] The last sentence is a playful but not wholly unfounded reference to the danger of overdiagnosis, a common problem with sense-based diagnostic techniques.

Improved skill in diagnosing pulmonary tuberculosis by means of mediate auscultation was a narrow but not insignificant gain for a medical trainee. Auscultation was still *the* method of diagnosing pulmonary tuberculosis. It was all-important for a tuberculosis specialist and valuable for anyone who came into regular contact with suspected cases of pulmonary tuberculosis. The latter group included practically all rural and urban medical officers and school medical officers, as well as many private practitioners.[32] Piispanen, who had a busy general practice in her hometown of Kuopio from 1908 onwards, wrote to her friend Viva Lagerborg (1871–1941) that she was "glad to have been in Nummela, for lung examinations are legion here and tuberculosis is rampant."[33] Mediate auscultation retained its importance in tuberculosis medicine for some time to come, despite being complemented and partly surpassed by other diagnostic methods, such as tuberculin tests, bacteriological sputum analyses, and X-ray diagnostics.

The latter half of the 1920s saw the introduction of surgical and radiological methods to the sanatorium. The quotation by Loimaranta at the beginning of this chapter indirectly refers to the significance of this step by defining the traditional sanatorium in terms of what it still *lacked* in the 1910s.[34] While these novelties did not significantly improve the patients' overall chances of survival, they did influence sanatorium life and learning in other ways. They made sanatoria more hospital-like and enhanced the status of the specialty, thus making the sanatorium more attractive as a clinical training ground and as a place of work.[35] The step towards the "technologization" of the sanatorium exemplifies, on a small scale, the way in which, in the words of George Weisz, "specialization has simultaneously produced and been the product of the massive changes that have created high-technology 'biomedicine' practised in hospitals."[36]

From the 1920s to the 1950s, all surgical operations used in treating pulmonary tuberculosis were variants of collapse therapy: the idea was to speed up the healing process by putting the tuberculous lung to rest. The immobilization had the added benefit of making the patient less contagious. Here, I will discuss only the least invasive and the most common form of collapse therapy, artificial pneumothorax (AP). The first experiments with therapeutic AP had taken place in the 1880s, and the first Finnish AP had been performed in 1908, but the method became a staple part of sanatorium treatment only during the latter part of the 1920s. In AP, the diseased lung was collapsed by introducing gas into the pleural cavity by means of a hollow needle, which was connected by a flexible tube to a simple device consisting of an air-filled tank, a valve, and a manometer. As the air in the pleural cavity would gradually be absorbed by the tissue and the lung would resume its original form, the procedure needed to be repeated regularly, usually once every 1–3 weeks. The recommended treatment time was 2–5 years.[37]

From the late 1920s to the early 1950s, "the pneumo" was the most important specific therapeutic skill that a medical apprentice learned in the sanatorium. It was the only surgical procedure routinely performed by tuberculosis physicians (rather than surgeons) and very much a part of sanatorium training. The fact that AP became hugely popular, despite a lack of conclusive evidence as to its therapeutic efficiency, may indeed have something to with the needs of clinical training (cf. the prophylactic appendectomies that were undertaken to give surgical apprentices the opportunity to practise[38]). The novice started by observing the procedure and perhaps operating the machine. The next step was to do a refill under supervision. For an undergraduate, this step was important enough to be recorded in a letter or a diary.[39] A more seasoned apprentice would carry out refills without supervision. Hagar Vaher (1898–1982) contentedly reported to a friend that "[t]he follow-up pneumos of Old Halila are my sole responsibility, so I can really get to know this form of treatment."[40]

Radiological methods gained ground in sanatoria around the same time as AP. Nummela Sanatorium got an X-ray machine in 1912 and Takaharju in 1914. The early machines were only suited for fluoroscopy, i.e. real-time imaging. Because of the high cost of film, fluoroscopy remained the rule and radiography the exception, even after the machines came fitted with a camera.[41] X-ray examinations became more common as equipment grew smaller, cheaper, and more accurate, and as sanatorium physicians became more adept at reading the images. In the 1920s and 1930s, when radiological know-how was still a rare commodity in Finland, sanatorium physicians would often go to Germany to learn the craft. Radiology was listed as a subsidiary specialization in 1931, but it took time for such professional subgroups as radiologists, radiographic nurses, or technicians to form. During the period we are looking into, many of the most experienced radiologists would have been found among tuberculosis physicians.

Mastery of AP and radiological methods was increasingly useful also outside the sanatorium. A physician needed these skills in general and, above all, in dispensary practice. Due to the broad political consensus concerning the need to tackle the tuberculosis issue, tuberculosis outpatient services, centred on dispensaries, spread quickly after the mid-1920s.[42] As already mentioned, AP required regular refills and an overall treatment time that was much longer than the average sanatorium stay. Therefore, this form of treatment could not have become as popular as it did without the existence of a support network of dispensaries and outpatient clinics that owned an AP machine and employed a physician who knew how to use it. The spread of X-ray diagnosis and AP went hand in hand, as fluoroscopic guidance made AP safer. An investment in one of these techniques could thus be used to justify an investment in the other. Above all, radiological diagnostics significantly facilitated case-finding, which was the core task of the dispensary physician. By making diagnostics more reliable, X-ray machines also improved the public image of dispensaries. All tuberculosis dispensaries, both urban and rural, were equipped with X-ray equipment by the mid-1930s.[43]

The beginning of the third phase, that of the central sanatorium, coincides with the greatest turning point in the history of tuberculosis, the introduction of effective chemotherapeutic medication between 1948 and 1952. The medication changed the character of "the tuberculosis issue," patients' prospects, and also the outlook of the sanatorium. It did not do these things overnight, however, and the whole of the 1950s can be regarded as a transition period. According to Håkan Hellberg (b. 1937), who was a clinical apprentice in Meltola Sanatorium in the mid-1950s, sanatorium medicine was "still a mixture of old and new" and "the atmosphere in the tuberculosis sanatorium often vacillated between hope and despair." Hellberg describes the changes:

> With effective use of new tuberculosis medication, advanced thorax surgery, and other forms of modern medical care, the treatment time in hospitals and controlled open care was reduced, [and] not only the treatment of tuberculosis as such, but also the inner world of the sanatorium changed. Fewer younger patients, no open-air rest hours in the halls, and a different social and psychological climate among patients contributed to this fundamental change; and summer trainees would learn more of modern medicine during their visits to Meltola.[44]

The central task of the sanatorium trainee was now to learn to administer the new industrially produced drugs. This could be challenging. Efforts at medication were complicated by the novelty of the very concept, the cost of the drugs, the side effects, and the problem of resistance, which was tackled by means of drug combinations. During this period of profound and rapid changes, a trainee could not always count on finding effective clinical guidance. Senior members of the profession had been educated during the pre-antibiotic age, and while some of them were able to keep themselves well-informed (often with the help of their international networks) during the therapeutic revolution, others were not.[45] For instance, a senior physician might prescribe new chemotherapeutic drugs in ineffective doses. Hellberg provides an example: "when summer trainees, with new experiences from the university clinics raised the penicillin dose from 3 x 15 000 units to 3 x 75 000 units [sic!], it was returned to the lower level during the chief physician's next ward round."[46] As late as 1957, a sanatorium physician recalls, "We had not yet learnt the right way to administer tuberculosis medicines."[47]

The introduction of effective tuberculosis chemotherapy did not immediately make tuberculosis sanatoria redundant, as tuberculosis experts agreed that the treatment, which was expensive, long-term, and difficult to administer, could be successfully carried out only in the controlled sanatorium environment. This way of thinking changed in the early 1970s,[48] when ambulatory medication became the norm and the sanatorium lost its raison d'être.

THE SANATORIUM EXPERIENCE

A trainee entering a sanatorium in the mid-1950s had more to do, and more to learn, than her early-twentieth-century predecessor. Whereas Suoma Loimaranta felt that she learnt little that was specifically medical in Takaharju in the 1910s, Håkan Hellberg observed that there was "more of modern medicine" on offer in Meltola in the 1950s than there had been before. But the sanatorium never lost all its idiosyncratic features, and the way that trainees described their personal sanatorium experiences in letters and reminiscences displays remarkable continuity from one decade to another. This shared "sanatorium experience" is rooted in the special nature of the institution and in the fact that the trainee did not just visit the sanatorium, but also lived there, usually for several months at a time.

Newcomers often felt they had entered a world of its own, an environment clearly different from other institutions of care, and especially from the busy university clinics. They marvelled at the isolated and self-sufficient nature of the institution, and especially at the slow pace of sanatorium life, which left them with an unexpected amount of free time.[49] Marja-Liisa Paljakka, a 1950s summer candidate, wrote that "the most peculiar thing was the conception of time in the sanatorium. After the hectic term, I had expected more action."[50]

The social world of the sanatorium was both hierarchical and communal. The chief physician was at the top and the undergraduate trainee at the bottom of the medical hierarchy. Patients and students referred to the former in their letters and reminiscences as "the Emperor," "the Pharaoh," or "the demi-god," while the latter was known as "the slave."[51] At the same time, there was a strong sense of community, of being in the same boat, a feeling that was enhanced by the physical isolation and the long treatment times. With relatively little to do and nowhere to go, cohabitants became important to one another in a way they did not at most other sites of clinical training. Especially young doctors willingly spent much of their free time with the patients, and some of them felt that interesting patients – not cases, but personalities – were among the things that made sanatorium life palatable. Paljakka grew especially attached to the small patients of the pediatric ward.[52]

From one decade to another, sanatorium trainees also appreciated the fringe benefits: free food and lodgings, and the opportunity to recover from the hardships of the academic year in beautiful and salubrious surroundings.[53] Medical people shared the widespread and deep-seated conviction that it was unhealthy, even downright dangerous, to spend the summer in town. Sanatoria were not only far removed from urban centres but had also been built in places that were considered especially health-promoting. The age-old belief in the healing power of the natural environment may have been on the wane but it was not extinct. One subgroup in particular was anxious to benefit from the environment: undergraduates and graduates with tuberculosis or suspected tuberculosis. Prior to the chemotherapeutic age, their number was considerable, and they often gravitated towards sanatoria. Training or working in a sanatorium, they did not need to worry about infecting their patients, they could benefit from the healthy environment, and they could earn a living and/or gain clinical experience without overexerting themselves. Sometimes a doctor turned into a patient and never left the sanatorium alive.[54]

Learning in sanatoria was very much through apprenticeship. Trainees picked up what they could by following senior members of the staff on their rounds, by listening to their discussions during meals and coffee breaks, and by observing and taking part in medical examinations and procedures.[55] Feedback, if there was any, was personal and immediate. What trainees learned, and how they experienced the learning process, depended greatly on the personal predilections and competencies of the senior staff. Trainees' letters are more likely to contain complaints than compliments. Hagar Vaher, who sought specialist experience in Halila in 1929, noted with dismay that "the senior physicians have absolutely no inclination to talk about pulmonary tuberculosis and its treatment. If one ever has the audacity to disturb them with a question, then the answer is so curt that one loses any desire to discuss the matter further. I will not benefit from my stay here as much as I could."[56] Göta Tingvald had a similar experience in Takaharju: "I get constantly humiliated by patronizing smiles when I try to start a [professional] discussion."[57]

These citations remind us that the sanatorium trainee experience (like the student experience in general) was gendered. The fact that Vaher and Tingvald were women may go some way in explaining their perfunctory treatment. Both men and women autobiographers agree that teachers and supervisors treated women differently, although most men and some women regarded the differential treatment as a benign cultural reflection of the natural course of things rather than as something that might actually disadvantage women.[58] Gender could also override professional hierarchies: female sanatorium trainees and physicians spent much of their free time with the female nurses rather than their male colleagues, and they often lodged in the nurses' quarters. Male trainees were also allowed diversions – notably bouts of heavy drinking – that would not have been tolerated in women.[59]

Another theme present in autobiographical texts and egodocuments from one decade to another is the nagging suspicion that sanatorium medicine is not exactly "real medicine" and that the sanatorium is too much a place of its own to be able to impart lessons useful in the outside world. A candidate returning from Takaharju in 1905 commented, "Life there is more like being at a folk high school [*kansanopisto*] than a hospital."[60] Paljakka summed up the narrative of her summer in Kinkomaa Sanatorium in the 1950s with the following words: "Eventually the summer was over. It felt as if the other people from my year had been doing work that is 'more real'. The summer was nevertheless a unique experience for me."[61]

CONCLUSIONS

The twentieth-century sanatorium was both central and marginal as a site of medical instruction. It was central in numerical terms, given that a considerable proportion of the medical workforce turned to sanatoria for specialist training. It was marginal geographically, being located far from the urban centres and the university, and initially also in the sense of being regarded as a medical backwater, distant from the most dynamic streams of academic medicine. Sanatoria became gradually better integrated with the rest of the health services. Sanatorium skills became more numerous, variegated, and "exportable." During the time of the traditional sanatorium, sanatorium medicine and clinical training was highly context-dependent, the treatment being provided as much *by* as *in* the sanatorium. The environment itself was seen as the primary healing agent, and there was thus little that was specifically medical that could be applied elsewhere. During the second period, internal changes (the introduction of novelties such as artificial pneumothorax and radiological diagnostics) and external changes (the needs of the expanding primary care network) made sanatorium training less context-dependent and more broadly useful. The third period saw the introduction of chemotherapeutic medication and an assortment of new diagnostic tools and procedures. Clinical training offered in sanatoria was no longer exclusively focused on the treatment and diagnosis of tuberculosis – a development that would make the impending transformation of the tuberculosis specialist into a specialist in respiratory disease less painful.

Egodocuments, in particular, suggest that medical students' "sanatorium experience" remained remarkably similar through the decades. This reminds us that the students' experience is not exhaustively or perhaps even primarily determined by the specific information and skills acquired, but is also predicated on the physical and social characteristics of the learning environment. In the case of sanatorium medicine, this experience was influenced by the location, natural environment, architectural features, and temporal and social order – all features that diverged from the primary learning environment, the university clinic. Thinking about sanatoria encourages us to de-centre twentieth-century medical education away from its long-standing focus on universities and medical schools and to consider other sites of training too.

ACKNOWLEDGMENT

This research was funded by the Academy of Finland, grant no. 259547.

NOTES

1   Suoma Loimaranta-Airila, "Pari muistelmaa Takaharjun parantolasta 1911–14," 1, unpublished manuscript, Helsinki University Museum (henceforth HUM), Helsinki.

2   Women have written only 23 of the 146 published book-length autobiographical works on my list. 11 of the 23 focus on the authors' work abroad and do not shed much light on Finnish medical education. Large thematic life-writing collections are something of a Finnish speciality (see Vento, "Folklore Activities"). I have made use of two health-related collections. First is *The Collection Competition for Sanatorium Tradition* (henceforth ST). The collection was organized in 1971 and brought in almost 10,000 pages of tuberculosis-related recollections. Second is *Memories of Medical Work* (henceforth MW), which comprises 1,500 pages and 75 contributions, was collected in 2004, and was written almost exclusively by doctors. These materials are held by the Folklore Archive of the Finnish Literature Society (henceforth FLS), except for the Swedish-language entries of MW, which are at the Folk Culture Archive of the Society for Swedish Literature in Finland (henceforth SSL), Helsinki.

3   Books focusing on teaching hospitals include Lawrence, *Charitable Knowledge*; Reinarz, *Health Care*; Waddington, *Medical Education*; Rosner, *Medical Education*. Studies encompassing student experiences include Crowther and Dupree, "The Invisible Practitioner"; Waddington, "Mayhem and Medical Students"; Kelly, "Irish Medical Student Culture." Jonathan Reinarz's 2005 paper on medical museums ("The Age of Museum Medicine") is particularly pertinent here, as it investigates a site of medical instruction that was once important

but has since disappeared from medical education and also largely from historical sight.

4   Kelly, *Irish Medical Education*, 136. On the importance of the hospital for teaching and the formation of professional identity, see also 106, 117, 127, 128. Kelly remarks that the student has been largely absent from the history of Irish institutions (105) and Hanley extends this criticism to the history of medical education in general ("Review," 888).

5   The authoritative history of the University of Helsinki has been written by a team of historians led by Matti Klinge, *Helsingin yliopisto*. For the University of Tampere, see Kaarninen, Harjula, and Sipponen, *Murros ja mielikuva*; for the University of Kuopio (now part of the University of Eastern Finland), Vuorio, *Lentoon*; and for the University of Oulu, Salo, *Pohjoinen*.

6   Aalto, "Ilman kollegiaalisuutta" and *Medisiinarit*; Dhondt, "Transnational Currents"; Hakosalo, "Coming Together," "Elin och Ille," "Modest Witness," "'Our Life Work,'" and "The Ryti Case."

7   For example, papers published in the special issue of *Medical History* 59, no. 3 (2015).

8   A comprehensive list of publications on the history of tuberculosis would be very long indeed. The following books discuss sanatoria as part of tuberculosis history: Bryder, *Below the Magic Mountain*; Smith, *The Retreat of Tuberculosis*; Ott, *Fevered Lives*; Bates, *Bargaining for Life*; Feldberg, *Disease and Class*; Rothman, *Living in the Shadow of Death*; McCuaig, *The Weariness*; Dormandy, *The White Death*; Jones, "Captain of All These Men of Death"; Lerner, *Contagion and Confinement*; Bynum, *Spitting Blood*. Stacie Burke's *Building Resistance* focuses on a sanatorium. *Tuberculosis Then and Now*, edited by Flurin Condrau and Michael Worboys, contains a useful review of tuberculosis historiography ("Tuberculosis and Its Histories") by Lynda Bryder and the two editors, and a chapter on the historiography of sanatoria by Condrau ("Beyond the Total Institution"). For a comparison between Germany and Britain, see Condrau, *Lungenheilanstalt und Patientschicksal*; and for Scandinavia Puranen, *Tuberkulos*; Blom, *Feberens ville rose* and "Contagion and Cultural Perceptions"; Ryymin, *Smitte, språk og kultur*. Studies focusing on Finnish tuberculosis history include Härö, *Vuosisata* (the history of the Finnish Anti-Tuberculosis Association); Nenola, *Parantolaelämää*; Jauho, *Kansanterveysongelman synty*; Järvelä, "A Genealogy of the Tuberculosis Sanatorium"; and my papers "A Twin Grip" and "Tubipommi." Tuberculosis is discussed as part of the broader history of Finnish public health in Tiitta, *Collegium medicum*; Harjula, *Hoitoonpääsyn* and "Citizenship and Access."

9   On the questionable therapeutic efficiency and the different functions of the sanatorium, see Bryder, *Below the Magic Mountain*, 67–9; Condrau, "Beyond the Total Institution," 76; Worboys, "The Sanatorium Treatment," 47;

Ott, *Fevered Lives*, 150–1; Rothman, *Living in the Shadow*, 194; Jauho, *Kansanterveysongelman*, 242–3. Contemporary tuberculosis experts were quite open about the poor therapeutic efficiency of the sanatorium and evoked its importance in curtailing infection by means of confinement and education. Savonen, "Minkätähden," 212–13; Buhre, *Till styrelsen*, 13; Neander, *Folksjukdomen*, 103.

10   Aalto, "Ilman kollegiaalisuutta," 78–9; Kauttu et al., *Kunnanlääkärin työ*, 108–9.

11   Custers and ten Cate, "The History"; Sjöstrand, "Läkarnas," 339.

12   Cf. Kelly, *Irish Medical Education*, 127.

13   "Nikkanen" 59, Poijärvi 20, Aitamäki 120 in ST; Kallio, *Osallistumiseni*, 39; Olin, *Muistelmia*, 38. Göta Tingvald to Margit Hildén, 29 June 1924 (Pär Österberg's Archive, Case 57, SSL).

14   Custers and ten Cate, "The History," S51.

15   Strömberg, "Ylioppilaat," 316; Dhondt, "Transnational Currents," 710.

16   On rural medical officers, see Hakosalo, "Lääkäri."

17   Dhondt, "Transnational Currents," 704; Kauttu and Kosonen, *Suomen Lääkäriliitto*, 207; Aalto, *Medisiinarit*, 52; Aalto, "Ilman kollegiaalisuutta," 89–90; The Proceedings of the Medical Faculty, 11 March 1913 § 1 (University of Helsinki Archives, henceforth UHA, Ca53).

18   Cf. Custers and ten Cate, "The History," S49.

19   Residents were called "assistant physicians" (*apulaislääkäri*) in Finland, but I will use the more familiar "resident" here.

20   On the development of specialist training and regulation in Finland, see Kauttu and Kosonen, *Suomen Lääkäriliitto*, 93–4; Ilmolahti, "Lääkärit," 338.

21   Ilmolahti, "Lääkärit," 337; Susitaival, *Suomen Lääkäriliitto*, 84–5; Kauttu, Reinilä, and Voutilainen, *Kunnanlääkärin*, 109; Kauttu and Kosonen, *Suomen Lääkäriliitto*, 258; Aalto, "Ilman kollegiaalisuutta," 89–90; Hartiala, *Polkuni*, 58–60; Kallio, *Osallistumiseni*, 73; Reenkola, *Mammanpojasta*, 182.

22   Säynäjäkangas and Kuoppala, "Suomen keuhkolääkäriyhdistyksen," 194.

23   Kauttu and Kosonen, *Suomen Lääkäriliitto*, 174, 216; Ilmolahti, *Lääkärit*, 338–9; Haavio-Mannila, *Lääkärit*, 7.

24   Robert Elmgren (the chief physician of Halila Sanatorium) to Hilda Elmgren, 1 November 1925, 20 May 1928, 20 December 1931; Robert Elmgen to Elin Elmgren, 21 May 1938 (Elmgren Family Archive, Cases 6 and 9, Finnish National Archives (henceforth FNA); Göta Tingvald Hannikainen (the chief physician of Muurola Sanatorium) to Margit Hildén-Österberg, 23 March 1959 (Per Österberg's Archive, Case 57, SSL).

25   Weisz, *Divide and Conquer*, xix, 44–5, 50, 106.

26   Cit. Säynäjäkangas and Kuoppala, "Suomen keuhkolääkäriyhdistyksen," 188. Italics mine.

27   Proceedings of the Medical Faculty, 4 May 1926 § 1 (UHA Ca56);
      "Proceedings of the Board of the Finnish Anti-Tuberculosis Association,"
      11 April 1945 § 12 (The Archive of the Finnish Lung Health Association,
      Helsinki).

28   On the low status of the specialty, see e.g. Venho, "Keuhkolääkärin," 182,
      183; Säynäjäkangas and Kuoppala, "Suomen keuhkolääkäriyhdistyksen,"
      194. On women in the specialty, Haavio-Mannila, *Lääkärit*, 7; Anni
      Seppänen, "Naislääkärin mahdollisuuksista sodanjälkeisessä jälleenrakennus-
      työssä," an unpublished speech given in September 1946 (Anni Dagmar
      Seppänen's Archive, Case 4, FNA). Cf. Elston 1986, *Women Doctors*, 236, 340.
      On the two female physicians-in-chief, Hakosalo, "En vacker kvinnogärning."

29   Tiitta, *Collegium*, 161–2.

30   Eva Piispanen to Viva Lagerborg, sometime between November 1907 and
      February 1908 (Rolf Lagerborg's Archive, Case B91, Manuscript Collection
      of the Library of Åbo Akademi University, Turku).

31   Göta Tingvald to Margit Hildén, 1 August 1923 (Pär Österberg's Archive,
      Case 57, SSL).

32   Göta Tingvald to Margit Hildén, 9 January 1922 (Pär Österberg's Archive,
      Case 57, SSL.

33   Eva Piispanen to Viva Lagerborg, 6 June 1908 (Rolf Lagerborg's Archive,
      Case B91, Manuscript Collection of the Library of Åbo Akademi University,
      Turku).

34   Aitamäki 957, 959; Jääskeläinen 15; Kumpulainen 2; Heino 39;
      Tuberkuloosi- ja keuhkovammaliiton aineisto 155 in ST.

35   The consequences of the arrival of surgical methods in sanatoria are
      discussed in e.g. Bryder, *Below the Magic Mountain*, 173–84; Condrau, "Beyond
      the Total Institution," 87, 77, 92; Ott, *Fevered Lives*, 148–9; Bynum, *Spitting
      Blood*, 146, 156–7.

36   Weisz, *Divide and Conquer*, xi.

37   On the discovery of AP and its introduction to Finland see Elmgren,
      "Keuhkotaudin hoitamisesta"; von Bonsdorff, *Nummela sanatorium*, 13–14;
      Seppänen, *Kertomus*, 17. On AP in the international context, see for instance
      Bryder, *Below the Magic Mountain*, 173–6; Bynum, *Spitting Blood*, 153–5.

38   Kyllikki Ohela in MW 617.

39   Göta Tingvald to Margit Hildén, 3 July 1923 (Pär Österberg's Archive,
      Case 57, SLL.); Maija-Liisa Paljakka in MW 713; Lahesmaa, *Pikkupojasta*, 135.

40   Hagar Vaher to Alli Wiherheimo, 27 September 1929 (Alli Wiherheimo's
      Archive, Case 1126, FLS).

41   Härö, *Vuosisata*, 92–3; Piikamäki 3–4 in ST; Lahesmaa, *Pikkupojasta*, 135.

42   Finnish tuberculosis dispensaries were standalone institutions, independent of sanatoria, and staffed by a tuberculosis physician and one or more nurses.

43   "Proceedings of the Board of the Finnish Anti-Tuberculosis Association," 2 December 1935 § 14 (Archives of the Finnish Lung Health Association, Helsinki). On the positive effect of X-ray equipment on the public image of dispensaries, see Qvarnström, "Perhetarkastukset." On the usefulness of radiological skills in rural practice, see Carl-Gustaf Gröndahl in MW 38, 71.

44   Hellberg in MW (Swedish), 36.

45   Positive examples are cited by Achté, *Lääkärikoulussa*, 69; and Lahesmaa, *Pikkupojasta*, 193.

46   Hellberg in MW (Swedish) 35.

47   Lahesmaa, *Pikkupojasta*, 172.

48   Kuoppala, *Kylmäkääreistä*, 50.

49   Suoma Loimaranta-Airila, "Pari muistelmaa Takaharjun parantolasta 1911–14," 4 (unpublished manuscript, HUM); Selma Lilius to Lilli Lilius, 18 April 1905 (Selma Rainio's Archive, Case 2, Archive of the Finnish Missionary Society, FNA); Hellberg in MW (Swedish) 224–8.

50   Paljakka in MW, 1713.

51   Göta Tingvald Hannikainen to Margit Hildén-Österberg, 28 June 1961 (Pär Österberg's Archive, Case 57, SSL); Aitamäki 76, 169; Mäki-Petäjä 20 in ST.

52   Patients often wrote that the sanatorium community (in which they explicitly included the staff) was like "one big family." See e.g. Jänesniemi 15; Torvela 1; Korhonen 11 in ST. Göta Tingvald to Margit Hildén, 5 August 1929 (Pär Österberg's Archive, Case 57, SSL); Suoma Loimaranta-Airila, "Pari muistelmaa Takaharjun parantolasta 1911–14," 1 (unpublished manuscript, HUM); Robert Elmgren to Inez Elmgren, 10 April 1907 (Elmgren Family Archive, FNA); Paljakka 712, 715, 717 in MW.

53   Suoma Loimaranta-Airila, "Pari muistelmaa Takaharjun parantolasta 1911–14," 1 (unpublished manuscript, HUM); Göta Tingvald to Margit Hildén, undated, 1922, and 3 July 1923 (Pär Österberg's Archive, Case 57, SSL).

54   Robert Elmgren often discusses his numerous tuberculous junior physicians in his letters; see e.g. Robert Elmgren to Hilda Elmgren, 18 September 1922, 16 August 1925 (Elmgren Family Archive, Case 6, FNA).

55   On the lack of systematic clinical teaching, see e.g. Kallio, *Osallistumiseni*, 154.

56   Hagar Vaher to Alli Wiherheimo, 27 September 1929 (Alli Wiherheimo's Archive, Case 1126, FLS).

57   Göta Tingvald to Margit Hildén, 1 August 1923 (Pär Österberg's Archive, Case 57, SSL).

324   Heini Hakosalo

58   E.g. Göta Tingvald to Margit Hildén, 10 October 1925 (Pär Österberg's
     Archive, Case 57, SSL); Nenola, *Parantolaelämää*, 125; Kerppola, *Ammattini*, 17;
     Achté, *Lääkärikoulussa*, 21.
59   Paljakka in MW, 712, 714; Hagar Vaher to Alli Wiherheimo, 27 September
     1929 (Alli Wiherheimo's Archive, Case 1126, FLS); Dominique, "Kvinnans,"
     174.
60   Selma Lilius to Lilli Lilius, 18 April 1905 (Selma Rainio's Archive, Case 2,
     Archive of the Finnish Missionary Society, FNA).
61   Paljakka in MW, 718.

BIBLIOGRAPHY

Aalto, Sari. "'Ilman kollegiaalisuutta ei ole lääkäreitä.' Lääkäriyhteisö ja ammatti-
    kunnan kulttuuriin kasvaminen." In *Vapaus, terveys, toveruus. Lääkärit Suomessa 1910–*
    2010, edited by Samu Nyström, 52–157. Helsinki: Suomen Lääkäriliitto, 2010.
– *Medisiinarit, ammattiin kasvaminen ja hiljainen tieto. Suomalaisen lääkärikoulutuksen murroksen*
    vuodet 1933–1969. PhD thesis. Helsinki: Helsingin yliopisto, 2016.
Achté, Kalle. *Lääkärikoulussa Paasikiven aikaan*. Helsinki: Recallmed, 1993.
Bates, Barbara. *Bargaining for Life: A Social History of Tuberculosis 1876–1938*.
    Philadelphia, PA: University of Pennsylvania Press, 1992.
Blom, Ida. "Contagion and Cultural Perceptions of Accepted Behaviour:
    Tuberculosis and Venereal Diseases in Scandinavia c. 1900 – c. 1950." *Hygiea*
    Internationalis 6, no. 2 (2007): 121–33.
– *Feberens ville rose. Tre omsorgssystemer i tuberkulosarbeidet 1900–1960*. Bergen, Norway:
    Fackförlaget, 1998.
Bonsdorff, Axel von. *Nummela sanatorium. Årsberättelse om sjukvården för år 1909*. Helsinki,
    1910.
Bryder, Linda. *Below the Magic Mountain: A Social History of Tuberculosis in Twentieth-*
    Century Britain. Oxford, UK: Clarendon Press, 1988.
Bryder, Linda, Flurin Condrau, and Michael Worboys. "Tuberculosis and Its
    Histories: Then and Now." In *Tuberculosis Then and Now: Perspectives on the History of*
    an Infectious Disease, edited by Flurin Condrau and Michael Worboys, 3–23.
    Montreal, QC, and Kingston, ON: McGill-Queen's University Press, 2010.
Buhre, Bertil. *Till styrelsen för Svenska Nationalföreningen mot tuberkulos. Vördsamt memorial*
    angående general plan för Nationalföreningens verksamhet under den närmaste tiden.
    Stockholm: Svenska nationalföreningen mot tuberkulos, 1904.
Burke, Stacie. *Building Resistance: Children, Tuberculosis and the Toronto Sanatorium*.
    Montreal, QC, and Kingston, ON: McGill-Queen's University Press, 2018.
Bynum, Helen. *Spitting Blood: The History of Tuberculosis*. Oxford, UK: Oxford
    University Press, 2012.

Condrau, Flurin. "Beyond the Total Institution: Towards a Reinterpretation of the Tuberculosis Sanatorium." In *Tuberculosis Then and Now: Perspectives on the History of an Infectious Disease*, edited by Flurin Condrau & Michael Worboys, 70–99. Montreal, QC, and Kingston, ON: McGill-Queen's University Press, 2010.

– *Lungenheilanstalt und Patientschicksal: Sozialgeschichte der Tuberkulose in Deutschland und England im späten 19. und frühen 20 Jahrhunderten*. Göttingen, Germany: Vandehoeck & Ruprecht, 2000.

Condrau, Flurin, and Michael Worboys, eds. *Tuberculosis Then and Now: Perspectives on the History of an Infectious Disease*. Montreal, QC, and Kingston, ON: McGill-Queen's University Press, 2010.

Crowther, Anne, and Marguerite Dupree. "The Invisible Practitioner: The Careers of Scottish Medical Students in the Late-Nineteenth Century." *Bulletin of the History of Medicine* 70 (1996): 387–413.

Custers, Eugène, and Olle ten Cate. "The History of Medical Education in Europe and the United States, with Respect to Time and Proficiency." *Academic Medicine* 93 (2018): S49–S54.

Dhondt, Pieter. "Transnational Currents in Finnish Medical Education (c. 1800–1920), Starting from a 1922 Discourse." *Paedagogica Historica* 48, no. 5 (2012): 692–710.

Dominique, Elisabeth. "Kvinnans plats i utbildningen och forskningen." In *Kvinnor i vitt. Om kreativitet på universitetssjukhus*, edited by Birgitta Evengård, 167–79. Stockholm: Bonniers, 1998.

Dormandy, Thomas. *The White Death: A History of Tuberculosis*. London: Hambledon Press, 1999.

Elmgren, Robert. "Keuhkotaudin hoitamisesta keinotekoisen pneumotoraksin avulla." *Duodecim* 25, no. 1 (1909): 1–14.

Elston, Mary Ann. *Women Doctors in the British Health Services: A Sociological Study of Their Careers and Opportunities*. PhD thesis. Leeds, UK: University of Leeds, Department of Sociology, 1986. http://etheses.whiterose.ac.uk/247/.

Feldberg, Georgina D. *Disease and Class: Tuberculosis and the Shaping of Modern North American Society*. New Brunswick, NJ: Rutgers University Press, 1995.

Haavio-Mannila, Elina. *Lääkärit tutkittavina. Sosiologinen tutkimus Suomen lääkärien ammattiin liittyvistä tavoitteista ja niiden saavuttamisesta*. Helsinki: Helsingin yliopisto, 1964.

Hakosalo, Heini. "Coming Together: Early Finnish Medical Women and the Many Levels of Historical Biography." In *Biography, Gender, and History: Nordic Perspectives*, edited by Erla Hulda Haldorsdottir, Tiina Kinnunen, Maarit Leskelä-Kärki, and Birgitte Possing, 209–30. Turku, Finland: k&h, 2016.

– "Elin och Ille. Syskon, kön och medicinsk karriär i det tidiga 1900-talets Finland." *Historisk Tidskrift för Finland* 100, no. 2 (2015): 125–60.

– "'En vacker kvinnogärning': Rita Gripenberg ja Muurolan parantola." In *Lisää tällaista! Marianne Junilan juhlakirja*, edited by Heini Hakosalo, Seija Jalagin, and Tiina Kinnunen, 145–60. Oulu, Finland: Oulun historiaseura, 2015.

– "Lääkäri, yhteisö ja yhteiskunta. Katsaus lääkäriprofession historiaan Suomessa." *Lääketieteellinen Aikakauskirja Duodecim* 126 (2010): 31–8.

– "Modest Witness to Modernization: Finland Meets Ovamboland in Mission Doctor Selma Rainio's Family Letters, 1921–32." *Scandinavian Journal of History* 40, no. 3 (2015): 298–331.

– "'Our life work': Professional Women and Christian Values in Early 20th-Century Finland." In *Between Ancestors and Angels: Finnish Women Making Religion*, edited by Terhi Utriainen and Päivi Salmesvuori, 83–102. New York: Palgrave Macmillan, 2014.

– "The Ryti Case: Language, Gender and the Rules of the Game in Finnish Academic Medicine in the 1920s." *Scandinavian Journal of History* 37, no. 4 (2012): 430–60.

– "Tubipommi ja rautlasi. Emotionaalisia esineitä 1900-luvun alkupuolen suomalaisissa tuberkuloosiparantoloissa." *Historiallinen Aikakauskirja* 114, no. 2 (2016): 165–76.

– "A Twin Grip on the National Disease: Finnish Anti-Tuberculosis Associations and Their Contribution to Nation-Formation (1907–17)." *Journal of Finnish Studies* 21, no. 1–2 (2018, special issue: *The Making of Finland: The Era of the Grand Duchy*): 208–36.

Hanley, Anne. "Review of Laura Kelly, *Irish Medical Education and Student Culture, c. 1850–1950* (Liverpool University Press, 2017)." *Social History of Medicine* 31, no. 4 (2018): 888–90.

Harjula, Minna. "Citizenship and Access to Health Services: Finland 1900–2000." *Social History of Medicine* 29, no. 3 (2016): 573–89.

– *Hoitoonpääsyn hierarkiat. Terveyskansalaisuus ja terveyspalvelut Suomessa 1900-luvulla.* Tampere, Finland: Tampere University Press, 2015.

Härö, Sakari. *Vuosisata tuberkuloosityötä Suomessa. Suomen tuberkuloosin vastustamisyhdistyksen historia.* Helsinki: Suomen tuberkuloosin vastustamisyhdistys, 1992.

Hartiala, Kaarlo. *Polkuni tieteen turuilla. Lääkärin ja tiedemiehen näkökulmasta.* Porvoo, Finland: Werner Söderström Osakeyhtiö, 1979.

Ilmolahti, Oona. "Lääkärit ja lääketaidon kokemus." In *Vapaus, terveys, toveruus. Lääkärit Suomessa 1910–2010*, edited by Samu Nyström, 330–425. Helsinki: Suomen Lääkäriliitto, 2010.

Järvelä, Simo. "A Genealogy of the Tuberculosis Sanitarium: The Methods of Knowledge Production and Care-Giving in a Finnish Sanitarium for Pulmonary Tuberculosis in 1932–1960." *Sosiologia* 42, no. 4 (2005): 275–87, 349.

Jauho, Mikko. *Kansanterveysongelman synty. Tuberkuloosi ja terveyden hallinta Suomessa ennen toista maailmansotaa.* Helsinki: Tutkijaliitto, 2007.

Jones, Greta. *"Captain of All These Men of Death": The History of Tuberculosis in Nineteenth and Twentieth Century Ireland.* Amsterdam: Rodopi, 2001.

Kaarninen, Mervi, Minna Harjula, and Kauko Sipponen. *Murros ja mielikuva. Tampereen yliopisto 1960–2000.* Tampere, Finland: Tampereen yliopisto & Vastapaino, 2000.

Kallio, K.E. *Osallistumiseni elämään. Kirurgin muistelmat.* Helsinki: Otava, 1973.

Kauttu, Kyllikki, and Tapani Kosonen. *Suomen Lääkäriliitto 1910–1985.* Helsinki: Suomen Lääkäriliitto, 1985.

Kauttu, Kyllikki, Anna-Maria Reinilä, and Antero Voutilainen. *Kunnanlääkärin työ ja elämä.* Helsinki: Suomen Lääkäriliitto, 1983.

Kelly, Laura. *Irish Medical Education and Student Culture, 1850–1950.* Liverpool, uk: Liverpool University Press, 2017.

– "Irish Medical Student Culture and the Performance of Masculinity, c. 1880–1930." *History of Education* 46, no. 1 (2017): 39–57.

Kerppola, Irma. *Ammattini on lääkäri.* Helsinki: Arvi A. Karisto, 1971.

Klinge, Matti. "Yliopisto ja virkamieskorkeakoulu." In *Keisarillinen Aleksanterin yliopisto 1808–1917*, edited by Matti Klinge et al., 333–417. Helsinki: Otava, 1989.

Klinge, Matti, et al. *Helsingin yliopisto 1640–1990 I–III.* Helsinki: Helsingin yliopisto, 1987–1990.

Kuoppala, Janne. *Kylmäkääreistä keuhkolääketieteeksi. Suomen keuhkolääkäriyhdistys ja keuhkolääketieteen kehitys 1900-luvulla.* MA thesis. Oulu, Finland: University of Oulu, History of Sciences and Ideas, 2016. http://jultika.oulu.fi/files/nbn-fioulu-201605051648.pdf.

Lahesmaa, Risto. *Pikkupojasta keuhkolääkäriksi.* [Turku, Finland: Author,] 2004.

Lawrence, C.S. *Charitable Knowledge: Hospital Pupils and Practitioners in Eighteenth-Century London.* Cambridge: Cambridge University Press, 1986.

Lerner, Barron. *Contagion and Confinement: Controlling Tuberculosis along the Skid Road.* Baltimore, MD: The Johns Hopkins University Press, 1998.

McCuaig, Katherine. *The Weariness, the Fever and the Fret: The Campaign against Tuberculosis in Canada, 1900–1950.* Montreal, QC: McGill-Queen's University Press, 1999.

Neander, Gustaf. *Folksjukdomen tuberkulos och dess bekämpande.* Stockholm: Albert Bonniers Förlag, 1928.

Nenola, Aili. *Parantolaelämää. Tuberkuloosipotilaat muistelevat.* Helsinki: Keuhkovammaliitto, 1986.

Olin, T.E. *Muistelmia.* Porvoo, Finland, and Helsinki: WSOY, 1970.

Ott, Katherine. *Fevered Lives: Tuberculosis in American Culture since 1870.* Cambridge, MA: Harvard University Press, 1996.

Puranen, Britt-Inger. *Tuberkulos. En sjukdoms förekomst och dess orsaker. Sverige 1750–1980.* Umeå Studies in Economic History 7. Umeå, Sweden: Umeå Universitet, 1984.

Qvarnström, E. "Perhetarkastukset tuberkuloositapausten toteamiskeinona." *Tuberkuloosilehti* 8, no. 3 (1932): 111–15.

Reenkola, Mies. *Mammanpojasta naisten mieheksi. Muistelmia gynekologin oppivuosilta.* Helsinki: Weilin + Göös, 1976.

Reinarz, Jonathan. "The Age of Museum Medicine: The Rise and Fall of the Medical Museum at Birmingham's School of Medicine." *Social History of Medicine* 18 (2005): 419–37.

– *Health Care in Birmingham: The Birmingham Teaching Hospitals, 1779–1939.* Woodbridge, UK: Boydell Press, 2009.

Rosner, Lisa. *Medical Education in the Age of Enlightenment: Edinburgh Students and Apprentices, 1760–1826.* Edinburgh: Edinburgh University Press, 1991.

Rothman, Sheila M. *Living in the Shadow of Death: Tuberculosis and the Social Experience of Illness in American History.* Baltimore, MD, and London: The Johns Hopkins University Press, 1994.

Ryymin, Teemu Sakari. *Smitte, språk og kultur. Tuberkulosarbeidet i Finnmark.* Oslo: Scandinavian Academic Press, 2009.

Salo, Matti. *Pohjoinen alma mater. Oulun yliopisto osana korkeakoululaitosta ja yhteiskuntaa perustamisvaiheista vuoteen 2000.* Oulu, Finland: Pohjois-Suomen historiallinen yhdistys, 2003.

Savonen, Severi. "Minkätähden keuhkotautikuolevaisuus Suomessa on niin korkea?" *Tuberkuloosilehti* 5, no. 4 (1929): 210–21.

Säynäjäkangas, Olli, and Janne Kuoppala. "Suomen keuhkolääkäriyhdistyksen vaiheita." In *Keuhkosairauksien uusi historia. Tuberkuloosista se alkoi,* edited by Olli Säynäjäkangas, 185–209. Rovaniemi, Finland: OMS Kirjatuotanto, 2015.

Seppänen, Väinö. *Kertomus Takaharjun keuhkotautiparantolan toiminnasta 10-vuotiskautena 1.10.1903 – 31.12.1912.* Helsinki: [Duodecim], 1913.

Sjöstrand, Nils O. "Läkarnas grundutbildning 1800–1977." In *Ett sekel med läkaren i fokus. Läkarförbundet 1903–2003,* edited by Nils O. Sjöstrand, 329–49. Stockholm: Sveriges Läkarförening, 2003.

Smith, F.B. *The Retreat of Tuberculosis, 1850–1950.* London: Croom Helm, 1988.

Strömberg, John. "Ylioppilaat." In *Keisarillinen Aleksanterin yliopisto 1808–1917,* edited by Matti Klinge et al., 277–332. Helsinki: Otava, 1989.

Susitaival, Paavo. *Suomen Lääkäriliitto. Finlands Läkarförbund 1910–1960.* Helsinki: Suomen Lääkäriliitto, 1960.

Tiitta, Allan. *Collegium medicum. Lääkintöhallitus 1878–1991.* Helsinki: Lääkintöhallitus, 2009.

Venho, Kari. "Keuhkolääkärin työnkuvan muuttuminen – niin kuin minä sen koin." In *Keuhkosairauksien uusi historia. Tuberkuloosista se alkoi,* edited by Olli Säynäjäkangas, 181–4. Rovaniemi, Finland: OMS Kirjatuotanto, 2015.

Vento, Urpo. "The Folklore Activities of the Finnish Literature Society." Folklore Fellows, 6 July 2009. http://www.folklorefellows.fi/the-folklore-activities-of-the-finnish-literature-society/.

Vuorio, Kaija. *Lentoon. Kuopion yliopiston neljä vuosikymmentä.* Kuopio, Finland: Kuopion yliopisto, 2006.

Waddington, Keir. "Mayhem and Medical Students: Image, Conduct and Control in the Victorian and Edwardian London Teaching Hospitals." *Social History of Medicine* 15 (2002): 45–64.

– *Medical Education at St. Bartholemew's Hospital, 1123–1995.* Woodbridge, UK: Boydell Press, 2003.

Weisz, Georg. *Divide and Conquer: A Comparative History of Medical Specialization.* Oxford, UK: Oxford University Press, 2006.

Worboys, Michael. "The Sanatorium Treatment for Consumption in Britain, 1890–1914." In *Medical Innovations in Historical Perspective,* edited by John V. Pickstone, 47–71. New York: St Martin's Press, 1992.

13

Looking Around: The Architecture of Medical Education

Annmarie Adams

This chapter explores the architectural history of medical education. While architectural historians have analyzed hospital design as an index of changing ideas in medicine, relatively few have looked at buildings for medical education. Pointing to the value of architecture as a source in the history of medical education, historian James Hopkins describes such buildings as a "crucial site in producing the dominant cultural values and practices of medicine."[1] Architecture for medical education illustrates concepts "drawn together by the design and construction of the building and incorporated into its physical form."[2] Focusing on McGill University and on two of its distinctive buildings, I carefully deconstruct how architecture reveals changing priorities in the medical curriculum, relationships in and outside medicine, and the culture of medical education. By situating architecture at the centre of historical inquiry, rather than as context, we get a sharper view of the values articulated by a medical school at specific moments in time and in relation to wider cultural values.[3]

McGill University in Montreal is an ideal case study for an investigation of the architecture of medical education. Founded in 1823 as the Montreal Medical Institution and incorporated into McGill University six years later, it was the first medical faculty in Canada. Just as McGill's early medical curriculum influenced other Canadian medical schools,[4] its buildings were also influential models. Two of these structures, the "Strathcona" and the "McIntyre" as they are known, are still in use as medical school buildings and figure prominently today in the overall identity of the university.[5]

The Strathcona and the McIntyre differ radically in their origins and architectural designs. The McIntyre Medical Building (Figure 13.1) is a cylindrical tower sitting on an elevated, paddle-shaped podium, on a steep site. It was designed by modernist, Montreal-based architects Marshall & Merrett in 1965. At its opening in 1966, McGill principal H. Rocke Robertson described it as "a complete break with Tradition."[6] The Strathcona Building

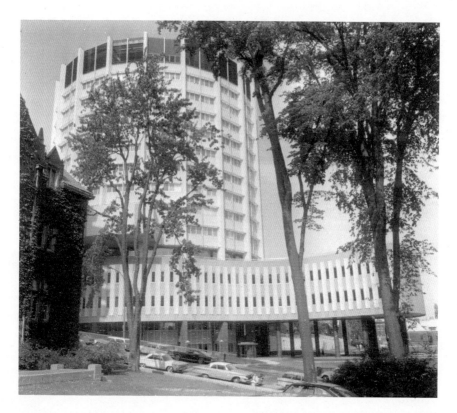

Figure 13.1 | The McIntyre Medical Building, McGill University, Montreal, 1966.
(NFOE Inc.)

(Figure 13.2), on the other hand, has the opposite relationship with tradition. Neo-classical in its inspiration, it relies on historical precedents for a more conservative expression. Like the McIntyre, it occupies a steep site, which can complicate the cross-section of any building, sometimes necessitating staggered entrances on different floors to accommodate a slope. Both buildings illustrate brilliant responses to context. Finally, each McGill building can be read as the architectural parallel to an influential public report. The Strathcona Building was constructed at the time of the Flexner Report of 1910, whereas the Royal Commission on Health Services' report of 1964 appeared just before the McIntyre opened. In the approach taken in this chapter, both reports serve as useful snapshots of medical education for their respective eras.

   Both buildings figure prominently in the university's public image. For example, advertisements for Expo 67, the popular world's fair held in Montreal to

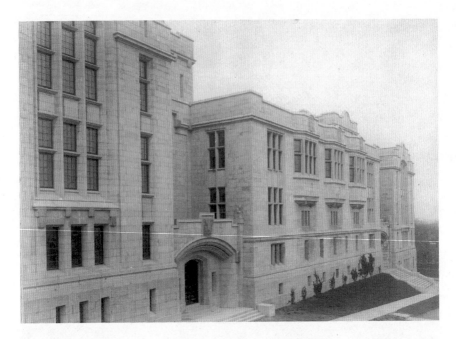

Figure 13.2 | The Strathcona Medical Building, elevation to campus, McGill University, Montreal, 1911. (Photographer unknown, McGill University Archives, PL007346)

celebrate Canada's centennial, featured the McIntyre in the foreground. Even today, photographs taken from Mount Royal, a natural mountain and park designed by renowned landscape architect Frederick Law Olmstead and widely considered to be the heart and soul of Montreal, often include the McIntyre.[7] The Strathcona Building, too, is once again the object of attention as it occupies a key component of McGill University's plan to reuse the now-empty Royal Victoria Hospital, perhaps as a gateway or threshold to the project.

Even beyond the boundaries of the university, medicine and medical education are important in Montreal. The urban history of medicine reflects Montreal's unique situation as a multilingual metropolis with strong historic ties to the scientific and medical traditions of Scotland, which are perhaps most evident in medicine.[8] The Montreal-based careers of world-famous physicians such as Norman Bethune and William Osler, for example, are foundational in the historical literature of Canadian medicine. L'Université de Montréal, located across Mount Royal from McGill, also has a medical faculty, founded in 1843. The celebrated architect Ernest Cormier designed an innovative, combined school-hospital for the Francophone university in 1927, one of only a handful of its kind in North America.[9] Mount Royal and its immediate surroundings are home to a remarkable collection of medical facilities, roughly forming a ring or a circle around the mountain, including the now-empty Hôtel-Dieu de Montréal, the Royal Victoria Hospital (colloquially known as the "Royal Vic"), the McIntyre, the Montreal General Hospital, and the Université de Montréal campus.

What does architecture tell us about medical education? Whereas social and cultural histories of medicine and medical education typically rely on textual or non-visual evidence, the built environment can reveal much about the unwritten priorities of medicine. The site plans of buildings for medical education, for example, show the changing importance of professional education in a city and/or on a campus. The relationship of a medical school to a hospital is clearly communicated in its architectural history. The arrangement of spaces, in general, can reveal what happened where, and who saw what. Design decisions, legible in archival drawings, reflect and shape the medical curriculum, illustrating the varying importance of educational components such as research, dissection, display, reading, lecturing, and discussion. Social hierarchies among faculty and students are legible in floor plans – needless to say, the dean, professors, and students occupy different places, reflecting their relative positions – as are the influences of other countries, traditions, universities, and disciplines. The McIntyre is "international" in its modern style, purposefully departing from the look of its close neighbours at McGill, while the Strathcona expresses a European lineage, especially Scottishness. Such bold assertions are not often articulated in written sources and underline the importance of architecture as a primary source.

Architecture for medical education after World War II shows how medical education looked outside itself to far-reaching and even radical cultural references to strengthen its modernist, global rise in importance. Such extroversion counters many cultural histories of medicine that look at sources produced by and for the profession of medicine rather than at general trends in cultural history for evidence. Finally, and with regards to the title of this contribution, "Looking Around," this work is about "looking" at medical education buildings and comparing them to other relevant building typologies. As the reader will note, the tone of this chapter is sometimes conversational, as if we are looking together, akin to a guided visit to the buildings under study. The overall discovery that emerges from this methodology of informed, visual observation is that researchers need to move across time periods and building types in order to unpack architectural meaning. "Looking around," then, refers to the *round* shape of the McIntyre, the primary case study examined in this chapter, but also emphasizes the importance of really *looking*, of *looking* back, and of visual evidence in general, as cues to historical meaning.

THE MCGILL CONTEXT

The McIntyre Medical Building was constructed in 1965, when the Faculty of Medicine was already almost 150 years old. It was McGill University's third purpose-built medical building. The first, "Old Medical" (Figure 13.3), had been designed in 1872 by architects Hopkins & Wily, with significant interior additions by Andrew Taylor in 1885, 1893, 1894, 1897, and sometime after 1901. Tragically and dramatically, Old Medical was destroyed by fire in 1907. McGill's second medical building, the 1911 Strathcona Medical Building, is the work of architects Brown & Vallance, a firm responsible for public buildings across Canada. These two older buildings are relatively rich in primary source materials, including original drawings and photographs. In this chapter they serve as comparative, historical examples to elucidate the design intentions of the much later McIntyre Building.

Additionally, these two early buildings are good examples of the common types identified by architectural historian Katherine L. Carroll in her PhD dissertation, "Modernizing the American Medical School, 1893–1940: Architecture, Pedagogy, Professionalization, and Philanthropy" (Boston University, 2012), and subsequent publication.[10] Carroll proposes three types in her survey of American medical schools after 1893: the institute; the single-building facility for preclinical studies, adjacent to a hospital; and the unified medical school-hospital. For Carroll, the institute type was best illustrated by Harvard's U-shaped quadrangle of medical buildings constructed c. 1906, reflecting the block system curriculum (each subject taught in a compressed time period). She argues that the influence for this distinctive ensemble of isolated pavilions came from Germany, mostly via doctors who had studied there. While McGill University's Old Medical roughly corresponds to Carroll's first type – it was an isolated pavilion with no partner buildings – the Strathcona was clearly designed as a single building with important connections to a nearby hospital, the Royal Vic. The Strathcona thus illustrates Carroll's second type, the isolated building for preclinical studies adjacent to a hospital. These two early McGill case studies thereby illustrate how trends in American medical education architecture also pertained to Canadian university buildings.

With Carroll's American research in mind, let's take a closer look at the McGill buildings. The original Old Medical was a five-bay, classical greystone building, almost like a Palladian villa. Andrew Taylor's 1901 extension was massive, creating a looming presence behind the original pavilion. Taylor's addition is in lighter stone and is wider and taller than the original building, demonstrating a decidedly layered approach to architectural growth (in other words, the fact of the addition is very evident). Cornice lines between the old and new buildings correspond. The plan of Old Medical,

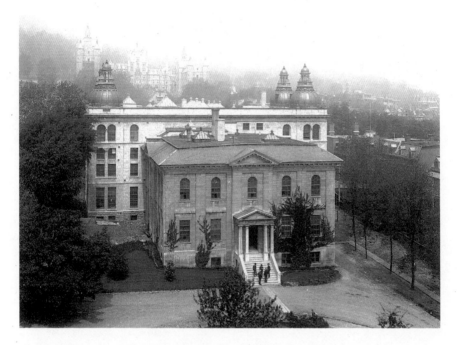

Figure 13.3 | Aerial photograph of Old Medical, McGill University, Montreal, c. 1900, showing additions. (VIEW-3619, Notman Photographic Archives, McCord Museum, Montreal)

with its various additions, is basically a central hall plan, with a generous widening of the corridor in the central section, and eight freestanding columns (Figure 13.4). The silhouette of the building, particularly its addition, was highly unusual, with four spherical domes rising from the corners of the rectangular pavilion.

The dramatic fire that destroyed Old Medical on 16 April 1907 drew extensive media coverage, including in the *New York Times*. Part of the drama was that there were two fires at McGill within a short period. On 5 April 1907, the nearby Engineering building was completely destroyed. The news that some artifacts from Old Medical survived made the place seem even more heroic. The library came through, but the medical museum was lost: "the museum, one of the best on the continent, was destroyed," reported *The Gazette*.[11] Certain specimens, however, unexpectedly survived, adding to the drama. Chief among these specimens was the Holmes heart, a single-ventricle heart autopsied by Andrew F. Holmes, who eventually became dean of Medicine in

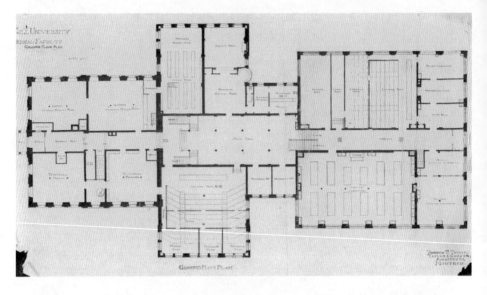

Figure 13.4 | Ground floor plan of Old Medical and additions, included in course calendars from the Medical Faculty. (McGill University, *Faculty of Medicine Annual Calendar: Sixty-Ninth Session, 1901–1902* [Montreal: Gazette Printing Co., 1901], Osler Library of the History of Medicine, McGill University)

1824. It is still one of the university's most precious artifacts. As a result of these two uncanny situations, Old Medical has a ghostly, mythical presence in the university's history (Figure 13.5).

The replacement building thus grew out of these extraordinary circumstances, plus it was "heroically" sponsored by benefactor Donald Smith, 1st Baron Strathcona and Mount Royal. Everything about it was highly visible. The design was chosen in an architectural competition. The site was strategically located between the university and the Royal Victoria Hospital (opened in 1893), which Strathcona had also supported. Carroll highlights the link to the hospital as a key component of her second type. The Strathcona's program also aligned with this type: it was compact, with laboratories, library, museum, and accommodation for administration. Carroll stresses that the hospital link enabled coordination in medical education; the linked design made students understand the branches of medicine as parts of a whole.[12] And she says most American medical schools opted for this type, which was praised by Abraham Flexner, author of the famous 1910 report that came to shape medical education in the twentieth century.[13]

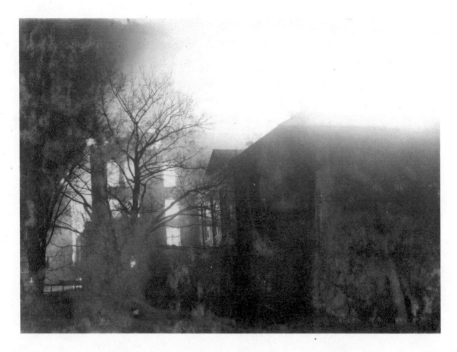

Figure 13.5 | During the fire at the Medical building, McGill University, Montreal, 1907. (MP.1994.15.1.3, McCord Museum, Montreal)

Because the Strathcona design was chosen through an architectural competition, there are rich archival documents illuminating its history and meaning. Eight firms were invited to submit drawings. Montreal architects Brown & Vallance won the competition.[14] The competition brief had defined the functional program and the schedule of floor areas that architects were to address. Five hundred thousand dollars was mentioned as an expenditure and Montreal limestone, "greystone" as it is known locally, was suggested as a facing material. The winning scheme was E-shaped in plan (Figure 13.6), with a medical museum at its centre. The arrangement of the building pays homage to the nearby hospital, whose pavilion plan had a similar footprint, maximizing ventilation in high-density wards. The design of the plan also addresses the university, as the museum and atrium occupy the end of an important north-south axis, roughly parallel to University Street, which continues to serve as the eastern border of the campus, more or less. "The design of Messrs. Brown & Vallance, as already mentioned is the only one which quite emphatically selects the University grounds as its principal relationship," reported a journalist in the *Canadian Architect and Builder* of 1907.[15]

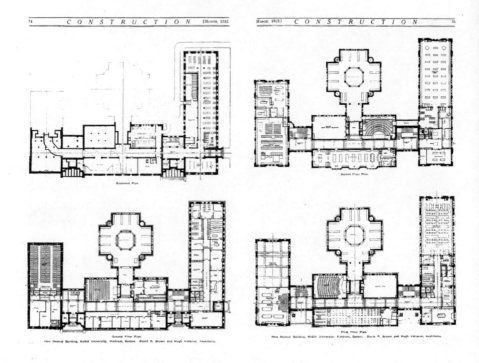

Figure 13.6 | Four floor plans of Strathcona Building, McGill University, Montreal, designed by Brown and Vallance. (*Construction* 5, no. 4 (March 1912): 54–5)

There is a popular belief among members of the medical community at McGill that the Strathcona Building turned its back on the hospital. Don Boudreau, respirologist and associate professor in the Department of Medicine, says many of his colleagues understood this as a gesture of dis-respect. Evoking an image of the building as an assembly of body parts, he recounts:

> Its posterior faced the RVH. The front side and the back side of the building evoke decidedly different emotions. The front has the two main entrances; these are ornate and open. They sport spectacular stairs; these are welcoming. The back is bleak and dingy; there are no doors or other ways in. Walking in the back of the building, between the east wing and the anatomy museum in the centre or between the west wing and the museum, is very much like walking in the armpits of the Strathcona. One does not wish to linger there. The two wings of the Strathcona,

like giant arms, are most certainly not arms that jut out to the Vic in an embrace. Rather they seem to be making the statement, in solid grey stone: keep your distance. The new medical school, by presenting uninviting physical facets, was a constant reminder to the "RVH medical tribe" that they were uninvited on the slopes of Mount Royal. The rump of the Strathcona building has exclaimed to its neighbor, in no uncertain terms: "Up yours."[16]

Neurologist Liam Durcan concurs: "the Strathcona being designed with its entrance towards campus and away from the Royal Vic as a deliberate affront to the hospital represent – even if misinformed – a fairly widely held idea among the medical community."[17]

While the siting and massing express these strong attitudes to the nearby hospital, what does the plan of the building tell us about what happened inside? The plan of the Strathcona shows the prominence of particular disciplines in the medical curriculum of 1911, such as anatomy, which occupies the whole east wing of the new structure. Especially prominent is the dissection lab (Figure 13.7), a monumental space measuring 88' x 40', almost ecclesiastical in its cross section, with a long-span, vaulted ceiling. In its massive expanses of glass and the exposed concrete ribs of the ceiling, however, it even looks vaguely industrial. In plan, the dissection lab reaches northward, towards the hospital on Pine Avenue, the source of cadavers. There was a tunnel beneath Pine Avenue, joining the Strathcona and the Royal Vic, but there is no evidence that bodies were transported below the street. By the 1920s, in any case, many went across University to the morgue and/or autopsy room in the Pathology Institute and then presumably made their way to Strathcona and even to the specimen jars in Maude Abbott's famous museum, which occupied the symbolic heart of the Strathcona Building.[18]

The Strathcona is also the original location of the world-famous Osler Library, opened in 1929, which was eventually relocated to the McIntyre Medical Building in the 1960s. Osler bequeathed his personal collection of books to McGill, "to be enshrined ... [with] a casket containing his heart."[19] Inspired by the historic importance of the library, architects Nobbs & Hyde designed an exquisite three-bay shrine for the books, distinguished by oak shelves with glass doors and stained-glass windows. The arrangement of the library was axial, with a clear focus on the shrine of Osler's remains located under a bronze portrait panel of the famous physician by Frederic Vernon, with a "secret receptacle." The books were carefully positioned, with Osler's own writings on one side of the room, facing those by others he so admired. Nobbs & Hyde took advantage of a barrel-vaulted, skylit room that already existed in the Strathcona, but decorated the cornices with the initials W.O.

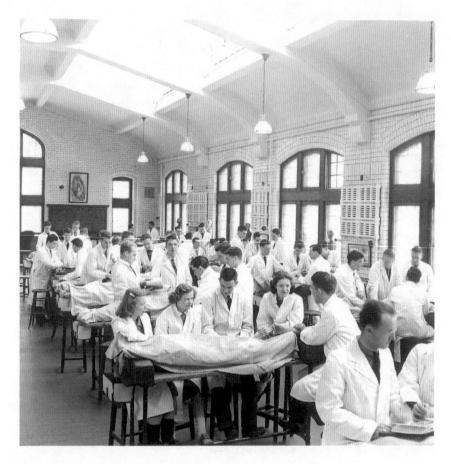

Figure 13.7 | Medical students in a laboratory doing dissections, Strathcona Medical Building, 1947. (Photograph by National Film Board, McGill University Archives, PR026766)

and added a collection of Kazak rugs. As Nobbs wrote in a loving description of the room for *The Journal of the Royal Architectural Institute of Canada* in 1930: "Here, as elsewhere, the intention has been to do things simply and solidly, in the hope that all may go on growing old together gracefully."[20]

The Strathcona Building is a good representation of the place of medicine following the influential Flexner Report, produced in 1910. There is no hard evidence that buildings being planned at the time of Flexner's fieldwork, however, were directly influenced by the publication. While Carroll never comes out and says such buildings were shaped by the report, she notes that this type, the isolated university pavilion, was twice as popular as the others with medical colleges at the time. Whether architects were aware of Flexner's research ahead of the publication of his report in 1910 is difficult to know. More evident, in light of the report's findings, is that Flexner's criticisms had architectural implications. At least three of Flexner's recommendations were strongly architectural or were related to planning. He said, for example, that medical schools had to be well-equipped; that they needed control of teaching hospitals; and that they needed funds to purchase land, construct buildings, and pay salaries.[21] Historians of medicine, notably Kenneth M. Ludmerer, have shown that the Flexner Report reduced the number of medical schools and raised standards. In general, its main influence on medical school architecture was that it standardized medical education (it would thus follow that buildings for medical education would become more alike, at least in plan) and especially that it established the university as the ideal site for training doctors. The report also resulted in increased mobility for doctors and students, who could now move between programs and institutions more easily. Ludmerer, however, notes that many of Flexner's points in the report were already in motion before the appearance of the publication: "there is little doubt that the extraordinary development of medical education that occurred in the years immediately following the report would have occurred without this catalyst," he says.[22] With regards to McGill's place in the influential report, Flexner paid "three short visits to the eight Canadian schools" in March, May, and October of 1909; these are summarized in seven pages at the end of his report, which came out in April 1910. Medical historian Jacalyn Duffin has argued that the *Canadian Medical Association Journal* (*CMAJ*) was "a nationalistic response to the Flexner report of the previous year." Duffin notes that Flexner assessed McGill and the University of Toronto relatively favorably, "if not perfect."[23]

OTHER CANADIAN EXAMPLES

McGill's Strathcona Medical Building is an excellent example of a whole cluster of Canadian buildings purposefully designed for medical education about the time of World War I. These buildings, in general, looked like non-medical university and school architecture. Like schools, these medical education buildings featured low-rise and horizontal massing, multiple entries to a *piano nobile*, and generous spaces for vertical and horizontal circulation. The locations of libraries, classrooms, and offices were easy to read from the exterior. Many institutions in the pre–World War II era drew on classical prototypes, identifiable by their symmetrical arrangements, monumental centralized entrances, elaborate window surrounds and moldings, and use of expensive materials such as stone.

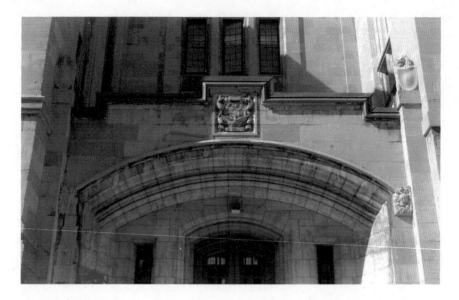

Figure 13.8 | Southeast entry of the Strathcona Building, showing medical imagery. (Photograph by Magdalena Milosz)

What truly distinguished medical education buildings from other university pavilions and schools was their unique programs, which included specialty spaces such as laboratories, accommodations for animals, and sometimes medical museums for teaching. All these medical spaces required elaborate preparatory areas, not always visible to users. For example, anatomy labs required morgues and special entrances; animals needed spaces for caretaking, feeding, cleaning, and dissection. Like museums today, medical museums sported special display spaces, custom furniture, and security details, but also required massive amounts of hidden storage.

Even in the spaces that were more visible, such as lecture halls, the buildings' medical mandates were legible. For example, many medical classrooms had large (i.e., not portable) illustrations on the walls, for constant reference during classes. Some early-twentieth-century medical buildings included custom symbolic exterior decoration, expressing the function of the interiors to passersby and users. For example, the Strathcona Medical Building's southeast entrance features McGill's coat of arms with two Rods of Asclepius, symbolizing medicine. Carved skulls surrounded by oak leaves and maple leaves prefigured the monumental dissection room and medical museum inside, both of which showcased dead bodies (Figure 13.8).

MCINTYRE MEDICAL BUILDING

The most recent building at McGill designed and constructed for general medical education is the McIntyre Medical Building (originally known as the McIntyre Medical Sciences Building), which opened in March 1966. At first glance it appears to be architecturally different in every possible way from the Strathcona. The major differences are the building's anticipation of arrival by automobile, its vertical rather than horizontal form, and a functional program based on styles of learning, rather than by medical disciplines. The Strathcona had been designed with mostly local materials and cultural references, while the McIntyre was designed according to international material and cultural references. Despite these significant differences, the buildings share characteristics. Both are carefully sited to bridge the university and nearby hospitals, both enjoy high visibility, both buildings contain important interiors that are legible from outside (lecture halls and library), and both are designed to accommodate a particular model of the curriculum.

The McIntyre Building was constructed at some distance from its predecessor, on the western edge of campus on a massive, sloping site between Peel and Drummond Streets, descending from Pine Avenue towards Doctor Penfield Avenue (formerly McGregor) (Figure 13.9). This site was strategic in that it was midway, or close to midway, between the Royal Victoria Hospital and the Montreal General Hospital, which had moved to its current site on Mount Royal, just west of McGill's campus, in 1955. This strategic location equidistant from the hospitals was noted in a speech at the building's opening: "a site which is particularly appropriate since it lies between the Montreal General Hospital and the Royal Victoria Hospital in close proximity to McGill itself."[24] The two McGill teaching hospitals were notoriously competitive, so building the medical school at the midway point was calculated and the three buildings – the medical school and the two hospitals – worked as a network until the Royal Victoria closed its doors and moved to a new site in 2015.

Additionally, in contrast to the low-rise, horizontal, classically inspired design of the Strathcona Building, the McIntyre Medical Building was a gleaming, modernist tower. At 311,620 square feet, it accommodated 10 per cent of the whole university.[25] Today, it is still the tallest building at McGill and distinctive in the skyline, due to its cylindrical massing. From below, it dominates the skyline, even masking parts of the outline of Mount Royal. From above, as has been mentioned, it occupies the foreground of many views from Mount Royal to downtown Montreal, the St Lawrence River, and beyond. Significantly, it opened at precisely the same time as three other new buildings at the university, two of which were dedicated to science: the adjacent Stewart Biological Sciences Building, the Otto Maass Chemistry Building, and a new

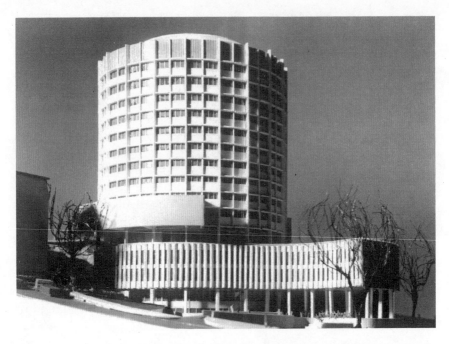

Figure 13.9 | Architectural model of the McIntyre Medical Building, 1966, showing the slope of the site between Pine and Doctor Penfield Avenues. (NFOE Inc.)

Student Union.[26] The massive Stewart Biological Sciences Building of 1965, just to the south of the McIntyre Medical Building, by architects Dobush, Stewart and Bourke, features precast concrete panels in an L-configuration, surrounding a block with two large theatres. Fleming and Smith's Otto Maass Chemistry Building, at the corner of Sherbrooke and University Streets, is four enormous blocks of Queenston limestone, a decidedly conservative choice in 1964–66 when most buildings of this size and style would have been concrete. Like the McIntyre, both these buildings for science integrate teaching and research spaces through architectural form.[27]

A significant difference between the McIntyre Medical Building and its predecessors, Old Medical and the Strathcona, was its program. Whereas the two older buildings showcased teaching and display, the planning of the McIntyre brought together research and teaching, through the design and locations of laboratories and classrooms. Dean Ronald V. Christie exclaimed at the opening, "Teaching and research have become inseparable."[28] At many medical schools by the 1960s, teaching was based more on problem-solving and teamwork,

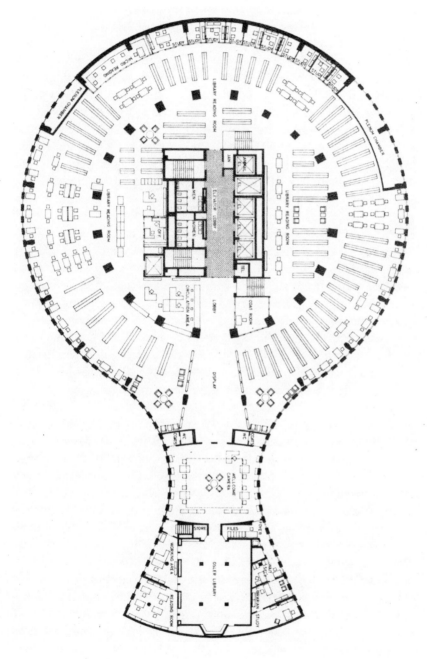

Figure 13.10 | Marshall & Merrett Architects, third-floor plan of the McIntyre Medical Building; the section protruding from the circle contains the Osler Library and cantilevers over a two-way driveway. (NFOE Inc.)

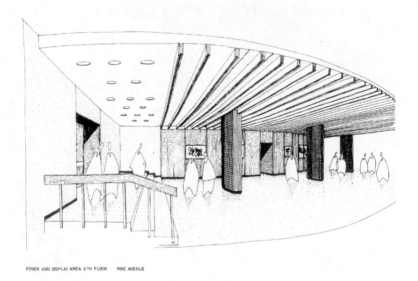

FOYER AND DISPLAY AREA 6TH FLOOR   PINE AVENUE

Figure 13.11 Marshall & Merrett Architects, perspective view of the McIntyre Medical Building's sixth-floor entrance foyer from Pine Avenue. (NFOE Inc.)

rather than comprehensive knowledge or rote learning. Even by the time of the Flexner Report, it was recognized that doctors needed to be problem-solvers and critical thinkers, rather than keepers of encyclopedic knowledge.

Dean Lloyd Grenfell Stevenson, a medical historian and the youngest dean ever at thirty-eight when Cyril James appointed him in 1956, oversaw the construction of the McIntyre Building.[29] Although essentially a modernist tower, crucial to the project was the inclusion of the historic Osler Library, lovingly transferred piece by piece from the by-then-historic Strathcona Building, and inserted in a special location on the third floor (Figure 13.10). From plans dated October 1962, we know that the other floors of the building accommodated the following, roughly moving from the lower floors upwards: lobby, mechanical, offices, library, cafeteria, auditoria, research labs, research spaces, teaching labs, animal quarters, and more mechanical. The building was designed principally by architects Janet Leys Shaw Mactavish and Dorice Brown Walford of the Montreal firm Marshall & Merrett. Mactavish had designed Stirling Hall at Queen's University and specialized in school design.[30] Walford was project manager of the Bell Telephone pavilion at Expo

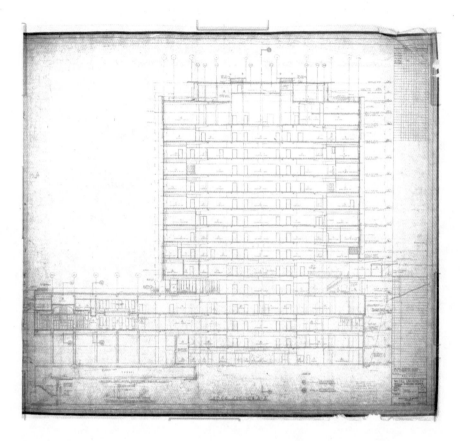

Figure 13.12 | Marshall & Merrett Architects, section of the McIntyre Medical Building, showing cantilevered section over the driveway at left and entrances on fifth and sixth floors at right, 1962. (NFOE Inc.)

67 and designed the addition to the Allan Memorial Institute, almost adjacent to the McIntyre site.

The distinctive massing of the McIntyre, its roundness and its height, were intended to signal a new era in medicine. The McIntyre is a sixteen-storey tower dominated by a round floor plan and a complex vertical circulation system. Its proportions are not unlike a beer or other food can, an aspect not lost on generations of students, who have invented comical nicknames for the building. Its steep site enabled the architects to provide staggered entrances on the first and sixth floors (Figure 13.11). Between these points of entry, on the third and fourth floors, the library occupies a paddle-like or tail-like

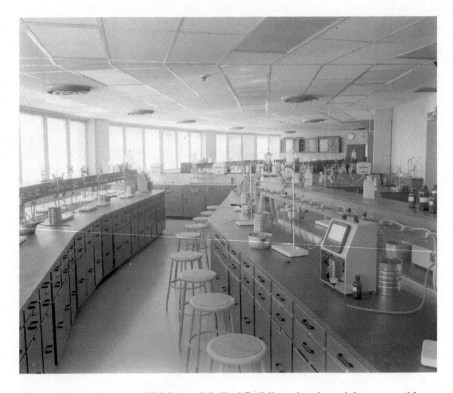

Figure 13.13 | Interior of McIntyre Medical Building, showing a laboratory with continuous windows. (NFOE Inc.)

section that protrudes southward, cantilevered over the two-way driveway, almost like a massive car port – a very popular feature in residential design in the post-war era (Figure 13.12). On these floors, the plans of the building resemble a giant spoon. It is difficult today to appreciate the sheer sculptural power of the building, especially this panhandle section, as it is now crowded out by new construction, but in its day the McIntyre was highly visible from below and from many other vistas. It functioned as what architects would call a "midspace object," deriving its meaning from its recognizable silhouette and isolation from adjacent buildings.

This isolation was purposeful and symbolic, speaking to the special significance of medicine at the university. Like many other twentieth-century towers, the McIntyre was intended to serve as a sign in the landscape. It makes us think about Roland Barthes's analysis of the Eiffel Tower, a classic essay by the influential French philosopher. He famously called the Parisian landmark

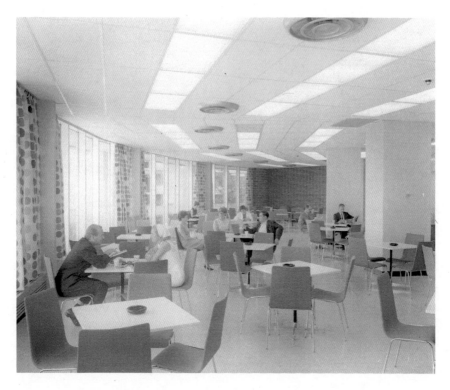

Figure 13.14 | Interior of McIntyre Medical Building, showing the fifth-floor cafeteria with floor-to-ceiling windows. (NFOE Inc.)

an "utterly useless monument." Still, he notes the unifying power of the tower: "that simple line whose sole mythic function is to join, as the poet says, base and summit, or again, earth and heaven," as well as the differences in experiencing it from outside and from within: "it becomes a lookout in its turn when we visit it ... the tower is an object which sees, a glance which is seen."[31]

The McIntyre Building was also a place *from which* to see, underlined by its round form. Archival photographs show laboratories with continuous windows, providing students with panoramic views of the campus and city. The cafeteria on the fifth floor, for example, also had floor-to-ceiling windows, framed with stylish curtains (Figures 13.13, 13.14). "Hardly a right angle," said one journalist, quoting the director of the building Murray Saffran. "The circular design ... is more than a clever aesthetic gimmick ... The design makes it possible for most of the human working areas such as laboratories and office to have outside exposure."[32]

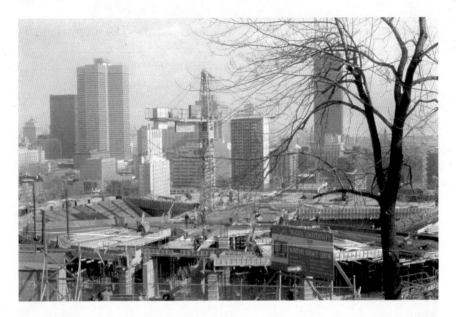

Figure 13.15 | The McIntyre Medical Building under construction, with Place Ville Marie in the left background. (NFOE Inc.)

Its presence was amplified by the immediate history of its empty grounds. The name McIntyre comes from the site itself: CPR founder Duncan McIntyre's residence, Craguie, had once occupied the ten-acre lot, before being demolished in the 1930s. His family donated the land to McGill in 1947 and the site had been called McIntyre Park before the construction of the McIntyre Building. The construction process itself attracted great attention and was documented closely by photographers. Many of these construction shots capture another fashionable and iconic tower, Place Ville Marie, designed by I.M. Pei and Henry N. Cobb (Figure 13.15). Built in 1962, it was cruciform in plan, and was at the time the tallest building in the Commonwealth. A swanky dance club called Altitude 737 perched on top; it is ironic that the building was as famous for having a large percentage of its space underground.[33]

Just as the key document for understanding the Strathcona is the Flexner Report, here the important document is the 1965 report of the Royal Commission on Health Services, sometimes called the Hall Commission after its chairman Justice Emmett M. Hall. He was appointed by the Diefenbaker government in 1961 to carry out the Royal Commission, which eventually recommended the national adoption of Saskatchewan's model of public health insurance. The main conclusions of the Commission, including a 277-page report on medical education in Canada, were that more physicians were needed.[34] As a consequence, new schools were established at McMaster University (Hamilton, Ontario), the University of Calgary, and Memorial University (St John's), and in Quebec the development of the Université de Sherbrooke was accelerated. With regards to architectural history, some of these had cutting-edge, fashionable buildings. Other schools, occupying older buildings, were urged to modernize. Following the Hall Commission, there was a new emphasis on research and theoretical grounding. Additionally, students demanded a medical school curriculum that was relevant to contemporary practice, and in the post-report era, they were exposed to patients in their first year, rather than in year three. Basic science labs were reduced and/ or eliminated. The new curriculum was called the "systems" approach and taught body systems in integrated blocks to showcase diagnosis and treatment, rather than from the disciplinary perspective. Seminar rooms were favoured over lecture theatres with static images. The most radical Canadian example of this new style of school was McMaster University. Its program emphasized problem-solving and teamwork and taught the skills needed to solve problems, rather than comprehensive knowledge. What was the architecture of this visionary, systems approach to medical education?

The design of the McMaster University Health Sciences Centre was the epitome of the new era in medical education. Built in 1968–72 and designed by Craig, Zeidler and Strong Architects, it was touted as a revolution in hospital design.[35] Unlike the McIntyre, to be fair, it was a hospital, not a medical school. And the hospital was a megastructure, an example of plug-in architecture, with no evident hierarchies, and clear vertical service cores. In a nutshell, its architecture was all about integration through technology. McMaster was the vision of Harry Thode, as the "first purpose-built medical facility in the world to attempt through design to ... spatialize medical interdisciplinarity."[36] The building was all about creating a close relationship between patients and researchers, with emphasis on horizontal circulation, allowing users to "walk" the institution. The design had an association with urban plazas and streets, enabling accidental meetings. Architectural historian Thomas Strickland has noted the importance of the lobby design at McMaster, especially designed to make health care services appear accessible.[37]

Like McMaster, the McIntyre was a utopian vision for teaching medicine. It showcased a futuristic, media-savvy society and also used architecture to "normalize" medical care, suggesting links to non-medical environments such as office buildings, world's fairs, and urban theatres. The elevator core, for example, was the building's heart, like an office building. Also drawing on the architectural language of the corporation were the elegant entrances, especially from Pine Avenue. For that upper entrance, on the building's sixth floor, the architects designed an elegant cantilevered entry roof which, like those of many apartment houses, reached out and brought in pedestrians, in addition to protecting them from inclement weather. Once inside, visitors saw the lobby spread out before them, showcasing art, furniture, and a rather stunning open stair. Additionally, the elegant entrance to the large auditorium and the "information booth" just inside the sixth-floor entrance were reminiscent of the ticket counters of 1960s urban theatres such as Place des Arts. One journalist even noted the beauty of the entrance at night, an uncommon observation for university buildings.[38] Significantly, the McIntyre also included 450 indoor parking spots, anticipating arrival by automobile. Such design features gave a sense of luxury and control to the building's visitors and everyday users, with cultural references outside of medicine itself. The Department of Pharmacology delivered a statement at the opening of the building, affirming that "the spacious lecture theatres, demonstration rooms and libraries (both Medical and Departmental) now available have contributed greatly to increased academic enthusiasm in both students and teachers."[39] Dean Christie described the building as a "rare combination of beauty and efficiency," with no reference whatsoever to medicine.[40]

A significant symbolic meaning of the McIntyre, deriving from its architectural design, was the concept of oneness and/or the wholeness of medicine.[41] Such expression depended on the idea of connection: connecting body parts, but also in real terms the linking of medical teaching to research. The roundness of the tower showed medicine as unified, with research and teaching as coordinated and harmonized parts. Unlike in the period before World War II, for example, where basic science departments such as Anatomy or Histology occupied distinctive and purpose-built suites of rooms, departments in the McIntyre basically looked the same. They blended together in a "seamless" architecture with few corners or ends, like infinite space. This illusion of infinity was one of the reasons that similarly round forms were popular for the design of planetariums. A journalist reporting on the opening said "the circular tower reminds one of the scientific advances of the last 30 years" and noted "electronic apparatus which make fact of yesterday's science fiction."[42] Note that the architects of the McIntyre Building also used the circular massing for the physics building at nearby Queen's University, illustrating that to them roundness symbolized science, not just medicine.

Montrealers were particularly design-savvy around the time of Expo 67, which boasted the power of architecture to bring people together. Man and His World, on a 1,000-acre site, included the construction of the metro system and 90 themed and national pavilions. International architects, given free rein, designed exuberant and structurally revolutionary pavilions, separated

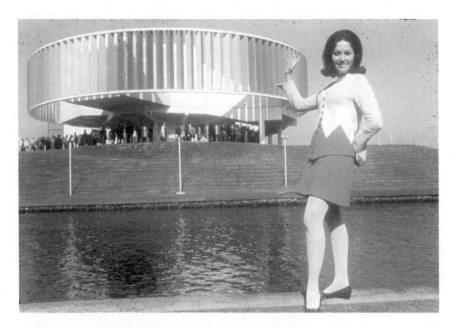

Figure 13.16 | A model presenting the Kaleidoscope Pavilion at Expo 67.
(Expo 67 Meredith Dixon Slide Collection, McGill University Library)

from each other. Expo buildings offered Montrealers and all visitors potent examples of in-between spaces, crowd control, the use of film and media simulation, multi-speed movement, car-free public space, and many other unprecedented design features.

Although Expo 67 hosted a medical pavilion, two other buildings are more relevant to the design of the McIntyre: Buckminster Fuller's American pavilion and Kaleidoscope. Designed by University of Waterloo Institute of Design, Kaleidoscope had 112 fins painted in a spectrum of colours, appearing to change colours (Figure 13.16). The intention was techno-savvy and something of a simulation, long before its time. Visitors to Kaleidoscope were intended to experience a "day" in 12 minutes, from sunrise to nightfall, through colour. One visitor captured the experience thus: "Man and Colour was the deceptively simple title of the show. Mirrors reflecting pulsing lights into infinity created a vision of space seemingly drawn from the imagination of Albert Einstein. Unaware though I was of the visit of La Scala and the Vienna State Opera to Place des Arts under the aegis of the World Festival of Entertainment, I could claim at least exposure to the avant-garde music of

R. Murray Schafer through Kaleidoscope."[43] Buildings like this thus made visitors feel worldly and sophisticated, demonstrating the power of technology to transport us to faraway, even imaginary, places. This architecture made us feel things in new ways. Such was the design context of the McIntyre Building, which featured an electrically shielded room to permit electrophysiological study of single nerve and muscle cells, an electron microscope lab, computer facilities, and a sterile room for skin-graft experiments.[44] The emphasis was on spinning, turning, on a world without ends or at least corners.

Round hospitals also enjoyed a decade or so of popularity about the time of the construction of the McIntyre, and provide clues to its meaning. A round plan was an attractive choice for hospital administrators because of the perceived reduction in distances for circulation, especially for nurses. Yale–New Haven Hospital's Memorial Unit undertook a study of the efficiency of round hospital plans. Published in Thompson and Goldin's survey of the building type in 1975, a chapter entitled "The Yale Traffic Index" tested thirty inpatient units according to efficiency, privacy, and size, showing that size and privacy had no impact on efficiency: it was *design* that mattered, with three circular wards ranking the highest. McIntyre Building architect Janet Mactavish had conducted a similar study of school arrangements and designed several circular schools in the mid-1950s, experimenting with how the shape affected circulation patterns.[45]

The architects of the McIntyre were likely aware of the popularity and success of circular hospitals. A notable example is the Medical Office Building for Kaiser Foundation Hospitals with Kaiser Aluminum Dome, designed by Clarence W. Mayhew.[46] A hospital that truly resonates with the design of the McIntyre is the Kaiser Foundation Hospital in Panorama City, designed in 1962.[47] Also not round but boasting a centralized plan is Bertrand Goldberg's Prentice Women's Hospital in Chicago, a nine-storey quatrefoil tower on a rectangular five-storey podium, with nursing stations in a central core and patients in the four lobes, opened in 1975.

The architects of the McIntyre also looked outward. For example, Marina City in Chicago, an apartment building also by Bertrand Goldberg constructed in 1959–68, and the Capitol Records Building in Los Angeles, designed by Welton Becket and Associates in 1956, share formal characteristics with the McIntyre and round hospitals. These distinctive circular silhouettes, like that of the McIntyre, served as modernist beacons in their respective contexts. The circular shape made them unique and thus recognizable at a distance. All these circular buildings expressed the utopian notion of oneness or wholeness. Architecture thus linked medical education to a larger cultural context of the 1960s. Circular imagery was also very popular in painting, sculpture, fashion, symbols of space flight, and even transportation.

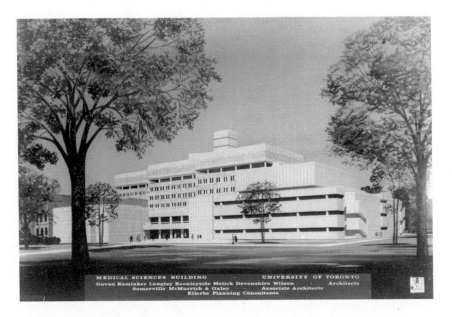

Figure 13.17 | Perspective view of Medical Sciences Building, University of Toronto. (University of Toronto Archives, A2012-0009/057(11), Division of Advancement and Communications Fonds)

Certainly there were other ways to design a medical school. "Med Sci" at the University of Toronto, designed at the same time as the McIntyre and finished in 1969, couldn't be more different from the building at McGill University. Architect Peter Goering opted for an eight-storey, nearly window-less concrete box (Figure 13.17). Its artfulness, however, was in a series of precast concrete panels by artist Robert Downing. According to Scott Sorli, the panels may have been "randomly (if unintentionally so) installed by the construction crew and were also one of the first Canadian examples of a rain screen system."[48] The University of Toronto building was more in the tradition of Brutalism than the so-called International Style, a mode popular in the post-war period that emphasized democratic processes, freedom of speech, material honesty, and sheer strength. In constructing its new medical education building, McGill University could have opted for a Brutalist monument, as is evidenced by the nearby Stephen Leacock Building, designed by ARCOP in 1965, an outstanding example of Brutalist architecture featuring precast, load-bearing concrete panels. Instead, the university opted for a very different expression for medical education.

CONCLUSIONS

Our tour has taken us through nearly a century of medical education by *looking around* archetypal medical buildings. As we have seen, the massing, siting, form, and disposition of medical education buildings enabled strategic relationships to the university and hospital contexts. Our example from pre–World War I shows the university's allegiance to Scotland through its choice of architectural style and materials. The building's location and design communicated mixed messages about the relationship with a nearby hospital. Additionally, the architectural evidence points to the significance of disciplinary boundaries in medical education at this time, including the major role of dissection and book-learning in medicine. In the early twentieth century, the medical museum was also at the heart of the educational enterprise. After World War II, however, the cultural references were more international and looked outside medicine. The modern medical-education tower was a place to see and a place from which to see other buildings. It integrated research and teaching through design and technology. Post-war architecture for medical education was savvy and even fashionable. It communicated a unifying message to constituents about medicine. At the same time, we have seen the potential for architecture to illustrate ideals articulated in major reports on medical education, in this case the influential Flexner Report and Hall Commission. Most importantly, looking around architecture for medical education shows how medicine, as an academic discipline, has reached outward for inspiration, linking faculty and students to a realm outside itself.

ACKNOWLEDGMENTS

I gratefully acknowledge the research assistance of McGill students and recent graduates Fiona Kenney, Ipek Mehmetoglu, Magdalena Milosz, Jennifer Phan, Philippe Saurel, and Cigdem Talu. Students in the Med 4 "Architecture + Medicine" selective, winter 2018, produced inspirational assessments of the McIntyre Building. Special thanks to Masa Fukushima at NFOE Inc. architects, who provided access to drawings and photos of the McIntyre Building. McGill librarian Jennifer Garland was super helpful, as always. Leïla Rached-d'Astous won a Hannah Summer Studentship, sponsored by the Associated Medical Services Inc. Her work on this topic benefited my research.

NOTES

1   Hopkins, "The (Dis)assembling of Form," 25.

2   Ibid., 29.

3   Ibid., 52.

4   Waugh and Bailey, "Medical Education."

5   During the writing of this chapter, the McIntyre Building was damaged in a fire on 13 July 2018, and was temporarily closed; see "Update."

6   "Speech by Dr. H. Rocke Robertson on the Occasion of the Opening of the McIntyre Medical Sciences Building," 4, 23 March 1966, McGill University Archives.

7   A good example from Expedia is "Mount Royal Park," https://www.expedia.ca/Mount-Royal-Park-Ville-Marie.d507156.Vacation-Attraction (accessed 18 September 2018).

8   Hornstein, "The Architecture of the Montreal Teaching Hospitals," 13–25.

9   Gournay, "L'Architecture Hospitalo-Universitaire" and "The Work of Ernest Cormier at the Université de Montréal."

10   Carroll, "Modernizing the American Medical School, 1893–1940" and "Creating the Modern Physician."

11   "M'Gill Again Victim from Fire," *The Gazette*, 16 April 1907, 4.

12   Carroll, "Modernizing the American Medical School, 1893–1940," 61.

13   Flexner, *Medical Education in the United States and Canada.*

14   The firms were Brown & Vallance, Finley & Spence, W. & W.S. Maxwell, Ross & Macfarlane, Robert Findlay, Marchand & Haskell, Saxe & Archibald, and Hogle & Davis. "McGill Medical Building Competition," 143.

15   Ibid., 143.

16   Don Boudreau, email message to author, 30 November 2018.

17   Liam Durcan, email message to author, 30 November 2018.

18   On the medical museum in the Strathcona Medical Building, see Adams, "Designing the Medical Museum," 177–81, and "Encountering Maude Abbott," 7–10.

19   Nobbs, "Bibliotheca Osleriana," 204.

20   Ibid., 204.

21   Ludmerer, *Learning to Heal,* 177.

22   Ludmerer, "Understanding the Flexner Report," 195.

23   Duffin, "Did Abraham Flexner Spark the Founding of *CMAJ*?" 811.

24   "Mr. Chancellor, Mr. Principal, Members of the Board of Governors, Members of Senate, Ladies and Gentlemen," undated speech, McGill University Archives. I am grateful to medical student Leila Rached-d'Astous for uncovering the speeches and newspaper articles cited here.

25   D.B. MacFarlane, "New Buildings Ready for Fall," n.p.

26 Ibid.

27 There is scant literature on the architecture of science education. See Forgan, "The Architecture of Science and the Idea of a University," 405–34. The classic reference is Galison and Thompson, eds., *The Architecture of Science*.

28 Ronald V. Christie, "The McIntyre Medical Sciences Building is a superb contribution," undated and untitled speech, 3, McGill University Archives.

29 Bates, "Obituary: Lloyd Grenfell Stevenson," 205.

30 Adams and Tancred, *'Designing Women,'* 75.

31 Barthes, "The Eiffel Tower," 124.

32 "New Science Unit Not For 'Squares,'" *Montreal Gazette*, 3 September 1965.

33 For more on the monument, see Vanlaethem et al., *Place Ville Marie*.

34 MacFarlane et al., *Medical Education in Canada*.

35 Strickland, "Passive and Active," 204.

36 Ibid., 210.

37 Ibid., 217.

38 "New McGill Medical Tower Ties Tradition, Technology," *Montreal Star*, 10 November 1965.

39 "re: Department of Pharmacology, McIntyre Medical Sciences Building," 10 January 1966, 2, McGill University Archives.

40 Ronald V. Christie, "The McIntyre Medical Sciences Building is a superb contribution," undated and untitled speech, 4, McGill University Archives.

41 For discussions on the relation of holism and medicine, see Lawrence and Weisz, eds., *Greater than the Parts*.

42 "New McGill Medical Tower Ties Tradition, Technology," *Montreal Star*, 10 November 1965.

43 Kaptainis, "Expo 67."

44 "Physiology at McGill was first taught," undated, 3, McGill University Archives.

45 Adams and Tancred, *'Designing Women,'* 75.

46 I am grateful to PhD student Gina Page for alerting me to this work.

47 "Kaiser's Geodesic Dome Clinic," https://kaiserpermanentehistory.org/latest/kaisers-geodesic-dome-clinic/ (accessed 12 October 2016).

48 Sorli, "Medical Sciences Building," 154.

BIBLIOGRAPHY

Adams, Annmarie. "Designing the Medical Museum." In *Healing Spaces, Modern Architecture, and the Body*, edited by Sarah Schrank and Didem Ekici, 171–85. London: Routledge, 2017.

– "Encountering Maude Abbott." *Feminist Encounters: A Journal of Critical Studies in Culture and Politics* 2, no. 2 (2018).

Adams, Annmarie, and Peta Tancred. '*Designing Women': Gender and the Architectural Profession*. Toronto: University of Toronto Press, 2000.

Barthes, Roland. "The Eiffel Tower." *AA Files* 64 (2012): 112–31.

Bates, Donald G. "Obituary: Lloyd Grenfell Stevenson." *Canadian Bulletin of Medical History* 5, no. 2 (16 December 2016): 205–6.

Carroll, Katherine L. "Creating the Modern Physician: The Architecture of American Medical Schools in the Era of Medical Education Reform." *Journal of the Society of Architectural Historians* 75, no. 1 (March 2016): 48–73.

– "Modernizing the American Medical School, 1893–1940: Architecture, Pedagogy, Professionalization, and Philanthropy." 2 parts. PhD diss. Boston, MA: Boston University, 2012.

Duffin, Jacalyn. "Did Abraham Flexner Spark the Founding of CMAJ?" *CMAJ* 183, no. 7 (19 April 2011): 811–13.

Flexner, Abraham. *Medical Education in the United States and Canada: A Report to the Carnegie Foundation for the Advancement of Teaching*. 1910. Facsimile reprint New York: Arno Press, 1972.

Forgan, Sophie. "The Architecture of Science and the Idea of a University." *Studies in History and Philosophy of Science* 20, no. 4 (1989): 405–34.

Galison, Peter, and Emily Thompson, eds. *The Architecture of Science*. Cambridge, MA: MIT Press, 1999.

Gournay, Isabelle. "L'Architecture Hospitalo-Universitaire: Le Tournant des Années 20." *Journal of Canadian Art History* 13, no. 1 (1990–91): 26–43.

– "The Work of Ernest Cormier at the Université de Montréal." In *Ernest Cormier and the Université de Montréal*, edited by Isabelle Gournay, 58, 67–70. Montreal, QC: CCA, 1990.

Hopkins, James. "The (Dis)assembling of Form: Revealing the Ideas Built into Manchester's Medical School." *Journal of the History of Medicine and Allied Sciences* 75, no. 1 (January 2020): 24–53.

Hornstein, Shelley. "The Architecture of the Montreal Teaching Hospitals of the Nineteenth Century." *Journal of Canadian Art History* 13, no. 1 (1990–91): 13–25.

Kaptainis, Arthur. "Expo 67: 50 Years Later Still an Expression of the Human Spirit." *Montreal Gazette*, 13 June 2017.

Lawrence, Christopher, and George Weisz, eds. *Greater than the Parts: Holism in Biomedicine, 1920–1950*. New York: Oxford University Press, 1998.

Ludmerer, Kenneth M. *Learning to Heal: The Development of American Medical Education*. New York: Basic Books, 1985.

– "Understanding the Flexner Report." *Academic Medicine* 85, no. 2 (2010): 193–6.

"McGill Medical Building Competition." *Canadian Architect and Builder* 20, no. 8 (August 1907): 143–4.

MacFarlane, J.A., R.C. Dickson, Roger Dufresne, Harold Ettinger, John F. McCreary, and J. Wendell Macleod. *Medical Education in Canada*. Ottawa: Royal Commission on Health Services, 1965.

Nobbs, Percy Erskine. "Bibliotheca Osleriana – McGill University, Montreal." *The Journal of the Royal Architectural Institute of Canada* 7, no. 6 (June 1930): 204–5.

Sorli, Scott. "Medical Sciences Building, Toronto's Largest Modern Sculpture." In *Concrete Toronto: A Guidebook to Concrete Architecture from the Fifties to the Seventies*, edited by Michael McClelland and Graeme Stewart, 154–9. Toronto: Coach House Books, 2007.

Strickland, Thomas. "Passive and Active: Public Space at the McMaster Health Sciences Centre, 1972." In *Healing Spaces, Modern Architecture, and the Body*, edited by Sarah Schrank and Didem Ekici, 203–23. London: Routledge, 2017.

"Update: Fire Damages McGill University's McIntyre Medical Building." *Montreal Gazette*, last modified 15 July 2018. https://montrealgazette.com/news/local-news/fire-at-mcgills-mcintyre-medical-building.

Vanlaethem, France, Sarah Marchand, Paul-André Linteau, and Jacques-André Chartrand. *Place Ville Marie: Montreal's Shining Landmark*. Montreal, QC: Québec Amérique, 2012.

Waugh, Douglas, and Patricia G. Bailey. "Medical Education." In *The Canadian Encyclopedia*. Last modified 11 March 2016. https://www.thecanadianencyclopedia.ca/en/article/medical-education/.

14

Bodies in Bits: Historicizing Anatomy's Digital Turn

Jenna Healey

In 1969, a South African anatomy lecturer described his first encounter with computer-assisted instruction (CAI) during a tour of Cornell Medical School in New York City. The computer, a collaboration between the Department of Anatomy and the International Business Machines Corporation (IBM), was too impractical for widespread use: it took over 300 hours, and thousands of dollars, to program a single hour of curriculum. And yet, the lecturer noted "with some alarm and apprehension," the machine "may eventually put [anatomists] out of business."[1]

The lecturer's early digital encounter foreshadowed a contentious contemporary debate within anatomy education, one that pits cadaver against computer. Dissection has been a pedagogical mainstay of Western medical education for hundreds of years. Defenders of the practice often invoke this historical legacy to argue that dissection is fundamental for the education and professionalization of future physicians.[2] While curricular hours dedicated to dissection have been on the decline since the early twentieth century, the computer has been singled out as a unique technological threat to dissection's central place in medical education, although there are as yet very few instances in which digital anatomy has successfully displaced dissection in an educational setting.[3]

This chapter historicizes this debate by asking when, how, and why computers were integrated into the anatomy lab. The introduction of CAI into medical education dates back to the 1960s, when several American medical schools experimented with integrating computers into the classroom. The Lister Hill National Center for Biomedical Communications, founded as a division of the National Library of Medicine (NLM) in 1968, promoted educational computing on a national scale by organizing conferences, compiling resources, and funding the development of an experimental CAI network. This chapter is one of the first scholarly attempts to account for the integration of CAI in medical education.[4] Anatomy is an excellent case study for this purpose, as it was the subject most frequently targeted as a site of curricular innovation. The focus on the United States reflects the outsized role of the NLM in promoting CAI, though the trend was visible in other Western countries, including Britain and Canada.

The chapter's argument is twofold. First, I will argue that CAI was developed in response to a growing temporal crisis within medical education. The post-war explosion of biomedical research strained an already crowded curriculum, and gross anatomy courses became an obvious target for freeing up curricular space. CAI was just one of several instructional technologies introduced during the 1960s that promised to make anatomy more efficient. The first anatomy software contained no images; its purpose was to automate the delivery of content. This history challenges the conventional framing of computerized anatomy as the enemy of dissection, instead suggesting that the computer was introduced to enable students and faculty to make the most of their time at the dissecting table. That the digital turn in anatomy predated the development of image-intensive software packages by several decades also undermines the assumption that the computerization of anatomy was an inevitable outcome of technological progress, as it is so often portrayed. Instead, digital anatomy can be traced back to the concerted efforts of a small group of reformers, who embraced the technology as the solution to a very particular set of curricular challenges.

Second, I situate anatomical software in a long line of educational technologies – such as illustrated anatomical atlases, waxes, preserved specimens, and papier-mâché manikins – that have offered either an alternative or a supplement to dissection as a way of knowing. Scholars have written extensively and eloquently about the production, use, and circulation of anatomical illustrations and models.[5] Following their methodological lead, I will take software seriously as an object of material culture, an approach that is also inspired by the emerging field of software studies.[6] By studying early examples of anatomy software, I seek to understand how the body was translated and transformed in digital space, and in so doing make a case that digital models are both distinct and worthy of study.

After a brief overview of the shifting status of gross anatomy within medical education, the narrative shifts to the post-war period, a moment of reckoning for departments of anatomy. The first section of the chapter will suggest that closed-circuit television, programmed learning, and CAI were all part of the same experimental impulse that sought to make teaching anatomy more efficient. I will then trace how federal funding supported the integration of CAI into medical schools, including the first computer-assisted course in gross anatomy without dissection in 1971. The final section of the chapter will explore the development of image-intensive anatomical software in the 1980s and 1990s. While digital anatomical images are now ubiquitous, the creation of a computerized cadaver posed significant creative and technical challenges. In addition to the well-known Visible Human Project, initiated by the NLM in 1989, this chapter presents the history of two other projects, ElectricCadaver and A.D.A.M. (Animated Dissection of Anatomy for Medicine), which each developed their own unique approaches to digitizing the body. The widespread availability of anatomical software has instigated yet another period of reflection and reform for anatomists who continue to grapple with the shifting status of gross anatomy as a cornerstone of medical education.

GROSS ANATOMY IN THE MEDICAL SCHOOL CURRICULUM

While the publication of Andreas Vesalius's *De humani corporis fabrica* in 1543 ushered in a new scientific fashion for human anatomy, it wasn't until the eighteenth century that dissection became an essential component of medical training. Proprietary anatomy schools, such as those operated by famous anatomists William and John Hunter in London, provided students with ample opportunity to dissect, a hands-on education that prepared students for surgical careers. Early American medical schools, founded by physicians trained in the Hunterian tradition, similarly placed dissection at the centre of their curricula.[7]

During the nineteenth century, the experience of dissection "was more prominent in the education of American doctors than any time before or since."[8] The possession of anatomical knowledge set orthodox physicians apart from their competitors in a crowded medical marketplace. Dissection was understood to be at once an important scientific activity and a powerful rite of passage that bordered on the taboo.[9] American medical students posed for photographs around the dissecting table, a genre that hinted at dissection's social function as well as its importance for the formation of professional identity.[10] Student demand for cadavers often outstripped supply, and grave robbing was widespread.[11] Medical schools sought to attract students by amassing impressive anatomical collections, but these museums were used primarily as an adjunct to dissection.[12] Only by obtaining first-hand knowledge of the body could medical students hope to gain access to the profession.

The turn of the century was a time of crisis for anatomy. The rise of new experimental sciences such as bacteriology threatened the subject's dominance in medical education as well as its status as a research discipline.[13] Anatomists, eager to defend their territory, sought to shift the rhetoric surrounding dissection. Instead of emphasizing the affective or professional aspects of dissection, a new generation of scientifically minded anatomists argued that gross anatomy was necessary because the subject prepared students not for the clinic, but for the laboratory. This emphasis on scientific values – objectivity, discipline, and precision – reflected a broader effort to modernize medical education as reflected by the Johns Hopkins model and the publication of the Flexner Report in 1910. That anatomical knowledge might be clinically useful was somewhat beside the point.[14]

This reframing of dissection as a scientific exercise meant that gross anatomy emerged from this period with its curricular status mostly intact. While the average number of hours dedicated to gross anatomy did decrease significantly in the early decades of the twentieth century, from 549 hours in 1909 to 338 hours in 1940, most educators acknowledged that anatomy provided an "underlying foundation for the student's future training and experience."[15] In his 1940 report on the state of American medical education, Herman Weiskotten described an ideal anatomy curriculum that placed a premium on first-hand experience, supplemented by lectures, museum material, and x-ray films where necessary.[16]

It wasn't until after the Second World War that medical education would go through another upheaval analogous to the Flexner-era reforms. New developments in the basic sciences, particularly in the field of molecular biology, demanded more instructional time. A move towards specialism further compounded curricular crowding.[17] At the same time, post-war population growth had created an unprecedented demand for physicians.[18] Fourteen new medical schools opened in the United States, while sixty-four of the eighty-eight existing American schools increased the size of their classes.[19] The looming physician shortage also meant that educators were loath to extend the length of the curriculum. In short, educators were expected to teach more material to more students in less time, a challenge that called for the elimination of all non-essential curricular content.

While no subject was safe from these cuts, gross anatomy was the most obvious target for reform. Gross anatomy still occupied an average of 330 hours of curriculum time, usually concentrated in the first two years.[20] As administrators scrutinized the curriculum for nonessential content, gross anatomy almost always ended up in the crosshairs, "a convenient whipping boy" for the administrative agenda.[21] A 1966 survey by the American Association of Anatomists found that since 1960, one-fifth of all surveyed anatomy departments had already shortened their gross anatomy courses, while an additional third had plans to do so in the near future. In comparison to other basic science disciplines, the Association concluded that "it is apparent that anatomy has been and will be subject to the greatest impact of curricular changes."[22]

In response to these new pressures, departments of anatomy across the country launched a number of curricular experiments throughout the 1960s and 1970s designed to make anatomical instruction more efficient. It is not a coincidence that many of these experiments flourished at newly opened American medical schools, where instructors were free from the twin burdens of tradition and inertia. In keeping with a post-war spirit of technological optimism, experimental programs often integrated cutting-edge instructional technologies such as closed-circuit television, programmed learning, and computer-assisted instruction. Perhaps counterintuitively, these innovations were introduced not to displace dissection, but to preserve it, by outsourcing the transmission of anatomical facts to allow for more time in the anatomy lab.

THE EXPERIMENTAL CLASSROOM

Peering into the experimental classrooms of the post-war period provides insight into how post-war educators imagined technology might transform student learning. Given the visual nature of anatomical learning, it is perhaps not surprising that new audiovisual aids would be integrated into gross anatomy classrooms. The use of film in medical education dates back to the late nineteenth century; by the 1960s, almost every medical school in the United States reported using film as an educational tool.[23] But film was not an overwhelmingly popular method for teaching anatomy. A prerecorded dissection offered little advantage over the study of prepared specimens, models, or even a textbook. Watching a film was ultimately a passive activity, an aid to student learning but no substitute for the hands-on nature of dissection.

Television, however, was perceived very differently. In the 1950s, anatomists were drawn to closed-circuit television as a tool that could promote interactivity in the anatomy lab. Closed-circuit television offered more than a new mode of visual representation: it reconfigured the gross anatomy lab both spatially and temporally. As John Huber, chair of the Department of Anatomy at Temple University, explained it during a conference on the use of audiovisual aids in medical education in 1967: "closed-circuit television can bring happenings, either live or on tape, to large audiences."[24] For Huber, the most exciting feature of closed-circuit television was magnification. An instructor might demonstrate a new dissection technique or point out the features of a prepared specimen, and "every individual in the audience has the equivalent of a front row seat."[25] Huber provided the example of a gross anatomy lab in which one group of students has located an unusual anomaly during the course of their dissection. Instead of students crowding around the dissecting table to jockey for a good look, a closed-circuit setup allowed for every student to participate from their own position in the lab.

Reconfiguring the gross anatomy lab using television was also promoted as a time-saver for the overworked instructor. At the Florida College of Medicine, an administrative edict in 1965 mandated that gross anatomy be reduced from 300 hours to 120 hours, collapsing what had traditionally been a two-year course into one. Faced with this time crunch, instructors sought to design an experimental course that would "fit these requirements without handicapping the students."[26] Closed-circuit television was used to present prosections to the entire class, so that material could be covered at a faster rate. Instructors reported that students were generally enthusiastic about this form of teaching, despite the school's lack of funds for colour televisions. The only stumbling block was that "the ineptness and inexperience of the faculty prevented utilization of this medium's complete potential."[27] Closed-circuit television was similarly integrated into the first-year curriculum at the new School of Medicine at the University of Kentucky, which opened in 1956. Each laboratory session was accompanied by live demonstrations by the instructor, broadcast on closed-circuit televisions. Instructors at the University of Kentucky argued that this method freed the instructor to then circulate through the laboratory to answer questions, instead of performing the same demonstration over and over.[28]

In both cases, the use of closed-circuit television went hand in hand with the use of prosected specimens. Perhaps in embracing an experimental approach, instructors felt less beholden to the tradition of full-body dissection. Neither school did away with dissection completely, but rather contained it or shifted it later in the curriculum. The University of Florida instructors concluded that "by employing prosected demonstration material and modern techniques of mass media presentation, and by discarding the idea that individual dissection of the whole cadaver is mandatory for learning, it has been found that an effective short course in human gross anatomy is feasible."[29]

Programmed instruction was another technology presented as a timesaver in the anatomy lab. The brainchild of psychologist B.F. Skinner, the method was inspired by his research on operant conditioning. In a 1956 paper, Skinner described a system "in which students were exposed to course material in small, incremental steps via frames presented in a box-like apparatus."[30] Every few frames, students would be asked a question to assess their understanding of the material, providing feedback in real time. Programs could be either linear or branched, the latter taking different paths depending on student input.

So-called "teaching machines" became popular at all levels of education, though they were not without their critics. Skeptics scoffed at the concept of a robot teacher, arguing that such a method was dehumanizing and denigrated the bond between teacher and student. Skinner insisted that his system was never meant to replace teachers, but rather to save instructors from the task of preparing and presenting content, thus freeing up time for individualized instruction.[31] Like closed-circuit television, programmed instruction was promoted as a technology that could help teachers make better use of their time, especially as class sizes continued to increase.

A long-standing critique of traditional gross anatomy courses was that too much time was wasted on the rote memorization of anatomical facts.

Programmed instruction offered a solution. While not as popular as the use of closed-circuit television – only sixty-four of eighty-four medical schools reported the use of programmed instruction, and only seven extensively – it appealed to instructors who needed to convey a large amount of material as efficiently as possible.[32] In part, the method was attractive because it did not require the use of specific equipment. Although there were teaching machines purpose-built for the method, programs written for medical students were often presented on paper, with each page representing a "frame" in Skinner's teaching box.

The University of Kentucky, which had already bucked tradition with its use of prosection and closed-circuit television, was also one of the first schools to integrate programmed instruction into its gross anatomy course. Faculty members designed two simple linear programs, using paper and pencil, to teach first-year anatomy students basic terms of orientation and motion. Students generally responded well to the program, though they complained the method was somewhat repetitive. Indeed, it was noted that over ten per cent of students had left their programs blank or less than half completed. Programmed instruction, it seemed, did little to solve the perennial problem of student disengagement.[33] At the University of Iowa, the introduction of programmed anatomy was found to save both time *and* money: on average, students spent 75 fewer hours studying anatomy in their first semester with comparable results, which translated to an estimated cost savings of $1.25 an hour. The programmed curriculum was ultimately adopted by physical therapy, dental, physician assistant, and graduate programs within a year of its introduction in the medical school.[34]

By the early 1970s, medical students across the United States were already trading in their scalpels for screens, and their textbooks for "programs." These new approaches, of course, were not immune to criticism. Hilliard Jason, a prominent medical educator who consulted with the federal government on instructional technologies, described a "country-wide spirit of change" that was both "promising and worrisome."[35] A bad lecture was not made better when it was broadcast on a television screen, and by lending the gloss of innovation to outdated methods, instructional technologies threatened to further perpetuate ineffective pedagogy. Roger Crafts, the chairman of the Department of Anatomy at the University of Cincinnati, echoed Hilliard's concerns. "If it is found by reliable tests that shortcut methods such as TV, movies, programmed learning, prosections, or the use of previously dissected material or museum specimens are effective in reaching stated goals as the customary method of dissecting," Crafts argued, "we should immediately adopt them." But until such a time, traditional courses in gross anatomy needed to be "conserved," as "it is this course in the medical curriculum among all others that ... is being curtailed to an absurd degree."[36] The battle over the future of anatomy education, and the place of technology within it, was already well under way.

COMPUTING IN THE GROSS ANATOMY LAB

As educators debated the merits of closed-circuit television or programmed learning, a new and potentially more radical technology appeared on the scene. Hot on the heels of the teaching machine, by the late 1960s the computer had become the newest darling of educational technologists. Emerging out of wartime research, the computer's military applications were already widely known. Military officials, eager to justify their enormous investment in computing, were actively seeking civilian applications, and medicine and education became major targets for computerization.[37] But as historian Joseph November has argued, there was nothing inevitable about the adoption of computers by biologists and physicians.[38] In fact, for every enthusiastic early adopter, there were many more naysayers who thought computers too expensive, too complex, or simply unnecessary for pedestrian tasks. While it is tempting to assume that the integration of computers into medical classrooms was the obvious outcome of technological progress, teleological narratives tend to obscure how the "groundwork for computerization was laid decades before computers became small, fast, and inexpensive."[39] The early history of computing in medical schools reveals how a pre-existing enthusiasm for reform accelerated the introduction of CAI.

In the United States, the federal government played a central role in the introduction of computers into medical education. Driven by Cold War anxieties about maintaining American scientific superiority, as well as general optimism about the growth of the biological sciences, Congress dedicated $50 million of emergency funding to the National Institutes of Health (NIH) in 1959 to discover and support new applications for computing within medicine.[40] The first "Conference on the Use of Computers in Medical Education," held in April 1968 at the University of Oklahoma Medical Center, was co-sponsored by the US Department of Health, Education, and Welfare, the Public Health Service, and the Bureau of Health Manpower. At the outset of the conference, a statement from the Surgeon General asserted that such a meeting was "not merely timely; it is of the highest urgency."[41] Later that year, the Lister Hill National Center for Biomedical Communications was established as a branch of the NLM. One of the Lister Hill Center's first projects was to collaborate with the American Association of Medical Colleges to establish a network for schools to share the CAI programs they had developed.[42]

While computers would have eventually found their way into medical schools without state support, there is no question that the financial and administrative might of federal agencies accelerated the development of CAI. Between 1968 and 1978, the federal government provided $5.4 million in funding to promote CAI in medical schools, which accounted for sixty per cent of all available funding, including money donated by private foundations and industry. Of that federal money, over fifty per cent went directly to American medical schools to purchase equipment and conduct experiments in CAI.[43]

In the years that followed the initial conference on CAI, computers began to appear in medical schools all around the country. A survey conducted in the fall of 1972 noted that forty of ninety-five medical schools surveyed in the United States and Canada had adopted CAI to some degree, while an additional thirty-one schools planned to purchase a computer in the near future. Over half of these schools purchased an IBM 360/67, a mainframe computer that was part of the company's enormously successful System/360 line. On average, between one and four terminals used to access the mainframe computer were placed in libraries or purpose-built computer labs.[44] For faculty who had previously worked with programmed instruction, the continuity with CAI was obvious. But unlike the simple, linear instructional programs that were printed on paper, computer programs could contain complex branching structures that were responsive to student input. In this sense, CAI was a logical extension of an existing pedagogical trend to transform rote learning into an interactive experience tailored to the individual learner.

The Experimental CAI Network, launched by the Lister Hill Center in July 1972, boasted ninety-five member institutions, a majority of which were medical schools.[45] The network offered a variety of CAI programs, including clinical simulations, dosage calculators, and directed independent study units designed to be integrated into the curriculum. In its first year of operation, the network was entirely subsidized by the NLM, at a rate of $18.78 an hour (a sum that would exceed $100 in 2020). In subsequent years, schools were expected to contribute at least part of the cost, up to $5 an hour.[46]

On the surface, that so many schools joined the network and invested in the necessary hardware indicated a widespread enthusiasm for computerization among medical educators. But observations on the ground revealed that the response was more ambivalent than the numbers might suggest. A report on the first two years of the Experimental CAI Network described widespread faculty resistance, or even hostility, towards the project. At the University of Rochester, demonstrations for faculty were met "with varying degrees of interest but as yet little commitment"; at the Hahnemann Medical College, fewer than ten faculty members agreed to attend a demonstration.[47] At the University of Southern California, faculty members complained that the programs were "dehumanizing" and full of factual errors, though the faculty who took the time to attend demonstrations reportedly "liked the programs and found them stimulating."[48]

In contrast to the skepticism of faculty, medical students expressed near-universal enthusiasm for CAI. Students, especially those in pre-clerkship, were the heaviest users of the network.[49] Given that most CAI programs were extra-curricular, the hours logged by students were entirely voluntary. When certain schools sought to terminate their membership in the network due to rising costs, students were "invariably vociferous in their objections."[50] Students at the Medical College of Virginia, for example, started a petition after the school cancelled its subscription. Comments on the petition included: "It was very, very useful to help develop clinical judgments"; "There was much valuable information in that computer"; "It combined enjoyment with learning"; and "We were going to be married!" (a tongue-in-cheek declaration of affection between student and computer).[51] When faculty at UCLA decided against integrating CAI into the curriculum, students accused them of being "behind the times."[52] While it seems possible that novelty played some role in student interest, the sustained use of the resource indicated that students found real value in computer study.

Browsing a list of the network's programs reveals that educators imagined applications for the computer in every area of medicine, including gross anatomy. A 1972 survey identified seventeen different computer programs designed to teach gross anatomy, by far the most popular application within the basic sciences.[53] Upon first glance, it seems somewhat surprising that gross anatomy would be a popular subject for CAI. While anatomical reformers had embraced other instructional technologies, they were primarily audiovisual. Even paper-based instructional programs could integrate illustrations and diagrams. But what could a computer, with a text-only terminal, offer to a discipline that was overwhelmingly visual? Just like closed-circuit television and programmed instruction, computerized anatomy was never meant to replace traditional approaches, but to improve upon them. By taking on the chore of didactic instruction, the computer freed instructors to use all of their curricular hours at the dissecting table.

The Ohio State University Medical Center was at the cutting edge of CAI and dedicated significant resources to its development.[54] The very first program designed at Ohio State was titled GANAT 1 (Gross Anatomy Self-Evaluation Exercise). Co-authored by faculty members and medical students, GANAT 1 was introduced into an experimental anatomy curriculum at Ohio State in 1967.[55] The program offered students an opportunity to independently review and test their anatomical knowledge. GANAT 1 was one of the most heavily used programs on the experimental network, and in 1973 became a required component of the anatomy curriculum at the Medical College of Wisconsin, with apparent success: students who used GANAT 1 scored significantly higher on the National Board Examination than those who had completed a more conventional lecture-based course.[56]

Following the integration of CAI into the Ohio curriculum, Emory University launched a five-year NIH-funded experiment in their own first-year gross anatomy program.[57] Beginning in the 1971–72 academic year, freshman medical students at Emory were divided into two groups. The control group completed the school's conventional course in gross anatomy, which included both lectures and the dissection of a whole cadaver. The experimental group was taught gross anatomy using computers and other multimedia technologies, forbidden from so much as picking up a scalpel. The Emory program went further than the curricular experiments of the 1960s, which relied heavily on prosected specimens but still offered opportunities for dissection. Emory's decision to eliminate dissection entirely in favour of a computerized approach was so novel as to be newsworthy, with an announcement appearing in newspapers across the country.[58]

A typical day in the Emory gross anatomy lab might have looked something like this: after starting the session off with a film or a slide-tape, a group of students proceeded to study at one of five computer terminals, while others "met with the instructor around prosected specimens for intense demonstration tutorials and oral quizzes."[59] The custom-built computer program took on much of the work of didactic instruction; branching sequences of questions allowed students to work at their own pace. The computer recorded the number of incorrect responses, as well as the time between responses, useful data for tracking student progress. Ultimately, a series of examinations, both internal and external, demonstrated that there was no statistically significant difference in student learning between the two groups, seemingly validating a dissection-free approach.

When Emory faculty published the results of this study in the *Journal of Medical Education*, Bernard Panner, a professor of pathology at the University of Rochester, described his reaction to the paper as "intense."[60] Panner rejected Emory's program as a faddish experiment, a misguided attempt to cater to a generation of screen-happy students who had "taught itself to read by watching 'Sesame Street.'"[61] Dissection cultivated discipline, teamwork, and the "joy of discovery," Panner argued, an experience that computerized instruction could never replicate. Panner needn't have worried; despite the study's positive findings, the experiment had little discernible impact on pedagogical practice at Emory or elsewhere. At the end of the 1970s, CAI was still in its infancy, and the use of computers in medical education was limited to a small cadre of early adopters. But after nearly two decades, experimentation with new instructional technologies was beginning to feel a lot like the status quo. The computer was not yet popular or powerful, but it had already made significant inroads into the anatomy lab.

CADAVERS ON SCREEN

Technological developments in the 1980s saw computers become smaller, faster, and more affordable than their predecessors. As the price of microprocessors fell, compact personal computers were marketed to consumers for the first time. Graphical user interfaces (GUIs) were user-friendly and allowed the display of images in addition to text.[62] Long gone were the days of the bulky mainframe and the text-only terminal – the computer was now a visual medium. Anatomy educators had already acknowledged the computer's potential to enhance anatomical learning, but the expanded graphical capabilities of the personal computer opened up a new world of pedagogical possibilities.

The first attempt to transform a computer into a cadaver actually predated the introduction of GUIs. The University of Wisconsin Anatomy Computer System, developed in 1969, was a joint project of the department of computer science and the university medical centre. With the goal of modelling "gross objects of the physical world," the project was, at its core, an experiment in computing that just happened to have a medical application.[63] Uploading a human body into a machine required programmers to convert body components into numeric expressions, which was achieved by overlaying cross-sectional anatomical images of the male torso with a three-dimensional matrix. These images were repurposed from an atlas of cross-sectional anatomy, first printed in 1911, which was based on classroom dissection of "fifty negro subjects" at the Anatomical Department at St Louis University.[64] Like many other American medical schools, it appears that St Louis University obtained a suspiciously disproportionate number of African-American cadavers for use in their anatomy program.[65] By selecting this particular text, the programmers directly encoded the racist history of American anatomy into the first digital model of the human body.

Each block of the coordinate grid was given a coded descriptor, which allowed the computer to identify which anatomical features were present in each section of the image. Based on this data, the user of the program was able to ask the computer questions. The questions ranged from the very simple "Are you aware of body component x?" to "What is dorsal to the prostate gland 764?"[66] The computer's answers could be quite detailed; for example, it could tell the user that the spleen was part of the hemic system, as well its size, volume, and the bodily components that surrounded it. While the authors described the work as "seemingly trivial in its results," they envisioned a program that could "communicate not just through written language, but by using visual display and photographs presented to a user as object images for interactive communication."[67]

This dream of an interactive digital cadaver would not be realized for another two decades. But what was clear, even as early as 1969, was that building a three-dimensional model of the body presented a technical challenge that demanded creativity as well as interdisciplinary collaboration. Proposed in 1989, the NLM's Visible Human Project (VHP) is perhaps the most famous attempt to digitize the human body. The VHP was a logical extension of the NLM's role as a facilitator of biomedical computing and CAI. Given the advance of both imaging and computing technologies, the NLM anticipated a demand for high-quality digital medical images. The stated purpose of the VHP was not to create software for educational purposes, but instead to create a digital image library that could then be utilized for a wide variety of medical applications.[68]

Work on the VHP got underway in 1991 with the opening of the Center for Human Simulation at the University of Colorado. Two cadavers – one male and one female – were cryogenically frozen and imaged using a magnetic resonance imaging (MRI) machine and a computer tomography (CT) scan. The bodies were then fitted into a dissection or "milling" device, sliced into one-millimeter cross-sections, and photographed.[69] Taken together, these images allowed for a complete digital reconstruction of the body. The model of the male cadaver, known as the "Visible Man," became available on the World Wide Web in 1994.[70]

The VHP attracted a significant amount of attention, both public and scholarly.[71] There are several explanations for this, including the spectacular nature of the images, the gruesome method of their creation, and the controversial selection of executed felon Joseph Jernigan as the first "Visible Man."[72] The sensational aspects of the VHP, however, have overshadowed contemporaneous and, perhaps, more mundane attempts to build a digital model of the human body. The remainder of this chapter will examine the history of two such projects – ElectricCadaver and A.D.A.M. Both projects predated the VHP and deployed very different approaches to digitizing the human body, revealing a diversity of material practices and institutional approaches in the creation of early anatomy software.

ElectricCadaver was developed at Stanford University Medical Center by hand surgeon Robert Chase and physician Steven Freedman.[73] In 1986, Freedman was a recent graduate of medical school who was fascinated with the idea of developing an electronic textbook.[74] The electronic textbook would have all of the features of a traditional book with the addition of video, animations, and a search function. ElectricCadaver was developed using Hypercard, a "software erector set" released for the Apple Macintosh personal computer in 1987.[75] Using Hypercard, even a relatively inexperienced programmer could create a stack of digital cards containing text and graphics that could be linked using hypertext. This "dynamic cross-referencing system" allowed students to easily jump between related concepts, mimicking the non-linear nature of the learning process.[76]

What was novel about ElectricCadaver was the ability to interact with a digital model of the human body. A simple bitmapped line drawing of a man was displayed on the computer monitor. The user could click to zoom in anywhere on the body, displaying line drawings with increasing degrees of anatomical detail. On a television monitor next to the computer, high-quality photographs of prosected specimens would appear that corresponded to the line drawing on the screen.[77] This setup added a visual dimension that had been missing in previous CAI programs. Now, a student could simultaneously view descriptive text and high-quality anatomical images, side by side.

The photographs used in ElectricCadaver were the work of late anatomist David Bassett, whose stereoscopic atlas of human anatomy was considered to be a "definitive work" by many anatomists.[78] Bassett began work on the atlas in 1948 in collaboration with William B. Gruber, a photographer and inventor of the popular "View-Master" stereoscope. At this time, Bassett was a professor of anatomy at Stanford, and would spend weeks meticulously preparing specimens for Gruber to photograph. Every few weeks, Gruber would visit Bassett at home, photographing the specimens from slightly different angles to create the depth necessary for stereoscopic viewing.[79] The images were unique in that they were intended to be viewed in three dimensions from the outset, although this perspective could not yet be simulated digitally. Instead, the nearly 1,600 stereoscopic slides had to be photographed to create two-dimensional images that were then loaded onto a videodisc. Chase remained hopeful that the images could one day be digitized and viewed in three dimensions, as Bassett and Gruber had intended.[80] ElectricCadaver was used as an electronic textbook at Stanford shortly after its completion, though plans to widely distribute the software never materialized.[81] Perhaps its most significant legacy was the creation of SUMMIT (Stanford University Medical Media & Information Technologies), a unit within the Stanford Department of Anatomy that focuses on the development of new curricular technology.[82]

Unlike ElectricCadaver and the VHP, which were both academic ventures, A.D.A.M. originated in an unexpected place: the personal injury law firm. In fact, there were no physicians or anatomists involved in its creation. Instead, A.D.A.M. was the brainchild of Gregory M. Swayne, a medical illustrator, and Robert S. Cramer, Jr, an entrepreneur with a background in publishing.[83] In 1985, after completing a master's degree in medical illustration, Swayne realized there was an untapped market for medical illustrations to be used at trials, especially in personal injury cases. Swayne, along with Cramer, founded a company called Medical Legal Illustrations Incorporated. By all accounts, the company was a success, but by 1989 Swayne was looking for something new. A failed attempt at magazine publishing opened up the pair's eyes to the computer's graphical potential. Swayne, inspired by the transparent layers used to illustrate anatomy in medical encyclopedias, envisioned a computer program where the body could be similarly dissected, layer by layer.[84]

In late 1989, Swayne set out to create the thousands of detailed images that such a piece of software would require. After drawing the hand and foot, Swayne realized it would take more than a decade to carry out the project on his own, so he used the profits generated by his first company to hire a team of twenty illustrators to assist him. They worked out of A.D.A.M. Inc.'s Atlanta headquarters, where all of the rooms were given appropriate anatomical names (the bathroom was the "Kidney Room," Swayne's office the "Hypothalamus," and so on). The artists agreed on dimensions, style, and a colour palette in order to give A.D.A.M., the software's five-foot-ten namesake, a uniform appearance. At least ten anatomical works, as well as anatomists at Emory, were consulted during the illustration process.[85] The fact that A.D.A.M. had many creators, all drawing on different sources, made him the first true digital cadaver: a composite body who was purpose-built for the virtual realm.

While A.D.A.M. was a commercial success, it was not widely adopted in medical schools. This was due, in part, to the cost of the software. Depending on configuration, A.D.A.M. was priced between $500 and $2,300, an expense that was prohibitive for many schools.[86] Marketing claims that A.D.A.M. was "the Gray's Anatomy of the 21st century" and would enable students to "dissect without cadavers" also seemed to rub medical educators the wrong way.[87] When British medical students were given the opportunity to try A.D.A.M. in 1994, they reported that the program was "fun" and would be useful as a study tool. According to their professor, however, "they all agreed no computer program would replace the hands-on experience of dissection."[88]

What these short histories of the VHP, ElectricCadaver, and A.D.A.M. demonstrate is that the creation of digital tools for anatomical education was neither inevitable nor fast; it required as much ingenuity and craft as the elaborately illustrated anatomical text or carefully sculpted wax model. Whether it was the repurposing of older images, a team of illustrators building a body from scratch, or the use of imaging technology to scan the human body, anatomical software has a material history all its own.

CONCLUSIONS

By the late 1990s, the successful commercialization of anatomy software prompted a new wave of soul-searching among anatomists, what could be characterized as a third period of crisis in American anatomy education analogous to the Flexnerian and post-war-era reforms.[89] Ironically, much of this discussion took place online, with anatomists using listservs and discussion forums to debate the fate of dissection in a digital world.[90] Countless articles on digital anatomy appeared in medical journals as well as the popular press, with most suggesting dissection was "on its way out."[91]

But by presenting dissection as a casualty of the computer, these narratives obscure the early history of digital anatomy as well as critiques of dissection that significantly predated the Internet era. A number of concurrent trends during the 1960s and 1970s – including changing funerary practices, the introduction of body donation programs, and a cultural backlash against the medical profession – renewed conversations about the affective dimensions of dissection. Critics of the practice argued that dissection was damaging to the emotional socialization of medical students, fostering "detached concern" and hindering the development of empathy.[92] Interestingly, as digital tools for teaching anatomy became more powerful, defenders of dissection often inverted these critiques by placing a positive emphasis on the emotional dimension of interacting with a cadaver. If dissection could be dehumanizing, computerized anatomy was even worse, as it decentred the body – and the patient – entirely.[93]

Anatomists have also expressed skepticism that two-dimensional images displayed on a screen could ever be an adequate substitute for the hands-on experience of dissection. This argument echoes a centuries-old debate about the relative merits of tactile and visual knowledge in learning anatomy. Advocates of dissection have long been skeptical of visual aids, such as preserved specimens or frozen sections, as insufficient for truly knowing the body.[94] But as the early history of anatomy software reveals, computer anatomy was never intended to be a replacement for dissection. Instead, it was a technological response to a very specific set of curricular challenges. By making the transmission of anatomical facts more efficient, instructors could make the most of their time in the anatomy lab. That the use of anatomical software significantly predates the development of sophisticated digital imagery forces a re-evaluation of popular narratives that present computerized anatomy as an existential threat to dissection, as opposed to a good-faith attempt to adapt to a new curricular reality.

Indeed, despite the proliferation of narratives pitting computer against cadaver, dissection as a pedagogical practice remains alive and well. Computers may not be the future of anatomy, as so many have predicted, but they have become a significant part of its history. A material history of computerized anatomy places software in a long tradition of crafting three-dimensional models of the body and, in so doing, undermines a narrative that positions the computer as an unprecedented or radical threat to anatomical tradition. Fifty years after the first computer was installed in an anatomy lab, A.D.A.M. can take its place alongside *Gray's Anatomy* in the history of medical education.

NOTES

1 Maclay, "Correspondence: Additional Medical Schools," 1120.

2 See, for example, Aziz et al., "The Human Cadaver in the Age of Biomedical Informatics"; McLachlan et al., "Teaching Anatomy without Cadavers"; and Scheckler, "It's More than a Computer Can Deliver."

3 Rizzolo and Stewart, "Should We Continue Teaching Anatomy by Dissection When …?"

4 November, *Biomedical Computing*; Prentice, *Bodies in Formation.*

5 Berkowitz, "The Beauty of Anatomy"; Dacome, *Malleable Anatomies*; Lamb, "Model Behaviour"; Maerker, *Model Experts*; Richardson, *The Making of Mr. Gray's Anatomy*; Sappol and the National Library of Medicine, *Dream Anatomy.*

6 Ensmenger, "Software as History Embodied"; Fuller et al., eds., *Software Studies.*

7 Blake, "Anatomy"; Sappol, *Traffic of Dead Bodies*, ch. 2.

8 Warner and Edmonson, *Dissection*, 8.

9 Ibid.; Sappol, *Traffic of Dead Bodies*; Warner and Rizzolo, "Anatomical Instruction."

10 Warner and Edmonson, *Dissection.*

11 Blake, "Anatomy," 37–8; MacGillivray, "Body-Snatching in Ontario"; Richardson, *Death, Dissection and the Destitute*; Sappol, *Traffic of Dead Bodies*, ch. 3.

12 Sappol, *Traffic of Dead Bodies*, 276.

13 Warner and Rizzolo, "Anatomical Instruction."

14 Blake, "Anatomy," 41–3; Hildebrandt, "Lessons to Be Learned from the History of Anatomical Teaching in the United States"; Warner and Rizzolo, "Anatomical Instruction," 408.

15 Bardeen, "Report of the Sub-Committee on Anatomy," 434; Council on Medical Education, *Medical Education in the United States*, 119, 123.

16 Council on Medical Education, *Medical Education in the United States*, 119–27.

17 Ludmerer, *Time to Heal*, ch. 11; Educational Affairs Committee, "Curriculum, Faculty, and Training in Anatomy," 956.

18 Bane, *Physicians for a Growing America.*

19 Educational Affairs Committee, "Curriculum, Faculty, and Training in Anatomy," 956.

20 Hoerr, "The Role of the Anatomical Disciplines," 14.

21 Stokes, "A Critical Evaluation of Research and Teaching in Anatomy," 978.

22 Educational Affairs Committee, "Curriculum, Faculty, and Training in Anatomy," 959.

23 Essex-Lopresti, "Centenary of the Medical Film," 819–20; Creer, "Use, Abuse and Misuse of Teaching Films," 1090; Jason, *Instructional Technology in Medical Education*, 24.

24 Huber, "Intramural Closed-Circuit Television Teaching," 1106.

25 Ibid., 1107.

26 Callahan and Gavan, "A Course in Gross Anatomy," 1107.

27 Ibid., 1110.

28 Benton and Cotter, "Seven Years' Experience," 1102.

29 Callahan and Gavan, "A Course in Gross Anatomy," 1114.

30 Rutherford, *Beyond the Box*, 27.

31 Ibid., 28–9.

32 Jason, *Instructional Technology in Medical Education*, 24.

33 Peck and Benton, "The Introduction of Programmed Instruction," 766.

34 Moffat, "Programmed Learning in Gross Human Anatomy," 973–8.

35 Jason, *Instructional Technology*, 6.

36 Crafts, "Conservation of Our Gross Anatomy Courses," 71.

37 Van Meer, "PLATO"; November, *Biomedical Computing*, ch. 2.

38 November, *Biomedical Computing*, Introduction.

39 Ibid., 8.

40 Ibid., 7.

41 United States Department of Health, Education, and Welfare, *Proceedings [of the] Conference on the Use of Computers in Medical Education*, 16.

42 Wooster, "An Experiment in Networking."

43 United States Congress Office of Technology Assessment, *Computer Technology in Medical Education and Assessment*, 23–4.

44 Brigham and Kamp, "The Current Status of Computer-Assisted Instruction," 278–9.

45 Rubin et al., *Evaluation of the Experimental CAI Network*, 6.

46 Wooster, "An Experiment in Networking," 334.

47 Rubin et al., *Evaluation of the Experimental CAI Network*, 13–14.

48 Ibid., 26.

49 Ibid., 15.

50 Ibid., 12.

51 Ibid., 31–2.

52 Ibid., 30.

53 Brigham and Kamp, "The Current Status of Computer-Assisted Instruction," 278.

54 Weinberg, "CAI at the Ohio State University College of Medicine (1973)," 299–305.

55 Ibid., 302.

56 Rubin et al., *Evaluation of the Experimental CAI Network*, 48–9.

57 Jones et al., "Evaluation of a Gross Anatomy Program without Dissection," 198–205.

58 E.g. "Anatomy by Computer," *The Hartford Courant*, 1 September 1971; "Computerized Anatomy," *Los Angeles Times*, 9 March 1975.

59   Jones et al., "Evaluation of a Gross Anatomy Program without Dissection," 199.

60   Bernard Panner, "Anatomy without Dissection," 623.

61   Ibid.

62   Campbell-Kelly et al., *Computer*, ch. 10.

63   Fiege Jr. et al., "An Experimental Anatomy Computer System," 373.

64   Ibid., 375; Eycleshymer and Schoemaker, *A Cross-section Anatomy*, xiv.

65   Halperin, "The Poor, the Black, and the Marginalized as the Source of Cadavers in United States Anatomical Education"; Washington, *Medical Apartheid*, ch. 5.

66   Fiege et al., "An Experimental Anatomy Computer System," 375–6.

67   Ibid., 379.

68   Ackerman, "Accessing the Visible Human Project."

69   Ackerman, "The Visible Human Project," 504–11; Waldby, *The Visible Human Project*, 12.

70   Cartwright, "A Cultural Anatomy of the Visible Human Project," 22.

71   Ibid.; Stern, "Dystopian Anxieties"; Waldby, *Visible Human Project*; Van Dijck, "Digital Cadavers." The Visible Human Project also received extensive coverage in the news media. See "The Visible Man"; Van, "The World's Fair of Anatomy"; Brown, "Not Just Any Cadaver Would Suffice"; "Cybercadavers"; Dowling, "How One Death Row Prisoner Found Afterlife on the Internet."

72   Cartwright, "A Cultural Anatomy"; Brown, "Not Just Any Cadaver Would Suffice."

73   Chen, "Medical Students to Study Anatomy with Computer Cadavers"; "The Electric Cadaver," 14; Freedman and Chase, "Electriccadaver," 1021–3.

74   "The Electric Cadaver," 14; Zagari, "The Electric Cadaver," 781.

75   Wooley-McKay, "Hypercard – What Is It?" 34.

76   "The Electric Cadaver," 14.

77   Freedman and Chase, "Electriccadaver," 1021.

78   Bassett, *A Stereoscopic Atlas of Human Anatomy*; "Computer Corpse for Students Cuts Down on Dissection," 38.

79   Chase, "The Wonderful Legacy of David L. Bassett," 153; John Schwartz, "The Body in Depth."

80   Chase, "The Wonderful Legacy of David L. Bassett," 155. In 2008, the Bassett collection was made available online by Silicon Valley Company eHuman, which as of 2020 has used the images to create three-dimensional virtual reality products, primarily for dental students. White, "Dazzling Dissection Images from Famed Bassett Collection Now Online"; eHuman Digital Anatomy, https://ehuman.com.

81   Altman, "Computers Create Electronic 'Cadavers' For Anatomy Lessons."

82   "Fact File Q&A: SUMMIT."

83   A.D.A.M., "The Birth of A.D.A.M. Software Inc."

84 Deriso, "The Genesis of A.D.A.M.," 12.

85 Ibid.

86 Seymour, "A.D.A.M. (Animated Dissection of Anatomy for Medicine)," 88.

87 Kristmundsdottir, "A.D.A.M. (Animated Dissection of Anatomy for Medicine)," 748.

88 Ibid.

89 Prentice, *Bodies in Formation*, ch. 2.

90 Paalman, "Why Teach Anatomy?" 1–2; "Virtual Issue: Dissection and Anatomy Education."

91 Zugler, "Anatomy Lessons, A Vanishing Rite for Young Doctors." See also Noonan, "Is the Cadaver Dead?"; Dotinga, "Med Schools Cut Out Cadavers"; Aziz et al., "The Human Cadaver in the Age of Biomedical Informatics"; Reidenberg and Laitman, "The New Face of Gross Anatomy"; McLachlan et al., "Teaching Anatomy without Cadavers."

92 Warner and Rizzolo, "Anatomical Instruction," 409.

93 Flack and Nicholson, "What Do Medical Students Learn from Dissection?"; Dyer and Thorndike, "Quidne mortui vivos docent?"

94 Al-Gailani, "The 'Ice Age' of Anatomy and Obstetrics."

BIBLIOGRAPHY

A.D.A.M. "The Birth of A.D.A.M. Software Inc." Archived 23 October 1996. https://web.archive.org/web/19961023201355/http://adam.com:80/adaminfo.html.

Ackerman, Michael J. "Accessing the Visible Human Project." *D-Lib Magazine* 1, no. 4 (1995).

Al-Gailani, Salim. "The 'Ice Age' of Anatomy and Obstetrics: Hand and Eye in the Promotion of Frozen Sections around 1900." *Bulletin of the History of Medicine* 90, no. 4 (2016): 611–42.

Altman, Lawrence. "Computers Create Electronic 'Cadavers' for Anatomy Lessons." *New York Times*, 6 September 1988.

Aziz, M. Ashraf, et al. "The Human Cadaver in the Age of Biomedical Informatics." *Anatomical Record* 269, no. 1 (2002): 20–32.

Bane, Frank. *Physicians for a Growing America: Report of the Surgeon General's Consultant Group on Medical Education.* Public Health Service Publication No. 709. Washington, DC: Government Printing Office, 1959.

Bardeen, C.R. "Report of the Sub-Committee on Anatomy to the Council on Medical Education of the American Medical Association. April, 1909." *The Anatomical Record* 3, no. 7 (1909): 415–39.

Bassett, David Lee. *A Stereoscopic Atlas of Human Anatomy.* Portland, OR: Sawyer, 1952.

Benton, R., and W. Cotter. "Seven Years' Experience with an Approach to a 'Vertical' Curriculum in Gross Anatomy." *Journal of Medical Education* 43, no. 10 (1968): 1098–1105.

Berkowitz, Carin. "The Beauty of Anatomy: Visual Displays and Surgical Education in Early-Nineteenth-Century London." *Bulletin of the History of Medicine* 85, no. 2 (2011): 248–78.

Blake, J.B. "Anatomy." In *The Education of American Physicians: Historical Essays*, edited by Ronald Numbers, 29–47. Berkeley, CA: University of California Press, 1980.

Brigham, Christopher R., and Martin Kamp. "The Current Status of Computer-Assisted Instruction in the Health Sciences." *Journal of Medical Education* 49, no. 3 (1974): 278–9.

Brown, David. "Not Just Any Cadaver Would Suffice." *The Washington Post*, 13 January 1999.

Callahan, W., and J. Gavan. "A Course in Gross Anatomy." *Journal of Medical Education* 43, no. 10 (1968): 1105–14.

Campbell-Kelly, Martin, et al. *Computer: A History of the Information Machine*, 3rd ed. New York: Westview Press, 2013.

Cartwright, Lisa. "A Cultural Anatomy of the Visible Human Project." In *The Visible Woman: Imaging Technologies, Gender, and Science*, edited by Paula Treichler, Lisa Cartwright, and Constance Penley, 21–43. New York: NYU Press, 1998.

Chase, Robert A. "The Wonderful Legacy of David L. Bassett." *Clinical Anatomy* 5, no. 2 (1992): 151–5.

Chen, Frank. "Medical Students to Study Anatomy with Computer Cadavers." *The Stanford Daily*, 8 February 1989.

"Computer Corpse for Students Cuts Down on Dissection." *New Scientist*, 2 June 1988.

Council on Medical Education. *Medical Education in the United States 1934–1939: Prepared for the Council on Medical Education and Hospitals of the American Medical Association*. Chicago, IL: American Medical Association, 1940.

Crafts, R. "Conservation of Our Gross Anatomy Courses." *Journal of Medical Education* 43, no. 1 (1968): 70–2.

Creer, P. "Use, Abuse and Misuse of Teaching Films." *Canadian Medical Association Journal* 98, no. 23 (1968): 1090–4.

"Cybercadavers: Slices of Life on the Internet." *The Globe and Mail*, 26 October 1996.

Dacome, Lucia. *Malleable Anatomies: Models, Makers, and Material Culture in Eighteenth-Century Italy*. Oxford, UK: Oxford University Press, 2017.

Deriso, Christine Hurley. "The Genesis of A.D.A.M." *Medical College of Georgia Today* 24, no. 1 (Fall 1995): 10–12.

Dotinga, Randy. "Med Schools Cut Out Cadavers." *Wired*, 19 May 2003.

Dowling, C. "How One Death Row Prisoner Found Afterlife on the Internet." *Life*, February 1997, 40–7.

Dyer, George S.M., and Mary E.L. Thorndike. "Quidne mortui vivos docent? The Evolving Purpose of Human Dissection in Medical Education." *Academic Medicine* 75, no. 10 (2000): 969–79.

Educational Affairs Committee, American Association of Anatomists. "Curriculum, Faculty, and Training in Anatomy." *Journal of Medical Education* 41, no. 10 (1966): 956–64.

"The Electric Cadaver." *Byte*, August 1988.

Ensmenger, Nathan. "Software as History Embodied." IEEE *Annals of the History of Computing* 31, no. 1 (2009): 86–8.

Essex-Lopresti, Michael. "Centenary of the Medical Film." *The Lancet* 349, no. 9055 (1997): 819–20.

Eycleshymer, Albert Chauncey, and Daniel Martin Schoemaker. *A Cross-Section Anatomy*. New York and London: D. Appleton, 1911.

"Fact File Q&A: SUMMIT." *Stanford Hospital and Clinics Medical Staff Update* 24, no. 9 (October 2000).

Fiege Jr., Reynold H., et al. "An Experimental Anatomy Computer System." *Computers and Biomedical Research* 2, no. 4 (1969): 373–84.

Flack, Natasha A.M.S., and Helen D. Nicholson. "What Do Medical Students Learn from Dissection?" *Anatomical Sciences Education* 11, no. 4 (2018): 325–35.

Freedman, Steve Jay, and Robert A. Chase. "Electriccadaver: A Dynamic Book of Human Structure and Function." In *Proceedings of the Annual Symposium on Computer Application in Medical Care*, 1021–3. Washington, DC: IEEE Computer Society Press, 1989.

Fuller, Matthew, Roger F. Malina, and Sean Cubitt, eds. *Software Studies: A Lexicon*. Cambridge, MA: MIT Press, 2008.

Halperin, Edward C. "The Poor, the Black, and the Marginalized as the Source of Cadavers in United States Anatomical Education." *Clinical Anatomy* 20, no. 5 (2007): 489–95.

Hildebrandt, Sabine. "Lessons to Be Learned from the History of Anatomical Teaching in the United States: The Example of the University of Michigan." *Anatomical Sciences Education* 3, no. 4 (2010): 202–12.

Hoerr, N.L. "The Role of the Anatomical Disciplines in Medical Education." *Journal of Medical Education* 31 (1956): 7–24.

Huber, J.F. "Intramural Closed-Circuit Television Teaching: Pre-Clinical Uses." *The Canadian Medical Association Journal* 98, no. 23 (1968): 1106–9.

Jason, Hilliard. *Instructional Technology in Medical Education*. Washington, DC: Office of Education Bureau of Research, 1970.

Jones, Nobert A., et al. "Evaluation of a Gross Anatomy Program without Dissection." *Journal of Medical Education* 53, no. 3 (1978): 198–205.

Kristmundsdottir, F. "A.D.A.M. (Animated Dissection of Anatomy for Medicine). CD-ROM Program." *British Medical Journal* 309, no. 6956 (1994): 748.

Lamb, Susan. "Model Behavior: A Material Culture Approach to the History of Anatomy Models." In *Building New Bridges*, edited by J. Keshen and S. Perrier, 29–48. Ottawa: University of Ottawa Press, 2005.

Ludmerer, Kenneth M. *Time to Heal: American Medical Education from the Turn of the Century to the Era of Managed Care.* Oxford, UK: Oxford University Press, 1999.

MacGillivray, Royce. "Body-Snatching in Ontario." *Canadian Bulletin of Medical History* 5, no. 1 (1988): 51–60.

Maclay, Charles. "Correspondence: Additional Medical Schools." *South African Medical Journal* 43 (1969): 1120.

Maerker, Anna. *Model Experts: Wax Anatomies and Enlightenment in Florence and Vienna, 1775–1815.* Manchester, UK: Manchester University Press, 2011.

McLachlan, John C., et al. "Teaching Anatomy without Cadavers." *Medical Education* 38, no. 4 (2004): 418–24.

Moffat, D. "Programmed Learning in Gross Human Anatomy." *Journal of Medical Education* 49, no. 10 (1974): 973–8.

Noonan, David. "Is the Cadaver Dead?" *Newsweek*, 23 June 2002.

November, Joseph. *Biomedical Computing: Digitizing Life in the United States.* Baltimore, MD: JHU Press, 2012.

Paalman, Mark H. "Why Teach Anatomy? Anatomists Respond." *The Anatomical Record* 261, no. 1 (2000): 1–2.

Panner, Bernard. "Anatomy without Dissection." *Journal of Medical Education* 53, no. 7 (1978): 623–4.

Peck, D., and R. Benton. "The Introduction of Programmed Instruction into a Gross Anatomy Course by Means of 'Unit Programming.'" *Journal of Medical Education* 45, no. 10 (1970): 760–9.

Prentice, Rachel. *Bodies in Formation: An Ethnography of Anatomy and Surgery Education.* Durham, NC: Duke University Press, 2013.

Reidenberg, Joy S., and Jeffrey T. Laitman. "The New Face of Gross Anatomy." *The Anatomical Record* 269, no. 2 (2002): 81–8.

Richardson, Ruth. *Death, Dissection and the Destitute.* Chicago, IL: University of Chicago Press, 2000.

– *The Making of Mr. Gray's Anatomy: Bodies, Books, Fortune, Fame.* Oxford, UK: Oxford University Press, 2008.

Rizzolo, Lawrence, and William B. Stewart. "Should We Continue Teaching Anatomy by Dissection When …?" *Anatomical Record* 289B, no. 6 (2006): 215–18.

Rubin, Martin L., Beverly Hunter, and Marilyn Knetsch. *Evaluation of the Experimental CAI Network (1973–1975) of the Lister Hill National Center for Biomedical Communications, National Library of Medicine, Final Report. No. ED-75-1.* Alexandra, VA: Human Resources Research Organization, 1975.

Rutherford, Alexandra. *Beyond the Box: B.F. Skinner's Technology of Behaviour from Laboratory to Life, 1950s–1970s.* Toronto: University of Toronto Press, 2009.

Sappol, Michael. *A Traffic of Dead Bodies: Anatomy and Embodied Social Identity in Nineteenth-Century America.* Princeton, NJ: Princeton University Press, 2002.

Sappol, Michael, and the National Library of Health. *Dream Anatomy.* Bethesda, MD: US Department of Health and Human Services, National Institutes of Health, National Library of Medicine, 2006.

Scheckler, William. "It's More than a Computer Can Deliver: Gross Anatomy – A Rite of Passage and a Right to Learning." WMJ-MADISON- 102, no. 2 (2003): 10–11.

Schwartz, John. "The Body in Depth." *The New York Times*, 22 April 2008.

Seymour, Anne K. "A.D.A.M. (Animated Dissection of Anatomy for Medicine)." *Bulletin of the Medical Library Association* 81, no. 1 (1993): 88–9.

Stern, Megan. "Dystopian Anxieties versus Utopian Ideals: Medicine from Frankenstein to the Visible Human Project and Body World." *Science as Culture* 15, no. 1 (2006): 61–84.

Stokes, J. "A Critical Evaluation of Research and Teaching in Anatomy." *Journal of Medical Education* 40, no. 10 (1965): 978–9.

United States Congress Office of Technology Assessment. *Computer Technology in Medical Education and Assessment.* Washington, DC: US Government Printing Office, 1979.

United States Department of Health, Education, and Welfare. *Proceedings [of the] Conference on the Use of Computers in Medical Education, Apr. 3–5, 1968.* Oklahoma City, OK: University of Oklahoma Medical Center, 1968.

Van Dijck, José. "Digital Cadavers: The Visible Human Project as Anatomical Theater." *Studies in History and Philosophy of Science Part C* 31, no. 2 (2000): 271–85.

Van Meer, Elisabeth. "PLATO: From Computer-Based Education to Corporate Social Responsibility." *Iterations: An Interdisciplinary Journal of Software History* 2, no. 1 (2003): 1–22.

Van, Jon. "The World's Fair of Anatomy." *Chicago Tribune*, 29 November 1994.

"Virtual Issue: Dissection and Anatomy Education." *The New Anatomist (Part B of The Anatomical Record)* 281B (2004). Archived 5 December 2004. https://web.archive.org/web/20041205183948/http://www.wiley.com/legacy/products/subject/life/anatomy/dissection.html.

"The Visible Man." *The Economist*, 19 October 1996.

Waldby, Catherine. *The Visible Human Project: Informatic Bodies and Posthuman Medicine.* London and New York: Routledge, 2000.

Warner, John Harley, and James M. Edmonson. *Dissection: Photographs of a Rite of Passage in American Medicine, 1880–1930.* New York: Blast Books, 2009.

Warner, John Harley, and Lawrence J. Rizzolo. "Anatomical Instruction and Training for Professionalism from the 19th to the 21st Centuries." *Clinical Anatomy* 19, no. 5 (2006): 403–14.

Washington, Harriet. *Medical Apartheid: The Dark History of Medical Experimentation on Black Americans from Colonial Times to the Present.* New York: Doubleday Books, 2006.

Weinberg, Armin D. "CAI at the Ohio State University College of Medicine (1973)." *Computers in Biology and Medicine* 3, no. 3 (1973): 299–305.

White, Traci. "Dazzling Dissection Images from Famed Bassett Collection Now Online." *Stanford Report*, 20 February 2009.

Wooley-McKay, Dorothy. "Hypercard – What Is It?" *Computers in Life Science Education* 5, no. 5 (1988): 34.

Wooster, Harold. "An Experiment in Networking: The LHNCBC Experimental CAI Network, 1971–1975." *Journal of the American Society for Information Science* 27, no. 5 (1976): 329–38.

Zagari, Martin. "The Electric Cadaver." *JAMA (Pulse Medical Student Supplement)* 261, no. 5 (1989): 781–3.

Zugler, Abigail. "Anatomy Lessons, A Vanishing Rite for Young Doctors." *New York Times*, 23 March 2004.

PART FOUR

Professional Identities: Gender, Emotions, Performance

15

Emotions and the Irish Medical Student, c. 1840–1940

Laura Kelly

In his 1957 memoir *Surgeon's Journey*, J. Johnston Abraham, who studied at Trinity College Dublin in the 1890s, vividly recalled commencing his medical education:

> So, at the age of eighteen, I was ready and eager to plunge into the work that was to train me for the career I had been thinking of ever since I was a little boy. All I had been doing up to now was in anticipation of this; and the Head decided I was to sit for the next entrance examination to the University. This was in October, during the first week of Michaelmas term; I knew that on passing it my whole future depended, and I was therefore nervously excited.[1]

Like many other Irish doctors' memoirs published in the twentieth century, Abraham's is filled with the common tropes of a lifelong ambition to study medicine, the knowledge of the importance of hard work to success in medical study, and the emotions of nervousness and excitement about what lay before him. Emotions are dotted throughout Abraham's memoirs. He later describes feeling "thrilled" passing by the gates of Trinity College, knowing that he would soon be a student there, before discussing his shyness and nervousness meeting the college registrar, Anthony Traill, his sense of unease in entering the dissecting room for the first time, and his happiness upon beginning his hospital experience.

As well as being described in emotional terms, beginning medical school marked an important transition from boyhood to adulthood for some students. R.W.M. Strain, a student at Queen's University Belfast, who began his first year of medical school in 1924–25, explained that "the school cap which generations of Inst. boys had worn with the peak screwed deliberately over the right ear was no longer appropriate, and went to the dust bin … instead, my

old friend Joe Gray and I purchased rather woolly felt hats, and we knew that
school days were gone."[2] As well as this, such accounts are further complicated
by the tendency among doctors and medical students of the past to describe
their student days and experiences in nostalgic terms.

In her ground-breaking article on the history of emotions in 2002,
Barbara Rosenwein put forward the concept of "emotional communities."
She described these as being the same as social communities such as families,
neighbourhoods, and guilds, with the difference being that the "researcher
looking at them seeks above all to uncover systems of feeling."[3] Through leaving behind the 'grand narrative' that had dominated emotions scholarship,
Rosenwein proposed that "the new narrative will recognise various emotional
styles, emotional communities, emotional outlets, and emotional restraints
in every period, and it will consider how and why these have changed over
time."[4] As Jan Plamper and Keith Tribe assess in their introduction to the history of emotions, "the conception of emotional communities is an attractive
way of approaching the way in which emotional bonds are formed and reproduced."[5] Rosenwein has also encouraged historians to think about reading for
"silences." Some texts are "unemotional in tone and content" and she argues
that these are just as important as "overtly emotional texts."[6] For instance, in
the case of texts produced by medical students and former medical students,
a lack of expressed emotion around a topic, such as one's first entrance to the
dissecting room, does not necessarily mean that the student did not experience
emotions around this event in his or her medical studies. Rather, a silence
around this could imply a desire to present an heroic front.

To date, historians of the medical profession and medical education have
been reluctant to apply methodologies from the history of emotions to their
work.[7] Michael Brown's recent chapter on surgery and emotion in the era
before anaesthesia in Britain is an important intervention. Brown illustrates
how "compassion and emotional expression played a surprisingly important
role in shaping the cultures of early nineteenth-century operative surgery as
well as the identities of its practitioners."[8] Moreover, Brown points to evidence
to suggest that surgeons continued to describe their work in emotional terms
into the 1900s.[9] John Harley Warner and Lawrence J. Rizzolo's historical
overview of anatomical instruction in the United States from the nineteenth to
the twenty-first centuries highlights the emotional intensity of the practice of
dissecting in the nineteenth century and how the practice was viewed to have
a potentially hardening effect on students' emotions.[10] While there have been
numerous studies of medical education in a range of geographical settings,
the voices of students themselves have often been absent.[11] Moreover, historians have not approached the history of medical education from a history of
emotions perspective. This chapter seeks to redress this balance through an

exploration of the experiences of Irish medical students from the late nineteenth to early twentieth centuries. Through doing so, it also speaks to the themes of the subsequent chapters in this subtheme, which include gender, performance, and professional identity.

As Rosenwein has argued, the study of emotional communities does not claim to show definitively how an individual felt in a certain situation; however, it can "help us to understand how people articulated, understood, and represented how they felt."[12] Through an examination of a range of sources, this chapter aims to interrogate the meaning of emotion in students' accounts of their experiences, as well as answering Rosenwein's call for historians utilizing her methodology to employ a diverse range of sources. This chapter therefore draws on a diverse variety of primary source material, including student diaries, student magazines and newspapers, novels about medical student life, professors' addresses, and doctors' memoirs.[13] Student magazines are useful in illuminating what it was like to be a student in the nineteenth and twentieth centuries. Written by students for students, they give us an engaging view of their day-to-day life.[14] Doctors' memoirs can also be used to reveal memories of and emotions associated with student days, and can help to highlight the power of collective memory. As Maurice Halbwachs has suggested, "an individual's memory is always situated within a collective or group consciousness of an event or experience," meaning that "individual memory is a part or even an aspect of group memory." Such collective memories, it could be said, helped to define who was a member of the profession and who was not.[15]

This chapter will explore three key themes: the link made between happiness and industry in advice given to Irish students in the nineteenth century, the tension between published and private accounts, and finally, the dissecting room and hospital as emotional sites. Ultimately, it will illustrate how shared emotions helped to cement a collective identity among Irish medical students, and examine the value of a history of emotions approach to the history of medical education.

MEDICAL STUDY, HARD WORK, AND EMOTIONS

From the eighteenth century, Dublin developed into a major centre of medical education, and by the 1850s there existed a large number of teaching hospitals and medical schools.[16] Dublin achieved international renown in the first half of the nineteenth century for its system of bedside clinical teaching, which was made famous by Robert Graves and William Stokes, physicians at the Meath Hospital. Graves, Stokes, Abraham Colles, and others generated an exceptional reputation as a result of their "exceptional personal skills of rigorous observation, forensic investigation and a humane patient-centred ethic."[17]

On the strength of the reputation of Graves and this group of fewer than a dozen practitioners who were famed for their teaching and advocacy of new medical instruments such as the stethoscope, the city of Dublin "shifted from its old dependence on universities abroad for medical education (in Scotland, the Netherlands and France) to becoming a centre in its own right."[18] By the mid-1850s, students had several options for medical study in Ireland. These included Trinity College Dublin (founded in 1592), the Royal College of Surgeons in Dublin (1784), the three Queen's Colleges in Cork, Galway, and Belfast (1845), the Catholic University School of Medicine in Dublin (1854, later University College Dublin), or one of several private medical schools, which were primarily located in Dublin. Women began to enter some Irish medical schools as students from the 1880s, and by 1904, women were able to enter all of them.[19]

The university played a significant role in providing students with a sense of identity. As Tomás Irish has suggested, universities, in a sense, may be described as families.[20] Students had a limited choice of colleagues and lived and socialized with members of the same group, in the same way that family members do, while the university community became a surrogate family.[21] In addition, kinship could be established not only through membership of the university, but also through university societies and sports clubs.[22] This resulted in "an intimate network of men who were friends, enemies, and many shades in between, but inextricably linked by this association for the rest of their lives."[23] A student's first day at medical school in the period in question usually began with attendance at an introductory lecture, which formed part of their initiation and at which students were acquainted with the hallmarks of Irish medical professional identity. Writing about his first day in a letter to a friend, Patrick McCartan, a student at University College Dublin in 1905, remarked, "I attended my first lecture at the University to-day and enjoyed it. Of course it is not very important as the real work only begins on Nov 2nd."[24]

The inaugural lecture was an important social occasion for members of the medical profession and was usually attended by members of the medical community, friends of the professor, and medical students who were now seen as being part of this medical community. Introductory lectures given at medical schools generally took the form of advice from a senior member of the profession to students. Lectures generally followed a similar pattern, usually referring to the necessity of proper study habits, the importance of a good preliminary education, and the expectations for student conduct. In a 1907 account in the student magazine, Q.C.C., from the perspective of a first-year medical student, the introductory lecture was described in the following way:

We are to remember that we are young men preparing for a profession, men standing on the shore of the boundless ocean of medical knowledge, men imbued with high aims, elevating thoughts and noble aspirations, whose ambition must be to follow in the footsteps of the great and good and stand out as the beacon-lights in the dark by-ways of existence.[25]

Medical students were, as this account satirizes, often warned of the great responsibility of their chosen career path. As John Harley Warner has outlined, introductory lectures at medical schools, like presidential addresses to medical society meetings and medical theses, were responsible for setting exemplars for the medical profession and outlining the traits that were desirable for physicians to possess.[26] Inaugural addresses often drew attention to important medical issues of the day, while also sometimes outlining the course of study that was to follow.[27] The importance of camaraderie to students' mental well-being was highlighted, and contemporary professors believed that the fostering of friendship among students was crucial to students' happiness. Alexander Fleming, professor of materia medica at Queen's College Cork, provided the introductory address to medical students there at the opening of the 1850–51 session. In his speech, which outlined advice ranging from the importance of industry to a strong preliminary education, Fleming also suggested that students should "cherish a good understanding among yourselves."[28] The significance of the emotional community is evident in Fleming's address. In his words:

The present is probably the best opportunity that you will ever enjoy of sowing the seeds of genuine friendship, by which you will secure happiness not only for the time of your studies, but lay up a store for after life.[29]

In Fleming's view, the bonds formed in university could be drawn upon later in life. Indeed, as Crowther and Dupree have argued in their study of medical students at the University of Glasgow and the University of Edinburgh in the nineteenth century, "the power of friendship could be a considerable asset in later careers, but even among students who had scarcely known one another at university, the shared experiences became a kind of passport, useful in all kinds of circumstances."[30]

The path of medical study was viewed as a difficult one and the trope of the doctor as soldier was often utilized by Irish professors in these addresses.[31] Henry Curran, speaking to students at the Carmichael School of Medicine in 1858, referred to the occasions "of darkness, hesitation, or faintheartedness" that students would experience "on the score of duty," but suggested that later on students would, "like a conqueror on the battle field, survey the scenes of your early struggles, strewn with the remains of rebellious desires," and feel noble and proud for having gained victory over themselves.[32] Students at the Richmond Hospital were told by Dominic Corrigan in 1858 that they should possess "steadiness, attention, propriety of conduct, good temper, and kindliness of disposition and manner in dealing with the sick."[33] This is the type of doctor that medical schools were trying to promote in the period. It is a predominantly "masculine" image, and from the late nineteenth century very few references were made to women doctors or the type of characteristics they should possess, even though women had been admitted to take the licences of the King and Queen's College of Physicians in Ireland from 1877, and the degrees of Irish medical schools from the mid-1880s and early 1890s. Industry, perseverance, and earnestness were also regularly put forward as important traits. G.T. Hayden, lecturer of anatomy and physiology, in an introductory address to his students at the Original School of Medicine, Peter Street, in 1840, for instance, directly linked such traits to personal happiness:

It has been amply proved by observation and experience, that the nearest approach to happiness in this life, will be found in the daily occupations of a successful struggler guided by judgement, perseverance and industry – requisites much more essential for professional success than great talents and towering genius.[34]

Indeed, this was recognized by some students themselves. Speaking to his fellow students in 1868, William Battersby, a student at Trinity College Dublin, at a meeting of the Dublin University Medico-Chirurgical Society, put forward the idea that students should focus on their role in alleviating "the misery and sickness of mankind" rather than on earning for themselves a "handsome fortune." Such a focus, he believed, would allow students to "find real wisdom, true happiness."[35]

Industry was often portrayed in inaugural addresses in contrast with idleness, which Arthur Wynne Foot in 1873 described to students as being "a moral syphilis, a swinish malady."[36] Hard work was viewed as important more generally in the Victorian period. For instance, Samuel Smiles, a British reformer, who had originally started his career studying medicine at the University of Edinburgh, put forward his doctrine of "self-help" in 1845, which placed emphasis on personal attributes such as perseverance, determination, and diligence in attaining success.[37] It is clear that, as Keir Waddington has argued, medical schools played a central role in inculcating professional ideals of diligence and hard work.[38]

Irish professors linked hard work in one's student days and subsequent career and a sense of purpose with the achievement of happiness. Speaking to students at the Ledwich School of Medicine in 1873, Arthur Wynne Foot explained:

> Most unhappy of all men is the man who has no fixed and definite object in life, who cannot tell what he is going to do, who has got no work cut out for him in this world, and who drifts purposeless along the stream of time, without rudder or compass, till he is beached on some sand-bank – solely useful as a warning to others not to imitate his courses.[39]

Similarly, speaking to students at St Vincent's Hospital in 1899, Richard Tobin stated that

> To work hard is the great pleasure of life, but the work must be con-genial and not beyond one's powers. One man will be happiest in the routine of military service; another in country practice where the strain is rather physical than mental; a third will delight in the keen contest of the metropolis, and in its difficulties find wholesome stimulation … the out-come of the difficult curriculum you have successfully traversed is a certain amount of medical knowledge, but still better, a trained state of mind – a capability of making the mind do what you set it to do. This is the most valuable possession, but one most easily squandered. He who cherishes it is pretty sure not only of success, but of happiness.[40]

Setting one's mind to a key goal and hard work were therefore seen as import-ant traits, not just for achieving success in the medical profession in Ireland, but in order to attain happiness in one's personal life. Members of the medi-cal profession do not appear to have been concerned about the potential for medical students to over-exert themselves. However, this was a major argu-ment against the entry of women to the medical profession, most notably by British psychiatrist Henry Maudsley and American doctor Edward Clarke.[41] As Cohen has shown, there was little concern about overstrain in young men in the period, as it was believed that boys were safe from overuse of mental energy because of a belief in their tendency towards "healthy idleness."[42]

PUBLIC AND PRIVATE EMOTIONS

Emotions permeated each aspect of medical study. The first day at medical school was often described by students and former students as a nerve-racking one. Writing in 1933, James Lloyd Turner Graham, for instance, explained:

Arose at 7:30. Went into lectures in the College of Surgeons. Felt very nervous going in as I did not know what to do but I got out all right. I met a fellow I had been in school with [from] whom I got all my news.[43]

Conversely, in some published accounts, students tended to be more positive in reflecting on their medical school days. One student writing in 1917 in *R.C.S.I.: Students' Quarterly*, the magazine of students at the Royal College of Surgeons explained, "Ours was a happy existence," and wrote, "When I look back now in fancy and call to mind that dull October day on which I listened to my first lecture, and entered the dissecting room with the shyness of a novice – a feeling of sadness, of longing for the vanished past – comes over me."[44] Similarly, R.W.M. Strain remarked, "our student days, though clouded by the usual preoccupation with examinations, were happy days."[45] Ken O'Flaherty, who was a student at University College Dublin in the 1940s, commented in his memoirs, "the long haul of seven years from the billboard in Harcourt Road to the conferring photograph on the steps of Earlsfort Terrace has left me with many happy memories."[46] However, in private, unpublished accounts, students could reflect on their negative emotions. For instance, James Little, a Dublin medical student in the 1850s, recalled retrospectively in his diary that he believed he had been "studying hard" because he stayed up late "writing out notes of lectures and consulting two or three books I had brought from Armagh with me," yet he believed "it would have been better if I had led a regular student life and not chalked out an impossible mode of study for myself."[47] As a result of his focus on working hard, and owing to his personal sense of awkwardness, Little felt that he missed out on the benefits of friendship that came from socializing with fellow students:

A country lad and a country lad who had been kept by himself and in seclusion I felt rather afraid at William Stephen's [his lodgings] and among the medical students and I rather think did awkward things without being aware of it – however the Stephenses were so very kind that I soon felt at home – I didn't mix with other medical students but studied alone – this may have kept me from dissipation but I would not advise such a course.[48]

Others were more explicit in writing about negative emotions. Alexander Porter, for instance, a medical student from a farming family in Co. Down, regularly wrote of his feelings of sadness in his diary in the 1860s. In January 1864, Porter became ill with a headache, and began "to fear that it is perhaps some obscene heart affection brought on by hard study."[49] The following day, he wrote, "Not recovering and having stopped eating I am thinking if I would happen to die then people would say I had killed myself studying which I would not like."[50] Physical ailments brought about from medical study were not unusual among medical students. In 1832, English surgeon and pioneer in the field of occupational health Charles Turner Thackrah (1795–1833) drew attention to the physical and mental health problems posed by medical study. As well as complaints of the stomach and bowels, pulmonary consumption, and the effects of wounds incurred during dissection, he also wrote about the "anxiety of mind" that medical students were prone to suffer from. Thackrah described this as "that sense of responsibility which every conscientious practitioner must feel, – the anxious zeal, which makes him throw his mind and feelings, into cases of especial danger or difficulty, – break down the frame, change the face of hilarity to that of seriousness and care, and bring on premature age."[51] The following month, Porter wrote that he was "getting on very slowly" with his anatomy study and that his "spirits are rather low."[52] In April, he wrote, "Still at Surgery and get on least middling. I feel very low spirited. I feel as if I would not care if I were dead."[53] Porter placed significant pressure on himself to succeed in his medical studies and find a career. Following the death of his father in the 1850s, he felt responsible for his younger siblings, and this appears to have been a major reason for these feelings of despondency. On 21 April 1864 he wrote, "I don't see any use in me living," but remarked that he was "too great a coward" to drown himself and that the need to put his younger brother in comfortable circumstances meant that "it is worthwhile to live for that if for nothing else. Put your trust in Providence and keep your powder dry!"[54]

Such depictions of unhappiness as a result of the pressures of medical study also appear in the contemporary student press and novels. In a 1905 edition of the student newspaper *St. Stephen's*, a poem was published entitled "The Song of the Bones," which depicted a student "sat in his lonely flat," studying for his second-year exam until he fell asleep, whereupon a group of skeletons began to creep over his bedclothes.[55] In *The Lion's Whelp*, a novel about student life in Belfast in the early twentieth century, Dan Nevin, a medical student, says to his friend Todd, "Look here, you fellows, come for a walk … You, Todd, you look miserable from pounding at books; you will be sick, and probably attain to celestial honours long before you reach the University exam."[56] Similarly, a 1907 piece in *Q.C.C.* magazine painted a rather unhappy picture of "the medicus" as a result of his studies:

Slinking along, its head sunk upon its breast, wrapped in gloom. No matter how blue the sky, or how brilliant the sunshine, the library or dissecting room is never without its baleful presence. Burdened with books, it takes its solitary way.[57]

Students such as James Lloyd Turner Graham, who attended the Royal College of Surgeons, reflected privately on this, and the pressure he felt leading up to his exams. Writing in his diary in April 1935, Graham explained:

> I am beginning to feel nervous about my exam. I shall have to keep my nose down. I am so terribly lazy that I feel I can never start. Stayed in all evening.[58]

An abundance of nervousness could potentially have disastrous consequences for a student's career. One tale published in *R.C.S.I. Students' Quarterly* in 1917 told the story of a "chronic" medical student and acted as a warning to students about the dangers of too much study to one's mental health. The student in question had been studying medicine for seventeen years. At first, the student had been "an earnest worker" and bought and read all of the textbooks that his professors suggested. However, he soon took on the advice of "grinders" instead of following that of his professor. He was soon reading "books, more books, different books" but struggled to take in the information from them, and instead of learning anything his "head was muddled with an incoherent jumble of different doctrines," ultimately rendering him incapable of study. The student wrote: "This torment preyed on my spirits so much that I became utterly unable to study, and for a time was threatened with a nervous breakdown. In my final year I ceased to struggle. I was overwhelmed by the mass of literature constantly accumulating and sank under the tide."[59] Instead, the student began to associate with a group of friends "that lived solely for pleasure" and began to attend card parties, race meetings, and drinking, ending up as a "chronic" medical, a student who took longer than the prescribed years to complete their studies and pass their examinations.[60]

Moreover, an absence of emotions, or emotional detachment, can also be telling. As sociologist Sharon R. Bird has surmised, emotional detachment, when combined with detachment and competitiveness as part of the process of homosociality, helps to perpetuate hegemonic masculinity.[61] This is telling in the case of accounts by Irish women doctors and medical students, where there is a tendency not to reveal emotions felt either at the time or looking back. For instance, published memoirs by women doctors such as Joyce Delaney, Clair M. Callan, and Beulah Bewley tend to avoid discussing emotions, while the women authors of available private memoirs, similarly, tend to not express feelings in the same way that memoirs by male students and doctors do.[62] While autobiographies written by women allow researchers to interrogate their experiences and permit women's voices to be heard, in the case of memoirs written by Irish women doctors, the silences around emotions perhaps indicate an attempt to come across as emotionally detached. A key argument against women studying medicine in the nineteenth century was that women were too emotional to be good doctors. A letter entitled "A lady on lady doctors" which appeared in the *Lancet* in 1870, for instance, commented that women were lacking "the coolness and strength of nerves" required of a doctor, and that "the constitutional variations of the female system, at the best are uncertain and not to be relied upon."[63] As Michael Brown has shown for the nineteenth century, "certain members of the medical profession invoked and elaborated visions of masculinity framed by war, heroism, and self-sacrifice."[64] The inaugural addresses given at Irish medical schools exemplify this. For instance, speaking to students at the Adelaide Hospital, Dublin, in 1889, Kendal Franks (1851–1920), senior surgeon, declared:

> The world expects that the medical man will not fail in the hour of need, and it is so accustomed to find that he can be relied upon, that any failure on his part is heavily visited. It expects that in sudden emergencies he will be calm; that when others have lost their heads, he at least will be cool and collected; that he not only will know what to do, but will be prepared to do it, whatever the risk to himself may be. When infection is rife, and friends and relatives have deserted the sufferers, the doctor must show no fear.[65]

Such images of the heroic doctor were commonplace in inaugural addresses to medical students at Irish institutions in the nineteenth century in an attempt to encourage "manly" ideals. Franks presents the doctor as the epitome of strength and composure, with the ability to make quick and rational decisions without trepidation. Students were required to possess "steadiness, attention, propriety of conduct, good temper, and kindliness of disposition and manner in dealing with the sick."[66]

EMOTIONAL SPHERES OF LEARNING

In this final section, I wish to explore two of the key sites of medical education, the dissecting room and the hospital, and the emotions that these particular spaces produced in students. As Anne Digby has argued, "medical schools helped individuals internalise a medical culture and so construct a professional identity, not least by supplying role models of how doctors might present themselves to the world, providing templates for how things should be done, and indicating how situations could be tackled without losing face."[67] They imbued students with a sense of identity and status, and additionally resulted in the creation of robust networks not only between students, but also between students and their professors.[68] Without doubt, out of all of the spheres of learning, it is the dissecting room and the hospital that are described in emotional terms in student recollections, magazines and memoirs – other sites of learning such as the lecture theatre, laboratory, and library do not have the tendency to be recalled in emotional language. For medical students, therefore, the dissecting room and hospital, and the shared emotions produced by each of these places, helped to cement a student's sense of emotional community. Students dissected together and, when gaining their clinical experience, often walked the wards together. Unlike other facets of their learning experiences, these were the two main ones that helped to bond students together and cement their sense of identity.

The dissecting room, and one's first entrance into it, was usually described by students and doctors recalling their experiences in fearful terms. As Michael Sappol has shown, American doctors in the first half of the nineteenth century embraced narratives concerning anatomy in order to forge a sense of collective identity.[69] For many medical students, the first entry to the dissecting room was a nerve-racking moment and the first time they had seen a corpse. William M. Hunter, who studied at Queen's College Belfast in the 1890s, for instance, wrote about his first day in the dissecting room in the following way:

> My first day in the Dissecting Room was pretty nerve racking. I will always remember the first time I saw so many dead bodies in different degrees of dissection. The first incision I made in the skin of a dead body was never forgotten.[70]

Similarly, a student writing in the student magazine *Q.C.C.* in 1907 described the dissecting room as "that bane and antidote of students … the chamber of horrors of the popular imagination is no ordinary room – it is a sanctuary with an atmosphere, and that not by any means an odoriferous one."[71] Fear and trepidation were commonly associated with one's first experience in the dissecting room, and numerous pieces, both fictional and non-fictional, in the student press outline the nervousness associated with this task. In a poem published in the *R.C.S.I. Students' Quarterly* in 1917, one student described his first time in the dissecting room in the following way:

> When first the budding student goes
> To the dissecting room, his nose
> By odours strange is greeted:
> And as he wears his new white clo'es
> And stares at all around, his pose
> Proclaims a mind unseated!

...While round about on tables lie
The subjects on which bye and bye
His skill will be directed.
On them he casts a nervous eye,
And firmly he resolves to try
And keep his thoughts connected.[72]

This poem, like many accounts in Irish doctors' memoirs, highlights the emotion of fear and the nervousness associated with dissection for the first time, which caused the student to feel unsettled. John Lyburn, a student at Trinity in the 1920s, remarked that his first entrance to the dissecting room "was a bewildering, even nauseating sight ... for this was the first time I had ever seen a dead man without apparel, and now for the first time I gained an impression of the magnificent architecture of the animal and human body."[73] An interesting visual representation of these emotions appeared in *Galway University Magazine* in 1922–23. A cartoon entitled "Nightmare of a medical student after his first visit to the Anatomy Dept" depicts a frightened, sweating medical student in his pyjamas, looking in terror at a dismembered cadaver lunging towards him with a scalpel.[74] Most doctors' memoirs recall the visceral nature of the dissecting room and its effect on their senses, noting, in particular, the smell. Robert Blackham, a student at the Ledwich School in Dublin in the late 1880s, recalled the anatomy room as a "long, ill kept apartment, cold and draughty in the winter and hot and stuffy in the summer session. The lighting was from flaring batswing gas burners. The floors were dirty and the smell from the 'subjects' was often overpowering."[75] R.W.M. Strain, a student at Queen's University Belfast in the 1920s, wrote in his memoirs: "When you go into the dissecting room with its unforgettable odours of formalin and strong carbolic soap you start a study that sets you apart from all the other Faculties. You get over the shock of the bodies." For Strain, "it was good to have the baptism over. It is quite a landmark."[76] In G.M. Irvine's novel *The Lion's Whelp*, the dissecting room at Queen's was described as "a long, foul-smelling, ill-kept room, poorly equipped for the purpose of teaching anatomy. Along each side were arranged six tables, on each of which lay a dead body, or the remains – more or less scant – of a dead body with one or more of the limbs removed, or extensively mangled ... the whole place looked horrible, smelt horribly."[77]

The language used by students in the dissecting room seems to denote an attempt at detachment from the grim reality of their subject. An article in *Q.C.B.* magazine in 1900, which discussed the different types of students at the university, presented a grim depiction of the typical second-year medical student: "his conversation makes one's blood run cold with its allusion to 'taking off a leg' or 'finishing an arm.'"[78] The use of such language perhaps indicates an attempt to come to terms with the disturbing nature of their new subject.

Gearoid Crookes, a student in the 1930s, wrote of his first experiences of the dissecting room in his second year of medical study:

> The scene had changed significantly from theory to practice. We learnt to talk of our subjects as "stiffs" and to grow an outer carapace making us seem indifferent to the handling of mortality, though indeed our skins were thinner than they seemed. As each new intimate dissection became necessary, behind the flippant speech we would grit our teeth, swallow hard, and get on with the newly presenting task.[79]

Some students never overcame the overwhelming feelings they experienced in the dissecting room.[80] A notable example of a medical student who gave up his studies due to a dislike of dissection is Charles Darwin, who studied at the University of Edinburgh Medical School in 1825, before changing his path and moving to the University of Cambridge in 1828.[81] Darwin wrote of his studies in anatomy while at medical school: "The study of anatomy disgusted me."[82] Such feelings were not unusual. Almost a hundred years later, in November 1911, Patrick Gallagher, a student at Queen's College Galway, wrote to the registrar of the university to ask whether he could switch to an Engineering degree. "My reason in changing is simply because I find it extremely difficult to remain for even a short time in the Anatomy room and I am afraid I could not endure to dissect a body."[83] For other students, however, once they had overcome the initial fear and repugnance of dissection, the practice of anatomy became an enjoyable experience, and one that was recorded in a more positive way. J. Johnston Abraham, for instance, a student at Trinity College Dublin in the 1890s, wrote in his memoirs:

> I soon found I liked dissecting. Anatomy had a fascination for me. I worked at it and enjoyed it. There is a scientific pleasure in making neat preparations. One forgets one is dealing with the human body. There is also an artistic satisfaction in making a good dissection that stimulates one to work hard. I did work hard and I was pleased in consequence to find in my second year that I had been appointed a "prosecutor," that is, one whose dissections are used by the Professor to lecture upon.[84]

In stark contrast, the hospital was often written about in more positive terms. Gentlemanly conduct in the hospital was seen as essential and professors advised on proper behaviour. As Brown has shown for the early nineteenth

century, the ideal surgeon was expected "to be a man of feeling."[85] Such ideas
persisted into the late nineteenth century, and students undertaking their clinical experience were encouraged to consider appropriate behaviour and emotions. For example, speaking to students in 1858, Dominic Corrigan stated
that they required "far more than mere professional knowledge" and advised
them to ensure they possessed the qualities of "steadiness, attention, propriety
of conduct, good temper, and kindliness of disposition and manner in dealing
with the sick."[86] Similarly, Charles Benson, speaking to students at the City
of Dublin Hospital in 1859, encouraged them to think about their patients'
feelings. He told students to

> avoid every thing that might offend the delicacy or wound the feelings, of
> the unhappy sufferers, or put them to any unavoidable pain … In dressing
> your patient, or questioning him about his complaint, or taking notes of
> his case, I would say, in the words of a little poem: "Speak kindly to thy
> fellow-man, lest he should die, while yet thy biter accents wring his heart
> and make his pale cheek wet." Recollect that he is really a brother in
> affliction, and that he has the same feelings that you have yourself.[87]

Benson here encouraged students to speak in a kindly manner to their patients
and to draw on their own empathy in their manner. In the same way, Edward
Hamilton, speaking to students at the Richmond, Whitworth and Hardwicke
Hospitals in 1856, advised them that

> [k]nowledge alone is not sufficient, a medical man must have manners,
> morals, and feeling; in some rare instances extraordinary talents may have
> made a way without these, but more commonly taken has been lost for the
> want of them.[88]

In 1885, he warned students to "avoid the temptation to levity," stressing
that students would be "surrounded by the sick and the dying, who watch
with bated breath each event of our visit, and scan with feverish curiosity
the countenance of their attendant, trying to read their fate in every shade
which passes over his features. Scenes like these are ill-suited to the rib-
ald jest, the merry jibe, or the ill-timed practical joke."[89] Yet, in contrast
to the gentlemanly conduct expected of students on the hospital wards,
some Irish students recalled in their memoirs the ritual humiliation that
they sometimes experienced from their clinical professors. Joyce Delaney,
a female student at University College Dublin in the 1940s, recalled the
following experience of clinical training at St Vincent's Hospital under surgeon Harry Meade:

Chivalry went by the board as people pushed and shoved to get into a strategic position around the patient's bed. Harry usually shoved the bed forward and stood behind the patient, arms resting on the bedhead. There was a great art in getting correctly placed. You didn't want to get too close in case Harry concentrated on making you the butt of his scathing tongue but on the other hand you wanted him to see you because he always favoured "regulars" when it came to the examination, figuring that whatever their knowledge or lack of it at least they showed good taste![90]

Nevertheless, the student's first day at the hospital undertaking clinical experience tended to be characterized in happy terms. One student writing for *St. Stephen's* student newspaper in 1905 described this as follows:

How shall I ever forget my first entrance to a General Hospital! And, apropos of that, what pleasure, what wealth, what happiness can equal the student's joy on the first day he possesses a stethoscope? A stethoscope! His own!! His very own!! In the privacy of his own room he tests his own heart-beat, and although he can distinguish nothing in the confused thumping conveyed to his ear, he smiles with the smug self-satisfaction of a man who owns something from the possession of which his fellows are debarred.[91]

For this particular student, clinical experience and ownership of a stethoscope, "something from the possession of which his fellows are debarred," enabled him to feel like part of the medical profession, and thus to feel joy. Similarly, J. Johnston Abraham, who trained at Trinity College in the 1890s, explained how the hospital work helped to make him feel more positive about his medical training, following a period of doubt over whether he was suited to the profession:

Accepting Dowden's advice to carry on, I started hospital in my second year, according to the Dublin custom. Immediately I was happier. I began to see how the preliminary lectures I had been attending – Anatomy, Chemistry, Physics, Botany, Zoology, Histology and Physiology, all a bit wearisome at times except Anatomy, Botany and Zoology – were essential if one was to understand the nature of disease and the methods of combating the ills that man, and especially woman, had to suffer. I knew I had found my vocation.[92]

Similarly, John Biggart, a student at Queen's who started his clinical experience at the Royal Victoria Hospital in the early 1920s, remarked, "for the first time we felt that we were really becoming engaged in our profession. I suppose for most of us it meant something to do with patients and their ailments, and we had a rather mystical conception of what the doctor could do." He recalled one of his greatest difficulties being "the overcoming of the shyness of bodily and physical intimacy ... yet somehow or other, almost unconsciously, we slowly acquired the art of medicine."[93] John Lyburn, who studied at Trinity College, remarked on his amazement as he witnessed his first surgical operation.[94] Through writing about their experiences in these spheres of learning in emotional language, Irish medical students further reinforced the importance of these spaces as rites of passage and ultimately as fundamental to their sense of professional identity.

CONCLUSION

Taking Ireland as a case study, this chapter has explored representations of emotions in sources created by professors and students at Irish medical schools in the nineteenth and early twentieth centuries. It is clear that the history of emotions approach offers much to the history of medical education and encourages us to think further about uncovering student experiences, such as one's first entry to the dissecting room or hospital. Yet, this is not without a caveat. As Lynn Abrams has suggested, "while memory for an emotion-inducing event might be quite accurate in terms of information, memory for the emotion felt at the time is likely to be inaccurate or at least very difficult to articulate."[95] However, the representation of the emotion felt is just as important, and these shared emotions and experiences helped Irish doctors to cement a sense of emotional community. Through undertaking these experiences which produced memorable emotions, medical students came to feel part of a group. While this chapter has only touched on a few aspects of this theme, it is clear that an emotional history approach to the study of medical education has much potential for future research. Future studies might consider emotions surrounding romance and relationships formed in medical student days, or the emotions of international medical students at Irish institutions. The silences in some medical students' accounts and doctors' memoirs could also be given more attention. Given that emigration was an integral part of the experiences of Irish medical students in the past, the emotions associated with this could also be a useful avenue of exploration.

It is clear that the study of medicine provoked a range of emotions in students, from nervousness at one's first day, to fear in the dissecting room, to happiness and joy at one's first time in the hospital setting. Indeed, emotions were also an integral part of the advice given by professors to medical students at Irish universities. Professors encouraged students to work diligently, for in this way they could secure happiness in their future careers. Additionally, students were also encouraged to possess empathy, to be "men of feeling" in their clinical encounters in the hospital. Encouraging students to be diligent in order to secure happiness and to think more about skills such as empathy and kindliness in the hospital setting may be viewed as part of a strategy to improve student behaviour in general. There are many accounts of bad behaviour among medical students in the early nineteenth century; from the late nineteenth century, however, as education became more regulated, student behaviour generally improved, and perhaps the incorporation of the language of emotions in introductory addresses may be viewed as part of a wider strategy to improve students' behaviour and to present members of the medical profession as gentlemanly. Nevertheless, it is clear that while publicly, in published memoirs, students tended to reflect on their student days in a positive light, in private diaries and letters, students expressed more negative emotions, such as unhappiness as a result of the pressures of medical study and over-work. Overall, these shared emotions, or shared representations of emotions, helped to bind students together and solidify their sense of professional identity.

ACKNOWLEDGMENTS

I am grateful to the Irish Research Council for funding the research on which this chapter is based. I would also like to thank Professor Jonathan Reinarz for his extremely helpful comments on an earlier draft of this chapter and the editors for their encouragement and feedback.

NOTES

1   Abraham, *Surgeon's Journey*, 38.
2   Strain, *Les neiges d'antan*, 4.
3   Rosenwein, "Worrying about Emotions in History," 842.
4   Ibid., 845.
5   Plamper and Tribe, *History of Emotions: An Introduction*, 70.
6   Rosenwein, "Problems and Methods in the History of Emotions," 19.
7   As Faye Bound Alberti has asserted, there has been limited attention paid to "the emotional engagement between the patient and his or her physician, the role of the physician's own emotions in diagnosis, prognosis and treatment." In Alberti, "Introduction: Emotion Theory and Medical History," xiv.
8   Brown, "Surgery and Emotion," 343.
9   Ibid., 344.
10 Warner and Rizzolo, "Anatomical Instruction," 403–14.

11 In recent years, studies of medical education have begun to address this gap in the historiography. Histories of medical education in Edinburgh and London have been joined by research on medical education and student experience elsewhere in Britain, America, and Europe. See for example: Lawrence, *Charitable Knowledge*; Rosner, *Medical Education in the Age of Enlightenment*; Heaman, *St. Mary's: The History of a London Teaching Hospital*; Reinarz, *Health Care in Birmingham*; Rosner, "Student Culture at the Turn of the Nineteenth Century"; Jones, "Montpellier Medical Students"; Bonner, *Becoming a Physician*; Waddington, *Medical Education at St. Bartholomew's Hospital*; Weatherall, *Gentlemen, Scientists and Doctors*; Kelly, *Irish Medical Education and Student Culture*.

12 Rosenwein, "Problems and Methods in the History of Emotions," n. 37, 11.

13 My methodology is also influenced by historians who have effectively utilized personal sources such as student diaries and letters and doctors' memoirs such as Warner, *The Therapeutic Perspective*; Rosner, "Student Culture at the Turn of the Nineteenth Century"; and Crowther and Dupree, *Medical Lives*.

14 See, for instance, Browne, "Squibs and Snobs."

15 Abrams, *Oral History Theory*, 95–6.

16 Jones and Malcolm, "Introduction," 1.

17 Dickson, *Dublin*, 313.

18 Ibid., 313.

19 For more on the history of women's entry to the medical profession in Ireland, see Kelly, *Irish Women in Medicine*.

20 Irish, "Fractured Families," 511.

21 Ibid., 511–12.

22 Ibid., 511–12.

23 Ibid., 512.

24 Letter from Patrick McCartan to Joseph McGarrity, dated 19 October 1905, [National Library of Ireland, MS 17,457/23(1)].

25 "Leaves from the Diary of a 'Gyb,'" 63.

26 Warner, *The Therapeutic Perspective*, 15.

27 Such lectures might be described as a ritual of admission and entering. Manning, *Rituals, Ceremonies and Cultural Meaning*, 8.

28 Fleming, "Queen's College Cork," 26.

29 Ibid., 26.

30 Crowther and Dupree, *Medical Lives*, 94.

31 Michael Brown's valuable work has highlighted the rhetoric of militarism and heroism that was an important part of physicians' writings in the nineteenth century. He has shown how "certain members of the medical profession invoked and elaborated visions of masculinity framed by war, heroism, and self-sacrifice." Brown, "'Like a Devoted Army,'" 592–622.

32 Curran, "The introductory lecture," 22.

33 Corrigan, "Introductory lecture," 10.

34 Hayden, "The medical profession," 24.

35 Battersby, "Medical education," 29.

36 Foot, "An introductory address," 17.

37 Goldthorpe, *Social Mobility and Class Structure in Modern Britain*, 3–4.

38 Waddington, "Mayhem and Medical Students," 47.

39 Foot, "An introductory address," 6.

40 Tobin, "Professional behaviour," 8.

41 Maudsley, "Sex in Mind and Education." Dr Edward Clarke's publication *Sex in Education; or, A Fair Chance for the Girls* (1873) questioned whether there was a role for women in the professions. Clarke argued that menstrual functions and co-education were incompatible for American girls, with too much education and mental exertion threatening their physical development, especially when this was undertaken during menstruation.

42 Cohen, "A Habit of Healthy Idleness," 27.

43 Diary of James Lloyd Turner Graham, 1933 [RCPI Heritage Centre].

44 "From the depths: a monologue – in one moan," *R.C.S.I. Students' Quarterly* 1, no. 4 (Christmas number, 1917): 71. [RCPI Heritage Centre, Kirkpatrick Collection: TPCK/6/7/12].

45 Ibid., 72.

46 O'Flaherty, *From Slyne Head to Malin Head*, 127.

47 Diary of James Little, [TPCK/6/5/10], RCPI Heritage Centre.

48 Ibid.

49 Diary entry for Alexander Porter, 20 January 1864, 26, Harry Ramsden Centre.

50 Ibid., 21 January 1864, 26.

51 Thackrah, *The effects of arts, trades and professions, and of civic states and habits of living, on health and longevity*, 175–6.

52 Diary entry for Alexander Porter, 26 February 1864, 42.

53 Ibid., 12 April 1864, 61.

54 Ibid., 21 April 1864, 65.

55 "The Song of the Bones by 'Innominatum,'" 199.

56 Irvine, *The Lion's Whelp*, 6.

57 "The Medicus," 5–6.

58 Diary of James Lloyd Turner Graham, 1935. [RCPI Heritage Centre].

59 "From the depths: a Monologue – in one moan," Kirkpatrick collection: Clubs and Associations TPCK/6/7/12, *R.C.S.I. Students' Quarterly* 1, no. 4 (Christmas number, 1917): 71.

60 Ibid., 71.

61 Bird, "Welcome to the Men's Club," 121–2.

62   See Bewley and Bewley, eds., *My Life as a Woman and Doctor*; Callan, *Standing My Ground*; Delaney, *No Starch in My Coat*. Private memoirs by Florence Stewart (a student at Queen's University Belfast in the late 1920s) and Emily Winifred Dickson (a student at the Royal College of Surgeons in the 1880s), for instance, are generally matter-of-fact in their description of their student days. Florence Stewart memoirs [PRONI D3612/3/1] and Emily Winifred Dickson papers [RCSI/IP/Dickson].

63   "Mater," "A Lady on Lady Doctors," 680.

64   Brown, "'Like a Devoted Army.'"

65   Franks, "Introductory address," 7.

66   Corrigan, "Introductory lecture," 10.

67   Digby, "Shaping New Identities," 20.

68   Loudon, *Medical Care and the General Practitioner*, 41, cited in Crowther and Dupree, *Medical Lives*, 2.

69   Sappol, "The Odd Case of Charles Knowlton," 460–98.

70   William M. Hunter, *Private Life of a Country Medical Practitioner*, 7. (Private memoir courtesy of the Hunter family.)

71   "Leaves from the Diary of a 'Gyb,'" 62–3.

72   "The Student's Progress," 5.

73   Lyburn, *The Fighting Irish Doctor*, 52.

74   "Nightmare of a medical student after his first visit to the Anatomy Dept."

75   Blackham, *Scalpel, Sword and Stretcher*, 31.

76   Strain, *Les neiges d'antan*, 8.

77   Irvine, *The Lion's Whelp*, 13.

78   "As others see us: the medical student [by a junior artsman]," 4.

79   Crookes, *Far Away and Long Ago*, 139.

80   Experiments involving vivisection in the nineteenth century also produced a similar response in some scientists, and emotions became central to debates around vivisection. See, for instance: White, "Sympathy under the Knife"; Mayer, "The Expression of Emotions in Man and Laboratory Animals."

81   See Browne, *Charles Darwin*, 56–61.

82   Ibid., 61.

83   Letter from Patrick Gallagher, 1911. [NUI Galway Special Collections: Bursar's Office collection: 7 Bursar's Correspondence: B/214].

84   Abraham, *Surgeon's Journey*, 47.

85   Brown, *Charles Darwin*, 336.

86   Corrigan, "Introductory lecture," 10.

87   Benson, "Address delivered to the students," 17.

88   Hamilton, "Richmond, Whitworth, and Hardwicke Hospitals," 5.

89   Hamilton, "Royal College of Surgeons Inaugural Address," 15.

90   Delaney, *No Starch in My Coat*, 19.

91 "First impressions," 194.
92 Abraham, *Surgeon's Journey*, 58.
93 Weaver, "John Henry Biggart," 6.
94 Lyburn, *The Fighting Irish Doctor*, 58.
95 Abrams, *Oral History Theory*, 95.

BIBLIOGRAPHY

Abraham, J. Johnston. *Surgeon's Journey: The Autobiography of J. Johnston Abraham*.
London: William Heinemann Ltd, 1957.

Abrams, Lynn. *Oral History Theory*. London: Routledge, 2010.

"As others see us: the medical student [by a junior artsman]." *Q.C.B.* 1, no. 2
(12 February 1900): 4.

Battersby, W. "'Medical Education,' an address delivered in the dining hall of Trinity
College at the opening meeting of the second session of the Dublin University
Medico-Chirurgical Society, November 27th, 1868 by the auditor W.E. Battersby,
B.A. Med. Sch." Dublin: M. & S. Eaton, 1868.

Alberti, Faye Bound. "Introduction: Emotion Theory and Medical History."
In *Medicine, Emotion and Disease*, edited by Faye Bound Alberti, xiii–xxviii.
Basingstoke, UK: Palgrave Macmillan, 2006.

Benson, Charles. "Address delivered to the students in the City of Dublin Hospital
on Tuesday, November 8th, 1859." Dublin: Fannin and Co., 1859.

Bewley, Beulah, and Susan Bewley, eds. *My Life as a Woman and Doctor*. Bristol, UK:
Silverwood Books, 2016.

Bird, Sharon R. "Welcome to the Men's Club: Homosociality and the Maintenance
of Hegemonic Masculinity." *Gender & Society* 10, no. 2 (April 1996): 121–2.

Blackham, Robert J. *Scalpel, Sword and Stretcher: Forty Years of Work and Play*. London:
Sampson Low, Marston & Co. Ltd, 1931.

Bonner, Thomas Neville. *Becoming a Physician: Medical Education in Britain, France,
Germany and the United States, 1750–1945*. Oxford, UK: Oxford University Press,
1995.

Brown, Michael. "Surgery and Emotion: The Era before Anaesthesia." In *The
Palgrave Handbook of the History of Surgery*, edited by T. Schlich, 327–48.
Basingstoke, UK: Palgrave, 2018.

– "'Like a Devoted Army': Medicine, Heroic Masculinity, and the Military Paradigm
in Victorian Britain." *Journal of British Studies* 49, no. 3 (July 2010): 592–622.

Browne, Janet. "Squibs and Snobs: Science in Humorous British Undergraduate
Magazines around 1830." *History of Science* 30, no. 3 (1992): 165–97.

– *Charles Darwin: Voyaging*, vol. 1. London: Random House, 2010.

Callan, Clair M. *Standing My Ground: Memoir of a Woman Physician*. Bloomington:
Archway Publishing, 2014.

Cohen, Michele. "'A Habit of Healthy Idleness': Boys' Underachievement in Historical Perspective." In *Failing Boys? Issues in Gender and Achievement*, edited by Debbie Epstein, Jannette Elwood, Valerie Hey, and Janet Maw, 19–34. Maidenhead, UK: Open University Press, 1998.

Corrigan, Dominic. "Introductory lecture, winter session 1858–9, Richmond, Whitworth and Hardwicke Hospitals." Dublin: J.M. O'Toole, 1858.

Crookes, Gearoid P. *Far Away and Long Ago: A Memoir*. Dublin: Tudor House Publications, 2003.

Crowther, Anne, and Marguerite Dupree. *Medical Lives in the Age of Surgical Revolution*. Cambridge: Cambridge University Press, 2007.

Curran, Henry. "The introductory lecture of the winter session 1858–59 delivered in the Carmichael School of Medicine on Tuesday November 2nd, 1858." Dublin: Browne & Nolan, 1858.

Delaney, Joyce. *No Starch in My Coat: An Irish Doctor's Progress*. London: Cox & Wyman, 1971.

Dickson, David. *Dublin: The Making of a Capital City*. London: Profile Books, 2014.

Digby, Anne. "Shaping New Identities: General Practitioners in Britain and South Africa." In *Medical Identities: Health, Well-Being and Personhood*, edited by Kent Maynard. New York: Bergahn Books, 2007.

"First impressions." *St. Stephen's: A Record of University Life* 2, no. 9 (December 1905): 194.

Fleming, Alexander. "Queen's College Cork, Faculty of Medicine, Session 1850–51, Introductory address on medical education with special reference to the course of study required for the degree of M.D. in the Queen's University, Ireland." Dublin: Hodges and Smith, 1850.

Foot, Arthur Wynne. "An introductory address delivered at the Ledwich School of Medicine, November 1st, 1873." Dublin: John Falconer, 1873.

Franks, Kendal. "Introductory address delivered at the opening of the session of 1889–90 at the Adelaide Hospital." Dublin: John Falconer, 1889.

Goldthorpe, John D. *Social Mobility and Class Structure in Modern Britain*, 2nd ed. Oxford, UK: Oxford University Press, 1987.

Hamilton, Edward. "Richmond, Whitworth, and Hardwicke Hospitals: Introductory address, delivered on the opening of the session, November 3rd, 1856." Dublin: J.M. O'Toole, 1857.

– "Royal College of Surgeons Inaugural Address, Session 1885–86." Dublin: Gunn & Cameron Printers, 1885.

Hayden, G.T. "The medical profession, as it was, as it is, as it ought to be; a lecture, introductory to the business of the Original School of Medicine, Peter-Street." Dublin: Fannin and Co, 1840.

Heaman, E.A. *St. Mary's: The History of a London Teaching Hospital*. Liverpool, UK: Liverpool University Press, 2003.

Irish, Tomás. "Fractured Families: Educated Elites in Britain and France and the Challenge of the Great War." *The Historical Journal* 57, no. 2 (June 2014): 509–30.

Irvine, G.M. *The Lion's Whelp*. London: Simpkin, Marshall, Hamilton, Kent & Co. Ltd, 1910.

Jones, Colin. "Montpellier Medical Students and the Medicalisation of 18th-Century France." In *Problems and Methods in the History of Medicine*, edited by Roy Porter and Andrew Wear, 57–80. London: Croom Helm, 1987.

Jones, Greta, and Elizabeth Malcolm. "Introduction: An Anatomy of Irish Medical History." In *Medicine, Disease and the State in Ireland, 1650–1940*, edited by Greta Jones and Elizabeth Malcolm, 1–20. Cork, Ireland: Cork University Press, 1998.

Kelly, Laura. *Irish Medical Education and Student Culture, c. 1850–1950*. Liverpool, UK: Liverpool University Press, 2017.

– *Irish Women in Medicine, c. 1880s–1920s: Education, Origins and Careers*. Manchester, UK: Manchester University Press, 2012.

Lawrence, S.C. *Charitable Knowledge: Hospital Pupils and Practitioners in Eighteenth-Century London*. Cambridge: Cambridge University Press, 1986.

"Leaves from the Diary of a 'Gyb.'" *Q.C.C.* 3, no. 3 (March 1907): 63.

Lyburn, John. *The Fighting Irish Doctor (An Autobiography)*. Dublin: Morris & Co., 1947.

Manning, Kathleen. *Rituals, Ceremonies and Cultural Meaning in Higher Education*. Westport, CT: Bergin & Garvey, 2000.

"Mater." "A Lady on Lady Doctors." *Lancet* (7 May 1870): 680.

Maudsley, Henry. "Sex in Mind and Education." *Fortnightly Review* 15 (1874): 466–83.

Mayer, Jed. "The Expression of Emotions in Man and Laboratory Animals." *Victorian Studies* 50, no. 3 (Spring 2008): 399–417.

"Nightmare of a Medical Student after His First Visit to the Anatomy Dept." *Galway University College Magazine* 2, no. 9: 1922–23.

O'Flaherty, Ken. *From Slyne Head to Malin Head: A Rural GP Remembers*. Letterkenny, Ireland: Browne Printers, 2003.

Plamper, Jan, and Keith Tribe. *History of Emotions: An Introduction*. Oxford, UK: Oxford University Press, 2015.

Reinarz, Jonathan. *Health Care in Birmingham: The Birmingham Teaching Hospitals, 1779–1939*. Woodbridge, UK: Boydell Press, 2009.

Rosenwein, Barbara H. "Problems and Methods in the History of Emotions." *Passions in Context* 1 (January 2010): 1–32.

– "Worrying about Emotions in History." *The American Historical Review* 107, no. 3 (June 2002): 821–45.

Rosner, Lisa. *Medical Education in the Age of Enlightenment: Edinburgh Students and Apprentices, 1760–1826*. Edinburgh: Edinburgh University Press, 1991.

– "Student Culture at the Turn of the Nineteenth Century." *Caduceus* 10, no. 2 (1994): 65–86.

Sappol, Michael. "The Odd Case of Charles Knowlton: Anatomical Performance, Medical Narrative, and Identity in Antebellum America." *Bulletin of the History of Medicine* 83, no. 3 (Fall 2009): 460–98.

Strain, R.W.M. *Les neiges d'antan: A Two-Part Story: Recollections of a Medical Student, the Queen's University of Belfast, 1924–30, and of a Houseman, The Royal Victoria Hospital, Belfast, 1930–31.* Truro, UK: R. Strain, 1982.

Thackrah, C. Turner. *The effects of arts, trades and professions, and of civic states and habits of living, on health and longevity: with suggestions for the removal of many of the agents which produce disease, and shorten the duration of life.* London: Longman, Rees, Orme, Brown, Green & Longman, 1832.

"The Medicus." *Q.C.C.* 3, no. 1 (January 1907): 5–6.

"The Song of the Bones by 'Innominatum.'" *St. Stephen's: A Record of University Life* 2, no. 9 (December 1905): 199.

"The Student's Progress." *R.C.S.I. Students' Quarterly* 1, no. 1 (February 1917): 5.

Tobin, Richard F. "Professional behaviour: an address delivered in St. Vincent's Hospital at the Opening of the Session 1898–1900." Dublin: John Falconer, 1899.

Waddington, Keir. "Mayhem and Medical Students: Image, Conduct, and Control in the Victorian and Edwardian London Teaching Hospital." *Social History of Medicine* 15, no. 1 (2002): 45–64.

– *Medical Education at St. Bartholomew's Hospital, 1123–1995.* Woodbridge, UK: Boydell Press, 2003.

Warner, John Harley. *The Therapeutic Perspective: Medical Practice, Knowledge and Identity in America, 1820–1885.* Princeton, NJ: Princeton University Press, 1997.

Warner, John Harley, and Lawrence J. Rizzolo. "Anatomical Instruction and Training for Professionalism from the 19th to the 21st Centuries." *Clinical Anatomy* 19 (2006): 403–14.

Weatherall, Mark W. *Gentlemen, Scientists and Doctors: Medicine at Cambridge, 1800–1940.* Woodbridge, UK: The Boydell Press, 2000.

Weaver, John A. "John Henry Biggart, 1905–1979: A Portrait in Respect and Affection: Presidential Address to the Ulster Medical Society, 1st November, 1984." *The Ulster Medical Journal* 54, no. 1 (April 1985): 1–19.

White, Paul. "Sympathy under the Knife: Experimentation and Emotion in Late-Victorian Medicine." In *Medicine, Emotion, and Disease, 1700–1950*, edited by Fay Bound Alberti, 100–24. Basingstoke, UK: Palgrave Macmillan, 2006.

16

Portrait of the Medical Student as a Young Man: Caricatures, Realism, and Airbrushed History, c. 1880–1920

Jonathan Reinarz

Given the title of this chapter, readers will be forgiven for thinking it deals with James Joyce and the medical world of early-twentieth-century Ireland. While it is about medical education and its depiction in literature, my appointed author is not Joyce, but Francis Brett Young (1884–1954), one of the most prolific and successful English authors of the first half of the twentieth century. The chapter's title, nevertheless, remains appropriate because Young, like Joyce, wrote an autobiographical novel, only, in his, Young recounts his time as a medical student in Birmingham, England. Equally unmistakable is Young's obsession with Joyce, who was hailed by literary critics in the first decades of the twentieth century. Although Francis Brett Young never achieved similar critical acclaim during his lifetime, he is a writer one cannot dismiss on grounds of literary merit alone. From a historical point of view, his novel *The Young Physician* (1919) remains valuable, for it provides unique insight into the world of medical education in Edwardian Britain, and the lives and experiences of medical students, as Thomas Bonner argued, continue to be understudied,[1] leaving many of them "silent consumers,"[2] absent from institutional histories. As I have argued elsewhere, Young's novels are among those rare sources that are both underused and contrast with medical schools' official records, many of which lost their "nineteenth-century colour and candidness" by the early twentieth century.[3]

Comparisons between Joyce and Brett Young are easily expanded. To begin with, Joyce's collected works, like those of many modernist writers, are preoccupied with the everyday events of daily life. As such, they describe the streets of Dublin in ways that allow readers literally to map the city as his characters wander its streets.[4] This preoccupation with realism is equally notable in the novels of Francis Brett Young, his main characters, like those of Joyce, often serving as fictional alter-egos. However, while Joyce was at the forefront of literary modernism, the few who still read Francis Brett Young are limited to those with a historical interest in the English midlands. During his life-time, Francis Brett Young established a reputation as a popular, middle-brow author, prominent enough to rank among the best-selling English authors in the 1920s and 1930s.[5] His novels sold in the tens of thousands and continue to stock the shelves of second-hand book shops in Britain today. His novel *Portrait of Clare* (1927), again incorporating an element of Joyce in its title, not only underscores his preoccupation with the Irish author, but demonstrated that Young's books could potentially sell more than one hundred thousand copies. Indeed, they were best-sellers of his time.

Although Young never attained the influence of Joyce, his oeuvre remains important. As David Cannadine argues most persuasively, they capture aspects of daily life in middle England, or its "atmosphere" during the early twentieth century.[6] As Ludmilla Jordanova has noted, fictional works are valu-able historical sources that chart "broad political and ideological shifts," and Young's similarly depict aspects of Victorian and Edwardian medicine, but also the ordinary, and always elusive, details of everyday life.[7] Without such documents, the story of medical education, for example, would remain a half-filled vessel, which Young literally fills with everything that is ordinarily left out of the official documents generated by administrators in higher educa-tion. *The Young Physician* is especially valuable in providing glimpses into the experiences of medical pupils in the British provinces, since much of the history of medical education has concentrated on capital cities such as Paris and London.[8] Roy Porter once reminded historians that there are certain sub-jects in medicine's past that are exceedingly difficult to recapture, and the medical student's story is as difficult to recover as that of the patient.[9] In this chapter, I will briefly attempt to present the equivalent of the "patient's view" for Edwardian medical students by relying on Young's work. What should immediately become apparent is the uncanny resemblance between the fic-titious world of *The Young Physician* and that of students at the University of Birmingham Medical School. That said, there are crucial ways in which the real and the invented diverge, one being the way in which medical students are represented compared to those who enrolled in other subjects in an industrial city such as Birmingham. Fortunately, by drawing on other sources, the ways in which Young's creativity occasionally led him to distort, or airbrush, the past should also become evident. I will therefore conclude by offering an alter-native image of the medical student, and this chapter will end with a caution on the way we employ literary sources in historical research.

Historians of medicine have been writing histories from below since at least the 1980s. In terms of medical education, some scholars have begun to concentrate less on the staff and syllabi than on students. Besides bringing women students into histories of medical schools, research has emphasized the importance of apprenticeship into the Victorian era,[10] but also the roles of practitioners, who occupied privileged positions in leading teaching hospitals in capital cities. While hospital staff determined what counted as appropriate medical knowledge, many struggled to encourage their pupils to adopt habits of appropriate professional behaviour. Students' identities may have changed by attending actual medical "schools," such as Guy's, Thomas's, or Bart's in London, but many noticeably lost the individual guidance previously offered by a master under the apprenticeship system of former times.[11] Between 1725 and 1815, approximately 11,000 medical students travelled to London, and concerns gradually arose because their reputation as drunken and disorderly scholars threatened to undermine the upright professional status claimed by their qualified instructors.[12] These anxieties shaped the ways in which students were described in the popular press, most often as men of low habits, famously parodied by Dickens in *Pickwick Papers* and in the pages of *Punch* magazine.

These caricatures were initially challenged by doctors, before medical school staff gradually introduced initiatives aimed at professionalizing medical students in these years. Keir Waddington has claimed that key structural changes actually led to significant transformations in the behaviour of students in the late Victorian and Edwardian periods. At St Bartholomew's Hospital Medical School these included the construction of student accommodation and the establishment of discipline committees, alongside the creation of sports teams and societies, the latter providing opportunities to develop teamwork and discuss coursework, rather than leaving students with time to explore the seedier side of London.[13] What reputedly emerged by the 1890s as a consequence was a more industrious medical student, with little time or interest in causing trouble inside or outside of medical school. The rest of this chapter aims to delve deeper into this story and question whether such representations were real, imaged, or airbrushed. Rather than merely re-examine the context of London, I will also explore this through the life of a medical student in the English provinces, and the industrial city of Birmingham in particular.

Francis Brett Young became a student at Birmingham Medical School soon after its Faculty of Medicine at the city's newly established university opened in 1900. Although attending a new school, Young was not new to medicine, both his father and grandfather having been medical practitioners.[14] Young, in turn, received what can only be described as a very privileged form of education, graduating from Epsom, among Britain's leading public schools, and one noted for training doctors.[15] Unfortunately, the death of his mother during his childhood not only mirrored the experience of James Joyce, but decisively changed the course of his life, as he recalled in his novels.[16] Equally crucial to his interrupted educational journey were his father's financial difficulties, which effectively dashed his dream to study literature at Oxford. Instead, he was encouraged to apply to the more affordable medical programme at Birmingham, beginning his studies at the new red-brick university in its second year of existence.[17] His ambitions thwarted, Young later described this episode in his novels; its influence on the way he depicted the midland city in his novels is perhaps predictable. If not the best ambassador for Birmingham, Young, as it turned out, was a very good medical student. He was awarded the Sands Cox Scholarship at the outset of his first year of study and finished his degree after four productive years.[18]

When Francis Brett Young decided that he would become a writer, he wrote about Birmingham and his experiences, not unlike another British author, David Lodge, in a later period. In the case of Brett Young's work, however, Birmingham is not Rummage, as Lodge disguised the city, but North Bromwich. Around 1911, while exploring the Severn River Valley and the countryside around Birmingham, he determined "to illuminate, by a number of sections through its social strata, a life of the western midlands during those impressionable years when I was best qualified to observe it."[19] One could argue that he was never really a creative writer, for, rather than invent people and places, he repeatedly drew on his midland experiences throughout his career. By the time Young was writing his last works, he was, according to some scholars, simply reproducing what were now familiar stories and scenarios from his earliest fiction. This aspect of his literary style, however, is what makes him so appealing to historians.

From the perspective of place, there is a geographical coherence between the settings of Young's novels and the contemporaneous West Midlands region. With even a rudimentary knowledge of its counties, readers can easily identify the invented towns in *The Young Physician*. In fact, by the 1930s, Young's works were republished with actual maps of the region because they corresponded so well with the world he "invented."[20] Neither are town names altered to an extent that would make them unrecognizable. For example, fictitious Dulston is actually Dudley; Halesby is Hales Owen, where Young was raised and later lived when attending medical school; and Wolverbury is clearly Wolverhampton, the industrial city to the northwest of Birmingham. These pseudonyms rapidly become familiar to anyone reading Young's works, for the region serves as the principal setting in nine of his thirty novels. With so much of *The Young Physician*'s plot unfolding on the streets of Birmingham, it is no surprise that the neighbourhoods of England's "Second City" also reappear, including Alveston (Edgbaston) and Sparkdale (Sparkbrook), along with actual thoroughfares.

If towns and neighbourhoods regularly reappear in Young's novels, so, too, does the world of medicine, including general practitioners, hospitals, and medical students. In *The Young Physician*, the main character is a medical student, Edwin Ingleby. Named after Birmingham's first lecturer in the diseases of women and children, Ingleby's views are recognizably Young's, including descriptions of Birmingham, which are disparaging. For example, on Ingleby's rail journeys from Halesby into North Bromwich, his descriptions radically change when he departs the midlands' leafy suburbs for its industrial capital. Trees and hills are gradually blotted out by "a hundred pit fires," slag heaps, "smoke-blackened walls," and "gloomy canal wharfs."[21] In general, Ingleby is critical of manufacturing towns. On one journey, he describes the way in which houses creep closer to the railway tracks as passengers approach cities, and gardens grow progressively smaller until there is no room for vegetation, "only for a patch of black earth occupied by lean cats, and posts connected by untidy pieces of rope on which torn laundry was hung out to collect the smuts or flap drearily."[22] His journeys into towns and cities usually conclude dramatically with a "sulphurous tunnel," with passengers "emerging amid acrid fumes."[23] The architecture of an industrial city such as Birmingham never impresses him; while grandiose, it stands out as dark and foreboding, and he instead emphasizes North Bromwich's "pretentious buildings."[24] The industrial townscape also comprises "a vast debris of rusty iron, old wheels, corroded boilers, tubes writhen and tangled as if they had been struck by lightning."[25] The "high clock tower of the Art Gallery" comes closest to being its sole redeeming feature, yet is tellingly described as "almost beautiful." North Bromwich, however, is little more than "endless mean streets of dusky brick houses with roofs of purple slate and blue brick footpaths."[26] In contrast to the clean air of the Severn Valley, its inhabitants are left to inhale "dust and an acrid smell as of smoking pit heaps."[27] In the eyes of a young man whose sights were originally set on the spires of Oxford, "the city of his dreams,"[28] North Bromwich was little more than a "sink of iniquity."[29]

The medical school, when Francis Brett Young enrolled at Birmingham, was based in Mason's College, a Victorian Science College in the city centre. Its departments were not relocated to the suburbs of Edgbaston until 1938, when a new medical school was built adjacent to the main university campus. Located next to the Town Hall and the Council House, the medical school is described as situated between a steam laundry and the office of a brass foundry, in reality one of Birmingham's main industries. In highlighting such trades, Young identifies the industrial wealth that allowed the city's leaders to build a medical school and university, but, as importantly, enabled its families, sometimes within a generation, to raise themselves from the ranks of shopkeepers and small manufacturers into an emerging professional "gentry." The steam laundry is therefore symbolic, for it is through the recently established university that the sons of industrialists figuratively wash off the grime in order to facilitate their social elevation. By identifying this process, Ingleby is determined to remind these families of their humble origins. Each attempt by Birmingham's inhabitants to invest in cultural pursuits is equally ridiculed by the medical student. For example, the three-day triennial music festival, which had funded local hospitals for over a century by the time Young began his studies, is regarded less as a sign of gentility than as another failed attempt by locals to attain social distinction. Ingleby suggests the town took to music in the way a boa constrictor eats its prey. Over a chaotic weekend, Birmingham's inhabitants are said to gorge themselves on musical performances before returning to their uneventful slumber for another three years when the process repeats itself.[30] Ingleby's disdain for the "smoky" "City of Iron" becomes apparent through many similar descriptions.[31]

Events in Young's novels also correspond with actual historical occurrences. For this reason, David Cannadine valued Young's novels when researching the decline of the English aristocracy, for he could literally trace the fortunes of the region's small gentry; by the late 1930s, the period marking the end of Cannadine's study, thirty-seven of forty-four local landed families had sold off their land holdings. Along with the aristocracy's decline, and the new industrial aristocracy's ascent, *The Young Physician* traces the rise of Birmingham's civic university, which was created in 1900 when its science and medical colleges merged.[32] Other details are as precise. Tuition fees, for instance, correspond with those advertised in contemporary prospectuses.[33] More interesting are descriptions not found elsewhere. For example, Young describes a public riot in North Bromwich mirroring an actual protest that occurred in 1904, when the forty-one-year-old radical Liberal politician David Lloyd George returned to Birmingham after having spoken out against the Boer War three years earlier.[34] Joining a crowd comprising largely workers in iron and brass, Edwin Ingleby notices a hostile group led by students, who surround the town hall, where the Welsh member of Parliament is scheduled to speak. Interestingly, within this phalanx of violent students, Ingleby recognizes several medical colleagues, who attempt to batter down the locked entrance to the Town Hall with "an immense beam of oak."[35] The suggestion in later years that Joseph Chamberlain sanctioned the actual riot lends further credence to newspaper reports that medical school staff periodically encouraged student misrule, not least when it supported their own social or political interests. The author further claims that the otherwise restrained Ingleby became so caught up in the melee that he would have "experienced a brutal satisfaction in seeing him torn limb from limb,"[36] adding emotional detail that has otherwise disappeared from the historical record.

While parents initially assumed Birmingham offered students a safer study environment than London, the city had its share of frivolity to distract students.

As a former medical student, Ingleby's father recognized the "many tempta-
tions for a boy his age," and, unlike some of the London schools, provincial ones
were not known for recreations such as sports. Birmingham had a literary society, of which Francis Brett Young was a co-founder; not surprisingly, Ingleby
joins this group, along with a small number of male students who aspired to
gentlemanly status and contrasted with the majority who were distinctly rough
around the edges. Ingleby had looked forward to the formalities of university
life, not least academic gowns, but these were uncommon in Birmingham,
where university governors had decided against imposing "the sight of such
an anachronism as academic dress on the streets."[37] To his disappointment,
students' gowns and battered mortarboards were therefore left in cloakrooms
and worn only on special occasions. Worse still, without a developed sporting
culture, provincial students appeared determined to burn off term-time stress
at a handful of annual events. The highlight of the social calendar was pantomime night, when students donned fancy dress and engaged in a night of
rowdiness. According to Young's novel, the medical school students, as during
the Lloyd George riots, took the lead in this night of debauchery that involved
two theatres, where students attended (and disrupted) performances *en masse*,
dressed as cavemen, cavaliers, and other carnivalesque characters. Regular
audiences were warned in advance to avoid the theatres on these nights, when
students interrupted performances to make presentations, along with the odd
inappropriate proposition, to the actors and actresses, and even taunt police
officers and overturn a cab in the post-performance hijinks.

As valuably, the novel explores the cross-section of students who entered provincial medical faculties, as opened in Birmingham, Bristol, Leeds, Liverpool,
Manchester, Newcastle, and Sheffield in these years. Apparent in the case of
Birmingham is that the student body, while diverse, was also divided. Although
the medical faculty's location in the centre of town, nearer its teaching hospitals, made practical sense, this affected relations between medical students and
those in other faculties. The non-medical students described by Ingleby are
generally regarded with some contempt. Much of this has to do with the circumstances that brought him to Birmingham, but matters were clearly aggra-
vated by the medical school's location; it remained distant from the rest of the
university until 1938, when the Edgbaston campus was finally completed.
This physical separation was further augmented by the social divisions recognized by Edwin. Birmingham's staff, like at other provincial medical schools,
was required to accept women as a condition of university status. In the years
when the novel is set, 169 of the 193 medical students were locals.[38] These
local youths were also joined by some older "seedy looking" men, practitioners who had previously qualified from the former medical school, but now
wished to return for a shorter period of study to gain a *university* degree in

order to upgrade their qualifications. Like these men, the non-medicals are almost unanimously (and dismissively) described by Ingleby as the aspiring sons or daughters of pawnbrokers, manufacturers, or shopkeepers. Few of the non-medicals ever associate with the former group and, as a result, the book's narrative concentrates exclusively on the experiences of medical students.

In Young's opinion, doctors had rarely been adequately treated in British literature, and to some extent, he personally rectified the perceived absence of fictional medical practitioners up to that time. His midland novels are also filled with broader medical themes. This is undertaken with his usual attention to detail – for example, employing professional and technical vocabulary that is not immediately accessible to lay members of the public. For instance, during Ingleby's pathology lessons, the novel's protagonist imagines the havoc that bacteria had inflicted on human bodies historically, and then outlines the actual methods he is being taught to isolate these fatal pathogens. Besides mentioning the organism of cholera and "the dreamy trypanosome," he recounts how he and his lab partner observed the "banded bacilli of tubercule, stained red with carbolfuchsin," terms that might have confused ordinary readers, before expanding on other accessible topics, such an illustrious line of TB's more famous victims, including Keats, Shelley, and Stevenson.[39]

The descriptions of medical practitioners in his novels, like Birmingham's districts and thoroughfares, are also based on Young's actual instructors, or practitioners he might have glimpsed on the corridors of the medical school, in the hospitals, or even on the city's streets during his years in Birmingham. Most are immediately identifiable, as Young only slightly altered names, with Charles Purslow, the assistant in gynaecology, becoming Jimmy Purswell, and professor of ophthalmology Hartley recognizable as Priestly-Smith, a midlands ophthalmologist of international renown. Less familiar individuals are also discernible, such as Lloyd Moore, fictionalized as professor of operative surgery Jordan Lloyd, whom Young's own fictional counterpart describes as "the outstanding surgical genius of the Midlands" and to whom Ingleby is attached as a surgical dresser in the novel. Initially said to speak an "unvarnished and foul" language, Moore is soon regarded as "the one man of unquestionable genius in the North Bromwich Medical School."[40] His shortcomings are quickly forgotten while Ingleby works alongside him in the casualty department, and it becomes clear that the surgeon's power of "diagnosis is a matter of inspired, unerring instinct," practically a "gift of the gods."[41] Under his tutelage, surgery appears exceedingly simple to Ingleby. Moore is also respected as a man of the people, who had fought his way "inch by inch into the honourable position that he held" in the profession. A man of "titanic energy," he had garnered the respect of colleagues, becoming "the general practitioner's friend," and, in the process, gained "the most interesting clinical material in the district." Moore is especially admired by his elderly female patients, who describe him to Ingleby as "the very image of Jesus Christ."[42]

When Young describes the dean of medicine, he similarly invokes the actual dean at the time, Bertram Windle, with his thin, fair hair and distinctive round, golden spectacles. The fictitious dean is an "Irish anatomist," while Windle also served as professor of anatomy at the newly established University Medical School, before eventually leaving Birmingham to become president of Queen's College Cork in Ireland halfway through Young's degree.[43] Interestingly, Windle would later become famous for vastly improving facilities for Cork's medical students, who previously inhabited what were described as very Spartan spaces. The common rooms, clubhouses, and canteens, among other facilities taken for granted by medical students in the later twentieth century, were absent from most Victorian medical schools. Prior to such developments, medical students congregated in porters' lodges, which doubled as lounges and second-hand shops. While at Birmingham, Windle already started to improve facilities. Although mediocre by today's standards, the disused workshops behind Mason's College were converted in the 1890s into what Young described as "a dismal chamber" in the basement of the school's cramped building.

In this "chamber," according to Young's narrative, medical students congregated with others not yet transferred to the new campus, drinking tea and eating "squashed-fly biscuits." In fact, Ingleby's pre-clinical years appear little more than a rotation between the lecture theatre, the dissecting room, and this social space. The history of the Newcastle Medical School refers to similar facilities, although accommodation and care for the students "was chiefly conspicuous by its absence."[44] While many schools were beginning to improve student facilities, most had some way to go before they could offer anything like what was available at the largest London schools. Not surprisingly, Ingleby regularly opts to visit Joey's, a local bar opposite the "Corinthian town-hall," where in his breaks he consumes "a quarter of the top of a cottage loaf, a tangle of watercress, a hunk of Cheddar cheese, and a tankard of beer," a combination known as "crust and bitter," for the sum of four pence.[45]

The years when Young studied in Birmingham were significant because women had only recently been admitted to the medical school. While their presence changed many aspects of the student experience, it was also described as sobering, with some emphasizing that women "civilised" the medical cohort at these institutions.[46] Although a single woman enrolled in the same year that Young commenced his studies in Birmingham, three others had entered the programme a year earlier.[47] The following year, another four women registered. Like the local shopkeepers' boys, with whom Ingleby did not mix, the sex division within the student body was marked. This was exacerbated by an age difference between the male and female students. Women were often several years older than the "boys" with whom they studied. In the case of the 1902 cohort, the eldest student, aged thirty-eight, was a woman.[48] As a result, those young men who commenced their studies, and perhaps hoped to meet a potential partner at university, had to seek one outside of the medical faculty or among the hospital's nursing staff. Indeed, Ingleby describes female medical students as having "insulated themselves with shapeless djibbehs of russet brown," and most "bunched back their hair in a manner ruthlessly unfeminine."[49] In contemporary photographs, they appear as mature students, and Ingleby states with conviction that "romance was not bound to emerge." Even if the women had been younger, the common study of a subject such as anatomy would, he claims, "have rubbed the bloom from any budding romance."[50] Similar frosty relations are alluded to in other historical studies of medical education.[51]

Given the centrality of anatomy in the medical curriculum – students at the time did little else during their first two years besides dissecting bodies – the dissection room features prominently in *The Young Physician*. Even if other subjects, such as chemistry and physics, were offered, lectures in the pre-clinical sciences made less of an impression on students. Besides finding them too near to the "desperate subject of mathematics," Ingleby finds "nothing romantic or human" in these subjects.[52] Dissection, on the other hand, was a formative moment in their educations, a "rite of passage," as other historians have appropriately described this aspect of medical training.[53] Located in the school's upper stories, the "irregular chamber" that comprised the anatomy theatre had an asphalt floor and a pungent scent of "unknown antiseptic" mixed with "ancient mortality." It was particularly "icy" in winter and described as a "Chamber of Horrors" by Ingleby and his classmates.[54] With students arriving in autumn, the cooler autumnal days ensured the necessity of commencing dissection soon after their arrival, beginning with the softer tissues, which the colder weather helped preserve. Each body was shared between two students, and anatomy partners had the choice of "an Upper or a Lower"; Edwin Ingleby is paired with Martin, a shrewd Celt, who opts for the Upper as he assumes there is "less fat and mess about it."[55] The Medical School Calendar of 1901 indeed confirms that the first-year anatomy course "deals with Osteology, Arthrology and the Anatomy of the *Upper and Lower Extremities.*"[56]

Young's narrative provides the reader with a valuable description of the anatomy teaching space. Besides its distinct size and shape, the room is filled with rows of zinc tables, each with a tin bucket at its head.[57] Open to students between 9am and 5pm during term,[58] it is largely abandoned on Ingleby's first visit after the inaugural anatomy lecture. On the four or five occupied tables, "subjects" are "sprawled on their faces" and draped in "coarse, unbleached calico."[59] As yet unappropriated, most are supported by a small metal platform "from which the heads rolled back," the limbs stretched out in a way that suggests "petrified agony."[60] Initially, Ingleby does not dare approach the corpses and stands in awe, while his dissection partner explains how these "withered," "toothless" mummies reached their "final indignity." They are, of course, paupers, Ingleby is told, unclaimed bodies from the city's workhouses pickled by the anatomy porters in vats stored in the school cellar. Besides injecting bodies with arsenic in order to preserve them, the porters "pump red paint into their arteries so that they're easier to dissect."[61] Like the porters, Ingleby grows used to the work and, instead of a dead man, sees only "a pathetic tanned skeleton ... from which all the humanity had shrunk away."[62] Among the unique insights included in Young's dialogue is the fact that students actually preferred older bodies because the muscles were "cleaner" and "subsequently less work."[63] Ingleby, like students before him, soon accepts "his new callousness," as conveyed in a particularly thoughtful paragraph, which presumably draws on Young's own experience of emotional adjustment. After some weeks, the sole objectionable feature of the dissection room according to Ingleby is its penetrating antiseptic odour, a scent he remains conscious of during his waking hours, whether on the train, at mealtimes, or "even in his sleep."[64]

Initially described as gloomy, the dissection room is made brighter by the students who populate it, and develop meaningful relationships during this formative educational experience, as well as the demonstrators, one or more of whom is always in charge of the room and ready to instruct.[65] Students inhabiting the room wear white overalls, joke, gossip, and smoke their pipes as they thumb "manuals of practical anatomy yellow with human grease."[66] According to the University of Birmingham's medical syllabus, each student was also issued with a guide explaining the "detailed working of the Department."[67] Although otherwise prohibited in the medical school, smoking was not only tolerated in the dissection room, but its stench convinced Ingleby of its necessity,[68] and reputedly helped to "ease the nerves."[69] Besides noting a student, in navy serge duffle coat, paired with "the correct red tie and a big orchid in his buttonhole" and smoking "an elaborate *meerschaum* pipe,"[70] this section of the novel also includes reference to an actual anatomical text; not surprisingly, it is a copy of *Gray's Anatomy* that is consulted by one of Ingleby's studious colleagues.[71] This section also conveys the important role of demonstrators in the delivery of teaching, not all of which was undertaken by the professors. Initially fascinated by a collection of coloured chalks upon entering the space, Edwin Ingleby and Martin grow to admire the demonstrators, who daily draw the various bodily tissues and systems on the black boards, and carefully illustrate with coloured chalk where muscles and tendons attach to bones. Demonstrators' names are prominent on the boards, but only one, Robert Moon, is named. Maintaining the day-to-day contact with students, some, such as Moon, are so good that they gradually make the professor look like a "dilettante." A "figure of romantic picturesqueness," who had acquired an unrivalled "familiarity with the dismembered fragments of humanity," Moon runs popular tutorials at which second-year students congregate at his feet "like the disciples of a Greek philosopher."[72]

After two years of lectures and practical work in the dissection room, and as at Birmingham, Ingleby first enters the two teaching hospitals with his cohort. Here, he joins the clinical teams, first as Lloyd Moore's surgical dresser, then as a physician's clerk. Lectures naturally continue, including in pharmacology, which Ingleby attends in his fourth year, but, again, these hardly feature in the book's narrative. Those serving as surgical dressers in one hospital later attend the other for their physician's training, or clerkship. In the novel, Birmingham's first teaching hospital, the Queen's Hospital, reappears as the Prince's Hospital. The latter is said to be located in the upper, "healthier part of the city," on "the fringe of the fashionable suburb of Alveston," but across the road from houses that had degenerated into "theatrical lodging houses" (and play an essential part in the closing section of the book, as will be discussed). In contrast, the hospital remains a "solid building of early Victorian red brick with a stern portico," much as the Queen's Hospital is depicted in contemporary images. Ingleby's claim that it treated half as many patients as its rival teaching hospital is again accurate, even noting the cab rank outside the building, as well as its 9am clinics. Among other details, he describes the military background of the hospital porter, the distribution of medicine and bandages in the casualty department, and even the hospital's smells.

The other teaching hospital is North Bromwich Infirmary, a fictionalized General Hospital, Birmingham. An impressive civic building, it is located in the middle of a slum, near the patients it was intended to serve in the lower, unhealthier part of the city. In Ingleby's opinion, this attenuated the building's grandeur, referring instead to its "terracotta arrogance." He also misses the "homely atmosphere" of the Prince's Hospital, where everything was familiar, in contrast to the Infirmary, which is twice the size of the other and has wards that are "colder and more formal," perhaps because its nurses are "drawn from a higher social strata."[73] Interesting too is Ingleby's reference to the hospital's "air that suffocated," for the windows of the actual General Hospital, on which it was based, did not open. In fact, it was one of the first British hospitals ventilated by the closed plenum air system when it opened in 1896, a feature that emphasized its advanced design, for air could be regulated and circulated more efficiently.[74] Ingleby, however, did not regard it

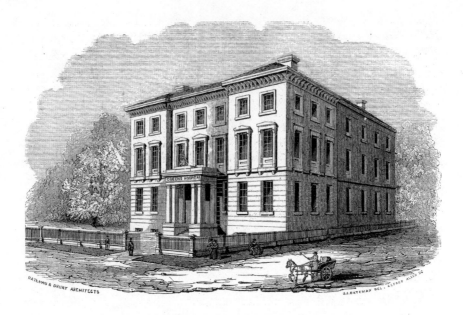

Figure 16.1 | The Queen's Hospital, Birmingham, at the time Francis Brett Young was studying medicine in Birmingham. (Wood engraving by A. Allen, 1903, private collection)

as the pinnacle of modernity. According to him, the forced system of ventilation filtered air until "it … lost all its nature," and he subsequently relishes each opportunity to escape to the countryside and "blow away the vapours of forced ventilation with Cotswold air."[75] When the governors of the actual hospital eventually became critical of the system, it was not because of concerns regarding air purity, but finances, as it consumed huge amounts of coal, the costs of which had grown fourfold and became prohibitive.[76] What historical studies have not communicated, but Ingleby does, is that the machine and its eight accompanying fans in the basement, which together circulated heated air through some 35,000 feet of steel tubing,[77] led the building to emit an audible, "melancholy groaning";[78] the sound made "the whole structure seem more like an artificial assembly of matter than a real hospital with a personality and a soul."[79]

Given Ingleby's initial depictions of Birmingham's industrialists and fellow students, his descriptions of hospital patients are considerably less disparaging. Unlike the hospital, the poor, sick inhabitants admitted to its wards have discernible personalities. While one might expect Ingleby to reduce them to an indistinct mass, his views grow tender, perhaps because the patients appreciate his developing medical skills. Among those arriving each day and filling the waiting rooms are

> old men whose skins were foul with the ravages of eczema and dirt combined; women, exhausted in middle age by child-rearing, and the accepted slavery of housework; sturdy mechanics who had been the victims of some unavoidable accident; pale young women, made anxious for their livelihood by illness that its conditions had caused, and, more terrible than all, the steady stream of wan, transparent children, the idols of maternal care, the victims of maternal ignorance.[80]

Ingleby throws himself into his clinical training with enthusiasm, often losing all sense of time. Gradually, the work is undertaken in a less confused manner, with dressings rarely ending up on the floor, applied more neatly, and he even grows accustomed to the hospital's smell. Although he recalls the names of few patients, relations between the students and patients grow more intimate. Ingleby is particularly flattered by their apparent trust in his nominal skills, and he gains confidence as a result. They respond to names such as "daddy," "granny," "Tommy," and "Polly," but to them, he is "Doctor." Besides giving Ingleby "a flush of gratification" deeper than he had ever known, it pleases him when his patients tell him that he dresses them more gently than the other staff in the casualty department. Emotions first aroused when learning about the TB bacillus in the lab soon re-emerge on the Infirmary wards when encountering phthisical patients. Invoking popular disease metaphors since explored by Susan Sontag, including the belief that those afflicted with consumption were refined and artistic,[81] Ingleby describes these patients as "creatures of intelligence," whose "eyes shone between their long lashes with a light that may have been taken for that of inspiration in those dead poets," including Keats and Shelley, who were similarly "banished" by the disease.[82] Such moments convince him that he has found his true vocation.

As with Ingleby's most memorable patients, there is a single non-medical student who stands apart from the crowd. On his first excursion to the medical school's café, Edwin Ingleby encounters Griffin, a fellow pupil from his boarding school, St Luke's, who enrolled at North Bromwich as a brewing student. In constructing this character, Young consciously drew on historical example, Birmingham having famously, and controversially, opened a School for Brewing, for which it was ridiculed nationally. In exchange for £28,000 from the Midland Association of Brewers, the university offered vocational courses in a department that would over time evolve into biochemistry. Governors also opened a Mining School when the university was inaugurated in 1900, as well as a Commerce Department specifically to support the needs of the regional economy. The arts, on the other hand, were little more than "a side-show" that was not taken seriously.[83] At the time, members of England's older, established universities satirized Birmingham's decision to offer practical instruction in such subjects. One Oxford pamphlet, for example, poetically lampooned these developments at provincial universities with the line "he gets a degree in making jam in Liverpool and Birmingham."[84] Unlike Ingleby, Griffin was destined to attend university in North Bromwich, for his uncle is one of the city's leading brewers and a university benefactor. Despite his unique persona and privileged background, Griffin is also intended to represent the "everyman" of Birmingham students, largely through his name, the griffin being the symbol of the University of Birmingham's Guild of Students. Like many other students Ingleby first encounters, Griffin is determined above all to have a good time at North Bromwich. Expelled from boarding school at the outset of the novel, and shamelessly in pursuit of the opposite sex, Griffin is the perfect brewing student given the department's early reputation.

While other students are drawn to excess, whether during riots or the pantomime, Griffin nevertheless manages to stand apart from the wider student body. Although initially bullied by Griffin at boarding school, Ingleby later befriends the brewing disciple, who no longer possesses "threatening physical superiority" and whose class background sets him apart from the average provincial student.[85] Seemingly less narrow-minded, Ingleby's classmates recognize Griffin's deviant nature and warn Ingleby against growing too close to "that pig of a brewer."[86] Griffin is variously described as a "bad hat," a "bad egg," a "nasty," "obscene" fellow, who will come to "a rotten sticky end."[87] He even dresses as Mephistopheles on pantomime night. Few readers will not recognize that things can only end badly for Griffin. From the first chapter, while at boarding school, he is described as "tall for his age" and heavily built, yet excused from sports because of his bad heart.[88] When it eventually ends fatally for Griffin in the novel's final pages, he is spotted by one of Ingleby's classmates in the lounge of the Grand Midland Hotel with Rosie Beaucaire, a pantomine actress (a contemporary euphemism for prostitute). Rosie has also recently charmed Ingleby, who, again, is unable to see what is obvious to others. While busy preparing for his final exams, Ingleby unknowingly allows his old rival to seduce his sweetheart. On discovering the rendezvous, Ingleby races to Rosie's lodgings in Prince Albert's Place and, hearing "the clock in the Art Gallery chime eleven," witnesses the couple's return after a night out. Initially overcome with fear, Ingleby grows incensed and confronts his adversary in Rosie's flat. A potentially violent face-off, however, quickly defuses as Griffin collapses, and dies, for the fray proves too much for his "rocky heart."[89]

Rosie begs Ingleby to depart (which he does), leaving the authorities to suspect the death was due to "natural causes."[90] In the next day's newspapers, the other students learn of Griffin's "sticky end," and, unaware of Ingleby's involvement in the episode, recount the details to the newly qualified doctor. With his reputation intact, Ingleby travels to Liverpool the following morning, presents himself at a shipping office, and sails off as the newly appointed medical officer on a ship bound for China.

While the novel ends here, this episode merely stimulated my interest to locate the inspiration for Griffin. On this occasion, it required greater effort, yet he appeared in the university archives in the form of Adrian Barry. Like so many other figures and features employed by Young in his literary works, Barry's resemblance to Griffin is uncanny. A former student at the University of Birmingham, Barry was originally from Tamworth, a town on the outskirts of Birmingham. Newspaper clippings from the 1910s in a faculty ledger reported his antics, such as being found drunk across the frame of his bicycle on more than one occasion.[91] From a family of not inconsiderable wealth, Barry reportedly received a public school education, and possessed a driver's licence at a time when few students drove. Each article repeated claims, much like Griffin's colleagues in the novel, that Barry was a troubled character who disgraced his profession through his antics. In 1913, a final article reports his death in a manner not dissimilar to that of the fictitious brewing student. Although started in 1911, Young's novel was interrupted by war, but was finished in 1918, by which time Barry's intrigues were available to the author. Like Griffin, on his last evening, Adrian Barry met an actress, Ethyl Clay, and, as significantly, the two reputedly met on Bull Street just before 11pm, the exact time when Edwin Ingleby hears the Art Gallery clock chime and spies Griffin and Rosie returning to her lodgings. On this occasion, Barry and Clay returned to Ethyl's home at 20 Belgrave Road, which, like Rosie's, was approximately a block away from the Queen's Hospital. Though not confronted by a fellow student, Barry complained of a "headache" and he was "snoring heavily" in Clay's bed, details which Young equally incorporates into the novel's narrative.[92] The following morning, Clay brought Barry breakfast in bed, but he remained asleep and unresponsive. Alarmed at the pallor of his face and unable to wake him, Clay called a doctor, who pronounced Barry dead on the scene, his death judged the result of "paralysis of the respiratory organs."[93] What Young failed to communicate to readers by the time he incorporated Barry into his story, however, was his true vocation. Instead of a brewing student, as the fictitious Griffin had become, Barry was in actual fact a medical student. While this detail may appear trivial to some of Young's readers, in the context of this chapter, it should be recognized as significant.

CONCLUSIONS

In recent years, historians have discovered sources that allow them to capture less familiar episodes in the history of medical education. These include works of fiction, including the novels of Francis Brett Young. While Young's writings have previously been identified as very faithful recordings of life in the English midlands, the pitfalls of using these sources have not yet been fully explored. Young's midland novels possess a recognized anti-Birmingham bias, yet most readers have been able to ignore such obvious prejudices and draw on the distinct regional atmosphere that infuses these novels. With this particular study, it is hoped that historians will recognize that it was not just the countryside that Young romanticized in his midlands-based writings. Although not regarded to have forged close links to his medical school cohort, it is clear that Young, like his fictional alter ego, Ingleby, became intensely loyal to his medical colleagues. I would also argue that this is best evidenced by his decision to edit out important details in *The Young Physician*, including reinventing Adrian Barry as Griffin, a contemptible brewing student, so as not to tarnish the reputation of fellow medics.

Of course, this was not unlike what was occurring elsewhere in the medical profession, as Waddington and others have argued for this same period. Young indeed admits to some professional "rustiness" among his cohort at medical school, but, according to his writings, there does not actually appear to be a charlatan among them by the time he commenced his studies in Birmingham.[94] Nevertheless, to comprehend fully such statements one must also consider the way in which Young internalized a shared medical culture during his Birmingham years, and, as Digby has claimed, actively constructed a professional identity, despite his initial feelings about studying in Birmingham.[95] Here, as at other provincial schools, students were shaped into medical gentlemen through their lectures, clinical work, and even societies, but the success of this process, or the ability to fully transform medical students from an "urban pariah to a hardworking individual training for a respectable profession," also often depended on certain details being pruned, or even purged, from official and even unofficial records, such as Young's semi-autobiographical novels.[96] At Birmingham, as at many other British medical schools, one would always find the "hearty perennials" (read: underachievers), but they likely survived longer at these institutions than most studies to date have acknowledged. After all, circumstances were unlike today, with each medical school receiving multiple applications for each available space. Young studied at a time when almost everyone who wanted to pursue a career in medicine, and could afford the tuition, gained a place at a school, regardless of age, academic performance, or character. It was only after the Second World War that staff and relevant committees at British medical schools actively began to eliminate the unprofessional and unproductive elements from provincial institutions. What played a more important role up until this time was the creative self-fashioning that was encouraged and clearly prevalent within the medical profession, even amongst those who, like Francis Brett Young, at first appeared less loyal to their colleagues. In this case, perhaps Young was also more creative than people have suggested.

NOTES

1   Bonner, *Becoming a Physician*, 7.

2   Waddington, "Mayhem and Medical Students," 45. One significant addition to this literature is Kelly's *Irish Medical Education and Student Culture*.

3   Reinarz, "Unearthing and Dissecting the Records of English Provincial Medical Education," 388.

4   Kiberd, *Ulysses and Us*, 10–12.

5   Hall, *Francis Brett Young*, 8.

6   Cannadine, *This Little World*.

7   Jordanova, *History in Practice*, 78.

8   See for example, Bonner, *Becoming a Physician*; Waddington, *Medical Education at St Bartholomew's Hospital*; Heaman, *St Mary's*.

9   Porter, "The Patient's View," 175–98.

10   Lane, "The Role of Apprenticeship in Eighteenth-Century Medical Education in England," 57–103.

11   Lawrence, "Charitable Knowledge."

12   Lawrence, "Anatomy and Address," 203.

13   Waddington, *Medical Education at St Bartholomew's Hospital*, 218–58.

14   Hall, *Francis Brett Young*, 42.

15   Aldrich, *School and Society in Victorian Britain*, 38.

16   Hall, *Francis Brett Young*, 32.

17   Ibid., 43.

18   Ibid., 158.

19   Cannadine, *This Little World*, 16.

20   Hall, *Francis Brett Young*, 86.

21   Young, *The Young Physician*, 117.

22   Ibid., 107.

23   Ibid.

24   Ibid., 238.

25   Ibid., 117–18.

26   Ibid., 118.

27   Ibid.

28   Ibid., 112.

29   Ibid., 155.

30   Ibid., 379.

31   Ibid., 230.

32   Ives, Schwarz, and Drummond, *The First Civic University*, 43.

33   *The Lancet*, 26 August 1911, 583–5.

34   Cregier, *Bounder from Wales*, 73.

35   Young, *The Young Physician*, 375.

36   Ibid., 373.

37   Ibid., 274.

38   University of Birmingham Cadbury Research Library (UBCRL), Student Register, 1892–.

39   Young, *The Young Physician*, 384.

40   Ibid., 363.

41   Ibid., 362–4.

42   Ibid., 364–5.

43   Taylor, *Sir Bertram Windle*, 246.

44   Turner and Arnison, *The Newcastle upon Tyne School of Medicine*, 111.

45   Young, *The Young Physician*, 274.

46   Kelly, *Irish Women in Medicine*, 178.

47   UBCRL, Student Register, 1892–.

48   Ibid.

49   Young, *The Young Physician*, 279.

50   Ibid.

51   Kelly, *Irish Women in Medicine*, 177–83.

52   Young, *The Young Physician*, 264.

53   Warner and Edmonson, *Dissection*; Kelly, *Irish Medical Education*, 135.

54   Young, *The Young Physician*, 264.

55   Ibid.

56   UBCRL, *Faculty of Medicine Syllabus, 1901–1902*.

57   Young, *The Young Physician*, 265.

58   UBCRL, *Faculty of Medicine Syllabus*, 277.

59   Young, *The Young Physician*, 265.

60   Ibid.

61   Ibid., 265–6.

62   Ibid., 266.

63   Ibid., 255.

64   Ibid., 269.

65   UBCRL, *Faculty of Medicine Syllabus*, 277.

66   Young, *The Young Physician*, 267.

67   UBCRL, *Faculty of Medicine Syllabus*, 324.

68   Young, *The Young Physician*, 271.
69   Kelly, *Irish Medical Education*, 143.
70   Young, *The Young Physician*, 267–8.
71   Ibid., 271.
72   Ibid., 311.
73   Ibid., 385.
74   Taylor, *The Architect and the Pavilion Hospital*, 200–10.
75   Young, *The Young Physician*, 393.
76   Reinarz, *Health Care in Birmingham*, 129.
77   Ibid., 128.
78   Young, *The Young Physician*, 385.
79   Ibid.
80   Ibid., 354.
81   Sontag, *Illness as Metaphor*, 28, 45.
82   Young, *The Young Physician*, 384, 387.
83   Ibid., 241.
84   Ives, *The First Civic University*, 143.
85   Young, *The Young Physician*, 280.
86   Ibid., 281.
87   Ibid.
88   Ibid., 10.
89   Ibid., 482.
90   Ibid., 483.
91   *Birmingham Daily Mail*, 17 September 1912; *Birmingham Daily Gazette*, 19 September 1912.
92   Young, *The Young Physician*, 478, 481.
93   *Birmingham Gazette*, 27 January 1913.
94   Hall, "Francis Brett Young's Birmingham," 360.
95   Digby, "Shaping New Identities," 20.
96   Waddington, "Mayhem and Medical Students," 63.

BIBLIOGRAPHY

Aldrich, R. *School and Society in Victorian Britain*. Abingdon, UK: Routledge, 2012.
Bonner, T.N. *Becoming a Physician: Medical Education in Britain, France, Germany and the United States, 1750–1945*. Oxford, UK: Oxford University Press, 1995.
Cannadine, D. *This Little World: The Value of the Novels of Francis Brett Young as a Guide to the State of Midland Society, 1870–1925*. Occasional Papers No. 4. Worcester, UK: Worcestershire Historical Society, 1982.
Cregier, D.M. *Bounder from Wales: Lloyd George's Career before the First World War*. Columbia, MO: University of Missouri Press, 1976.

Digby, A. "Shaping New Identities: Health, Well-Being and Personhood."
In *Medical Identities: Health, Wellbeing and Personhood*, edited by Kent Maynard,
14–35. New York: Berghahn Books, 2007.

Hall, Michael. *Francis Brett Young*. Bridgend, UK: Seren, 1997.

– "Francis Brett Young's Birmingham: North Bromwich – City of Iron." PhD thesis.
Birmingham, UK: University of Birmingham, 2007.

Heaman, E.A. *St Mary's: The History of London Teaching Hospital*. Liverpool, UK:
Liverpool University Press, 2003.

Ives, E., L. Schwarz, and D. Drummond. *The First Civic University: Birmingham,
1880–1980*. Birmingham, UK: University of Birmingham Press, 2000.

Jordanova, Ludmilla. *History in Practice*. London: Hodder Arnold, 2006.

Kelly, L. *Irish Medical Education and Student Culture, c. 1850–1950*. Liverpool, UK:
Liverpool University Press, 2017.

Kiberd, Declan. *Ulysses and Us: The Art of Everyday Living*. London: Faber and Faber,
2009.

Lane, J. "The Role of Apprenticeship in Eighteenth-Century Medical Education in
England." In *William Hunter and the Eighteenth-Century Medical World*, edited by W.F.
Bynum and R. Porter, 57–103. Cambridge: Cambridge University Press, 1985.

Lawrence, S. "Anatomy and Address: Creating Medical Gentlemen in Eighteenth-
Century London." In *The History of Medical Education in Britain*, edited by V. Nutton
and R. Porter, 199–228. Amsterdam: Rodopi, 1995.

Lawrence, S. *Charitable Knowledge: Hospital Pupils and Practitioners in Eighteenth-Century
London*. Cambridge: Cambridge University Press, 1996.

Porter, R. "The Patient's View: Doing Medical History from Below." *Theory and
Society* 14, no. 2 (1985): 175–98.

Reinarz, J. "Unearthing and Dissecting the Records of English Provincial Medical
Education, c. 1825–1948." *Social History of Medicine* 21, no. 2 (2008): 381–92.

Sontag, S. *Illness as Metaphor*. New York: Doubleday, 1990.

Taylor, J. *The Architect and the Pavilion Hospital*. Leicester, UK: Leicester University Press,
1997.

Taylor, M. *Sir Bertram Windle*. London: Longmans, Green and Co., 1932.

Turner, G.G., and W.D. Arnison. *The Newcastle upon Tyne School of Medicine, 1834–
1934*. Newcastle, UK: Andrew Reid & Co., 1934.

Waddington, K. "Mayhem and Medical Students: Image, Conduct, and Control in
the Victorian and Edwardian London Teaching Hospital." *Social History of Medicine*
15, no. 1 (2002): 45–64.

– *Medical Education at St Bartholomew's Hospital, 1123–1995*. Woodbridge, UK: Boydell
& Brewer, 2003.

Warner, J.H., and J.M. Edmonson. *Dissection: Photographs of a Rite of Passage in American
Medicine: 1880–1930*. New York: Blast Books, 2009.

Young, Francis Brett. *The Young Physician*. London: W. Collins Sons, 1930.

17

Failures and Alternative Paths:
Jessie White Mario and Women's Struggles to Obtain
Medical Education in Victorian England

Diana Moore

In August of 1856, twenty-four-year-old Jessie Meriton White (referred to throughout this chapter as Jessie White Mario, the name she used most frequently after her 1857 marriage) applied to King's College London to become a candidate for the degree of bachelor of medicine. White Mario planned to use this medical training as a nurse in the forthcoming battles of the Italian Risorgimento, a campaign to liberate the various states of the Italian peninsula from foreign and despotic governments and to create a unified and regenerated Italian state. When King's College rejected White Mario's application, she redirected her efforts to parallel work in the Italian propaganda campaign, lecturing, fundraising, translating, and working as a newspaper correspondent, before eventually fulfilling her dream of serving as a nurse in Italy throughout the 1860s. Both contemporaries and historians have recognized the important role White Mario played in the Risorgimento. While some accounts of her life briefly mention her rejection from medical school, they focus their attention on her accomplishments as a nurse, lecturer, journalist, biographer, and social scientist.[1] Despite her failure to obtain a medical degree, therefore, White Mario was undoubtedly a success.

In this chapter, I focus on the life of White Mario (1832–1906) as a case study to demonstrate the fierce resistance faced by women seeking standardized medical education in the mid-nineteenth century and how these women rebounded from rejection by educational and medical establishments, gathering knowledge where they could, often on the battlefields of Europe and North America. Moreover, for many of these women, the medical degree was not their ultimate goal and they refused to define themselves by their failure to obtain it. They sought education and certification as a means to fulfill diverse personal and professional goals, and when denied formal education pursued alternative paths to obtain knowledge and achieve their objectives.

Much of the historical literature on Anglo-American women in the medical profession in the nineteenth century has focused too heavily on institutional or legal changes, such as admission to medical school, or on select biographical figures who triumphed over their opposition and found success in recognized establishments. Popular figures in these types of work include Elizabeth Blackwell (1821–1910), who in 1849 became the first woman to earn a medical degree in the United States, and Florence Nightingale (1820–1910), who rose to prominence as a nurse during the Crimean War (1853–56) and afterward promoted the professionalization of nursing in Britain.[2] Although some scholars try to expand their scope by focusing on lesser-known figures, they still limit their study to those women who earned formal medical degrees and qualifications.[3]

I argue that this is a somewhat problematic approach for studying the history of women and other marginalized groups. The professionalization of medicine in the mid-nineteenth century was an intentionally exclusionary act designed to reinforce existing hierarchies and further deny the majority of the population respectability within the medical field. As historians of medicine, we must take care not to reinforce those structures of exclusion with our methodology. To achieve a more equitable history of medicine, we must look beyond those individuals who gained admittance to conventional institutions of medical education and acknowledge those who learned and practised standard medicine in alternative ways or who learned and practised alternative forms of medicine. By taking this approach, this chapter builds on existing scholarship discussing how marginalized groups found greater agency by working as midwives, as homeopaths, or in religious and charitable nursing organizations.[4]

This chapter also closely connects to the scholarship on female war nurses. These works argue that the exigencies of war allowed women to be active in the medical field in ways they could not during peacetime, and claim that the success of female nurses in wartime led to the recognition of nursing as a profession. Most of these works, however, focus on the twentieth century, and those that cover the nineteenth century centre their discussion on the Crimean War (1853–56) or the American Civil War (1861–65).[5] One notable exception is historian Anne Summers's 1988 monograph on British war nurses, which includes the mid-nineteenth-century wars of national unification and the Anglo-Boer War (1899–1902).[6] This chapter builds on these studies by showing how White Mario and women like her used their experiences as war nurses as alternative paths to medical education. I was also inspired by historian Kara Dixon Vuic's argument that war nurses were political agents and active participants in acts of war.[7] Like Vuic, I recognize that women's war experiences were frequently quite political rather than acts of disinterested humanitarian charity.

This chapter begins with an introduction to White Mario and the Italian Risorgimento, revealing her steadfast commitment to its ideals and her numerous contributions to the movement. The second section then examines her failed attempt to obtain formal medical education, while the third section demonstrates how as a war nurse she learned not only about anatomy and surgery but also the logistics of practising medicine. In the conclusion, I examine White Mario's accounts of her nursing and their strong political content. Throughout, I show that she never sought medical knowledge as an end in itself but continually used that knowledge to achieve her political goals. Overall, I argue that her work reveals a greater variety of reasons why women pursued medical knowledge in the nineteenth century.

To support my arguments, I use White Mario's own rich archive of personal letters, memoirs, biographies, and newspaper articles discussing her experience in nursing. I also utilize British newspapers and periodicals to emphasize the strong opposition White Mario and women like her faced in pursuing medical careers.

JESSIE WHITE MARIO AND THE RISORGIMENTO

Jessie White Mario was born Jessie Meriton White to a family of non-conformist middle-class shipbuilders in Portsmouth, England, who fostered her intellect. Taught to seek justice rather than propriety, White Mario was already pushing beyond the borders of a typical middle-class life and studying philosophy at the Sorbonne in Paris in the early 1850s when she developed an interest in the Italian Risorgimento.[8]

At that time, the Italian peninsula was politically divided into a series of moderate and conservative states. Nineteenth-century Italian nationalists fought to overcome these divisions and to reform, modernize, and unite the peninsula. On the left were the radicals, led by Giuseppe Mazzini (1805–1872) and Giuseppe Garibaldi (1807–1882), who organized uprisings and revolutions to bring about a unified and republican Italy. While Mazzini focused his efforts on propaganda, fundraising, and organizing revolutions, Garibaldi worked primarily in military campaigns for freedom not only in Italy, but also in South America throughout the 1830s and 1840s. For this, he earned the nickname "The Hero of Two Worlds." In 1848–49, Mazzini, Garibaldi, and other republicans staged nationalist revolts in Milan, Venice, and Rome to initial success but ultimate failure. Following these disappointments, radical republicans continued to organize small-scale revolts, while middle-class liberals, led after 1859 by prime minister of Piedmont Count Camillo de Cavour (1810–1861), worked through the channels of diplomacy and conventional warfare to bring about an Italian state in 1861 under the auspices of Piedmont's monarchy.

After participating in their failed revolutions, Italian patriots faced exile and many chose to live in Britain. There they developed close supportive friendships with British men and women who provided not only monetary aid but also key political support.[9] Members of the left wing of the Italian Risorgimento distinguished themselves through their purposeful cultivation of British women as political allies and supporters. Historian Lucy Riall has argued that Mazzini and Garibaldi were unique in their "political use of British women" at that time.[10] They welcomed in British women as collaborators and these women readily took up their invitation. Scholars such as Sarah Richardson, Maura O'Connor, and Anne Summers have argued that British women involved themselves in Italian Unification because it could arguably be construed as a part of the British Protestant "civilizing mission" and was thus a more acceptable outlet for their political ambitions.[11] Others have emphasized the ways in which Mazzini's feminism and promotion of universal egalitarianism and emancipation attracted strong-willed and independent women.[12]

White Mario went from an observer and intellectual supporter of the Risorgimento to one of its most active and dedicated participants after meeting Garibaldi in Paris in 1854. Inspired by their meeting, White Mario joined the Italian nationalist propaganda campaign upon her return to London, sending sympathetic letters and articles to the English press and translating Italian patriot and exile Felice Orsini's (1819–1858) memoirs into English.[13] Once she had established herself as a member of the Italian nationalist circles, she met Mazzini in 1856 and began a lifelong friendship.

From the beginning of her involvement White Mario used every tool at her disposal to aid the cause of Italian Unification and republicanism. She consistently participated in fundraising efforts, translated favorable articles for the English press, and even began a career as a journalist to further control the movement's narrative. From 1856 to 1862, she went on four separate lecture tours in Britain and the United States. In 1857, she travelled to Genoa under the guise of her journalistic career, while covertly participating in the organization of the failed Pisacane uprising. During the plotting, White Mario became close to fellow conspirator Alberto Mario (1825–1883), and though the pair were separated by their respective arrests following the failure of the uprising, they maintained their romance through letters and were married upon White Mario's release from prison that December.

In addition to her work as a writer, translator, lecturer, fundraiser, and conspirator, White Mario also acted as a nurse in the battles for Unification.

In her memoirs, White Mario recalled her initial promise to nurse Garibaldi and his troops and dated it back to the very beginning of her friendship with Garibaldi in 1854 when, "certain of being summoned to fight against the Austrians or lead the Italians in revolution, Garibaldi had obtained my promise to be the nurse of his wounded."[14] Fulfilling her promise, White Mario served as Garibaldi's nurse throughout the 1860s in his campaigns for full Italian Unification and republicanism.

She first and most famously acted as Garibaldi's nurse in his campaign of the Thousand that successfully linked Sicily and southern Italy to the northern territories and Piedmont, effectively creating an Italian state.[15] Risking arrest, White Mario and her husband Alberto Mario sailed to Sicily, arriving on 28 June 1860.[16] Though White Mario had not seen Garibaldi in years, he remembered her and her vow. She described the scene, saying, "The first time that I found him alone he said to me, alluding to an old promise – I have provided you with sufficient wounded to cure."[17] White Mario was a nurse first under Dr Pietro Ripari (1802–1885), the head of the ambulance service, and then under Dr Cesare Stradivari at Barcellona in the "Convent on the Hill," where many cases were gathered.[18] After the success of this campaign, Garibaldi became a national hero and White Mario a minor celebrity for her support of him and his soldiers.[19]

Though a unified Italian state emerged after Garibaldi's campaign in 1860–61, for many the dream of Italian unification was not complete. Two of Italy's most important cities, Rome and Venice, remained outside of its borders. Austria retained control of Venice while the Pope, supported by French troops, maintained his rule over the city of Rome. Garibaldi fought repeatedly to regain control of these territories, and each time White Mario provided her skills as a nurse. The first instance was in August of 1862 when Garibaldi attempted to conquer the city of Rome. Facing harsh pressure from the French, the Italian government opposed Garibaldi's attempt with a force of 3,500 troops. After his surrender, the state then arrested Garibaldi and imprisoned him in the fort of Varignano near La Spezia. During the suppression of this revolt, Italian troops shot Garibaldi twice, a light wound in his left thigh and a more serious wound in his right ankle.[20] Though she was not present in the initial revolutionary moment, White Mario later travelled to Varignano and nursed Garibaldi through his recovery.

She then provided more traditional battlefield nursing by working in the ambulance for Garibaldi's volunteer troops in Italy's 1866 war against Austria to regain control of Venice.[21] Though this was White Mario's first time serving as a nurse in a government-regulated army, the large number of Garibaldi's republican comrades in the volunteer unit ensured that she still held a position of respect and authority.[22]

In the autumn of 1867, after the liberation of Venice, Garibaldi once again raised a force of volunteer troops and attempted to take Rome. He marched into the Papal States, in the hopes that his actions would trigger popular or governmental support. Neither materialized, and the French defeated Garibaldi's forces in a minor engagement at Mentana on 3 November 1867. During this campaign, White Mario again served as a nurse for Garibaldi and his troops.[23]

White Mario finished her career as Garibaldi's war nurse during the Franco-Prussian War of 1870–71.[24] Due to his hatred for Emperor Napoleon III (1808–1873), Garibaldi had traditionally regarded the French as his enemies. After the defeat of the emperor, however, he became an ardent supporter of the French Third Republic and joined the primarily volunteer French Army of the Vosges. White Mario initially went to France as a newspaper correspondent, preferring to aid the cause of republicanism through her journalistic and propagandistic efforts, but when it became clear that the troops needed her medical services, she stepped in.

FAILURE TO OBTAIN FORMAL MEDICAL EDUCATION

By choosing to serve as a nurse for Garibaldi's troops, White Mario pushed against the boundaries of middle-class respectability. In the mid-nineteenth century, nursing outside of one's own family was only acceptable as a charitable and religious endeavour, particularly within a nursing sisterhood. The most famous of these sisterhoods was the German Kaiserswerth sisters (1836), but Britain also had its share, including the Catholic Sisters of Mercy (1827), the non-denominational Institution for Nursing Sisters (1840), and the Anglican Sisterhood of the Holy Cross (1845), Sisterhood of Mercy of Devonport and Plymouth (1848), and St John's House Training Institution for Nurses (1848).[25] Middle-class women also increasingly worked as volunteer nurses, managing paid nurses and promoting a new understanding of nursing as a respectable vocation for women grounded in ideals of domesticity, morality, and charity.[26] Hired or professional nursing, however, was quite unacceptable. According to historian Louise Fitzpatrick, hired nurses in the mid-nineteenth century in both Britain and America "had no training, were often very old or alcoholic, untidy, filthy, and in general viewed with distaste." She added that, "as a rule, middle-class American women did not practice nursing in the homes of others for pay."[27]

Wartime nursing fell somewhere in the middle of these two extremes in terms of its respectability. Prior to the Crimean War, only a few British women had worked as war nurses, and while some were able to portray themselves as devoted wives, military authorities and the British public tended to group these women alongside camp followers or the disreputable paid nurses.[28] The Crimean War and the activities of Florence Nightingale then radically changed the status of nursing in Britain. In October 1854, facing public outcry after newspapers reported on the poor medical treatment of British soldiers, British war secretary Sir Sidney Herbert sent Florence Nightingale and 38 other female nurses to the Crimea. By the war's end, the number of female nurses rose to over 200 and included 9 Anglican Sisters, 28 Roman Catholic nuns, 128 paid hospital nurses, usually of the working class, and 54 volunteer women, usually of the middle or upper classes.[29]

Another notable instance in which large numbers of women served as war nurses in the mid-nineteenth century is the US Civil War.[30] In both the Crimean and Civil Wars, nurses generally spent more time caring for men suffering from frostbite or sick from diseases such as diarrhea, dysentery, typhoid, pneumonia, erysipelas (a streptococcal infection), measles, smallpox, and general fever than treating wounds.[31] Both Union and Confederate women in the Civil War, however, worked closer to the front lines. Though they most frequently provided food and relief for the sick and wounded in field hospitals, they also encountered skirmishes and sometimes dragged men off active battlefields to attend to their wounds.[32]

Historian Anne Summers argued that when war became more of a general patriotic and civilian concern throughout the nineteenth century, support for it, including war nursing, became a more respectable option for women. Since the men who fought in the Civil War or with Garibaldi in Italy were national heroes fighting for ideals rather than social undesirables or cannon fodder, it was more acceptable for women to want to help care for them.[33] In her work, Summers notes how women such as Jessie White Mario served in the wars of Italian Unification and how other women, including Anne Thacker, Kate Nelligan, Florence Lees, Zepherina Veitch, Louise McLaughlin, and Emma Pearson, served in the Franco-Prussian War.[34]

Despite the somewhat controversial status of nursing, White Mario was determined to serve as a nurse to the best of her ability. As she explained, determined "to fit myself for the task, I now resolved to secure the best medical education possible."[35] Unfortunately, White Mario had few options open to her for formal nursing training. Middle-class women could only gain training through religious sisterhoods and White Mario was insufficiently comfortable with organized religion to take that approach. It was only after the Crimean War that Florence Nightingale, upset with the lack of training among her nurses, particularly the middle-class volunteers, set out to ensure that they were educated professionals rather than menial servants. Leveraging her fame, she developed the Nightingale Fund, an endowment of forty-four thousand pounds dedicated to the establishment of a training institution for nurses.[36]

The Nightingale Fund's first school did not open until 1860, however, and focused on training nurses to provide a sanitary and moral environment rather than on anatomical knowledge or surgical techniques.[37] After the Civil War, American doctors similarly recognized the necessity of setting up appropriate educational institutions for nurses, but these were not available to White Mario in 1856.[38]

Given the lack of nursing schools, White Mario turned to traditional medical schools. With the encouragement of Dr Little, Sir Benjamin Brodie, Sir Bence Jones, and other physicians, White Mario studied medicine at University College London.[39] In August 1856, two years after her fateful meeting with Garibaldi, she then applied to King's College, London for permission to become a candidate for the degree of bachelor of medicine. In response, the Senate of the London University submitted a case for the opinion of counsel questioning whether their charter would enable them to admit a woman.[40] After some consideration, King's College determined that White Mario was unable to sit the exam for the full degree. Recalling the decision in her memoirs, she wrote, "votes being numbered and not weighed, the authorities decided that the words 'British subject' referred to males only, and I was debarred from obtaining quality of treatment."[41] She frequently lamented her exclusion, complaining once to her friend and noted feminist Barbara Leigh Smith Bodichon (1827–1891) that in no case had she received "a logical response to my question: why cannot a woman study medicine?"[42] In another instance, she further questioned why "the examination of bodies of nude men in an anatomy lesson was irreconcilable with the respectability of a lady."[43]

Many newspapers found her unconventional decision to apply for medical school noteworthy and published articles announcing her request. These brief notices did not include much debate on White Mario's potential. I also found no similar set of articles following King's College's announcement that they had rejected her candidacy.[44] Nearly a year later, however, following White Mario's arrest in Genoa, the *Lancet* published an article claiming that the British medical schools had been correct in denying her application and should reject any similar application from a woman. It read, "We trust that the same course will be pursued wherever a woman, who fancies herself qualified for an M.D., because she has A Bee in her bonnet, seeks to enroll herself as a medical studentess; and to assume the academic cap and gown, far less becoming than the female articles of attire bearing the same names. For the request proves a lamentable deficiency of right judgment, the first essential in medical knowledge."[45] The article also argued that women who studied dissection would "violate every feeling of decency and propriety." Finally, it claimed that women could not be both mothers and doctors: "They cannot marry, since urgent cases of disease would require attention ... nor could a midwifery patient be deserted whilst Mrs. M.D.

tended her own sucking babe. If remaining single their position would be one that we should deeply regret to see assigned to any woman of high feeling or delicate nature." Many doctors shared this belief that women were not suited for medicine because their reproductive organs made them too distracted and emotional for proper scientific thought. Others claimed that women simply had smaller brains than men had and were not intelligent enough to act as doctors.[46] Finally, some opposed the admission of women into medical school because it would devalue a man's education.[47]

It was nearly impossible for a woman in Great Britain to become a doctor, particularly given the push towards the professionalization of the field in the 1850s, designed both to increase quality of service for patients and to ensure that doctors held a position of respect and authority within society. The Medical Act of 1858 decreed that all doctors required a licence or a medical degree from one of the nineteen registered bodies in Britain and Ireland to be listed on the newly created register of medical practitioners in the UK. The act also emphasized the standardization of medical qualifications from universities and established the General Medical Council of Medical Registration and Education to distinguish between qualified and unqualified practitioners. This professionalization excluded women, who generally lacked the necessary strenuous secondary education required to gain admittance into those schools. A clause in the Medical Act recognizing doctors who had practised in the UK prior to 1858, however, allowed Elizabeth Blackwell, an American who had earned her degree in New York State, to qualify, and in 1859 she became the first woman to appear on the register.[48]

White Mario's options for gaining a medical degree abroad were somewhat stronger but still quite limited.[49] Though a few Italian women in the eighteenth century had received medical degrees and practised medicine, few pursued medical careers in the nineteenth century.[50] Certain states, such as Austria, even forbade women from entering medical schools until the end of the century.[51] In France and Switzerland, women had some options, and in 1871 Mary Corinna Putnam Jacobi (1841–1906) became the first woman to matriculate at the École de Médecine in Paris. While attending lectures, however, she was required to sit in a separate chair near the lectern and to enter through a side door in deference to male sensibility.[52] In general, therefore, the outlook for women in medicine was poor.

AN INFORMAL AND PRACTICAL MEDICAL EDUCATION

Despite her best intentions to obtain formal training, White Mario gained most of her medical knowledge in the field. At the end of the first campaign in 1861, she said that she had "the sensation of having picked up a few words of a foreign language by ear and the conviction that all real drill and training had yet to come, to be gained by hard study of grammar and syntax."[53] She similarly described her work with her friend and compatriot Dr Agostino Bertani (1812–1886) in the campaign of 1866 as a learning experience.[54] Recalling her excitement at finding herself attached to the General Ambulance, White Mario explained that she was "thankful to get the chance of thorough drill and training, well knowing that it would be all work and no play, as Doctor Bertani was famed for being a strict disciplinarian."[55] By learning through practice, White Mario was like many other war nurses of her day. War service liberated those female nurses from traditional restrictions on their education and provided an alternate path for medical education.

Much of what White Mario learned through her practical education concerned the logistics and practicalities of battlefield medicine, such as how to best locate supplies and provisions.[56] Both on the front lines and in the hospitals, female nurses often assumed responsibility for maintaining supplies, running the kitchens, and feeding patients proper diets at regular intervals.[57] While some contemporaries downplayed the importance of this aspect of White Mario's work, she believed that providing food was a vital part of an army's process. Reflecting on her experience, she wrote, "I, during that march, wrote on my tablets what ever since I have had good reason to act upon: 'If you want to be in for the fray, to really succour the wounded, and not be voted back to the rear, then blamed for not being up to time, feed the hungry *un*wounded whenever you get a chance.'"[58]

Implicitly challenging the focus on anatomical or surgical knowledge as the key to medical care, White Mario emphasized the importance of the practical and mechanical aspects of wartime nursing, including horses, ambulance carriages, litters, and invalid chairs. In an article for *Fraser's Magazine*, she fondly remembered the horse she used during her campaigns with Garibaldi, noting, "many a wounded man has he borne, many a life has he saved by a timely lift. Indeed, I think it open to question whether quadrupeds do not play a more necessary part in ambulances than bipeds. The latter are always at hand; of the former the supply is as limited in volunteer ambulances at least, as 'the powers that be' can make it."[59] When recounting the war of 1866, she included an extensive description of the ambulance transport carriage designed by Bertani, indicating her interest and appreciation for the details of the design, as well as her belief that it might be of use for others. She also included a glowing review of Prussian hand litters, "which are the strongest, lightest, and most easily carried of any that I have ever seen."[60] The litters, she noted, were simply designed, adaptable, and lacked complicated parts that could easily break.

Her preference for logistics and planning notwithstanding, White Mario occasionally found herself participating in surgeries and amputations. In the campaign of 1861, she had to hold a twelve-year-old boy on her lap while his arm was removed.[61] This experience witnessing amputations and their consequences prompted White Mario to write fervently against their over-use. She likewise praised Bertani and his practice of "conservative surgery," for giving soldiers a chance at a more normal future. As an example, she told the story of a young boy whom Bertani saved from amputation through "a neat resection," and who afterwards barely limped. She added in her belief that "if on the field or nearest ambulance the question of primary or secondary operations were to be decided by men of experience and wisdom – instead of by the younger ones, always eager for practice and fearing to give nature a chance – many limbs would be spared now ruthlessly sacrificed."[62] White Mario also provided scientific reasoning for why an excess of amputations was troublesome. In one instance, she noted the high death rates for "thigh amputation in the upper third," adding that "during the Crimean war both the Russians and the French lost from 90 to 95 per cent. in primary thigh amputations."[63]

Not all of White Mario's medical experience or knowledge came from the frontlines. As previously discussed, Italian troops shot Garibaldi while halting his revolutionary attack on Rome in 1862. The wound in Garibaldi's ankle soon grew inflamed and Garibaldi's doctors struggled to locate the position of the musket ball before removing it in a carefully planned operation.[64] White Mario not only nursed Garibaldi before the operation and through his recovery, but also administered the chloroform during the surgery itself. In doing so, she acquired an in-depth knowledge of the complicated procedure.[65]

In a letter to the *Newcastle Courant*, White Mario revealed this knowledge and described how the doctors had used a probe to confirm that the ball was in the tibia and was operable. She gave a clear explanation of the probe, describing it as "a simple silver stem clasping a tiny ball of unpolished porcelain, which blackens on coming in contact with the lead."[66] Revealing a level of medical precision and understanding, she added that it penetrated the wound four centimeters before coming out "black with a substance which, subjected to chemical analysis, proved to be lead." After deciding on the position of the ball, the doctors prepared Garibaldi for surgery by enlarging the wound "by means of a sponge steeped in solution of gum arabic." The sponge, "pressed into the wound on Saturday night, when withdrawn on Sunday morning, brought with it a long slender splinter of bone about two centimetres in length." White Mario explained that Dr Zanetti then inserted pincers, clenched them, and removed the ball. Through this detailed description White Mario clearly demonstrated not only her personal proximity to the operation and her participation in it, but a level of scientific and medical understanding that went beyond what many contemporaries believed possible for a woman.

Her account was not primarily intended as a demonstration of her medical knowledge, however, but part of a larger campaign to restore Garibaldi's reputation. By vividly illustrating Garibaldi's suffering, she attempted to sway public opinion towards the revolutionary hero. At Aspromonte, Garibaldi had gone from a celebrated national hero to an enemy of the state, and White Mario felt a need to defend his actions as a just campaign for freedom and unity rather than a disorderly and disreputable riot or insurrection.

CONCLUSIONS

In the post-Unification period, White Mario worked primarily as a writer, producing newspaper articles and monographs celebrating the history of the Risorgimento and documenting the socio-economic struggles of the newly unified peninsula. She sometimes included descriptions of her nursing as part of a larger narrative but also published some accounts, including a series of articles published in *Fraser's Magazine* in 1877, focused primarily on her nursing experience.[67] Many other women, including Crimean War nurses Mary Stanley (1813–79), Fanny Margaret Taylor (1832–1900), Elizabeth Davis (1789–1860), and Martha C. Nicol, similarly published accounts of their experience.[68] Unlike White Mario, most of these Crimean War nurses did not discuss politics and focused instead on the ways in which nurses provided proper supplies, diet, and cleanliness to the wounded soldiers and defended the strong moral character of the volunteer nurses. According to historian Jane Schultz, forty-three women then wrote and sought publication of monographs detailing their experience as nurses during the American Civil War and others left smaller sketches published in independent commemorative volumes.[69] These Civil War narratives were more political and revealed strong partisan sentiments.[70] Emma Maria Pearson and Louisa Elisabeth McLaughlin also included strong statements of sympathy for the French in their narrative of nursing during the Franco-Prussian War.[71] White Mario was therefore neither the only woman to envision her nursing as part of a larger political movement, nor the only woman to document and publish an account of her nursing to serve a greater political purpose.

She was more consistently concerned about politics, however, than most other nurses. From the outset, her search for medical knowledge was in service of Italian Unification and her accounts of nursing always contained a strong political message and vote of support for left-wing Italian politics. In her first article on her nursing experience for *Fraser's Magazine*, for instance, White Mario lamented that Italians were forgetting the obstacles patriots faced in creating their new state. She wrote, "Unfortunately, we think, for the world, those Italians who have effected most for the liberation of their country rarely speak or write (now that Italy is free and united) of the dreary journey per-formed, the dangers and hardships encountered, the errors committed, the apparently insurmountable obstacles overcome, from the time when they first willed to be a nation until the goal was reached."[72] Even in an article explicitly about medical service, White Mario included a plea for the recognition of the revolutionary and radical contribution to Italian Unification.

By fully recognizing the importance of White Mario's political agenda, we uncover the relative unimportance of her rejection from medical school to her career. Though standard narratives that focus on the admission of women to organized medical or nursing schools would consider White Mario a failure, she would not have defined herself as such. As White Mario herself noted, when the pain of her rejection from the medical establishment was still fresh, "I wished you know for a profession, as a means to an end, rather than as an end in itself, as I am preparing myself for future work in Italy."[73] As her goal was never to be a medical professional, her failure to obtain a medical diploma or certificate, while temporarily distressing, was not devastating.

NOTES

1   There are numerous biographies of Jessie White Mario including: Daniels, *Jessie White Mario: Risorgimento Revolutionary*; Certini, *Jessie White Mario: Una giornalista educatrice*; Paolo Ciampi, *Miss Uragano*; Prisco, *Adorabile Uragano*; Alberti di Mazzeri, *Le donne di Garibaldi*; Bacchin, "Felice Orsini"; and Manica, ed., *Dalla questione meridionale alla questione nazionale*.

2   Boyd, "Florence Nightingale and Elizabeth Blackwell."

3   Stock, *Better than Rubies*; Bell, *Storming the Citadel*; Morantz, "Feminism, Professionalism, and Germs"; Bonner, *To the Ends of the Earth*; Furst, *Women Healers and Physicians*; Laura Kelly, *Irish Women in Medicine*. Occasionally these narratives are included within larger histories of science and medicine, such as Carpenter, *Health, Medicine, and Society in Victorian England*.

4   Maher, *To Bind up the Wounds*; Summers, "The Costs and Benefits of Caring"; Rafferty, *The Politics of Nursing Knowledge*; Fraser, *African American Midwifery*; Kirschmann, *A Vital Force*; More, Fee, and Parry, eds., *Women Physicians*; Rutherdale, ed., *Caregiving on the Periphery*; Nolte, "Protestant Nursing Care."

5   Fitzpatrick, ed., *Prologue to Professionalism*; Helmstadter, "Class, Gender and Professional Expertise"; Giesberg, *Civil War Sisterhood*; Schultz, *Women at the Front*; Maling, "American Nightingales."

6   Summers, *Angels and Citizens*.

7   Vuic, "Wartime Nursing and Power."

8   Daniels, *Jessie White Mario*, 5, 13–16.

9   Mack Smith, *Mazzini*; Isabella, *Risorgimento in Exile*; Bacchin, *Italofilia*.

10 Riall, *Garibaldi*, 343.

11 Richardson, "'Well-Neighboured Houses'"; O'Connor, *The Romance of Italy*; O'Connor, "Civilizing Southern Italy"; Summers, "British Women."

12 Falchi, "Democracy"; Falchi, "Beyond National Borders."

13 Bacchin, "Felice Orsini." A devout patriot, Orsini participated in the Roman Republic of 1848–49 and was later arrested by the Austrians in 1854. White translated Orsini's account of this arrest, imprisonment, and subsequent escape. In January 1858 Orsini attempted to assassinate French Emperor Napoleon III and was soon executed.

14 White Mario, *The Birth of Modern Italy*, 253.

15 Inspired by a local revolt against the Bourbon Kingdom of the Two Sicilies in 1860, Garibaldi and a small group of volunteer fighters sailed from Genoa for Sicily. After landing on 6 May, his underprepared and undersupplied forces marched across the southern kingdom, defeating Bourbon troops and cultivating popular support. By early September 1860 they had captured Naples, thereby placing all of southern Italy under Garibaldi's control. In response, Prime Minister Cavour sent Piedmontese troops south towards Naples and put pressure on Garibaldi to give up control of the south in favour of Italian unification. Garibaldi conceded to Cavour's demands and held plebiscites in late October in Naples and Sicily that led to the unification of the majority of the Italian peninsula under Piedmontese control.

16 Menghini, *La Spedizione Garibaldina*, 124.

17 White Mario, "Della vita di Alberto Mario," cvi–cvii.

18 White Mario, *The Birth of Modern Italy*, xxv. Barcellona Pozzo di Gotto, not to be confused with Barcelona, Spain, is a small town in northern Sicily near Messina.

19 Fazzini and Lucarelli, *Cortigiane ed eroine*, 182.

20 Duggan, *Force of Destiny*, 244–6.

21 Ibid., 249–53. After the outbreak of the Austro-Prussian War in 1866, Italy declared war on Austria on 20 June. Garibaldi served as head of the volunteer forces. Though the Italians did not fight well, the Prussians defeated the Austrians. As part of the armistice the Austrians ceded the Veneto to the French emperor, Napoleon III, who then gave it to the Italians.

22 Garibaldi, "Appendice: VIII," 314.

23 Duggan, *Force of Destiny*, 249–53.

24 As a result of the Franco-Prussian War, France was forced to remove its troops that had been guarding Rome, thereby allowing Italy to gain control of the city in September 1870.

25 Nolte, "Protestant Nursing Care," 167; Summers, *Angels and Citizens*, 19–20.

26 Summers, "The Costs and Benefits of Caring," 144–5.

27 Fitzpatrick, *Prologue to Professionalism*, 7.

28 It was only after 1838 that soldiers' wives were forbidden to attend male patients except with the previous sanction of the secretary of the state at war. Male orderlies, however, rather than wives or camp followers, nursed most wounded British soldiers. Summers, *Angels and Citizens*, 26–7.

29 Monteiro, "On Separate Roads," 522; Helmstadter, "Class, Gender and Professional Expertise," 31–2.

30 Schultz, *Women at the Front*, 17.

31 Maher, *To Bind Up the Wounds*, 110; Taylor, *Eastern Hospitals*, 64.

32 Schultz, *Women at the Front*, 39.

33 Summers, *Angels and Citizens*, 5–6.

34 Ibid., 139–41.

35 White Mario, *The Birth of Modern Italy*, 253.

36 Fitzpatrick, *Prologue to Professionalism*, 13. Though both the paid nurses and members of religious sisterhoods in the Crimean War had previous professional medical training, the volunteer nurses generally did not.

37 Monteiro, "On Separate Roads," 522; Carpenter, *Health, Medicine, and Society*, 168–9.

38 Schultz, *Women at the Front*, 170.

39 White Mario, *The Birth of Modern Italy*, 253, 259.

40 "Female Applicant for a Medical Diploma."

41 White Mario, *The Birth of Modern Italy*, 253.

42 Alberti di Mazzeri, *Le donne di Garibaldi*, 114. Among her other activities, Bodichon co-founded the *English Woman's Journal* in 1858 and later co-founded Girton College, the first women's college at Cambridge University, along with Emily Davies in 1869.

43 Prisco, *Adorabile Uragano*, 35–6.

44 "Female Applicant for a Medical Diploma"; "Daily and Periodical Press"; "Miscellaneous"; "Multiple News Items"; "Foreign Intelligence."

45 "Petticoat Physic."

46 Bonner, *To the Ends of the Earth*, 9.

47 "A Would-Be Female Bachelor."

48 Kelly, *Irish Women in Medicine*, 7. While Elizabeth Blackwell was admitted to Geneva Medical College in rural New York, the college saw her admission as an experiment, rather than a precedent, and did not admit any women after her.

49 Ibid., 7–8. Those degrees would also not qualify her for the Medical Register or allow her to practise medicine in Britain.

50 Campbell Hurd-Mead, *A History of Women in Medicine*, 509.

51 Bonner, *To the Ends of the Earth*, 8.

52 Ibid., 1–2.

53 White Mario, "Experience of Ambulances," 785.

54 A physician and patriot in the campaigns for Italian Unification, Bertani later served in the Italian parliament and was the political leader of the Extreme Left.

55 White Mario, "Experience of Ambulances – Part II," 58.

56 White Mario, "Experience of Ambulances," 779.

57 Nicol, *Ismeer*; Davis, *The Autobiography*; Monteiro, "On Separate Roads"; Summers, *Angels and Citizens*; Giesberg, *Civil War Sisterhood*; Giesberg, *Army at Home*.

58 White Mario, "Experience of Ambulances," 779.

59 Ibid., 780.

60 White Mario, "Experience of Ambulances – Part II," 63.

61 Mario, *The Red Shirt*, 39–40.

62 White Mario, "Experience of Ambulances," 776.

63 White Mario, "Garibaldi in France – Part II," 602–3.

64 Gregorovius, *The Roman Journals*, 170; Bent, *The Life of Giuseppe Garibaldi*, 208–9.

65 Doni, *Donne del Risorgimento*, 205.

66 "The Extraction of the Ball from Garibaldi's Wound."

67 White Mario, "Experience of Ambulances"; White Mario, "Experience of Ambulances – Part II"; White Mario, "Experience of Ambulances – Part III."

68 Summers, *Angels and Citizens*, 38; Taylor, *Eastern Hospitals and English Nurses*; Nicol, *Ismeer*; Davis, *The Autobiography*.

69 Schultz, 220. Some of these accounts include: Wormeley, *The Other Side of the War*; Woolsey, *Three Weeks at Gettysburg*; Woolsey and Woolsey Howland, *Letters of a Family*.

70 Schultz, *Women at the Front*, 212.

71 Pearson and McLaughlin, *Our Adventures during the War of 1870*. Pearson and McLaughlin also wrote an account of their work in Serbia with the Red Cross, *Service in Servia under the Red Cross*; Summers, *Angels and Citizens*, 139.

72 White Mario, "Experience of Ambulances," 768, 773.

73 Daniels, *Jessie White Mario*, 43.

BIBLIOGRAPHY

"A Would-Be Female Bachelor." *The Derby Mercury*, 13 August 1856, Issue 3381.

Alberti di Mazzeri, Silvia. *Le donne di Garibaldi*. Milan, Italy: Editoriale nuova, 1981.

Bacchin, Elena. "Felice Orsini and the Construction of the Pro-Italian Narrative in Britain." In *Britain, Ireland and the Italian Risorgimento*, edited by Nick Carter, 80–103. London: Palgrave Macmillan, 2015.

– *Italofilia: Opinione pubblica brittanica e Risorgimento italiano, 1847–1864*. Turin, Italy: Carocci editore, 2014.

Bell, E. Moberly. *Storming the Citadel: The Rise of the Woman Doctor.* Westport, CT: Hyperion Press, 1982.

Bent, Theodore. *The Life of Giuseppe Garibaldi.* London: Longmans, Green & Co., 1882.

Bonner, Thomas Neville. *To the Ends of the Earth: Women's Search for Education in Medicine.* Cambridge, MA: Harvard University Press, 1995.

Boyd, Julia. "Florence Nightingale and Elizabeth Blackwell." *The Lancet* 373, no. 9674 (May 2009): 1516–17.

Burgess, Major. "Recollection of the Red Cross." *The Illustrated Naval and Military Magazine* 1, no. 6 (1 December 1884): 410–19.

Campbell Hurd-Mead, Kate. *A History of Women in Medicine: From the Earliest Times to the Beginning of the Nineteenth-Century.* Haddam, CT: The Haddam Press, 1938.

Carpenter, Mary Wilson. *Health, Medicine, and Society in Victorian England.* Santa Barbara, CA: Praeger, 2010.

Certini, Rossella. *Jessie White Mario: Una giornalista educatrice: Tra liberalismo inglese e democrazia italiana.* Florence, Italy: Le lettere, 1998.

Ciampi, Paolo. *Miss Uragano: la donna che fece l'Italia.* Florence, Italy: Romano, 2010.

"Daily and Periodical Press." *The Newcastle Courant Etc.*, 22 August 1856, Issue 9478.

Daniels, Elizabeth A. *Jessie White Mario: Risorgimento Revolutionary.* Athens, OH: Ohio University Press, 1972.

Davis, Elizabeth. *The Autobiography of Elizabeth Davis: A Balaclava Nurse, Daughter of Dafydd Cadwaladyr.* Edited by Jane Williams. 2 vols. London: Hurst and Blackett Publishers, 1857.

Doni, Elena. *Donne del Risorgimento.* Bologna, Italy: Il Mulino, 2001.

Duggan, Christopher. *Force of Destiny: A History of Italy since 1796.* London: Penguin Books, 2008.

Falchi, Federica. "Beyond National Borders; 'Italian' Patriots United in the Name of Giuseppe Mazzini: Emilie Ashurst, Margaret Fuller and Jessie White Mario." *Women's History* 24, no. 1 (2015): 23–36.

– "Democracy and the Rights of Women in the Thinking of Giuseppe Mazzini." *Modern Italy* 17, no. 1 (January 2012): 15–30.

Fazzini, Gianni, and Caterina Lucarelli. *Cortigiane ed eroine: Storie di un altro Risorgimento.* Rome: EdUP, 2011.

"Female Applicant for a Medical Diploma." *The Bury and Norwich Post, and Suffolk Herald*, 13 August 1856, Issue 3868.

"Female Applicant for a Medical Diploma." *Hampshire Telegraph and Sussex Chronicle Etc.*, 16 August 1856, Issue 2967.

Fitzpatrick, M. Louise, ed. *Prologue to Professionalism: A History of Nursing.* Bowie, MD: R.J. Brady Co, 1983.

"Foreign Intelligence." *The Bristol Mercury*, 30 August 1856, Issue 3467.

Fraser, Gertrude Jacinta. *African American Midwifery in the South: Dialogues of Birth, Race, and Memory*. Cambridge, MA: Harvard University Press, 1998.

Furst, Lilian R. *Women Healers and Physicians: Climbing a Long Hill*. Lexington, KY: University Press of Kentucky, 1997.

Garibaldi, Giuseppe. "Appendice: VIII. Richiesta di assistenza, Salò, 23 June 1866." In *Epistolario di Giuseppe Garibaldi*, vol. 11: April–December 1866. Edited by Giuseppe Monsagrati. Rome: Istituto per la storia del Risorgimento italiano, 2002.

Giesberg, Judith Ann. *Army at Home: Women and the Civil War on the Northern Home Front*. Chapel Hill, NC: University of North Carolina Press, 2009.

– *Civil War Sisterhood: The U.S. Sanitary Commission and Women's Politics in Transition*. Boston, MA: Northeastern University Press, 2000.

Gregorovius, Ferdinand. *The Roman Journals of Ferdinand Gregorovius, 1852–1874*. Edited by Friedrich Althaus. Translated by Mrs Gustavus W. Hamilton. London: George Bell & Sons, 1907.

Helmstadter, Carol. "Class, Gender and Professional Expertise: British Military Nursing in the Crimean War." In *One Hundred Years of Wartime Nursing Practices, 1854–1953*, edited by Jane Brooks and Christine E. Hallett, 23–41. Manchester, UK: Manchester University Press, 2015.

Isabella, Maurizio. *Risorgimento in Exile: Italian Emigres and the Liberal International in the Post-Napoleonic Era*. New York: Oxford University Press, 2009.

Kelly, Laura. *Irish Women in Medicine, c. 1880s–1920s: Origins, Education and Careers*. Manchester, UK: Manchester University Press, 2013.

Kirschmann, Anne Taylor. *A Vital Force: Women in American Homeopathy*. New Brunswick, NJ: Rutgers University Press, 2004.

Mack Smith, Denis. *Mazzini*. New Haven, CT: Yale University Press, 1996.

Maher, Mary Denis. *To Bind up the Wounds: Catholic Sister Nurses in the U.S. Civil War*. New York: Greenwood Press, 1989.

Maling, Barbara. "American Nightingales: The Influence of Florence Nightingale on Southern Nurses during the American Civil War." In *One Hundred Years of Wartime Nursing Practices, 1854–1953*, edited by Jane Brooks and Christine E. Hallett, 42–57. Manchester, UK: Manchester University Press, 2015.

Manica, Giustina, ed. *Dalla questione meridionale alla questione nazionale: Leopoldo Franchetti, Sidney Sonnino e Jessie White Mario nei carteggi di Pasquale Villari (1875–1917): (Con documenti editi ed inediti)*. Florence, Italy: Edizioni Polistampa : Fondazione Spadolini Nuova Antologia, 2014.

Mario, Alberto. *The Red Shirt. Episodes*. London: Smith, Elder & Co., 1865.

Menghini, Mario. *La spedizione Garibaldina di Sicilia e di Napoli nei proclami, nelle corrispondenze, nei Diarii e nelle illustrazioni del tempo*. Turin, Italy: Società Tipografico-Editrice Nazionale, 1907.

"Miscellaneous." *The Ipswich Journal*, 23 August 1856, Issue 6120.

Monteiro, Lois A. "On Separate Roads: Florence Nightingale and Elizabeth Blackwell." *Signs* 9, no. 3 (Spring 1984): 520–33.

Morantz, Regina Markell. "Feminism, Professionalism, and Germs: The Thought of Mary Putnam Jacobi and Elizabeth Blackwell." *American Quarterly* 34, no. 5 (1982): 459–78.

More, Ellen Singer, Elizabeth Fee, and Manon Parry, eds. *Women Physicians and the Cultures of Medicine*. Baltimore, MD: Johns Hopkins University Press, 2009.

"Multiple News Items." *Dundee Courier*, 27 August 1856, Issue 2086.

Nicol, Martha C. *Ismeer, or, Smyrna and Its British Hospital in 1855. By a Lady*. London: James Madden, 1856.

Nolte, Karen. "Protestant Nursing Care in Germany in the 19th Century: Concepts and Social Practice." In *Routledge Handbook on the Global History of Nursing*, edited by Patricia D'Antonio, Julie Fairman, and Jean Catherine Whelan, 167–82. London and New York: Routledge, 2013.

O'Connor, Maura. "Civilizing Southern Italy: British and Italian Women and the Cultural Politics of European Nation Building." *Women's Writing* 10, no. 2 (2003): 253–68.

– *The Romance of Italy and the English Political Imagination*. New York: St Martin's Press, 1998.

Pearson, Emma Maria, and Louisa Elisabeth McLaughlin. *Our Adventures during the War of 1870*. London: R. Bentley and Son, 1871.

– *Service in Servia Under the Red Cross*. London: Tinsley Brothers, 1877.

"Petticoat Physic." *Hampshire Telegraph and Sussex Chronicle Etc.*, 25 July 1857, Issue 3016.

Prisco, Mario. *Adorabile Uragano: Dalle lotte Risorgimentali alla "Miseria in Napoli": La straordinaria avventura di Jessie White Mario*. Naples, Italy: Stamperia del Valentino, 2011.

Rafferty, Anne Marie. *The Politics of Nursing Knowledge*. New York: Routledge, 1996.

Riall, Lucy. *Garibaldi: Invention of a Hero*. New Haven, CT: Yale University Press, 2008.

Richardson, Sarah. "'Well-Neighboured Houses': The Political Networks of Elite Women, 1780–1860." In *Women in British Politics, 1760–1860: The Power of the Petticoat*, edited by Kathryn Gleadle and Sarah Richardson, 56–73. New York: St Martin's Press, 2000.

Rutherdale, Myra, ed. *Caregiving on the Periphery: Historical Perspectives on Nursing and Midwifery in Canada*. Montreal, QC: McGill-Queen's University Press, 2010.

Schultz, Jane E. *Women at the Front: Hospital Workers in Civil War America*. Chapel Hill, NC: University of North Carolina Press, 2004.

Stock, Phyllis. *Better than Rubies. A History of Women's Education*. New York: Putnam, 1978.

Summers, Anne. *Angels and Citizens: British Women as Military Nurses, 1854–1914*. London: Routledge & Kegan Paul, 1988.

– "British Women and Cultures of Internationalism, c. 1815–1914." In *Structures and Transformations in Modern British History: Essays for Gareth Stedman Jones*, edited by David Feldman and Jon Lawrence, 187–209. Cambridge: Cambridge University Press, 2011.

– "The Costs and Benefits of Caring: Nursing Charities, c. 1830–1860." In *Medicine and Charity before the Welfare State*, edited by Jonathan Barry and Colin Jones, 133–48. London: Routledge, 1991.

Taylor, Fanny Margaret. *Eastern Hospitals and English Nurses; The Narrative of Twelve Months' Experience in the Hospitals of Koulali and Scutari. By a Lady Volunteer.* 3rd ed. London: Hurst and Blackett Publishers, 1857.

"The Extraction of the Ball from Garibaldi's Wound." *The Newcastle Courant Etc.*, 5 December 1862, Issue 9806.

Vuic, Kara Dixon. "Wartime Nursing and Power." In *Routledge Handbook on the Global History of Nursing*, edited by Patricia D'Antonio, Julie Fairman, and Jean Catherine Whelan, 22–33. New York: Routledge, 2013.

White Mario, Jessie. *The Birth of Modern Italy: Posthumous Papers of Jessie White Mario.* Edited by Litta-Visconti-Arese. London: T. Fisher Unwin, 1909.

– "Della vita di Alberto Mario. Memorie." In *Scritti letterari e artistici di Alberto Mario*, by Giosuè Carducci. Bologna, Italy: Nichola Zanichelli, 1901.

– "Experience of Ambulances." *Fraser's Magazine* 15, no. 90 (June 1877): 768–85.

– "Experience of Ambulances – Part II." *Fraser's Magazine* 15, no. 91 (July 1877): 54–74.

– "Experience of Ambulances – Part III." *Fraser's Magazine* 16, no. 92 (August 1877): 247–65.

– "Garibaldi in France – Part II." *Fraser's Magazine* 16, no. 95 (November 1877): 602–18.

Woolsey, Georgeanna. *Three Weeks at Gettysburg.* New York: A.D.F. Randolph, 1863.

Woolsey, Georgeanna, and Eliza Woolsey Howland. *Letters of a Family During the War for the Union, 1861–1865.* New York: Printed for Private Distribution, 1899.

Wormeley, Katharine Prescott. *The Other Side of the War with the Army of the Potomac.* Boston, MA: Ticknor and Fields, 1889.

18

"Don't Tell Them You're Guessing":
Learning Obstetrics in Canadian Medical Schools,
c. 1890–1920

Whitney Wood

After receiving his MD from the University of Toronto in 1908, Abraham Isaac Willinsky accepted a position as a locum tenens (replacement physician) in Carp, Ontario, a rural community outside of Ottawa. Willinsky took over the practice of Dr Magee, a graduate of McGill University, whose reputation consistently rivalled that of his replacement's alma mater as Canada's "best" medical school in this period. Willinsky described their initial encounter years later. "What do you know about babies?" Magee immediately asked Willinsky, who replied sheepishly, "Well, I can recognize them." The novice's response reflected his self-confessed "greenhorn" status when it came to obstetrics and was met with the senior doctor's best advice when it came to obstetric cases. "If you run across something you don't recognize, never let on," Magee urged. "Don't tell them you're guessing."[1]

The most popular medical textbooks in use in Canadian medical schools at this time – written by a mix of Canadian, American, and British authors – stressed the need for specialists and general practitioners alike to be proficient in obstetrics. Yet students at a variety of Canadian schools routinely expressed the belief that they were instead expected to "bluff it out" when it came to attending deliveries. Medical curricula stipulated that students must attend a minimum number of deliveries to pass courses in obstetrics. Extant student narratives, however, call into question how strictly such requirements were enforced. As one student remarked, births considered successfully "attended" "counted if you got there in time to hear the first cry."[2] Professional outcry over the "crisis" in obstetrical training quickly escalated after the Flexner Report decreed in 1910 that at several Canadian schools "the very worst showing is in the matter of obstetrics."[3] Some schools quickly rebutted the claims made in Flexner's influential report in public forums including the *Canadian Medical*

Association Journal. On the whole, however, Canadian medical schools reacted with a host of post-Flexner educational reforms that augmented the place of physician-attended hospital births in the curriculum, and, in turn, raised the prestige of obstetrics as a medical specialty in early-twentieth-century Canada.

This chapter analyzes accounts of Canadian medical students and new practitioners to examine the state of medical education in obstetrics in turn-of-the-century Canada. It accomplishes this by comparative analyses of medical school calendars, journal articles, and a representative selection of popular medical textbooks published in the late nineteenth and early twentieth centuries. Physician N. Tait McPhedran has traced the broad contours of medical education in nineteenth- and early-twentieth-century Canada, and historians including R.D. Gidney, W.P.J. Millar, and Ruby Heap have conducted case studies of the education of medical students in the early twentieth century, focusing on the University of Toronto.[4] The development of medical education has also been addressed, to varying degrees, in institutional histories of individual medical schools. The broader history of obstetric education, however, remains largely unwritten. This is particularly true in the Canadian context, with the exception of Wendy Mitchinson's brief but illuminating sketch of the "uncertain world" of obstetric medicine and its practitioners in early-twentieth-century Canada, included in her groundbreaking study, *Giving Birth in Canada, 1900–1950*.

With the goal of strengthening these foundations, this chapter provides a complementary and critical focus on the relationship between medical education in obstetrics, on the one hand, and the construction of hierarchies of lay and professional knowledge, on the other. Such relationships shaped the interactions between physicians and the women they "confined." Despite often limited practical obstetrical training and knowledge, Canadian medical students received important lessons in professional conduct that allowed them to articulate and emphasize their expertise relative to that of their obstetric and gynecological patients. In addition to these disparities between experience/knowledge and expertise/authority, this chapter also critically examines the inherently gendered power dynamics found in doctor-patient encounters between an exclusively female patient population and a Canadian medical profession that was almost exclusively male.[5] While Canadian physicians disagreed in their interpretations and definitions of quality obstetric care, the historical record reveals a resounding consensus that the only qualified interpreter of the sights, sounds, and sensations of the birthing room was the licensed physician. This analysis shows how characteristics of obstetrical training – including, often, a lack thereof – in formal medical education markedly shaped subsequent medical practice, and especially how women were treated (both medically and socially) in the birthing room and beyond.

"THE VERY WORST SHOWING": OBSTETRIC EDUCATION IN TURN-OF-THE-TWENTIETH-CENTURY CANADA

In October 1874, an article published in the *Canada Lancet* asserted: "it has long been noted that success in midwifery paves the way for family practice, and serves indeed as the best foundation for the practitioner's success in life."[6] In the decades that followed, emerging leaders in this particular medical specialty, including University of Toronto professor of obstetrics Adam Wright, recognized that "the gratitude of obstetrical patients form[ed] the best sort of capital for medical practitioners," suggesting that obstetrical visits played a central role in a financially successful general practice, and offered a key way for doctors from a range of educational backgrounds to secure patients for life.[7] Despite these assertions, however, the subject had a limited place in Canadian medical school curricula until well into the twentieth century. While the most popular medical textbooks of the period stressed the need for specialists and general practitioners alike to be proficient in obstetrics, medical school calendars and student accounts suggest a different picture. Although the quality of instruction understandably varied, the ambiguities and uncertainties that surrounded obstetrical training did much to shape broader perceptions of pregnancy in late-nineteenth- and early-twentieth-century Canada.[8]

The roots of what historian Wendy Mitchinson refers to as the "uncertain world of obstetrics" in early-twentieth-century Canada can be traced back to the mid-Victorian period.[9] The nineteenth century saw the gradual disappearance of midwives in many, but not all, regions of British North America, as an increasingly organized and male-dominated medical profession lobbied against what they generally depicted as women's antiquated and "unskilled" provision of childbirth care. As physicians and professional medical organizations relied on legislative measures to ensure that midwives could no longer effectively replace their ranks, the female-dominated practice of midwifery was severely constricted, especially in urban areas, by the turn of the twentieth century.[10] This made the experience of giving birth in Canada, for many women, remarkably different from experiences in Britain, Ireland, and other European countries where midwives were a visible, active, and continuing part of the medicalization of childbirth.

At the same time, the nineteenth century saw a rapid growth in the educational opportunities available for men who wished to enter the medical profession. British North America's first medical education program was established in 1824 at the Montreal Medical Institution, and was formally recognized by McGill University five years later. The University of Toronto originally opened its medical school at King's College in 1843, but suspended formal classes after a decade. As was the case in Montreal, teaching duties were transferred to a selection of proprietary schools – Trinity Medical College, the Toronto School of Medicine, Victoria University (also known as Rolph's School), and Women's Medical College. Medical teaching at the University of Toronto resumed in 1887. By 1900, medical faculties existed at the University of Montreal, Laval University, Queen's University, Dalhousie University, the University of Western Ontario, and the University of Manitoba.[11] Individual requirements for admission varied widely, but no program required students to have a previous undergraduate degree. As late as 1910, the year of Abraham Flexner's landmark report, approximately ninety per cent of students entered medical education at the University of Toronto – by all accounts one of the more prestigious schools due to its minimum matriculation requirement – with no more than a high school education.[12]

As a result, Canadian medical students tended to be young, a characteristic that had bearing on schools' curricula and contributed to the ongoing place of liberal arts education, particularly in the first year of medical studies.[13] The student body at many institutions also tended to be a relatively homogenous crowd composed of sons of Canada's growing middle class, which was characteristically English-speaking, Protestant, and self-identified as white or Caucasian. The children of professionals and businessmen made up the largest groups.[14] Students who belonged to ethnic or visible minority groups were sometimes admitted to Canadian medical schools but faced particular discrimination.[15] Reflecting (and perhaps reinforcing) the gender and racial homogeneity of Canadian medical school classes, the majority of clinician-professors were also white men, hailing predominantly from the middle classes.[16]

By the first decades of the twentieth century, at Canada's most prestigious universities, Toronto and McGill, the four-year medical curriculum was divided into two fairly equal sections. The medical trainee's first two years were dedicated to laboratory sciences, with the final two years focused on clinical work "in medicine, surgery, and obstetrics."[17] When it came to learning obstetrics, the quality of instruction understandably varied from institution to institution, professor to professor, and even student to student. The expectations placed on future doctors were shaped, at times, by medical and cultural attitudes towards the bodies of the patients they would be expected to treat. William Victor Johnston (1897–1976) recalled, for example, during his time as a medical student at the University of Toronto in the early 1920s, overhearing one of his professors comment to a colleague, "that Johnston boy doesn't know very much, but he is going to [practise in] the north country, so I think I'll pass him."[18] With few practitioners choosing to practise in rural, remote, and northern areas, the presence of any doctor – including a mediocre one – would have been better than no physician at all. But with such statements, members of the faculty also perhaps implied that rural and northern bodies required a less adept practitioner than those in other geographical contexts. Regardless, Johnston recalled that such attitudes created an environment that allowed many students "to hang back and do nothing but listen" during periods of clinical instruction.

Throughout the late Victorian period, the place of obstetrics in Canadian medical schools was a source of ongoing discussion and, for many, of concern. Wendy Mitchinson has summarized the state of formal obstetric education in early-nineteenth-century Canada as "a confusing choice between apprenticeship (whatever this meant) and formal education, divided as it was among various competing proprietary schools and public institutions" that were located both within and outside of Canada. By the close of the century, much had changed, but anxieties surrounding the need for greater training persisted.[19]

These tensions led many new Canadian practitioners to travel abroad, seeking out training and apprenticeships. International educational experiences, disproportionately available to those hailing from well-off families, gave new Canadian practitioners the opportunity to work with some of the leading names in medicine, particularly when it came to training in midwifery and obstetrics. Kenneth Neander Fenwick, who earned his MD from the Royal College of Physicians and Surgeons in Kingston, Ontario, in 1871, and went on to become professor of obstetrics and diseases of women and children at Queen's University in the late nineteenth century, undertook post-graduate training at St Thomas' Hospital in London and travelled to New York for additional study.[20] Abraham Willinsky, whose account opened this chapter, travelled to Europe in fall 1909 to undertake a six-month post-graduate course at the Rotunda Hospital in Dublin, working towards a licentiate in midwifery (LM), based on the advice of a fellow doctor who told him, "If you're interested in babies, Dublin's the place," and assured him that the LM degree "meant something," perhaps suggesting the opposite for Canadian credentials.[21] At the Rotunda, he encountered other Canadian practitioners, and was quickly paired with a roommate who had come to study the LM after a period of teaching midwifery at McGill. Though his roommate "was like a boy let out of school" while in Dublin, making good use of the Guinness provided to Rotunda students in a dedicated common room and, as a result, missing "many of his calls," Willinsky was more than willing to take on extra cases for additional experience. By the end of the course, he recalled that he had attended "almost four times the number of deliveries required for the degree."[22]

Medical centres such as London and Edinburgh were the most common choices for additional study, reflecting, in part, the British credentials of many leading practitioners during this period.[23] Study in continental Europe, including destinations such as Paris and Vienna, represented another popular option.[24] By the first decades of the twentieth century, a growing number of Canadian practitioners sought out educational opportunities in the United States. Dr Wilfred Abram Bigelow, who had received his MD from Toronto in 1903, for example, recalled his habit of biannual American visits to "large surgical centres" in the first decades of the twentieth century, but remarked that he knew this was "more travelling than most of my Canadian associates managed at the time." His sense of unease about his own Canadian credentials may have fuelled his ongoing assessment of Toronto as a "stuffy and provincial medical school" lacking the research-driven focus and prestige of other institutions, a view that led him, even in the post–World War II period, to advise his son, "don't stay there after you graduate – go to the Mayo Clinic."[25]

Foreign credentials, particularly in post-graduate specialties such as obstetrics, remained commonplace well into the twentieth century. These reflected, in part, ongoing limitations in terms of the place of obstetrics in Canadian medical school curricula. In her study of obstetric technologies in the United States, Jacqueline Wolf argues that throughout the nineteenth century, the majority of American physicians "considered obstetrics a trivial sideline, unworthy of professional training, attention, and respect."[26] Across North America, it is clear that the emerging specialty was seen by many as less prestigious than surgery and other branches of medicine. As the professionalization of obstetrics continued in the second half of the nineteenth century, however, the subject came to occupy an increasing presence at Canadian medical schools.

Students at McGill and Queen's University were required to take "two full courses of six months each" in obstetrics and the diseases of women and children from the 1850s and 1860s onwards.[27] Until the early 1870s, McGill calendar listings for courses on midwifery specified that this instruction drew on "a series of drawings on a large scale," "humid preparations" of anatomical specimens,[28] "models in wax," and the use of "the artificial pelvis" or obstetric phantom or manikin. In the 1872–73 academic year, this description was amended to include clinical "cases in the wards of the Lying-in Hospital" as an additional means of instruction.[29] Midwifery lectures in the senior years were one hour long, interspersed with instruction in gynaecology on alternate days. Perhaps as a recognition of the shortcomings of instruction during the academic year, summer course offerings on obstetrics, "not mandatory but recommended," were available at the additional cost of $10 per class.[30]

While the use of obstetric phantoms continued,[31] the decades that followed saw a greater emphasis on the value of clinical instruction in obstetrics. In the 1890–91 academic year, McGill explicitly restated what appears to have been a long-standing requirement – that before a practitioner could receive a degree, "he must also give proof by ticket … of having attended at least six cases of labour."[32] These requirements, McGill students were reminded, were by no means as strict as the number of cases required to qualify for a licence in Great Britain.[33] By the first decade of the twentieth century, though standards varied from institution to institution, Canadian medical periodicals recorded that students in Great Britain required "personal attendance on about fifty cases each" to demonstrate proficiency in obstetrics. In North America, on the other hand, practitioners argued for the uniform enforcement of a six-case minimum.[34] At Canada's leading institutions, McGill and the University of Toronto, clinical teaching was increasingly recognized as "perhaps the most important element of medical education," though other more traditional teaching methods persisted.[35] Into the first decades of the twentieth century, all Toronto medical students were required to "attend" or "conduct" – both terms were used interchangeably – at least six labours by their fourth-year examinations, and were required to provide a certificate as proof that they had completed this requirement.[36] These guidelines continued until approximately 1913, when an additional year of clinical instruction in obstetrics was added; in 1924, the University of Toronto proclaimed the five-year curriculum "a thing of the past," and introduced a new requirement for six years of medical study.[37]

Officially, then, the place of obstetrics in Canadian medical schools increased during these critical post-Flexner decades. Student narratives and external assessments, however, suggest an alternative picture. These sources reveal ongoing discrepancies between institutional proclamations and assurances about the significance of obstetrics and medical graduates' ability – both perceived and actual – to manage births proficiently. Canadian medical experts such as Adam Wright asserted that it would take "an educated woman or man not less than four years to learn how to properly conduct a normal case of labour." As such, he concluded, deficits in student training remained a persistent source of anxiety.[38] Students were required to provide documentation of the deliveries they attended to fulfill curriculum requirements, but personal narratives call into question how strictly these guidelines were enforced. Students at the University of Toronto, for example, were required to attend six deliveries, but, as Willinsky recalled, the popular attitude among his classmates in the early 1900s was that this "attendance" "counted if you got there in time to hear the first cry."[39] The anxiety produced by the disconnect between attendance and experience was noted repeatedly in both student narratives and medical commentaries.

Calls to reform the Canadian medical school system – including education in obstetrics – were amplified with the publication of the Carnegie Foundation's *Report on Medical Education in the United States and Canada* in 1910.

This document, which quickly became known as the Flexner Report after its author, American education critic Abraham Flexner (1866–1959), directed the harshest criticisms at schools in the United States, commenting that the state of medical education north of the border "had never become so badly demoralized."[40] Flexner praised the trend at some Canadian schools to extend undergraduate programs to five years, and recognized McGill and Toronto graduates as possessing the ideal "self-supporting" temperaments for rural practice. Nevertheless, the report placed the two leading Canadian universities in the second division of medical schools, below American institutions that had higher entrance requirements.[41] Singling out the University of Western Ontario (now Western University), Flexner decreed that for Canadian schools, "the very worst showing [was] in the matter of obstetrics."[42]

Holding up clinical training above all other forms of instruction, Flexner questioned the value of lectures and existing teaching methods, including the obstetric phantom or manikin.[43] Out-patient work was framed as a particularly important part of the development of young physicians, but Flexner also lamented that the student trained fully in the field through out-patient work received "about the same training as a midwife."[44] Underscoring the combined value of classroom, clinical, and community training for the future doctor, Flexner drew a clear and hierarchical distinction between physician and non-physician care. The subsequent delineation between practical experience in midwifery and clinical training in obstetrics – and Flexner's positioning of the latter as integral to the scientific practice of "modern" medicine – centred gender as integral to the articulation of professional authority and expertise in the early-twentieth-century birthing room.

Despite attempts on the part of several Canadian medical schools to "brush off" some of the criticisms contained in the Report, medical education underwent significant reform in the post-Flexner years. After 1910, as Jacalyn Duffin argues, Canadian schools were "intent in emphasizing the high quality of their education, the rich opportunities for scientific and clinical learning, and increasingly careful selection of students."[45] Within a decade, clinical experience in obstetrics also became a more integral and entrenched part of medical school curricula.[46] In the years following the publication of the Flexner Report, the University of Toronto made its own reforms to emphasize the place of clinical instruction. An "entirely clinical" fifth-year course on obstetrics appeared on the calendar in 1913,[47] and clinical requirements continued to be more explicitly articulated in the years that followed. By 1920, students were required to submit certificates showing they had "conducted at least twenty labours under the supervision of the Head of Department of Obstetrics and Gynaecology" as a requirement for graduation.[48]

While Canadian medical students were required to attend an increasing number of deliveries in the years following the publication of the Flexner report, student comments, including Willinsky's caveat, call into question the extent to which these guidelines were enforced. Perhaps understandably, then, many young physicians felt thrown into obstetric practice. Working in a remote area of Parry Sound District with no guidance other than the "supervision" of a Sudbury doctor over a hundred kilometers away, Clifford Hugh Smylie, a graduate of the University of Toronto in the mid-1920s, recalled feeling as though he had been left to "sink or swim" in his obstetric cases.[49] William Victor Johnston expressed similar emotions in remembering the short time he spent as a student in the early 1920s assisting in the practice of an elderly doctor in Sprucedale, Ontario. After being sent to his first solo confinement by "horse and cutter" on the evening of his arrival and protesting that he had "never attended a confinement alone," his mentor assured him: "you can do better than anyone else … there is no one else there."[50]

Given their general lack of experience in obstetrics, many students found formal and informal internships under the supervision of trained physicians to be valuable sources of instruction.[51] Lessons in obstetrics, however, also came from other health practitioners. As an intern at Edmonton's Royal Alexandra Hospital in the early 1920s, Samuel Peikoff lamented his lack of experience, and recalled that during the first half of a semester spent interning in obstetrics (an experience which appears to have been atypical during this period), he had yet to witness a delivery, always arriving after the child was born.[52] After a slow start, Peikoff appealed to the head nurse of the maternity ward, a Miss Steward. Peikoff confessed his ignorance in the subject – "all I know is what I have read in books. I have never witnessed a delivery or brought a baby into the world" – and appealed to Steward for help. With her assistance, Peikoff went on to attend more than two dozen cases by the end of his internship, and later asserted that "without a doubt," his time working under Steward represented "the most practical and useful semester in my entire year."[53] Canadian medical students, then, could and did learn obstetrics from sources other than medical school faculty and professors. At the same time, however, future physicians were taught to carefully articulate their obstetrical expertise and authority relative to both their expectant patients and other birth attendants who may have been present in the delivery room.

PHYSICIANS, PATIENTS, AND THE PERFORMANCE OF MEDICAL EXPERTISE

The late nineteenth and early twentieth centuries marked a key moment in terms of both the professionalization of obstetrics and the medicalization of childbirth. During these transformative decades, older prejudices against a range of practitioners gradually gave way to growing respect for the "modern" and "scientific" medical professional, who was, increasingly, conceptualized as the licensed physician.[54] On their part, physicians appear to have been well aware of the need to reform – and later maintain – the image of the mainstream medical practitioner, and medical school instructors presented the future doctor with a range of lessons on professional conduct, in the hopes that these would enable him to articulate his expertise effectively in the birthing room.

Medical texts, published both within and outside of Canada and widely in use in Canadian schools, routinely placed emphasis on the same core set of professional standards that the medical student and young practitioner must develop. Well into the twentieth century, the majority of Canadian births continued to take place in the home,[55] often posing structural challenges to the authority that the medical profession was determined to monopolize. The majority of physicians, additionally, rarely saw their patients before they were summoned to the delivery. Despite the material realities of turn-of-the-twentieth-century obstetric practice, however, the most popular textbooks of the period instructed medical students to "always" examine their patients early in pregnancy to identify any abnormalities or potential problems.[56] In his 1908 text *The Principles and Practice of Obstetrics*, University of Toronto professor Adam Wright stated that "the accoucheur will generally have seen the patient before labour," and he recommended that future physicians make a point to carry out at least a week of daily post-natal visits, followed by visits every two to three days thereafter for the first three weeks of the post-partum period. Wright acknowledged that, compared to country and rural practices, "such directions apply especially to attendance on patients in cities or towns."[57] Ultimately, however, he called for patterns of physician-attendance at births that were beyond the reach of many Canadian women in the late nineteenth and early twentieth centuries.

Other texts offered a more realistic perspective. In his 1889 textbook, Kenneth Neander Fenwick of Queen's University appeared to be more aware of the reality that the first contact between the physician and his parturient patient often took place in the birthing room. He advised his students to, during delivery, "enquire into the history of the case, such as the length of previous labours, [the patient's] health during pregnancy, the number of previous pregnancies, whether she is now up to full time, when the pains began, as to their frequency and situation, and if the membranes have ruptured."[58] Many of these more rudimentary aspects of the patient's history would have, presumably, been addressed in any earlier visits had these taken place. Into the twentieth century, Canadian practitioners recorded that in many cases, the first point of contact between doctor and patient remained the birth itself. Clifford

Hugh Smylie recalled of his Parry Sound practice in the 1920s: "Rarely would I see a maternity case until I was called to deliver her, and then usually only after she had been in labour a long time, and the neighbor woman with her had decided something must be wrong."[59] The fact that physicians were regularly called at the last minute, particularly in cases that were perceived as problematic or abnormal, undoubtedly contributed to the predominance of increasingly pathological views of pregnancy and birth amongst Canadian practitioners.[60]

Often called into the homes of their expectant female patients on short notice during the labour process, Canadian physicians were, at times, unaware of the potential audiences they would encounter in the birthing room. On these occasions, doctors could be forced to articulate their obstetrical expertise relative to husbands, family members, friends, and other childbirth attendants, both midwives and, increasingly, nurses. These pressures were seen as having the potential to negatively affect the physician's practice, especially for beginners and young doctors lacking experience in obstetrics. In one 1912 text, then in wide use in Canadian medical schools, Barton Cooke Hirst, professor of obstetrics at the University of Pennsylvania, highlighted the "most unenviable frame of mind in the practitioner attending his first few cases of labour," fuelled by "the knowledge that his every movement is watched by critical friends or attendants of the patient, who possess, perhaps, just what he lacks – practical experience."[61] The presence of the patient's husband, in particular, had the potential to challenge gendered power dynamics in the birthing room. In his lessons to Toronto medical students in the early twentieth century, Wright identified this complication, pointing out that the presence of the husband during the first stage of labour sometimes represented "an intolerable nuisance" for the physician; fortunately, Wright went on to note, most husbands readily followed the doctor's advice and left the birthing room near the moment of delivery "without making any trouble."[62]

In reaction to, and anticipation of, the possibility of encountering an audience in the birthing room, experts in the emerging field of obstetrics increasingly argued that the medical practitioner's appearance and demeanor were integral components of both his professional identity and his reputation as a dependable birth attendant. Medical students were cautioned of the dangers of assuming "a tone of familiarity" with female patients that had the potential to be "construed into impertinence, or downright insult."[63] Students learned, however, that different categories of women demanded varying levels of courtesy and respect. Gunning Bedford, professor of obstetrics at the University of New York, described the proper method for turning back one's coat and shirt sleeve and pinning a napkin over the wrist prior to conducting a pelvic examination in his 1861 text. In noting that such a method was "more in keeping with neatness and refinement, two attributes always well appreciated in her physician by a delicate and cultivated female," he insinuated that well-to-do patients required greater respect than their working-class counterparts.[64] More broadly, Canadian medical students learned that gynecological examinations often posed a particular affront "to the sensibilities of the patient" and had "in many cases a bad effect on the nervous system," delaying the progress of labour. Professors asserted that experience, often lacking in new practitioners, represented the best safeguard against unnecessary and repeated physical examinations.[65]

LEARNING TO READ THE PARTURIENT PATIENT

The leading medical texts of the late nineteenth and early twentieth centuries demonstrate that pelvic examinations were a persistent source of anxiety for both practitioners and patients. Recognizing the clinical value of the exam for its diagnostic indication, doctors were advised to tactfully negotiate the complexities of administering a gynecological examination with the parturient woman. Adam Wright recognized that all pelvic exams were "more or less distasteful to the patient" but advised that some women experienced more discomfort than others. Wright described the "modern" practice of digital examination, in which the female patient adopted a recumbent position, as involving "an exposure so marked that the sensitive woman naturally shrinks from it."[66] This "modern" posture was contrasted with older, early-nineteenth-century methods, in which the physician knelt before a standing patient, performing a blind digital examination beneath her skirts in order to refrain from exposing her genitalia. By the close of the century, physicians widely recognized that the older method furnished "incomplete results" and was still "apt to offend sensitive patients." Subsequently, it fell out of use.[67]

The act of performing pelvic examinations also posed a potential threat to the professional image of the physician. Tactile examinations offered new practitioners unparalleled opportunities to learn about the bodies of their female patients, but when incorrectly performed, ran the risk of showcasing the ignorance – and shortcomings in the training – of the young physician. In his 1861 text, Bedford posed a cautionary question to medical students:

How are you to find the vagina? This may appear to you a very unnecessary question – but, gentle men, it is full of sterling import to you as practitioners. What would be the measure of your mortification if, in attempting an examination of this kind, the patient, after more than Christian forbearance, should exclaim, "Doctor, what are you about; do you not know better than that?" and you should discover that the rebuke

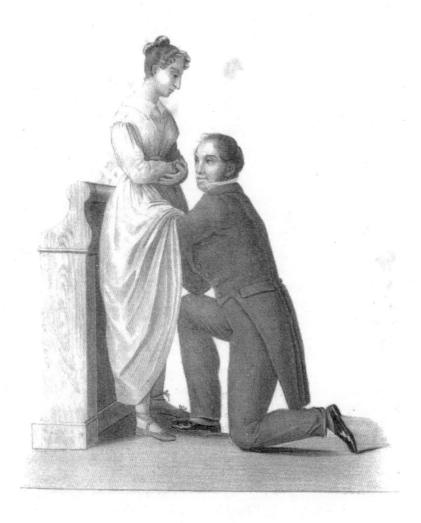

Touching, the female erect.

Figure 18.1 | Drawing illustrating early-nineteenth-century method of gynecological examination, in which the physician knelt before a standing patient, performing a blind digital examination beneath her skirts in order to refrain from exposing her genitalia. (J.P. Maygrier, *Midwifery Illustrated*, second edition [New York: Moore & Payne, 1833], plate 29.)

was prompted by the painful circumstance that, instead of the vagina, you had introduced the finger into the anus! And yet, gentlemen, strange as it may seem to you, this blunder has been committed, for want of proper knowledge, much to the chagrin of the practitioner, and the outraged feelings of the patient.[68]

Over the course of the following decades, medical education in obstetrics and gynecology underscored the value of tactile examinations, but students were regularly reminded that the practitioner must always give "the impression that he is thoroughly at home in his work." In his popular 1901 textbook, American physician Charles Reed cautioned the medical student that "if he betrays his inexperience by suddenness of movement, inexactitude of touch, or other evidence of the novitiate, his usefulness will be limited or destroyed."[69] For young practitioners, then, both personal pride and professional reputations were at stake when it came to learning proper examination practices.

Due in part to these ongoing tensions, coupled with an increasing recognition that frequent examinations during the first stage of labour were often a source of infection, medical professionals framed the "diminution in the number of necessary vaginal examinations" during confinements as "one of the great advances of modern midwifery." One 1911 text surmised that this progression was "only rendered possible by the possession of a certain degree of skill in the practice of abdominal palpation and auscultation, a skill which it is the duty of the student to acquire by practice on every available occasion."[70] As medical professionals placed increasing emphasis on the diagnostic value of a broader range of sensory interpretations of the female body, beyond those involving touch, new practitioners were expected to perform a broader and more systematic examination of the expectant patient, grounded in, in the words of British obstetrician J.S. Fairbairn's 1924 text, "the usual medical routine of inspection, palpation, percussion, and auscultation."[71] The modern obstetrician increasingly relied on a combination of tactile, visual, and auditory evidence to shape his understandings of the events taking place in the birthing room, most notably the progress of labour.

Long-standing anxieties surrounding the proper performance of pelvic examinations on female patients were rooted in the fact that physicians had long privileged touch as a means of uncovering information about the condition of the female body. In his mid-nineteenth-century text, American obstetrician Charles Meigs instructed medical students that "The Touch alone" would allow the practitioner to glean the necessary information required to accurately determine the progress of labour.[72] In his 1907 volume, J.C. Edgar, professor of obstetrics and clinical midwifery at Cornell University, emphasized the role of touch in diagnosing cases of uterine inertia. He advised students that a firm diagnosis was "readily made, as a rule, by palpation, which reveals the absence of a natural uterine action and the arrest of labor."[73] Charles Reed offered an even stronger assessment of the value of touch in turn-of-the-century obstetric practice, writing that "by far the most important method of investigation is the examination by the fingers and hands. The tactile sense is so acute, and may be so highly educated, as to supersede or take the place of every other method, provided one were limited to a single means of obtaining information."[74] By the first decades of the twentieth century, however, the emergence of new medical technologies including the vaginal speculum posed an increasing challenge to physicians' traditional reliance on touch, marking a growing trend of incorporating other sensory modalities – including sight and sound – into medical practice.[75]

Aside from the obvious utility of "hands-on" interpretations, future physicians were also taught to interpret the various sounds of labour. While recurring descriptions of the varying cries, groans, and grunts associated with distinct stages of labour are the most obvious example of this phenomenon,[76] doctors suggested that the experienced practitioner also drew information from more subtle auditory cues. The Scottish obstetrician William Smoult Playfair was one of several practitioners to describe uterine or placental souffle to his students. Pointing out the "peculiar single whizzing murmur," deeply affected by the uterine contractions during labour, that became "louder and more intense before the pain comes on, disappearing during its acme, and again being heard as it goes off," Playfair advised future practitioners that through the skill of auscultation – listening to the internal sounds of the body – they could obtain new knowledge about the experiences of their parturient patients.[77]

Reflecting what historian Joanna Bourke has identified as a broader nineteenth-century fixation on the "gestural languages" of pain,[78] Canadian medical students and physicians alike were urged to "cultivate their powers of observation," taking in the "expression, action, and demeanor" of the obstetric case. Upon entering the birthing room, Adam Wright advised his students to converse with their parturient patients "for a time on an ordinary topic." He continued:

While thus talking, the physician should watch the patient carefully (without, if possible, appearing to do so). He should see and hear as much as possible and thus get a fair idea as to her general condition and also as to the particular symptoms present at the time. One can thus generally obtain an almost exact knowledge as to the frequency and severity of her pains.[79]

By relying on a combination of their senses and new technologies – including, most significantly, the stethoscope, developed in France in the first half of the nineteenth century – rather than traditional tactile examinations, medical men gained what they saw as new objective and scientific knowledge about the bodies and births of their female patients.[80] This knowledge underscored the recurring emphasis on male physicians' professional expertise in the field of obstetrics, particularly when it came to distinguishing between "true" and "false" pains and determining the progress and efficiency of labour.

As early as the 1860s, practitioners asserted that a trained physician could interpret the pains of parturition, effectively distinguishing between "true" pains – "the offspring of a uterine contraction ... synonymous with the existence of labor" – and "false" or "spurious" pains, "the product of some cause entirely foreign to uterine connection."[81] The ability to tactilely read the female body, grounded in modern medical expertise and a knowledge of obstetrics and anatomy, was at the heart of this skill. By placing a hand on the abdomen or introducing a finger into the vagina, and feeling either the hardened uterus or the stiffened neck of the womb during a contraction, physicians were taught that they – and they alone – could establish the "legitimacy" of women's pains, and thus determine the efficacy or progress of labour. For late-Victorian obstetricians such as Gunning Bedford, this was objective medical science. He advised medical students: "there is no speculation here; it is a matter of fact, which you can ascertain for yourselves in the very first case of labor which may present itself to your observation."[82] The ability to make such distinctions was seen as crucial to the success of the modern obstetrician. Bedford cautioned the future physician that without the ability to discriminate and diagnose the true and spurious pains of labour, "he will be like a ship without its rudder; his progress will not only be uncertain, but will be unsafe, and sometimes indeed, disastrous."[83] As failure to recognize the "false" nature of the pains could lead one to anticipate the moment of delivery far sooner than could be reasonably expected, the young practitioner risked the patient's frustration and disappointment, along with potential embarrassment.

Adam Wright spoke at length on the physician's powers of observation. Stressing that "it is not easy to explain the difference between the *false* pains which occur so frequently during the latter part of pregnancy and the regular or *true* pains of labor," he underscored the expertise, authority, and professional status of the modern physician.[84] In contrast to the realities of obstetric education, the authors of medical texts confidently expressed the belief that, with the proper training, future practitioners would be able to effectively make these difficult divisions. Relying on new technologies coupled with this professional expertise, physicians positioned themselves as the arbiters of the distinction between "true" and "false" labour pains.[85] As traditional female-dominated cultures of social childbirth continued to decline over the course of the late nineteenth and early twentieth centuries, and more and more Canadian women knew little of what to expect during the birthing process, medical men became, in many cases, the sole interpreters of the events taking place in the birthing room.

Taking it upon themselves to tell the private, subjective, and personal stories of labour pain, physicians effectively appropriated certain aspects of the childbirth experience. Oftentimes, a key part of this appropriation involved the denigration of women's own narratives of bodily experiences such as pregnancy, accounts that physicians described, at times, as "opinions" rather than facts.[86] This denigration was inseparable from a broader cultural context that included literary expressions of women's growing frustrations with mainstream medicine. In the closing decades of the nineteenth century, these discontents were captured, most vividly, in Charlotte Perkins Stetson's "The Yellow Wallpaper" (1892), a short story in which Stetson (later Gilman) drew on her own experiences of being treated for neurasthenia by leading American expert Silas Weir Mitchell following the birth of her daughter in 1885 to detail her protagonist's decline under the many restrictions of the so-called "rest cure" and the constraints of the male-dominated medical establishment.[87] Into the first decades of the twentieth century, physicians increasingly positioned themselves as the key point of contact and source of knowledge when it came to all matters related to pregnancy and birth: future practitioners were taught to encourage expectant mothers "to come to him [the physician] whenever anything occurs to worry her, instead of taking advice from her women friends."[88] On some occasions, physicians were also advised to actively withhold knowledge – including, for example, information on the expected duration of labour – from their parturient patients.[89]

The justification for these decisions, based on the perceived authority and expertise of the obstetrician, went hand in hand with broader descriptions of the generally untrustworthy nature of the female patient. In several popular medical texts of the period, practising physicians warned their students of the problems that could arise from blindly trusting the women they treated. On the most basic level, for example, Wright suggested that the young doctor, in asking the patient about her pains, "without appearing to have any doubt on the subject … should try to satisfy himself that she is pregnant and try to ascertain whether she is in labor."[90] Recounting a case where he was "deceived" by a thirty-four-year-old unmarried female patient experiencing excessive menstrual bleeding, ultimately operating and removing both the ovaries and uterus, the latter of which contained a healthy fetus at roughly three months' gestation, Peikoff concluded that the medical practitioner "cannot always believe the patient's story when there is a possibility of pregnancy."[91]

Fairbairn made this point explicitly clear in his 1924 text. He advised future practitioners that "the patient's statements, particularly in those cases in which she may have some object in either concealing or feigning pregnancy, should be accepted with extreme caution."[92] In a number of ways, then, and drawing on a number of criteria, physicians expressed the belief that they were the most qualified interpreters of the bodies and reproductive health of their female patients.

CONCLUSION

As Kathryn Montgomery Hunter has argued, medicine is, at its core, "an interpretive activity ... the art of adjusting scientific abstractions to the individual case."[93] The clinical gaze – rooted in the professional expertise of the physician and bolstered by modern medical technologies that allowed the turn-of-the-twentieth-century practitioner to more effectively read the female body – transformed (and continues to transform) subjective, patient-narrated "medical symptoms," or accounts of pregnancy, pain, and the progress of labour, into observable "medical signs."[94] Canadian medical students, typically male in this period, were regularly taught that they could and should read clinical signs confidently in their interpretations of the condition (pregnancy), the progress and efficacy of labour, and, more generally, the bodies and health of all their female patients. Not surprisingly given the shortcomings and critiques of obstetrical training published by medical education reformers, countless young physicians who graduated during these transformative decades were less than confident, and many expressed anxiety about the vicissitudes of the birthing room. In order to gain hands-on experience and practical knowledge essential to a successful medical practice, these novice practitioners often were forced to seek out extracurricular internships or informal apprenticeships, which, in turn, informed and shaped their obstetric practices. The formal education future doctors received in Canadian medical schools, ultimately, performed a different function: the mostly-male student population internalized fundamental messages assuring them that the performance of professional identity and the articulation of obstetrical expertise were essential to a profitable medical practice because these distinguished the licensed physician from the midwife and, increasingly, from the maternity work of nurses, another group of practitioners determined to professionalize and expand their jurisdiction in this period. Forced to suppress doubts and anxiety about their lack of obstetrical knowledge, physicians routinely embodied this core educational message of professional and scientific authority in order to read and interpret the bodies and labour pains of their parturient patients. This convincing and powerful façade justified their role in the birthing room, and, fundamentally, contributed to the ongoing medicalization of childbirth in late-nineteenth- and early-twentieth-century Canada.

NOTES

1 Willinsky, *A Doctor's Memoirs*, 28, 33.

2 Ibid., 20–1.

3 Flexner, *Medical Education*, 117.

4 Gidney and Millar, "Medical Students," 29–52; Millar, Heap, and Gidney, "Degrees of Difference"; Gidney and Millar, *Professional Gentlemen*; McPhedran, *Canadian Medical Schools*.

5 Cheryl Krasnick Warsh shows that 1.76% of medical doctors in Canada were female in 1891; 2.7% of physicians were female in 1911, 1.8% in 1921, and 3.7% in 1941. See Krasnick Warsh, *Prescribed Norms*, 201.

6 "The Cultivation of Obstetrics," *Canada Lancet*, 58.

7 Wright, *A Text-Book of Obstetrics*, 85.

8 This statement is true for both physicians and the women they attended. This chapter focuses on the ways in which medical students and physicians approached the bodies and births of Canadian women, but Canadian women expressed their own fears and anxieties surrounding the many uncertainties associated with childbirth in the late nineteenth and early twentieth centuries, a transformative period in terms of the professionalization of obstetrics. These are explored in greater detail in Wood, "'When I Think of What Is Before Me, I Feel Afraid,'" 187–203.

9 Mitchinson, *Giving Birth in Canada*, 47–68.

10 Ibid., 72–7.

11 See McPhedran, *Canadian Medical Schools*.

12 Gidney and Millar, "Medical Students," 32.

13 Medical students at the University of Toronto had an average age of twenty in 1910 and nineteen in 1930. This age "affected everything from increased regulation over dissecting-room rule or classroom behaviour, to the structure of the program itself" (Gidney and Millar, "Medical Students," 33–4).

14 Gidney and Millar recall that at the University of Toronto, medical students were also more likely to come from urban rather than rural Ontario. "They were also overwhelmingly white, Protestant, and of British stock" (ibid., 37).

15 Though growing numbers of Jewish students were admitted to Canadian medical schools, including the University of Toronto, for example, they often faced a range of barriers in pursuing educational opportunities, including post-graduate internships. See also Duffin, "The Queen's Jews," 369–94.

16 Howard J. Alexander, who received his MD in 1925 from the University of Toronto, reported that at that institution, "all the professors were either English, Irish, or Scottish," and appeared to favour students from these backgrounds (Alexander, *56 Years in Medical Practice*, 14).

17 Flexner, *Medical Education*, 117.

18 In this environment, Johnston recalled that it was very easy for most students "to hang back and do nothing but listen" during periods of clinical instruction (*Before the Age of Miracles*, 15, 17).

19 Mitchinson, *The Nature of Their Bodies*, 24.

20 Kenneth Neander Fenwick, *Manual of Obstetrics, Gynaecology, and Pediatrics* (Kingston, ON: John Henderson & Co., 1889).

21 Willinsky, *A Doctor's Memoirs*, 35.

22 Ibid., 36–7.

23 Howard J. Alexander undertook post-graduate lectures in surgery in London (Alexander, *56 Years in Medical Practice*, 14). See also Peikoff, *Yesterday's Doctor.* Peikoff, who would receive his MD from the University of Alberta in the mid-1920s, went to Edinburgh. Professor John Clarence Webster trained in Edinburgh before being appointed lecturer in gynecology at McGill in 1896 (John Clarence Webster Fonds, P 011, Osler Library for the History of Medicine).

24 Willinsky, *A Doctor's Memoirs*, 24, 41–2, 105. Ontario-born Jack Elmer Harrison, who graduated with an MD from McGill in 1923, also undertook post-graduate training in Vienna, before going on to work as a senior obstetrician at Vancouver General Hospital and becoming associate professor in obstetrics and gynaecology at the University of British Columbia (Jack Elmer Harrison Fonds, P 173, Osler Library for the History of Medicine).

25 Bigelow, *Forceps, Fin & Feather*, xvii, 34, 41.

26 Wolf, *Deliver Me from Pain*, 20.

27 McGill University, 1852–1853 Academic Calendar, 8. Queen's University and College, Kingston, Faculty of Medicine Calendar, 1865–1866.

28 Over the course of the nineteenth century, "humid" or "wet" preparations of anatomical specimens were increasingly preferred over their "dry" counterparts, as they offered a better preservation of the colour, texture, and natural shape of body parts including the uterus. For more information see Alberti, "Anatomical Craft," 231–46.

29 McGill University Calendar, 1868–1869; 1872–1873, 10.

30 McGill University Calendar, 1879–1880, 33; 1884–1885.

31 McGill University Calendar, 1884–1885, 34; 1887–1888, 33, 57–8; 1890–1891, 48.

32 McGill University Calendar, 1890–1891, 38.

33 McGill University Calendar, 1889–1890, 49.

34 "The Present Status of Obstetrical Education in Europe and America," *Western Canadian Medical Journal* (WCMJ) 4, no. 6 (June 1910): 262, 274.

35 *University of Toronto Report of the Standing Committee of the Faculty of Medicine on the Subject of Hospital Facilities* (Toronto: Rowsell & Hutchinson, University Printers, 1892), 3–4.

36 See University of Toronto, Medical Faculty Calendar, Session 1889–1890, 51; Session 1915–1916, 39.

37 "Want Fewer Students Says Dean of Medicine," *Canadian Journal of Medicine and Surgery* 54, no. 2 (February 1925): 67.

38 Wright, *A Text-Book of Obstetrics*, 85.

39 Willinsky, *A Doctor's Memoirs*, 20–1.

40 Flexner, *Medical Education*, 326.

41 Ibid., 15, 24. The first division of schools required two or more years of college work for entrance; the second demanded graduation from a four-year high school or its equivalent; while the third "ask little or nothing more than the rudiments or the reconciliation of a common school education" (28).

42 Ibid., 117.

43 Ibid.

44 Ibid., 118.

45 Duffin, "The Queen's Jews," 373. See also Duffin, "Did Abraham Flexner Spark the Founding of CMAJ?" 811–13.

46 Jacqueline Wolf argues that in the United States, this process was complete by the 1920s. Wolf, *Deliver Me from Pain*, 23.

47 A fourth-year lecture course on obstetrics "illustrated by diagrams, lantern slides, and models" introduced students to physiology and management of normal and abnormal pregnancies, while the fifth-year course on obstetrics was "entirely clinical," consisting of "demonstrations on interesting and abnormal cases" (University of Toronto, Faculty of Medicine Calendar, Session 1913–1914, 71–2).

48 University of Toronto, Faculty of Medicine Calendar, Session 1919–920, 44; Session 1920–1921, 42.

49 Clifford Hugh Smylie, *Personal Memoirs*, Clifford Hugh Smylie Fonds, MU 2853, Archives of Ontario, 139, 154.

50 Johnston, *Before the Age of Miracles*, 14.

51 See Willinsky, *A Doctor's Memoirs*, 64–8.

52 Peikoff, *Yesterday's Doctor*, 3.

53 Ibid., 6–7.

54 For more on this process see Gidney and Millar, *Professional Gentlemen*.

55 In Ontario, for example, arguably the most "modern" and medicalized province, the majority of deliveries took place in the home until 1939. See Oppenheimer, "Childbirth in Ontario," 36–60.

56 J.M. Smith, "Lecture Notes on Obstetrics (as taken from Dr Meek or Dr Eccles)," University of Western Ontario, 1900, A00-194-01, Archives Research and Collections Centre, Western University.

57 Wright, *The Principles and Practice of Obstetrics*, 86, 153–4.

58 Fenwick, *Manual of Obstetrics, Gynaecology, and Pediatrics*, 61.

59 *Personal Memoirs*, Clifford Hugh Smylie Fonds, 154.

60 For more on this see Wood, "'Bound to Be a Troublesome Time,'" 35–55.

61 Hirst, *A Text-Book of Obstetrics*, 170.

62 Wright, *A Text-Book of Obstetrics*, 104.

63 Meigs, *Obstetrics*, 281.

64 Bedford, *The Principles and Practice of Obstetrics*, 198.

65 Edgar, *The Practice of Obstetrics*, 477.

66 Wright, *A Text-Book of Obstetrics*, 87–9.

67 Lusk, *The Science and Art of Midwifery*, 108.

68 Bedford, *The Principles and Practice of Obstetrics*, 99.

69 Reed, *A Text-Book of Gynaecology*, 39.

70 Jellett, *A Manual of Midwifery*, 189. See also Mitchinson, *Giving Birth in Canada*, 195–6.

71 Fairbairn, *Gynaecology with Obstetrics*, 36, 245.

72 Meigs, *Obstetrics*, 300. Capitalization of "The Touch" in the original text.

73 Edgar, *The Practice of Obstetrics*, 571.

74 Reed, *A Text-Book of Gynaecology*, 35.

75 See Yeniyurt, "When It Hurts to Look," 23.

76 See, for example, Fenwick, *Manual of Obstetrics, Gynaecology, and Pediatrics*, 43–4.

77 Playfair, *A Treatise*, 139. This emphasis continued into the early twentieth century. See Edgar, *The Practice of Obstetrics*, 124.

78 Bourke, *The Story of Pain*, 167.

79 Wright, *A Text-Book of Obstetrics*, 86. See also Hirst, *A Text-Book of Obstetrics*, 473.

80 See Duffin, *History of Medicine*, 287.

81 Bedford, *The Principles and Practice of Obstetrics*, 331.

82 Ibid., 330.

83 Ibid., 331.

84 Wright, *A Text-Book of Obstetrics*, 86.

85 Yeniyurt has argued that the speculum, for example, incorporated new parts of the female body into the "medical ocular economy." In order to appropriate the female patient's voice, the male physician "needed to literally look inside her to see what she could not tell him." Likewise, male obstetricians relied on technology – in this case, the stethoscope – to interpret (and legitimize) private and subjective experiences of pain. Yeniyurt, "When It Hurts to Look," 33.

86 Advising the future physician to inquire as to the number of former pregnancies on a first visit (often at the moment of birth) and to ask the patient if she had reached full term, Wright asserted that "she may think that she has or has not and will probably give her reasons for such opinions" (*A Text-Book of Obstetrics*, 87).

87 Stetson, "The Yellow Wallpaper," 647–57.

88 Williams, *Obstetrics*, 247.

89 In his 1888 text, Fenwick advised Canadian medical students, "if asked as to the duration of labour," to "be guarded and possibly ambiguous" (*Manual of Obstetrics, Gynaecology, and Pediatrics*, 61).

90 Wright, *A Text-Book of Obstetrics*, 86–7.

91 Peikoff, *Yesterday's Doctor*, 106.

92 Fairbairn, *Gynaecology with Obstetrics*, 109.

93 Montgomery Hunter, *Doctors' Stories*, xviii.

94 Malterud, "The (Gendered) Construction of Diagnosis," 275–86; Foucault, *The Birth of the Clinic*.

BIBLIOGRAPHY

Alberti, Samuel J.M.M. "Anatomical Craft: A History of Medical Museum Practice." In *The Fate of Anatomical Collections*, edited by Rina Knoeff and Robert Zwijnenberg, 231–46. Burlington, VT: Ashgate, 2015.

Alexander, Howard J. *56 Years in Medical Practice*. Compiled and edited by Frank Fubie. Tillsonburg, ON: Bennett Stationary, Ltd., 1981.

Bedford, Gunning S. *The Principles and Practice of Obstetrics*. New York: Samuel S. & William Wood, 1861.

Bigelow, Wilfred Abram. *Forceps, Fin & Feather: The Memoirs of Dr. W.A. Bigelow*. Altona, MB: Frieson & Sons, 1970.

Bourke, Joanna. *The Story of Pain: From Prayer to Painkillers*. Oxford, UK: Oxford University Press, 2014.

Duffin, Jacalyn. "Did Abraham Flexner Spark the Founding of CMAJ?" *Canadian Medical Association Journal* 183, no. 6 (2011): 811–13.

– *History of Medicine: A Scandalously Short Introduction*, 2nd ed. Toronto: University of Toronto Press, 2010.

– "The Queen's Jews: Religion, Race, and Change in 20th Century Canada." *Canadian Journal of History* 49 (Winter 2014): 369–94.

Edgar, J. Clifton. *The Practice of Obstetrics: Designed for the Use of Students and Practitioners*. Philadelphia, PA: P. Blakiston's Son & Co., 1907.

Fairbairn, J.S. *Gynaecology with Obstetrics: A Text-Book for Students and Practitioners*. Toronto: Oxford University Press, 1924.

Flexner, Abraham. *Medical Education in the United States and Canada: A Report to the Carnegie Foundation for the Advancement of Teaching.* Carnegie Foundation for the Advancement of Teaching, 1910.

Foucault, Michel. *The Birth of the Clinic: An Archaeology of Medical Perception.* New York: Pantheon Books, 1973.

Gidney, R.D., and W.P.J. Millar. "Medical Students at the University of Toronto: A Profile." *Canadian Bulletin of Medical History* 13 (1996): 29–52.

– *Professional Gentlemen: The Professions in Nineteenth Century Ontario.* Toronto: University of Toronto Press, 1994.

Hirst, Barton Cooke. *A Text-Book of Obstetrics.* Philadelphia, PA, and London: W.B. Saunders Company, 1912.

Hunter, Kathryn Montgomery. *Doctors' Stories: The Narrative Structure of Medical Knowledge.* Princeton, NJ: Princeton University Press, 1991.

Jellett, Henry. *A Manual of Midwifery for Students and Practitioners.* New York: William Wood and Company, 1910.

Johnston, William Victor. *Before the Age of Miracles: Memoirs of a Country Doctor.* New York: Paul S. Eriksson, Inc., 1972.

Lusk, William Thompson. *The Science and Art of Midwifery.* New York: D. Appleton and Company, 1888.

Malterud, Kirsti. "The (Gendered) Construction of Diagnosis: Interpretation of Medical Signs in Women Patients." *Theoretical Medicine and Bioethics* 20 (1999): 275–86.

McPhedran, N. Tait. *Canadian Medical Schools: Two Centuries of Medical History, 1822 to 1992.* Montreal, QC: Harvest House, 1993.

Meigs, Charles Delucena. *Obstetrics: The Science and the Art.* Philadelphia, PA: Blanchard and Lear, 1852.

Millar, Wyn, Ruby Heap, and Bob Gidney. "Degrees of Difference: The Students in Three Professional Schools at the University of Toronto, 1910 to the 1950s." In *Learning to Practice: Professional Education in Historical and Contemporary Perspective,* edited by Ruby Heap, Wyn Millar, and Elizabeth Smyth, 155–88. Ottawa: University of Ottawa Press, 2005.

Mitchinson, Wendy. *Giving Birth in Canada, 1900–1950.* Toronto: University of Toronto Press, 2002.

– *The Nature of Their Bodies: Women and Their Doctors in Victorian Canada.* Toronto: University of Toronto Press, 1991.

Oppenheimer, Jo. "Childbirth in Ontario: The Transition from Home to Hospital in the Early-Twentieth Century." *Ontario History* 75 (1983): 36–60.

Peikoff, Samuel S. *Yesterday's Doctor: An Autobiography.* Winnipeg: The Prairie Publishing Company, 1980.

Playfair, William Smoult. *A Treatise on the Science and Practice of Midwifery.* Philadelphia, PA: Henry C. Lea, 1876.

Stetson, Charlotte Perkins. "The Yellow Wallpaper." *New England Magazine* 11 (January 1892): 647–57.

Warsh, Cheryl Krasnick. *Prescribed Norms: Women and Health in Canada and the United States Since 1900*. Toronto: University of Toronto Press, 2010.

Williams, J. Whitridge. *Obstetrics: A Textbook for the Use of Students and Practitioners*. New York and London: D. Appleton and Company, 1931.

Willinsky, Abraham Isaac. *A Doctor's Memoirs*. Toronto: The MacMillan Company of Canada, Ltd, 1960.

Wolf, Jacqueline. *Deliver Me from Pain: Anaesthesia and Birth in America*. Baltimore, MD: Johns Hopkins University Press, 2009.

Wood, Whitney. "'Bound to Be a Troublesome Time': Canadian Perceptions of Pregnancy, Parturition and Pain, c. 1867–1930." In *Perceptions of Pregnancy from the Seventeenth to the Twentieth Century*, edited by Jennifer Evans and Ciara Meehan, 33–55. Basingstoke, UK: Palgrave Macmillan, 2017.

Wood, Whitney. "'When I Think of What Is Before Me, I Feel Afraid': Narratives of Fear, Pain, and Childbirth in Late-Victorian Canada." In *Pain and Emotion in Modern History*, edited by Rob Boddice, 187–203. Houndsmills, UK: Palgrave MacMillan, 2014.

Wright, Adam H. *A Text-Book of Obstetrics*. New York and London: D. Appleton and Company, 1908.

Yeniyurt, Kathryn. "When It Hurts to Look: Interpreting the Interior of the Victorian Woman." *Social History of Medicine* 27, no. 1 (2014): 22–40.

PART FIVE

History Matters:
Medical Practice and
Historical Thinking

19

Infiltrating the National Curriculum:
A Medical History Handbook for Medical Students

Frank Huisman

In 1948 George Rosen wondered: "Is the study of medical history only a fad ... and a mark of culture and intellectual refinement; or is it sufficiently important to be considered an essential element in medical education?"[1] His answer to this question was unequivocally the latter, even though he needed thirty-five pages to make this point: "When properly presented, medical history counterbalances the divisive effects of specialization, and helps the medical man to synthesize for himself an organic conception of medicine." In the discussion that followed his article, Erwin Ackerknecht said: "I am firmly convinced that I can contribute to making [my students] better doctors." Owsei Temkin concluded that although "the study of medical history *is* of value to medical education," there is "a great variety of opinions regarding when and where and by whom and in what form medical history should be taught."[2] In the decades that followed, much ink was spilt on these and similar issues: what is the value of medical history (instrumental or humanistic)? Who should be teaching it (clinicians or researchers; physicians or historians)? What should the curriculum contain (highlights or context)? When should medical history be offered (at the beginning or at the end of the curriculum)?[3]

Then Jackie Duffin entered the scene. After pointing out to the world how she had successfully infiltrated the medical curriculum of Queen's University in Kingston, Ontario, she published a handbook: the result of many years of hands-on experience.[4] Six years after she was invited to start a medical history course for undergraduate medical students, she decided to share her experiences in an article submitted to *The Journal of Medical Humanities*. She did not waste too much time on the eternal questions: why (to which she responded: "to foster critical thinking and to demonstrate that history is a research discipline"), who (difficult to answer, but competence matters), when ("there is no ideal time"), what ("there is no consensus ... as long as the information is accurate and relevant"), and how (the course should be taught "in real time" alongside the rest of the curriculum, and students should be evaluated). She quickly decided to become practical, fully realizing that the success or failure of any medical history program depends on institutional factors and personal creativity.[5] Therefore, she conceded, her approach should be considered more as an inspiration than as a blueprint to be emulated and followed. Because she also realized that a full-time medical history course would not be feasible at Queen's University, she decided that piggybacking it on medical courses was the best strategy: "I planned a little history of anatomy during anatomy; history of pathology in pathology; history of obstetrics in obstetrics, and so on," dreaming of "giving presentations under the rubric of the science disciplines, preceded and followed by professors wearing white coats who would give me credibility," hoping ultimately to have one question on every exam. Although she met with some resistance, gradually the barriers fell. Both students and faculty came to appreciate Jackie's teaching, and she was invited to serve as associate dean of Undergraduate Medical Studies and Admissions.

Just a few years later, Jackie presented her infiltrative approach in more detail in a handbook. As she pointed out on many occasions, a discipline lacking a handbook and examination is not taken seriously – neither by students nor by academic staff. But how to organize it? Until then, most handbooks were organized chronologically. In line with the above, she decided to arrange her material by medical discipline. Inspired by Cecilia Mettler's *History of Medicine*, she included chapters on the history of anatomy, physiology, pathology, pharmacology, obstetrics, and so on. Because the chapters were devoted to the various disciplines of medicine, they could be read in random order, depending on the specific requirements of the medical curriculum. Thirteen "disciplinary chapters" were preceded by a game called "Heroes and Villains in Medical History" and followed by a chapter on doing research in medical history. Both were intended to show that medical history is a research discipline like any other, requiring a critical attitude and sound methodology: "Medical history, like medical practice and medical science, is about questions and answers, evidence and interpretation," she argued.[6] In an article she later co-authored with David Jones, Jeremy Greene, and John Harley Warner, Jackie made the case for history in medical education.[7] It was necessary to do so, because they realized how much historians in medical schools found themselves competing with medical ethics and medical humanities. Although to the outsider these disciplines may seem similar, history, they argued, has something profoundly different on offer: "Historical analysis contributes essential insights to our understanding of disease, therapeutics, and institutions – things that all physicians must know in order to be effective, just as they must learn anatomy or pathophysiology."[8]

Over the course of the nineteenth and twentieth centuries, the rationale for teaching medical history to medical students – and hence the need for a specific type of handbook – changed profoundly in response to developments in medical research and the needs of the medical curriculum. Until the late eighteenth century, every university-trained physician was also a historian, shaping and articulating his professional identity by relating to specific predecessors from Hippocrates to the present. Around 1800, however, a new historical consciousness emerged in medicine, putting an end to this "doxographical" tradition. Kurt Sprengel famously embodied this new perspective. In *Versuch einer pragmatischen Geschichte der Arzneykunde*, he claimed that one can learn from the past to become a better physician with a sense of civic responsibility. On the one hand, history could teach students modesty and humility, while on the other, they learned that they stood on the shoulders of giants. Sprengel's "pragmatic" history was to remain influential until laboratory medicine caused a profound sense of discontinuity between medicine's past and present. Physician-historians such as Charles Daremberg and Carl Wunderlich used medical history to stress the revolutionary aspects of physiology and celebrate progress, but many others lost interest in history and focused on experimental and clinical research instead. By the end of the nineteenth century, Theodor Puschmann, Julius Pagel, and Max Neuburger grew concerned about the widening gap between science and the humanities, and they argued that medical history was capable of bridging this divide between "the two cultures." In the introduction to their *Handbuch der Geschichte der Medizin*, Neuburger and Pagel elaborated on their Hegelian views and the value of medical history. Like Sprengel, they wanted to integrate it in the medical curriculum, arguing that medical history could make students aware of the historical foundations of science and medicine and complete their education. Although their cultural approach was embraced by people such as William Osler, Henry Sigerist, and Owsei Temkin, medical history lost curricular ground almost everywhere, especially after the Second World War, when breakthroughs in biomedical research changed medicine and health care definitively. Medical educators increasingly deemed medical history obsolete and irrelevant.[9] The ideal of the scholarly Oslerian "gentleman-physician" had become a thing of the past, limited to small groups of loyal adherents to Osler's brand of medical humanism. After critics such as Michel Foucault, Ivan Illich, Thomas Szasz, and David Armstrong had pointed to the "medicalization" of society and the "dehumanization" of medical practice, a new brand of medical history came into being in the 1970s and 1980s: the social history of medicine. In 1997 Roy Porter – one of its champions – had the courage to write a medical history handbook again. In *The Greatest Benefit of Mankind* he pointed to the paradoxes of contemporary medicine. While on the one hand, it was "an enormous achievement," on the other, "its triumphs are dissolving in disorientation."[10] In an attempt to "rehumanize" medicine, he wanted to supply historical perspectives and material to inform intelligent discussion and policy-making. The past, Porter argued, could and should be made relevant to the present. Jackie Duffin agreed, and published her own handbook two years later.

I would like to thank Jackie for her profound insights, her pragmatic solutions, her feisty way of engaging with medical history, and for simply being there. In 2018, I co-edited *Leerboek medische geschiedenis* (*Handbook of Medical History*), published in Dutch and aimed at senior undergraduate medical students in the Netherlands.[11] As a tribute to Jackie, I would like to share our editorial team's insights into the thematic and didactic choices we made in producing the handbook.[12] Before doing so, I would like to provide some context.

THE DUTCH CONTEXT

In line with the article of Jones and Duffin et al., we believe that medical history has the potential of creating a sensitivity among medical students for the contingent nature of disease categories, for the constructed nature of medical knowledge, for the dynamic relationship between doctor and patient, and for power dynamics within health care. In a medical context, history should not be taught as a stand-alone course, nor as a goal in itself – it must be made relevant for the student to promote the realization that medicine and health care are not fixed entities or domains, but subject to constant change. We agree with Jones et al. when they write: "By showing the number of crucial insights that history can offer, it makes it more difficult for skeptics to dismiss history of medicine as window dressing for gentlemanly physicians."[13] There is a real need for medical history in the medical curriculum, we maintain, but it needs to be made manifest and official. There are two ways of accomplishing this: bottom-up, as Jackie did with her *local* approach, convincing each head of each clinical department at Queen's University to include history; or top-down, by trying to infiltrate the *national* medical curriculum. We set out to accomplish the latter by producing a handbook that is general enough to appeal to all medical programs in the country, but also flexible enough to adapt to local demands. While we believe in the global educational value of medical history, we were equally convinced that it must be context-specific. We decided, therefore, that our handbook needed to fit in with the Dutch context.

In the Netherlands, the end terms of the medical curriculum are stipulated by a document called the Framework for Undergraduate Medical Education (*Raamplan artsopleiding*), which has been in existence since 1994. The framework is issued under the auspices of the Dutch Federation of University Medical Centers (NFU) and inspected through site visits made by the QANU (Quality Assurance Netherlands Universities). Because the world undergoes continuous change (and with it, medicine), curricula must periodically respond and adapt. The framework was renewed in 2001 and again in 2009. In June 2020 a new edition was published.[14] Since its inception, the framework has been a crucial document for medical education, and, consequently, medical practice. Its legal context is the Law on the Professions in Individual Health Care (*Wet BIG*), which implies that medical certification is grounded in Dutch medical legislation. For some time now, it has been observed that medical education in the Netherlands has focused too much on the technicalities of biomedicine, disregarding the clinical and societal dimensions of medicine and health care. Having basic biomedical knowledge is no longer considered enough for modern physicians. The framework of 2009 called for more attention in the curriculum to social medicine (creating an awareness of health determinants), to translational medicine (bringing knowledge from the bench to the bedside), and to disciplines such as medical ethics, health law, and medical history. These calls, however, were stated in general terms. With regard to medical history, the framework stipulated only that students should be aware of the broad outline of the "history of scientific medicine." The eight University Medical Centers in the Netherlands[15] realized that, come accreditation time, a site committee would use the 2009 framework criteria to evaluate their curricula and that a bad evaluation would be very bad news indeed. However, the new terms related to medical history were so vague that they led to nothing in concrete terms. There was hardly serious attention devoted to medical history in any of the UMCs, and there was certainly no evaluation. Despite its official reinstatement in 2009, neither faculty nor students were taking much notice of medical history.

Thus, medical teaching in the Netherlands was in need of two things: a new framework stipulating the end terms of the medical curriculum with regard to medical history, and a handbook supplying the teaching material.[16] But in what order? Because a new framework was not due for another few years later, we decided to work on a handbook first. We would work on it with an awareness of the new framework, trying to get in contact with the framework committee as soon as it was installed. We also decided that rather than producing a single-authored handbook, as Jackie had done, we would publish an edited volume of units created by individual specialists in the field.

The three editors of the handbook (Harry Hillen, Eddy Houwaart, and I) started working on an outline. We made a list of chapter topics, we decided on the intended audience (advanced undergraduate medical students), and we chose the language (Dutch). In terms of didactics, we decided to link up to Canada's CanMEDS competency framework.[17] We then submitted our plan to the members of the national Working Group Teaching and Research Medical History to request feedback. The working group consisted of medical historians affiliated with both medical and humanities faculties.[18] We regarded their input as essential: first of all because of their expertise, but also because they were the ones that we hoped would eventually use our handbook to teach medical history. Their input turned out to be invaluable. While they agreed on audience and language, they made important suggestions with regard to existing chapters and suggested additional chapter topics. Perhaps most importantly of all, these expert reviewers suggested a way to organize the book into four parts.

It was never our intention to be comprehensive, nor did we want to teach history for its own sake. Rather, we were keen on using history as a tool to cultivate awareness and provide explanations of present conditions in the (Dutch) health care system. In contrast to Roy Porter (who organized his handbook chronologically),[19] and different from Jackie (who employed medical specialties as her organizational principle), we opted for a topical approach. Each of the chapters deals with an issue that we think is significant and relevant for all contemporary physicians. By historicizing and contextualizing those issues, we contribute to the reflectivity of physicians-to-be. Whether they like it or not, doctors must be able to take an informed and socially responsible stance towards lay responses to individual illness and epidemic disease; to the socially constructed character of disease categories (as they appear in the ICD and the DSM); to the double nature of medical technology; to funding rationales in health care systems; to alternative and complementary healing strategies; to patient autonomy and shared decision-making; to the protocolization and marketization of health care; and to the societal role of the medical profession itself. Of course history cannot offer blueprints for the present or the future, but by explaining to students how and why things developed as they did, we believe that medical history contributes to shaping reflective citizen-physicians – in other words, people who are biomedically educated as well as knowledgeable about the rights and duties of doctors, patients, and the state, and about the goals and limits of medicine.[20]

THE DUTCH HANDBOOK

Thanks to the feedback of several members of the working group (some of whom would later contribute to the handbook), we decided to organize the seventeen chapters into four parts: "Disease"; "Knowledge"; "Doctor and Patient"; and "Health Care and Society." Parts 1 and 2 speak to each other, as do parts 3 and 4. One could say that while part 1 ("Disease") deals with ontology, or with the object of medicine itself, part 2 ("Knowledge") focuses on epistemology, or the ways in which knowledge about disease is constructed from ideas. To be more specific: all five chapters of part 1 grapple with the elusive category of disease. They do so from the perspective of historical demography (testing the validity of Abdel Omran's theory of epidemiological transition for the Netherlands); cultural history (suggesting "paradigmatic" responses to disease from the Black Death to AIDS); philosophy (presenting the realist and the constructivist conceptions of disease); again philosophy (about the dualism between body and mind and about somatic symptom disorder); and historical anthropology (non-Western traditions vis-à-vis Western biomedicine). The five chapters of part 2 deal with different sites of knowledge that medicine has used over the course of time. Although these sites are presented in a loosely chronological way, they also present ideal types: every site produces its own way of knowing.[21] Thus, the chapter on "the library" discusses not only the physical setting, but also the textual character of medical knowledge (from Hippocrates to PubMed); whereas the chapter on "the clinic" shows how observation is the key to knowledge. The chapter on "the laboratory" explains how the authority of experimental research is not self-evident; and the next chapter points out how statistics attempted to "objectify" the body of the patient by using numbers on a population level. The final chapter clarifies how, in the twentieth century, doctors were no longer the only ones engaged in the creation of medical knowledge and began collaborating with mathematicians, IT specialists, and technicians in complex technological systems.

In a similar way, parts 3 and 4 speak to each other. While part 3 is on the micro dimension of health care, part 4 focuses on its macro dimension. The three chapters of part 3 examine what transpires in clinical encounters between doctor and patient. They deal with the doctor-patient relationship from various historical perspectives; with three medical thought styles (removing, treating, and supporting), using the case of cancer; and with the hospitalization of care (moving from offering *hospitalitas* in medieval asylums to medical treatment in the total medical institutions of the twenty-first century). Part 4 pans out to consider societal dimensions – in particular, the political economy of health care. Its four chapters examine the medical profession (using the three logics of Eliot Freidson as organizing principle[22]); the way citizenship is defined in public health arrangements (moving from the sanitary movement to new public health); the domain of mental health care (looking at the ways in which society has dealt with "marginal" people); and the way health care has been funded over time (taking Bismarck, Beveridge, and Enthoven as ideal typical sources of inspiration). After some time, finished chapters started to come in from contributors. Based on our editorial discussions, we asked authors to revise and submit a second version. The second versions were then sent to a selected pool of medical students from Utrecht and Maastricht who we knew were interested in medical history. We asked them to read the chapters carefully and critically, and to supply us with any and all feedback they thought could improve the handbook. The students turned out to be meticulous readers and provided us with much very good advice.

Every chapter starts with a brief vignette that is both medical and contemporary. Fully realizing that medical students are not naturally inclined towards history, we meant these stories to engage their interest in the subject matter for each specific chapter. The vignettes deal with a contemporary problem or a paradox to which students can relate, which has the effect of alerting them to an issue worth reflecting upon. We hope that by being sensitized in this way, they will be receptive to the subject matter of that particular chapter. To give just one example: the chapter on the medical profession opens with a letter to the editor in a leading Dutch national newspaper, published in 2016. The letter was written by a medical student and a PhD student in internal medicine. They voiced their concern that more and more students suffer from burn-out symptoms and depression, which ultimately may have detrimental effects on patient care. They describe high levels of anxiety and dissatisfaction among medical students caused by many bewildering scientific and political developments, yet they lack the time to reflect upon these important developments. Just a few decades ago, doctors enjoyed a great deal of autonomy. On the one hand, students worry that they are trained merely to become "managers in a white coat," and, on the other, they agree that there is no place for traditional hierarchical leadership in health care anymore. Modern doctors are expected to be self-reflective and transparent, acting responsibly with regard to the costs of health care. The chapter on the medical profession aims to amplify that awareness by explaining, first, how medical practice developed from Graeco-Roman holism to modern reductionism, and from medical anarchy to professional organization and even dominance. The paradox of our time is that science-based medicine can do more than ever, yet public suspicion of medicine and anxiety about health are greater than ever. At the same time, health care costs are rising exponentially. Drawing on the insights of Eliot Freidson, this chapter also invites students to think about the three logics that may be used to organize health care as a system: the logic of the profession, the logic of the bureaucracy, and the logic of the market. In the first case, doctors are in the lead; in the second case, bureaucrats using guidelines and protocols are the leaders; while, in the third, everything is left to market dynamics. Of course the three forms of logic represent ideal types that will never be found in their pure form in clinical practice, but we hope that this way of presenting history, context, and present issues together enables students to evaluate constructively the reasons protocols and health managers were introduced: to create accountability in the health care system and to put new governance structures in place, in response to new realities.

In the introduction to each chapter, the contemporary issue at hand is problematized and the periodization explained. We also indicate which CanMEDS competencies the chapter intends to address or train. In doing so, we hoped to make it easier for the framework committee to understand how medical history can contribute to the shaping of modern doctors. Every chapter also contains "frame texts" – small stories about people and concepts that we did not want to exclude, but that we felt would interrupt the flow of expositions and explanations. The handbook has frame texts about famous researchers and physicians (among them Hippocrates, Galen, Boerhaave, Frank, Bichat, Pasteur, Charcot, Osler, Einthoven, Halsted, Ehrlich, Bradford Hill, and Balint); about analytics and critics of medicine (Fleck, Foucault, Kuhn, Illich, and Freidson); and about relevant concepts (acupuncture, the birth of the clinic, reductionism, the Gaussian function, and the ICD). Every chapter opens with learning objectives (required by most medical schools for every educational intervention), and it closes with learning questions, the answers to which are found on the website that accompanies the handbook (each copy of the book contains a unique code that provides access to the website). Besides answers to the learning questions, additional teaching materials may be found there, organized by chapter, that approach topics from a different angle or elaborate further. Besides the digital version of the handbook, the website includes related YouTube videos, TED Talks, podcasts, online resources, and additional reading material in PDF format.

CONCLUSIONS

Jackie Duffin is right – a discipline lacking a handbook is not taken seriously. Like Jackie, we believe in the value of medical history in the medical curriculum. And, because a handbook (in Dutch) was lacking, we decided to create one. The *Leerboek medische geschiedenis* was presented in April 2018, at a conference to which not only colleagues were invited, but also deans and program directors of Dutch medical faculties. In the academic year 2018–19, the handbook was included in several medical curricula in the Netherlands. The next step was trying to convince members of the framework committee to include historical end terms – not in the vague and general way of the 2009 framework, but with adequate justice to the didactic and reflective potential of medical history. Ideally, revised historical end terms would reflect the structure of our national handbook and deal with: conceptions of disease (normal and pathological, body and mind); ways of medical knowing (the epistemological dynamics of the library, the clinic, the laboratory, statistics, and technological systems); the clinical context (doctor and patient, the hospital, treatment options); and societal structures (legislation, public health, the professions, health insurance).[23] The final step to be taken is to try and get the learning questions of the handbook included in the *Voortgangstoets*, or "progress test" – an exam at the level of the end terms that medical students are expected to do every year in order to track their learning progress. Once again, we agree with the soundness of Jackie's rationale: only material and knowledge that are tested are taken seriously. Therefore, it is essential to have history questions included in the national progress test.

Jackie Duffin's work on infiltrating the medical curriculum was an important source of inspiration as we conceived, compiled, and disseminated our handbook. While the above is intended as a tribute to Jackie and her passion for teaching through medical history, I hope to have contributed to the didactic thinking of other medical educators and historians as well.

NOTES

1   Rosen, "The Place of History," 594; Rosen, "Levels of Integration," 460–8.
2   Rosen, "Levels of Integration," 626 (Rosen), 627 (Ackerknecht), and 628 (Temkin).
3   Galdston, *On the Utility*; Blake, *Education*; Risse, "The Role"; Bylebyl, *Teaching the History of Medicine*; Prioreschi, "Does History of Medicine Teach Useful Lessons?"
4   Duffin, "Infiltrating the Curriculum"; Duffin, *History of Medicine*.
5   "I began to think that no single format could be perfect in every situation. Effective solutions depend on individual teachers and their institutions" (Duffin, "Infiltrating the Curriculum," 155–6).
6   Duffin, *History of Medicine*, 6.
7   Jones and Duffin et al., "Making the Case."
8   Ibid., 626.
9   Lammel, "To Whom Does Medical History Belong?"; Gourevitch, "Charles Daremberg"; Schmiedebach, "*Bildung* in a Scientific Age"; Fee and Brown, "Using Medical History to Shape a Profession"; Huisman, "Dialectics of Understanding," 18–21, 32–4.
10 Roy Porter, *The Greatest Benefit of Mankind*, 12, 718.
11 Hillen et al., *Leerboek medische geschiedenis*.
12 "We" are: Harry Hillen, emeritus professor of internal medicine and former dean of the Faculty of Health, Medicine and Life Sciences of Maastricht University; Eddy Houwaart, professor in the history of medicine of the Faculty of Health, Medicine and Life Sciences of Maastricht University; and the author of this chapter, professor in the history of medicine of the University Medical Center of Utrecht University.
13 Jones and Duffin et al., "Making the Case," 641.
14 Raamplan Medical Training Framework 2020, https://www.nfu.nl/sites/default/files/2020-08/20.1577_Raamplan_Medical_Training_Framework_2020_-_May_2020.pdf (accessed 29 November 2021).

15 Two in Amsterdam and one each in Groningen, Leiden, Maastricht, Nijmegen, Rotterdam, and Utrecht.

16 Since 1961, there had been a handbook written by Gerrit Arie Lindeboom, but it no longer meets modern standards. It had a chronological, positivist buildup and strove to be comprehensive without integrating principle. See Lindeboom, *Inleiding*. Before Lindeboom's handbook, medical history teachers in the Netherlands had relied on Dutch translations of handbooks by Emil Isensee, Heinrich Haeser, and Henry Sigerist. See Isensee, *Oude en middel-geschiedenis van de geneeskunde*; Haeser, *Leerboek van de geschiedenis der geneeskunde*; Sigerist, *Geneeskunde*.

17 The CanMEDS roles include: medical expert, communicator, collaborator, leader, health advocate, scholar, and professional. See http://www. royalcollege.ca/rcsite/canmeds/canmeds-framework-e (accessed 26 November 2021). For the historical context of the CanMEDS framework, see Duffin and Butt, "Educating Future Physicians."

18 Later its name was changed to "History, Health and Healing." It is now a recognized working group of the Huizinga Institute, the Dutch Research Institute and Graduate School of Cultural History: https://www. huizingainstituut.nl/working-group/history-health-and-healing/ (accessed 26 November 2021).

19 Porter, *The Greatest Benefit of Mankind*.

20 Huisman, "Creating Reflective Citizen-Physicians."

21 Cf. Pickstone, *Ways of Knowing*.

22 Freidson, *Professionalism*.

23 Just before this volume was taken to the press, the new Dutch framework was published. The framework committee had considered its task to formulate an answer to the question "What are the most important competencies that a doctor in 2025 must have?" In the crucial chapter on "Knowledge aspects" (4.2), it is stipulated that the newly graduated doctor must have an under-standing of the philosophical, ethical, and historical principles of medical treatment. This implies that the principles of a physician's actions "are based on the historical development of medicine and the manner of thinking about health and disease derived from it in the full scope of society." The newly graduated doctor should also be capable of putting "current thinking about disease and health in historical and lifespan perspective" (33, 69).

BIBLIOGRAPHY

Blake, John B., ed. *Education in the History of Medicine*. New York: Hafner Publishing Company, 1968.
Bylebyl, Jerome J., ed. *Teaching the History of Medicine at a Medical Center*. Baltimore, MD: Johns Hopkins University Press, 1982.

Duffin, Jacalyn. *History of Medicine: A Scandalously Short Introduction*. Toronto: University of Toronto Press, 1999.

– "Infiltrating the Curriculum: An Integrative Approach to History for Medical Students." *The Journal of Medical Humanities* 16 (1995): 155–74.

Duffin, Jacalyn, and Hissan Butt. "Educating Future Physicians for Ontario and the Physicians' Strike of 1986: The Roots of Canadian Competency-Based Medical Education." *Canadian Medical Association Journal (CMAJ)* 190, no. 7 (2018): E196–8.

Fee, Elizabeth, and Theodore M. Brown. "Using Medical History to Shape a Profession: The Ideals of William Osler and Henry Sigerist." In *Locating Medical History: The Stories and Their Meanings*, edited by Frank Huisman and John Harley Warner, 139–64. Baltimore, MD: Johns Hopkins University Press, 2004.

Freidson, Eliot. *Professionalism: The Third Logic*. Cambridge: Polity, 2001.

Galdston, Iago, ed. *On the Utility of Medical History*. New York: International Universities Press, 1957.

Gourevitch, Danielle. "Charles Daremberg, His Friend Émile Littré, and Positivist Medical History." In *Locating Medical History: The Stories and Their Meanings*, edited by Frank Huisman and John Harley Warner, 53–73. Baltimore, MD: Johns Hopkins University Press, 2004.

Haeser, H. *Leerboek van de geschiedenis der geneeskunde*. Translated by A.H. Israëls. Utrecht, Netherlands: Van der Post, 1859.

Hillen, H.F.P., E.S. Houwaart, and Frank G. Huisman, eds. *Leerboek medische geschiedenis*. Houten, Netherlands: Bohn Stafleu van Loghum, 2018.

Huisman, Frank. "The Dialectics of Understanding: on Genres and the Use of Debate in Medical History." *History and Philosophy of the Life Sciences* 27 (2005): 13–40.

– "Creating Reflective Citizen-Physicians: Teaching Medical History to Medical Students." In *Communicating the History of Medicine: Perspectives on Audiences and Impact*, edited by Solveig Jülich and Sven Widmalm, 18–42. Manchester, UK: Manchester University Press, 2020.

Huisman, Frank, and John Harley Warner, eds. *Locating Medical History: The Stories and Their Meanings*. Baltimore, MD: Johns Hopkins University Press, 2004.

Isensee, E. *Oude en middel-geschiedenis van de geneeskunde en hare hulpwetenschappen*. Translated by L. Ali Cohen. Groningen, Netherlands: Van Zweeden, 1843.

Jones, David, Jeremy Greene, Jacalyn Duffin, and John Harley Warner. "Making the Case for History in Medical Education." *Journal of the History of Medicine and Allied Sciences* 70 (2015): 623–52.

Lammel, Hans-Uwe. "To Whom Does Medical History Belong? Johann Moehsen, Kurt Sprengel, and the Problem of Origins in Collective Memory." In *Locating Medical History: The Stories and Their Meanings*, edited by Frank Huisman and John Harley Warner, 33–52. Baltimore, MD: Johns Hopkins University Press, 2004.

Lindeboom, G.A. *Inleiding tot de geschiedenis der geneeskunde*. Haarlem, Netherlands: Bohn, 1961.

Pickstone, John. *Ways of Knowing: a New History of Science, Technology and Medicine*. Manchester, UK: Manchester University Press, 2000.

Porter, Roy. *The Greatest Benefit of Mankind: A Medical History of Humanity from Antiquity to the Present*. London: Harper Collins, 1997.

Prioreschi, Plinio. "Does History of Medicine Teach Useful Lessons?" *Perspectives on Biology and Medicine* 35 (1991): 97–104.

Risse, Guenter B. "The Role of Medical History in the Education of the 'Humanist' Physician: A Reevaluation." *Journal of Medical Education* 50 (1975): 458–65.

Rosen, George. "Levels of Integration in Medical Historiography: A Review." *Journal of the History of Medicine* 4 (1949): 460–7.

– "The Place of History in Medical Education." *Bulletin of the History of Medicine* 22 (1948): 594–627, 627–9.

Schmiedebach, Heinz-Peter. "*Bildung* in a Scientific Age: Julius Pagel, Max Neuberger, and the Cultural History of Medicine." In *Locating Medical History: The Stories and Their Meanings*, edited by Frank Huisman and John Harley Warner, 74–94. Baltimore, MD: Johns Hopkins University Press, 2004.

Sigerist, Henry. *Geneeskunde: encyclopaedisch overzicht*. Translated by J.G. de Lint. Leiden, Netherlands: Stenfert Kroese, 1933.

20

Jacalyn Duffin:
A Scandalously Celebratory Essay on Her Scholarship

Susan Lamb

Since the 1980s, Jacalyn Duffin[1] has practised medicine and history simultaneously, and her scholarly corpus epitomizes the symbiotic relationship that she observes between these two practices. "The Hippocratic triangle of doctor, patient, and disease," she argues, "finds an analogy in the relationship between a historian, her sources, her audience, and the histories they build together."[2] Through this dual praxis Duffin has emerged as a superb mediator for two disciplines that each sometimes struggle to recognize what the other has to offer.

With this correlation between medical and historical practice as a foundation, Duffin also became an award-winning medical educator. This is why my co-editor, Delia Gavrus, and I chose the theme of medical education for a collection of historical scholarship produced in her honour. The impact of her research and character on the history of medicine, our shared discipline, inspired the following insights into both. Nevertheless, as promised in its title – an homage to Duffin's successful textbook – even this expanded consideration of her contributions remains unapologetically celebratory and one-sided.

Many of the case studies in this volume examine ways in which educational models and professional regulation shape processes of belonging in medicine, including who is permitted to belong at all. In addition to highlighting Duffin's professional trajectory and areas of expertise as a historian of medicine, I offer my observations on the compelling character of Duffin's scholarship and the scholar herself. In particular, I indulge my curiosity about her experiences of becoming a historian who is also a physician – especially as she navigated, contested, and examined disciplinary boundaries that she encountered in that process of belonging.

Raised in small-town Ontario, Duffin graduated in medicine from the University of Toronto and trained as a specialist in internal medicine and hematology in the 1970s. She then earned a doctorate in philosophy and history of science from the Sorbonne in Paris. Upon her return to Canada,

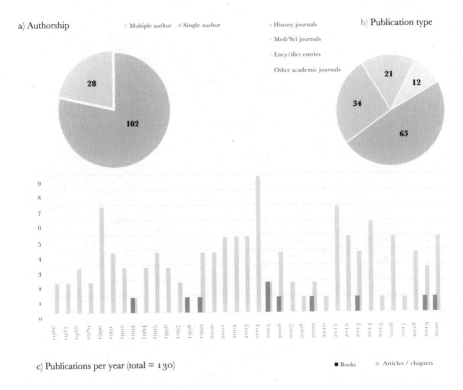

a) Authorship

Multiple author ▨ Single author

· History journals
· Med/Sci journals
· Ency/dict entries
· Other academic journals

b) Publication type

28

102

21

12

34

63

c) Publications per year (total = 130)

■ Books ▨ Articles / chapters

Figure 20.1 | Three graphic representations of Jacalyn Duffin's substantial scholarly corpus (1985–2020) according to a) authorship, b) publication type, and number of c) publications per year. Like most historians, most of her research is single-authored and published in history journals; a third of her corpus is collaborative and/or published in medical journals, which reflects the goals and expectations of a historian of medicine who works in clinical settings. (Data prepared by Serina Khater, MD, University of Ottawa, 2020)

she combined a post-doctoral fellowship in history of medicine with a part-time hematology practice at the University of Ottawa. She was appointed Hannah Chair of the History of Medicine at Queen's University in 1988, at that time one of just five such named professorships in Canadian medical schools endowed by the charitable trust Associated Medical Services (AMS). In addition to her research and teaching, Duffin continued to practise and teach clinical hematology. With its libraries and archives nestled close to its medical school and teaching hospitals, the Kingston campus on Lake Ontario was ideally suited to support a practitioner of both history and medicine.

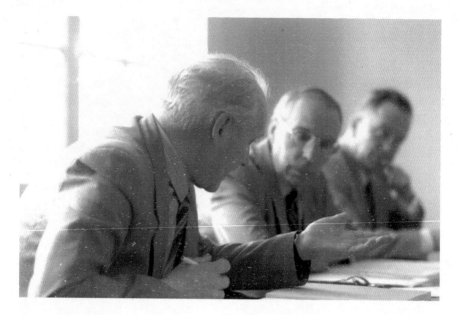

Figure 20.2 | Duffin's doctoral advisor was Mirko Grmek, seen here (in foreground, gesturing) with fellow examiners Jacques Roger and Roger Rullière at her thesis defense on 3 June 1985. (Photograph courtesy of J. Duffin)

Today Duffin's enormous contributions as a historian of medicine are recognized at home and internationally. She is a fellow of the Canadian Academy of Health Sciences and the prestigious Royal Society of Canada. She served as president of both the American Association for the History of Medicine (AAHM) and the Canadian Society for the History of Medicine (CSHM); on the Board of Curators for the Osler Library (McGill University); and as an International Advisor to the Wellcome Centre for the History of Medicine in London, England. In addition to numerous honours for teaching, writing, and advocacy, in 2019 the AAHM recognized her with its Genevieve Miller Lifetime Achievement Award and her fellow physicians inducted Duffin into the Canadian Medical Hall of Fame. She is always in high demand as a keynote speaker and pundit – due to her intellectual clout, certainly, but also her characteristic blend of candour, insight, and zeal. In 2020, she was inducted into the Order of Canada, a high civilian honour for extraordinary contributions to the nation.

Duffin's scholarly corpus reflects a range and depth that only a handful of historians of medicine achieve. To date, it comprises six monographs, three

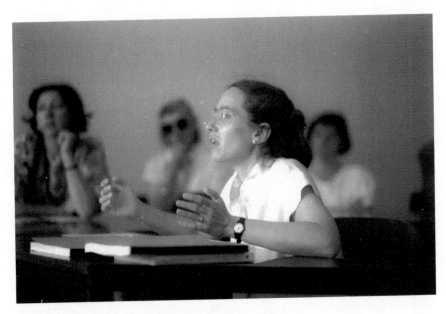

Figure 20.3 | Duffin defends her doctoral thesis at the Université Paris-Sorbonne in Paris on 3 June 1985. (Photograph courtesy of J. Duffin)

edited volumes, a textbook in its third edition, and over one hundred peer-reviewed articles and chapters (Figure 20.1). She is a specialist on nineteenth-century clinical medicine, medical epistemology, processes of scientific discovery, religion and medicine, and the politics of professional medicine and medical education. She has also produced important histories and collaborative research on palliative care, irritable bowel disease, Nobel Prize discoveries, visual culture in medicine, women in medicine, pharmacology, public health, shoe-fitting fluoroscopes, dementia, the CSHM, the founding of the *Canadian Medical Association Journal* (*CMAJ*), the digitalization of primary sources, psychiatry, water contamination in Indigenous communities, medical protest music, and sweating blood. This is still only a selective list.

Questions and answers, which abound in this volume, both motivate and delight its honoree. "The best reason for addressing a topic," Duffin declares, "is a passionate and personal desire to answer the question."[3] When the co-editors interviewed her for this volume (chapter 21), she told us that her scholarly curiosity is often piqued by a chance encounter with a manuscript or person, even a specimen. Her recent book on the Canadian scientific expedition to

Easter Island, *Stanley's Dream* (2019), resulted from just such serendipity in the archives. Other research projects have been inspired by her decades of clinical work and teaching. "I'm grateful for my patients and for my students," she explains; "both have asked me questions that ended up becoming major research projects."[4] The significance of her published work extends beyond its remarkable scope and substance.

Reading across her corpus while remaining attentive to her historical practices, one cannot escape Duffin's character as a scholar: constrained by her research question and evidence; liberated by a compulsive curiosity that questions boundaries; attuned to unexamined bias; allergic to injustice; and at once optimistic and critical, inclusive and irreverent. Though wide-ranging across subject, time, and space, her research is unified by an abiding attention to epistemologies of disease, compelling analyses and narratives, and a deft ability to marshal quantitative data in the service of humanistic inquiry. The corpus showcases Duffin's skill for bringing historical methods to bear on medicine, past and present. It also narrates some of the disciplinary tensions within the history of medicine during the previous four decades.

Duffin's scholarship also reflects the intellectual orientation of her famed thesis advisor, Mirko Grmek.[5] In our interview she recounts how a young hematologist from Toronto unexpectedly undertakes a PhD at the Sorbonne supervised by the eminent historian of medicine. Grmek believed that Duffin's training in internal medicine would enable her to make sense of the unstudied manuscripts of René Laennec in order to analyze Laennec's discovery of auscultation (facilitated, of course, by his iconic invention, the stethoscope). The manuscript evidence, recently catalogued by Grmek, comprised approximately ten thousand pages of lectures, clinical records, and scientific notes.[6] Also trained in medicine, Grmek had pursued graduate studies in science, and eventually a second doctorate in philosophy under the supervision of Georges Canguilhem. For Grmek, as Duffin wrote later in an obituary for her mentor, the historian's central task was "the question, the argument, and the evidence."[7] Among other important conceptual innovations, Grmek insisted that few diseases were actually new; rather, most were newly observed, depending on changing epistemological contexts. Every disease, he emphasized, represented an idea or argument.[8] Interested in intellectual history, he advised Duffin not to dwell on Laennec's life story or social contexts.[9] Her *thèse*, completed in 1985, was a meticulous reconstruction of Laennec's clinical activities, both technical and conceptual. The research clarified her subject's foundational contributions to the complex epistemological and structural transformations in nineteenth-century medicine that historians of medicine call, simply, the Paris Clinic.[10] During the public defense of her thesis, she wrote later, she suppressed laughter as she mused silently about what her Canadian medical colleagues might think of "me sitting there arguing about the implications of vitalism in post-Revolutionary France" with scholars at the Sorbonne.[11]

Upon her return to Canada, Duffin pursued a return to hematology, but encountered opposition. She found that her having become a medical historian triggered distrust among Ottawa hematologists. "These people who shared with me the nine years of training needed to become a blood specialist," she recounted later, "*they* did not view me as an equal, or a colleague."[12] She also accepted a post-doctoral fellowship under the direction of Toby Gelfand, the Hannah Chair at the University of Ottawa and a historian of French medicine. Gelfand became a valuable mentor, though initially he insisted that a historian could not also practise medicine.[13] Duffin forged ahead and eventually found a way to practise both, successfully, in Ottawa.

Duffin's initiation into professionalized history in North America in the late 1980s was also significant to her becoming the historian of medicine that this volume honours. The period was characterized by a groundswell of new social and cultural histories that decentred the discipline's long-standing focus on elite individuals (typically male), their political ideas (typically European), and their belief in inexorable progress (so-called Whig history). Using novel research methods and theories of historical interpretation, often drawn from sociology and cultural anthropology, many academic historians were committed to disrupting "great man" history. The decade was also characterized by fierce debates among historians about which methods and theories ought to prevail: political, sociological, post-structural, or post-modern (or some synthesis thereof). Historian Paula Fass later described it as a hostile yet exhilarating atmosphere.[14] The historiographical complexities of this "social-cultural turn" were generally unified, nevertheless, by efforts to amplify the voices of groups previously marginalized by history and recover the lived experiences of everyday people. Today, most historians recognize both the consequences of social structures *and* their constructed nature, especially as instruments of power and through language; and they acknowledge that "every social actor is embedded in a matrix of social relationships based on myriad categories of identity and power," as Nicole Eustace describes the post-modern development, of which the categories of race, class, and gender, she rightly points out, "are but the beginning."[15] Many historians, including Duffin, pay close attention to connections and disparities among these factors without committing to any single method or theory.

Within history of medicine, these developments played out in particular ways that shaped some of Duffin's early professional experiences and reactions to her work. Like colleagues in other subfields, historians of medicine were newly focused on understanding the consequences of medicine's social structures and power relationships for populations and patients, rather than the ideas of influential doctors or medical progress.[16] It was also during this period that scholars with graduate training in history increasingly displaced physicians as writers of medical history and editors of the field's journals (whereas its parent discipline, history, had professionalized in the nineteenth century).[17] In both content and professional practice, many historians of medicine felt strongly that the discipline needed to marginalize physicians. It was into this historiographical and professional context that Duffin entered in 1985.

Throughout the decade that followed her graduate training, remarkably, she simultaneously worked on biographies of two physicians. Both were white, male, and privileged, but they were otherwise very different. After a summary of each project's methods and conclusions, I discuss some of Duffin's responses to their reception. First, she set out to expand her research on Laennec's clinical and teaching activities with an analysis of his personal papers. Her examination reveals an inner consistency between Laennec's vitalistic science and his religious and political views. Duffin also shows that he conceived of his clinical practices, the diseases he defined and detected, even his stethoscope, all in physiological terms. His physiological investigations, moreover, had been distorted by later admirers who, to suit their own needs, rendered him the founder of anatomical medicine and a "champion of localism." These distortions, in turn, shaped how twentieth-century scholars viewed Laennec. "Most authors, including [Michel] Foucault," Duffin explains, "reduced Laennec to a pathologist who saw disease as the product of anatomical change." Critically, her analyses show that, while his techniques and discoveries had indeed reinforced the positivism that eventually characterized nineteenth-century medicine, Laennec himself rejected its reductionist epistemological implications. Her painstaking day-by-day examinations of Laennec's intellectual processes also explain how he employed diagnostic semiology to construct diseases.[18] "Laennec had to invent language to express the sounds and their anatomical significance, and once he possessed the words, the ideas became objects to be sought."[19] After misreadings by both admirers and historians, Duffin's research resituates the Paris clinician's paradigm-shifting discoveries within the context of his own era and experiences. She succeeds in her stated aim to put Laennec back into French medicine, and the new social history of French medicine into the life of Laennec. Indeed, she successfully arcs her analyses around both the social and cultural turns in history.[20]

During the same decade, Duffin located and gained access to the records of James Miles Langstaff, a general practitioner who trained and practised in Toronto in the second half of the nineteenth century. She was "in love with manuscripts and archives" and curious about how the disease concepts and clinical techniques of the Paris Clinic expressed themselves in everyday medical practices.[21] The private archive contained Langstaff's medical daybooks

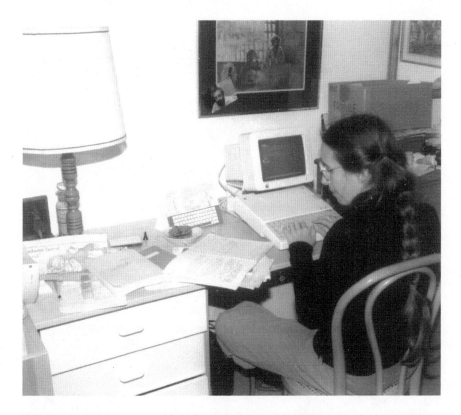

Figure 20.4 | Duffin became an early adopter of computational methods for histori-
cal research when she utilized an Apple IIC to compile and analyze manuscript data
for her doctoral thesis in the 1980s. (Photograph courtesy of J. Duffin)

and financial accounts for a forty-year period, but no personal papers or letters. Unlike Laennec, Langstaff was an "ordinary practitioner," Duffin reasoned, and might therefore function productively as a tool of microhistory,
a type of social analysis.[22] To make historical sense of the voluminous data,
Duffin became an early adopter of computational methods.

She built a database to detect patterns in Langstaff's record of births,
illnesses, treatments, innovations, unusual cases, payments, and expenses.
She was "awash in statistics" and she began to conceive of the project as "a
biography of a practice."[23] Once again, Duffin scrutinized quotidian mech-
anisms of medicine, both clinical and social, integrating the specific into
generalizable intellectual and sociological phenomena.[24] In addition to these
two commanding monographs, her research on Laennec and Langstaff led to

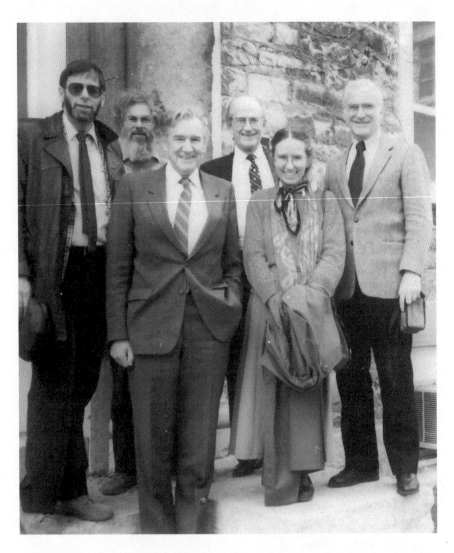

Figure 20.5 | Duffin occupied the Jason A. Hannah Chair in History of Medicine at Queen's University from 1988 to 2018. Soon after her appointment, she hosted the annual gathering of Ontario's then five Hannah Chairs, pictured here on the steps of Queen's Old Medical Building, from left to right: Toby Gelfand (University of Ottawa), Paul Potter (Western University), Donald R. Wilson (president of AMS), Robert Macbeth (CEO of Hannah Institute), Jacalyn Duffin (Queen's University), and Charles G. Roland (McMaster University). (Photograph courtesy of J. Duffin)

dozens of discrete studies on numerous aspects of nineteenth-century medicine, including professionalization, therapeutics, education, and women's
entry into the profession.[25]

Together, Duffin's monographs on Laennec and Langstaff offer detailed
insight into the full scope of organized medicine's transformation in the nineteenth century, from the construction of the clinical gaze in Paris to its bear-
ings on the structures of workaday medicine. The biography of a practice,
Langstaff: A Nineteenth-Century Medical Life, was published by the University of
Toronto Press in 1993. In 1998, *To See with a Better Eye: A Life of R.T.H. Laennec*
was published by Princeton University Press and received the Royal Society's
Hannah Medal, adjudicated by historians. Both biographies are compelling
works of history that clarify the technical and constructed origins of the disease model that dominates medicine to this day.

Yet, as Duffin recounted later, many historians and editors of academic
presses in the late 1980s dismissed her scholarship prematurely, sometimes
scornfully. Her decision to historicize these troubling experiences in peer-
reviewed commentaries became a recurring practice in her scholarship. It is a
mark of Duffin's humanist impulse to ask critical questions about constructed
and sociological phenomena, even those encountered during her own journey
of becoming a historian. I consider two examples, one professional and one
historiographical.

In 1988, Duffin's selection as Hannah Chair at Queen's University met with
resistance from the university's historians, who told her that a physician was
incapable of studying medicine's past objectively.[26] Throughout her career,
in fact, she encountered historians who dismissed clinician-written history as
"necessarily presentist, Whiggish, internalist."[27] Her choice to practise both
medicine and history, she told us in the interview, was unacceptable to many
historians. "I learned that really fast when I got back to North America," she
says of those early encounters at history of medicine conferences. "If I had
trouble making friends with historians, it was because of my MD."[28] In two
scholarly essays in 2004 and 2005, she addresses the "otiose debate over who
should do medical history and who does it best" (those with MDs or those
with PhDs).[29] Having devised ways to quantify and qualify whether clinician-
written histories share enough characteristics to constitute a genre, Duffin
determines they do not. She concludes, moreover, that *all* history is presentist
(as demonstrated, for example, by the activist motivations of many social and
cultural historians), and, furthermore, that physicians are undeniably preoccupied with progress (that is, always in search of better solutions to cure or
prevent suffering from illness).[30] Clinician-written history as something to be
scorned, she finally decides, is nothing more than a Vonnegutian granfalloon,
a "construct of would-be detractors who marshal it in service of a useless turf

war over who should be writing history."[31] Intent on exploring a related question, Duffin invited over twenty clinician-historians to interrogate how their own historical practice influences their clinical experiences. The resulting essays in *Clio in the Clinic: History in Medical Practice* (2005) showcase how "history provides a strong antidote to the arrogance that tracks medical life like an occupational hazard."[32] Over the arrogant protests coming from the direction of the Queen's History Department, the university's Faculty of Medicine appointed Duffin to its professorship in the history of medicine.

As she sought publishers for her books on Laennec and Langstaff in the 1990s, Duffin encountered another challenge to the validity of her scholarship on individual doctors. She later examined these experiences at a symposium on the history and poetics of scientific biography organized by Thomas Söderqvist. Unlike clinician-written history, biography is a bone fide genre, though, according to Söderqvist, one "despised and rejected" by academic historians.[33] Duffin recounts, for example, the reactions of editors at university presses to her research on Laennec. Market realities, one confessed, made academic biographies largely unpublishable. The problem, clarified another, was the focus on Laennec "the person" rather than using him as a "window to an age" (in fact, Duffin accomplishes this superbly) or as a vehicle for "demolishing the positivist approach to medicine and science" that Laennec's discoveries did so much to encourage (one of the book's most important revelations is that Laennec himself resisted that very positivism in clinical medicine).[34] One can only conclude, then, that Duffin was right: "My work had been put in a box before it had been read." The biography of Langstaff's medical practice faced its own challenges on the road to publication. An initial series editor, who had contracted the manuscript with the expectation of a short medical biography, balked upon receipt of Duffin's comprehensive microhistory based on numerical analyses and rescinded the offer to publish. Returned by mail, this time it was obvious that the manuscript had not been read. Eventually published with top university presses, Princeton and Toronto, she reflected a decade later: "Two editors took risks on me."[35]

Duffin's humanist impulse was triggered again. She wanted to know if – and if so, why – post-war historians had disowned biography. She frames her analysis around the notion that many committed social historians perceived it as a harmful weed ("une mauvaise herbe") in a methodological garden fertilized with theories.[36] Once again, she combines quantitative methods with a critical interpretation to show that academic biography's perceived utility did indeed diminish after the passing of the "great man" approach in humanities disciplines.[37] In Duffin's own estimation, by reorienting the history of medicine away from elite European physicians and towards the use of conceptual frameworks that dismantle structural and representational processes in medicine, historians in the 1960s, 1970s, and 1980s had rethought and revitalized our field for the better.[38] Their studies "provided more questions, and indeed *better* questions," for biographers.[39] Nevertheless, she insists that it is equally true that all individuals, even physicians, "transit through" the useful (but, ultimately, artificial) divisions that historians use such as nation-states, institutions, groups, geographies, ideas, or epistemes. Duffin resolves, therefore, that history of medicine must maximize its approaches, and that biography can serve as a means to test our models and concepts.[40] "Life writing provides us with vigorous specimens to challenge the formal garden of theoretical history," she contends. "There is art in cultivating weeds."[41]

Duffin entered our profession in the midst of an important disciplinary reformation that sought to redefine the role of medical doctors as both subjects and writers of history. As a result, she overcame some unexpected resistance to her belonging in the history of medicine because she was also a physician who conducted research on physicians. Reading across her corpus today, which includes the recent memoir "Mirko Grmek: mon maître" (2019), other factors also appear significant. First, training with Grmek in France in the early 1980s (and simultaneously co-parenting an infant and toddler), she was initially insulated from history's social-cultural turn. While Grmek acknowledged the relative importance of social structures, for example, he had cautioned that the "new" social historians tended to overestimate the influence of these forces external to medicine's ideas and science.[42] Nor did he urge his trainees to consider the new post-structuralist and post-modernist challenges to social history, including those of French intellectuals such as Foucault. "Grmek never told us much about [Foucault]," Duffin recalls, "and it wasn't until later that I realized that they had both been students of Canguilhem – and maybe rivals, in a sense."[43] She was initially puzzled when some of her early work submitted to North American journals was rejected based on its "internalist" perspective, and Grmek comforted her by explaining that she had "learned the profession of historian in old Europe."[44] All scholars are, in part, products of what we keep and discard from our advisors' partialities.

Second, then, it is clear that, early on, she internalized advice that she attributes to Grmek: "You must question the past on its own terms, accepting the judgment of no one – historical figure or historian – until you have checked everything."[45] One of the first historians Duffin challenged was Grmek himself when she returned to Paris on a research leave from Queen's determined to integrate Laennec's personal and social contexts into her initial work on his disease concepts. Grmek supported this rebellion by sharing his space and books at the Sorbonne.[46] Next was Toby Gelfand, who insisted that Duffin choose between history and hematology. She refused. Gelfand, she emphasizes, was otherwise engaged with and supportive of her research, especially

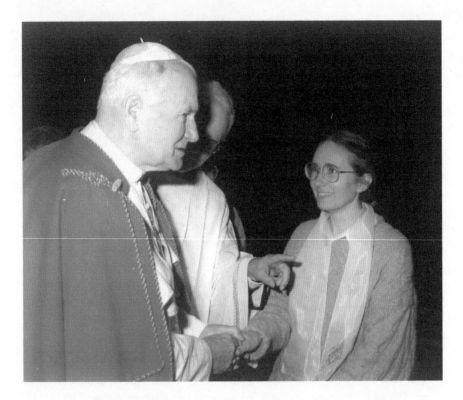

Figure 20.6 | Duffin was introduced to Pope John Paul II by Father Constanin
Bouchaud on 9 December 1990 at the canonization of Marie Marguerite d'Youville,
the first Canadian-born saint. The complementarity of Duffin's medical and historical practice was highlighted by her unplanned involvement in the canonization.
(Photo credit: Foto@VaticanMedia)

with a "crash course in social history" from a North American perspective.[47] Working with Gelfand "slowly led me to appreciate social history (and
Foucault!) more."[48] The narrative supplied by her corpus, however, makes this
point more forcefully.

Third, her earliest published research from the late 1980s makes it clear that
Duffin recognized the significance and utility of social and cultural approaches.
If and where they led to evidence-based answers for her research questions,
she drew on the insights and tools of "externalists." In 1987, she published
"The Great Canadian Peritonitis Debate, 1844–47" in the journal *Histoire
sociale / Social History*, for example, in which she effectively integrates analyses

of a "new" disease concept, clinical and post-mortem observations, political ideas, institutions, and contested medical identities – principally by exploiting primary sources produced by individual physicians.[49] In 1988, the year she was appointed Hannah Chair, the *Bulletin of the History of Medicine* – whose reviewers had rejected her research on Laennec only a year or so earlier – published "Vitalism and Organicism in the Philosophy of R.T.H. Laennec."[50] Her corpus reveals a scholar who is eager to adopt what is useful from fellow historians, both supporters and critics, but undeterred by either from answering well-defined research questions with sound evidence. If Duffin's own testing of professional and historiographical boundaries shaped much of her becoming a historian of medicine, so too did a chance encounter in her clinical practice.

Duffin's historical work on the interconnectedness of medicine and religion has earned her international recognition as a historian of medicine. The story of her foray into this area highlights her talent for translating curiosity into compelling research questions that are answerable by historical methods. In 1987, a hematology colleague asked Duffin to review a series of bone marrow samples and report her conclusions. She was not given any clinical details or justification for this "blind reading." The decade-old samples showed a course of acute myelogenous leukemia in a patient who, she reasoned, was certainly now dead since survival rates for the disease are measured in months. She submitted a comprehensive report that confirmed the fatal diagnosis, assuming her findings were part of a lawsuit. "The tribunal that questioned me was not juridical, but ecclesiastical," she wrote later of the exceptional experiences that followed.[51] Contrary to all scientific findings on the disease, the leukemia patient was not dead. The medical case, which now included Duffin's pathology report, eventually became part of a successful application to the Vatican by Canadian postulants who claimed that they had been miraculously cured by Marguerite d'Youville, founder of the Catholic order known as the Grey Nuns. Readers can learn more about her invitation to the canonization ceremony and introduction to Pope Jean Paul II in her scholarship, highlighted below, and in the interview that follows this chapter. Afterwards, she contemplated her own medical testimony, now deposited in the *Archivum Secretum Apostolicum Vaticanum*: "The historian in me recognized that one such file must exist for every saint canonized in modern times."[52] Tantalizing questions began to preoccupy her: "What diseases were cured, and did they change through time? How many miracles, like 'mine,' entailed cutting-edge science and the testimony of skeptical, even atheist, physicians like me?"[53] Still under the allure of manuscript evidence and determined to answer her questions, she began to conduct research in the Vatican Archives in two additional languages, Latin and Italian.

Manic Moments in Medical Education

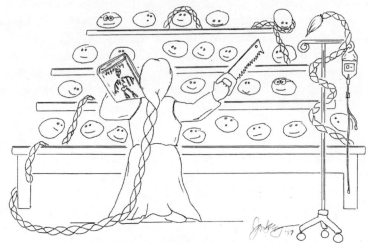

1996: Brave hematologist continues work as universal donor to
Queen's History of Medicine Curriculum.
Students beg for more!

Figure 20.7 | In 1997, medical student and cartoonist James Truong (Queen's MD, 1998) depicted Duffin as a brave "transfuser" of historical practice into the medical curriculum when he portrayed her as a "universal donor" complete with a caduceoid hair braid. (Image courtesy of J. Duffin)

While many scholars had used the Vatican's collections for historical research, Duffin was the first to survey systematically all the canonization miracles of the last three centuries. Again she relied on the computational power of databases. In *Medical Miracles: Doctors, Saints, and Healing in the Modern World* (2009) – which earned Duffin a second Hannah Medal – she identifies more than 1,400 miracles between 1588 and 1999, most of which involved incidents of recovery from illness or injury.[54] She examines the treatments and testimony of physicians, many of whom were "as baffled as herself" by phenomena they could not explain medically.[55] To qualify as miraculous, Duffin concludes, a cure required simultaneous recourse to both medical and religious systems of belief. "I never expected such reverse skepticism and emphasis on science within the church," she admitted later in an op-ed for the *New York Times* in 2016: physicians were necessary "as non-partisan witnesses and unaligned third parties" in order to corroborate the claims of hopeful postulants. Medicine today, the affirmed atheist insists, ought to handle patients' spiritual beliefs the same way. After all, she suggests, both the Vatican and the leukemia patient (who is still alive) construct the recovery as a miracle. "Why should my inability to offer an explanation trump her belief?" Duffin the physician asks. Like biomedicine's diseases, the historian concludes, miracles exist as ideas.[56] She extends her analyses of religious healing in numerous other articles and chapters, and, within the context of responses to medical orthodoxy, particularly among Catholic immigrants, in *Medical Saints: Cosmas and Damian in a Postmodern World* (2013).[57]

How diseases are constructed remains a cornerstone of Duffin's scholarship. Invited to give the Joanne Goodman Lectures at Western University in 2002, she chose to address the constructed nature of diseases in her three public lectures. Published under the delightful title *Lovers and Livers: Disease Concepts in History* (2005), Duffin's characteristically masterful combination of analysis and composition shows how "the observer" is involved in every component of disease construction.[58] Presumed causes, treatments, diagnostic signs, and outcomes are all necessarily filtered through "who gets to explain the illness, to write it down, to compose the disease concept."[59] Duffin returns to the power of diagnostic signs, so integral to her work on Laennec. In terms that are clear and compelling – not only to fellow humanists, but to health professionals and general audiences – her studies of the now-defunct but once-serious disease of lovesickness and the emergence of a new disease, hepatitis C, show how cultural histories and constructivist epistemologies matter to medicine today.

The notion that diseases, old and new, are ideas also figured prominently in Duffin's teaching in the medical curriculum at Queen's University. Teaching history to future physicians, she emphasizes, is not about drilling them on important people or famous discoveries. Rather, it encourages medical students to be skeptical about everything else they learn in medical school, and thereby prepares them for the reality that all knowledge may be subject to revision. In an important essay titled "A Hippocratic Triangle" (2004), she identifies correlations among historical thinking, clinical reasoning, and medical training to conclude that history is an instructive analogy for medicine: "The opinions of both doctors and patients about sickness and each other combine to make disease a socially and temporally contingent idea about suffering." Using the Hippocratic triangle of disease-patient-physician, medical students engage with how diseases are constructed.[60]

Countless former students, now physicians themselves, gleefully attest to her ability to situate medicine's past in ways that continue to help them make sense of complex issues in an ever-changing scientific, professional, and ethical medical landscape.[61] Duffin's teaching regularly induced her medical students to mobilize history to improve medicine. "If they see a problem in the present that they think needs to be fixed, and they're outraged by it," she explains in our interview, "they need to understand *why* it was once seen as a good thing." Recent examples include studies co-authored with students on mercury poisoning in Indigenous communities in Ontario and the need for essential medicines lists.[62] She shows how the ability to historicize is a valuable skill for future change-makers in medicine. In 2000, the Canadian Federation of Medical Students presented her with its Friend Award for outstanding student advocacy.

For three decades, she modelled her educational approach on the self-described goal of "infiltrating the medical curriculum" with the lessons and tools of history. At Queen's University Duffin successfully mapped over twenty hours of history teaching onto disciplinary areas such as anatomy, physiology, obstetrics, and pharmacology. She also views history as a means to subvert medicine's "hidden curriculum," in which medical students can feel tacit pressure to abandon empathy, cooperation, and humility in favour of diseases, procedures, and hierarchies.[63] She supports and disseminates her infiltrative model with an accessible and interdisciplinary textbook. Now in its third edition (and translated into Korean and Spanish), *History of Medicine: A Scandalously Short Introduction* is an invaluable reference for future doctors and historians.[64] In 2014, she teamed with members of an active network of educators who teach history in clinical settings to "make the case" for the inclusion of history in medical curricula. This instrumental scholarship provides advocates of humanities-based medical education with a series of compelling rationales and evidence – including Duffin's infiltrative approach – to lay before deans of medicine and other decision-makers.[65]

Her scholarly activities reveal a habit of advocacy and social justice within medicine and for patients. First, she has always delivered history and historical evidence directly to medics where they learn and practise. She published research on Langstaff, the Everyman general practitioner, for example, in the journal *Canadian Family Physician*.[66] In the *Journal of Thrombosis and Hæmostasis*, she explained to medical readers why characterizations of Christmas Disease have changed over time, from clinical recognition to molecular modelling.[67] In the *Canadian Medical Association Journal* (*CMAJ*), she asked (and answered): Why does cirrhosis belong to Laennec? Do practice guidelines cause drug shortages? Do humans really sweat blood? Why do we need essential medicines lists? And why does Vesalius still matter to medicine today? (co-written with fellow scholar and Duffin's daughter Dr Jessica Duffin Wolfe, who had once attended Grmek's seminars as a babe in arms).[68] Provocatively, in *Genitourinary Medicine*, she considered how the AIDS epidemic may have had a greater impact on the practices of historians than of public health authorities.[69] Duffin likewise invests in collaborative projects that bring together history and medicine in fruitful ways. Her co-authored examination of inflammatory bowel disease in the *Journal of Crohn's and Colitis* revealed a tale of two diseases, historically.[70] Duffin has also contributed her unique disciplinary perspective to several peer-reviewed papers on the relationships of music and dementia.[71] Within a few months of the 2003 SARS outbreak in Toronto, she convened a symposium that united key players in the medical and political response with historians of epidemics. The papers generated insightful comparative analyses that were co-edited by Duffin and Arthur Sweetman and published under the title *SARS in Context: Memory, History, Policy* (2006).[72] Most recently, she edited the memoirs of Polish-Canadian scientist and Holocaust survivor Halina Maria Czajkowska Robinson, whose laboratory observations led to the recognition of the first vinca alkaloid as a cure for childhood leukemia: *Heaven, Hell, and Purgatory: A Canadian Memoir of a Happy Polish Childhood, Nazi Horror, and Swedish Refuge* (2020).[73]

Advocacy and activism have long figured in Duffin's modus operandi. As a medical student at the University of Toronto in the late 1970s, she reveals in our interview, she advocated for curriculum change, including a new course on computers in medicine. Throughout her scholarly corpus, one feels a gravitational pull towards critical analyses of organized medicine. Using innovative methods, for example, she demonstrates how medical school tuition fees fluctuate according to political factors, not economic ones, that periodically reduce accessibility to affordable medical training.[74] In another study, she exposes the historical realities of admission quotas used by North American medical schools to discriminate against female and Jewish students.[75] Invited to join fifteen fellow female medical educators in 1996 to reflect on issues confronting women in the medical academy, Duffin wrote powerfully and honestly about how her experiences of full-time teaching and administration revealed to her the value of feminism, which she and her fellow female medical classmates in the 1970s had dismissed as no longer necessary. "I came to realize that feminism is a perspective that recognizes the *possibility* of discrimination on the basis of factors other than ability," she explains, "factors that may include gender, race, religion, sexual orientation, and privilege of birth."[76] When pundits blamed Canada's doctor shortage on the post-war "feminization" of medicine, Duffin and Meryn Stuart employed historical methods to show that the crisis had nothing to do with higher numbers of women physicians.[77]

Duffin's historical research on the Canadian health care system is yet another avenue for her advocacy. Her work illustrates how socialist ideals and medical expertise coalesced with popular movements and state and medical politics to lead to Canadian Medicare, and how these relationships continue

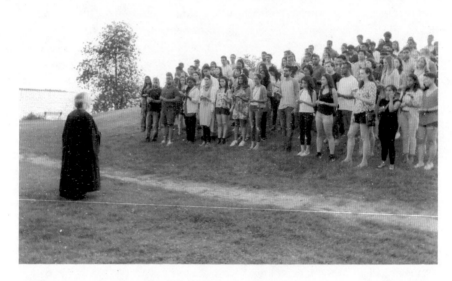

Figure 20.8 | Until her retirement from the Hannah Chair in History of Medicine in 2018, each September the first-year medical class at Queen's University invited Duffin to contextualize and then lead their collective recitation of the Hippocratic Oath – standing on the shore of Lake Ontario at sunset. (Photograph courtesy of J. Duffin)

to matter for the system today.[78] Her findings on medical tuition rates led to a request from the group Canadian Doctors for Medicare in 2009 to study the effects of the single-payer health care system on physicians' incomes. Lacking any direct source of data (doctors were and are conspicuously secretive about their earnings, she reminds us), Duffin devised and employed a painstaking research methodology that used census data and taxation statistics to create equal-dollar comparisons of incomes of average Canadian doctors and those of average Canadian citizens between the 1940s and 1990s. Her analyses show conclusively that medical incomes rose after the advent of Canada's single-payer system. When she tried to publish her findings in Canadian medical journals, however, physician-editors were uninterested in research that showed how Medicare had helped to raise doctors' revenues to the highest among Canadian professionals. Fortuitously in 2010, with Obamacare in its ascendance, her findings were published in the American journal *Health Economics, Policy and Law*, in part, the editors hoped, to provide its readers with a context for considering the financial boon for physicians that had followed the implementation of universal health coverage in Canada.[79]

Concurrent with the preparation of this essay, as Medicare turned fifty, Duffin continues to question the degree to which Canadian doctors have protected and championed it. Despite the centrality of universal health care to many Canadians' national identity, she finds that the country's medical profession has historically withheld support for the system due to continued concerns about loss of income and professional autonomy. Integrating sociological and biographical approaches, Duffin examines five small organizations of doctors that advocated to strengthen the system in order to improve health outcomes. "With each new crisis, another group of idealistic young doctors eventually stands up on behalf of patients to oppose their profession's grasping self-interest," she concludes. Sadly, she declares, these minority voices have always had to fight against their own profession, and take on "the personal risks that attend to speaking evidence to organized power."[80] Duffin herself spoke evidence to power when she was invited recently to share her research on Medicare with an audience of Canadian doctors and policy-makers. The historical evidence, she explained, contradicts the notion that medical incomes suffer under single-payer systems, and, furthermore, demolishes the assumption that the Canadian medical profession has lobbied on behalf of patients for a strong health care system. Her practice of history inexorably influences how she relates to her fellowship in medicine. She is embarrassed, she told her medical peers, when she hears them complain about their incomes. When fellow physicians claim their complaints about Medicare are about patient health, she added, "I cringe at the hypocrisy."[81] Duffin also uses her platform and tireless energy to publicize the reality of drug shortages in Canada, engaging in regular media appearances and running an activist website (www. canadadrugshortage.com).[82]

Jacalyn Duffin has answered questions big and small, quirky and controversial for four decades. "History is an art created by individuals," she says, and its beauty is in "the originality of their questions, and unique ways that they go about answering them."[83] Her corpus is comprehensive and rich, and, throughout, reveals the artisanal and the artful in Duffin's historical practice. Her exceptional contributions to the history of medicine and medical education not only merit celebration, they are instructive. Her scholarship reveals ways in which history of medicine relates to its subject matter, including the construction of disciplinary boundaries sometimes enforced to keep physicians at a distance. It also shows the utility of historical research and thinking to medicine, endowing some doctors with a ballast of relativism or humility, and perhaps disrupting arrogance and triumphalism among others. Always ready to pursue innovative research and never devoted to a particular method or theory, she has practised as a true student of Mirko Grmek to become a commanding historian of medicine in her own right. She belongs in history of medicine. Indeed, our discipline would not feel right without her.

Delia Gavrus and I are proud to have assembled this collection of original histories of teaching, learning, and belonging in medicine in honour of Jacalyn Duffin, and we commend her indefatigable and principled approach to our shared field. At age sixty-five, Duffin voluntarily transitioned to professor emerita by stepping down from the Hannah Chair at Queen's University. "I saw retiring as part of my duty as a scholar to make room for the next generation," she told a journalist, "but it didn't mean I had to shut up."[84] We are so pleased that is the case.

NOTES

1   Professor emerita, Queen's University, MD, PhD, FRCPC, FRSC, FCAH.
2   Duffin, "Hippocratic Triangle," 433.
3   Ibid.
4   Tribute video, 2019 Canadian Medical Hall of Fame Induction Ceremony. https://youtu.be/zODVa4vLwRs.
5   For a short biography of Grmek and critical appraisal of his contributions, see Méthot, "Mirko Grmek's Investigative Pathway."
6   Duffin describes her graduate training in Duffin, "Lighting Candles" and "Mirko Grmek, mon maître."
7   Duffin, "In Memoriam: Mirko Drazen Grmek."
8   See also Méthot, "Mirko Grmek's Investigative Pathway."
9   Duffin, "Mirko Grmek, mon maître."
10   Duffin, "Laennec: entre la pathologie et la clinique."
11   Duffin, "Lighting Candles," 35.
12   Ibid., 35.
13   Gavrus and Lamb, "Oral History with Jacalyn Duffin," ch. 21 in this volume.
14   Fass, "Cultural History / Social History," 40–1.
15   Eustace, "When Fish Walk on Land," 88. See also Hunt, *History: Why It Matters*.
16   For fuller discussions of these developments, see Linker, "Resuscitating the 'Great Doctor'"; Fee and Brown, "Using Medical History."
17   Burnham, *How the Idea of Profession Changed the Writing of Medical History*; Numbers, "History of American Medicine: A Field in Ferment."
18   Duffin, *To See with a Better Eye*; Duffin, "Cadavers & Patients"; Duffin, "Vitalism and Organicism; Duffin, "Medical Philosophy of R.T.H. Laennec."
19   Duffin, *To See with a Better Eye*, 147.

20 Duffin, "'La mauvaise herbe,'" 191.

21 Ibid., 191.

22 Duffin, *Langstaff*, 4–5.

23 Duffin, "'La mauvaise herbe,'" 191.

24 Ibid., 191.

25 For example, Duffin, "Vitalism and Organicism"; Duffin, "Sick Doctors: Bayle and Laennec"; Duffin, "A Rural Practice"; Duffin, "In View of the Body of Job Broom"; Duffin, "Great Canadian Peritonitis Debate"; Duffin, "Death of Sara Lovell"; Duffin, "Poisoning the Spindle."

26 Duffin, "Hippocratic Triangle," 438.

27 Ibid., 437.

28 Gavrus and Lamb, "Oral History with Jacalyn Duffin," ch. 21 in this volume.

29 Duffin, "Clio in the Clinic," 6. See also Duffin, "Hippocratic Triangle."

30 Duffin, "Hippocratic Triangle," 436–43.

31 Duffin, "Clio in the Clinic: An Introduction," 6.

32 Duffin, *Clio in the Clinic*, 10.

33 Söderqvist, "No Genre," 253.

34 Duffin quotes from the rejection letter she received in Duffin, "'La mauvaise herbe,'" 191.

35 Ibid., 189.

36 Ibid., 191.

37 Ibid., 186.

38 Duffin, "Clio in the Clinic," 5.

39 Duffin, "'La mauvaise herbe,'" 195.

40 Duffin, *To See with a Better Eye*, 4.

41 Duffin, "'La mauvaise herbe,'" 195.

42 Duffin, "Mirko Grmek: Mon maitre," 248. "Je découvris également qu'il éprouvait peu d'attrait pour l'histoire sociale de la médecine. Bien qu'il admit qu'on devait prendre en considération les forces extérieures, il croyait que les nouveaux (puisqu'ils étaient nouveaux, à l'époque) historiens sociaux avaient tendance à surestimer l'influence de ces forces, tout simplement parce qu'ils ne comprenaient ni la médecine, ni sa science." Author's translation. For Grmek and social history, see also Méthot, "Mirko Grmek's Investigative Pathway."

43 Duffin, "Mirko Grmek: Mon maitre," 246. "Grmek ne nous parla jamais beaucoup de lui, et ce n'est que plus tard que je réalisai qu'ils avaient tous les deux été des étudiants de Canguilhem – et peut-être des rivaux, dans un sens." Author's translation. For relations between Grmek and Canguilhem, see Klein, "Quelle place pour Mirko D. Grmek, élève de Georges Canguilhem dans l'historiographie médicale française?"

44 Duffin, "Mirko Grmek: Mon maitre," 251. "Je n'avais pas à rougir de l'épithète 'internaliste', puisqu'elle m'était donnée par 'les adeptes de la

"nouvelle" approche sociologique', ou pour avoir appris 'le métier d'historien dans la vieille Europe.'" Author's translation. Duffin cites a letter from Grmek to her, 2 June 1986.

45   Duffin, "Mirko Grmek: Mon maitre," 247. "Vous devez interroger le passé suivant ses propres conditions, en n'acceptant le jugement de personne – figure historique ou historien – avant d'avoir tout vérifié, disait Grmek." Author's translation. Given this imperative's strong resonance with how a clinician is trained to approach a difficult differential diagnosis, I suspect Duffin was already strongly inclined to approach historical evidence and literature similarly.

46   Ibid., 255.

47   Duffin, "Lighting Candles, Making Sparks," 36.

48   Duffin, "Mirko Grmek: Mon maitre," 250. "J'eus la chance de décrocher une bourse postdoctorale Hannah de trois ans avec Toby Gelfand, qui m'amena tout doucement à apprécier davantage l'histoire sociale (et Foucault!)." Author's translation.

49   Duffin, "Great Canadian Peritonitis Debate."

50   Duffin. "Vitalism and Organicism."

51   Duffin, "OP-ED: Pondering Miracles, Medical and Religious."

52   Duffin, *Medical Miracles*, 3–4.

53   Ibid., 3–4.

54   Ibid.

55   Duffin, "OP-ED: Pondering Miracles, Medical and Religious."

56   Ibid.

57   Duffin, *Medical Saints*; Duffin, "Hospitals of Rome/Apostolic Visit of 1825"; Duffin, "Miracles and Wonders; Duffin, "Parallels Between Medicine and Religion"; Duffin, "Doctor Was Surprised"; Duffin, "Medical Miracles and the longue durée."

58   Duffin, *Lovers and Livers*.

59   Ibid., 22.

60   Duffin, "Hippocratic Triangle," 434.

61   "Jacalyn Duffin Tribute Video – A Gift from Meds 2020." Posted by Hissan Butt, April 2017. https://youtu.be/fFo7tAgfvXI (accessed 12 August 2020).

62   Mosa and Duffin, "Mercury Poisoning"; Eom, Grootendorst, and Duffin, "Case for an Essential Medicines List."

63   See Duffin, "Infiltrating the Curriculum: An Integrative Approach"; Duffin, "Infiltrating the Curriculum: Triumphs and Disasters"; Duffin, "Hippocratic Triangle"; Duffin, "Why History of Medicine in the Undergraduate Curriculum."

64   Duffin, *History of Medicine*.

65   Jones et al., "Making the Case."
66   Duffin, "'They Fed Me.'"
67   Taylor, Duffin, et al. "Characterisation of the Original Christmas Disease."
68   Duffin, "Why Does Cirrhosis Belong to Laennec?"; Duffin, "Do Practice Guidelines Cause Drug Shortages?"; Duffin, "Sweating Blood"; Eom, Grootendorst, and Duffin, "Case for an Essential Medicines List"; Duffin and Duffin Wolfe, "The Annotated Vesalius."
69   Duffin, "AIDS, Memory and the History of Medicine."
70   Mulder, Duffin, et al. "A Tale of Two Diseases."
71   Vanstone, Duffin, et al. "Exceptional Preservation of Memory"; Duffin and Cuddy, "Music, Memory, and Alzheimer's Disease."
72   Duffin and Sweetman, eds., SARS *in Context.*
73   Duffin, ed., *Heaven, Hell, and Purgatory* (by Czajkowska Robinson).
74   Duffin, "A History of Medical Tuition."
75   Duffin, "CSHM/SCHM Presidential Address: The Quota."
76   Duffin, "Lighting Candles," 34.
77   Duffin and Stuart, "Feminization of Canadian Medicine."
78   Duffin, "The Guru and the Godfather"; Duffin and Falk, "Sigerist in Saskatchewan."
79   Duffin, "Doctors as Stewards of Medicare, or Not."
80   Ibid., 469.
81   Ibid., 465.
82   Duffin, "Drug Shortage"; Eom, Grootendorst, and Duffin, "Case for an Essential Medicines List"; Duffin, "Do Practice Guidelines Cause Drug Shortages?"
83   Duffin, "Hippocratic Triangle," 442.
84   Lisa Xu, "Retired Queen's Professor Inducted into Canadian Medical Hall of Fame," *The Whig Standard*, 16 May 2019. https://www.saultstar.com/news/local-news/retired-queens-professor-inducted-into-canadian-medical-hall-of-fame/wcm/64d6cbe6-f9a4-4f46-b8e9-5107f65c5a78/.

BIBLIOGRAPHY

Burnham, John C. *How the Idea of Profession Changed the Writing of Medical History.* *Medical History.* Supplement no. 18. London: Wellcome Institute for the History of Medicine, 1998.

Czajkowska Robinson, Halina Maria. *Heaven, Hell, and Purgatory: A Canadian Memoir of a Happy Polish Childhood, Nazi Horror, and Swedish Refuge.* Edited by Jacalyn Duffin. Toronto: Poison Spindle Press, 2020.

Duffin, Jacalyn. "AIDS, Memory and the History of Medicine: Musings on the Canadian Response." *Genitourinary Medicine* 70, no. 1 (1994): 64–9.

– "Cadavers & Patients: Laennec's Vital Principle and the Historical Diagnosis of Vitalism." In *Vitalisms: From Haller to the Cell Theory*, edited by Guido Cimino and François Duchesneau, 205–23. Florence, Italy: Biblioteca Di Physis 5, 1997.

– ed. *Clio in the Clinic: History in Medical Practice*. Toronto: University of Toronto Press, 2005.

– "CSHM/SCHM Presidential Address: The Quota: 'An Equally Serious Problem' for Us All." *Canadian Bulletin of Medical History* 19, no. 2 (2002): 327–50.

– "The Death of Sara Lovell and the Constrained Feminism of Emily Stowe." *Canadian Medical Association Journal (CMAJ)* 146, no. 6 (1992): 881–8.

– "Doctors as Stewards of Medicare, or Not: CAMSI, MRG, CDM, DRHC and the Thin Alphabet Soup of Physician Support." *Health Economics, Policy and Law* 13 (2018): 450–74.

– "The Doctor Was Surprised: Or, How to Diagnose a Miracle (Presidential Address to the AAHM)." *Bulletin of the History of Medicine* 81, no. 4 (2006): 699–729.

– "Do Practice Guidelines Cause Drug Shortages? The Historical Example of Beta-Blockers." *Canadian Medical Association Journal (CMAJ)* 191, no. 37 (2019): E1029–E1031.

– "Drug Shortage: Recent History of a Mystery (Salon)." *Canadian Medical Association Journal (CMAJ)* 184, no. 8 (2012): 1000.

– "The Great Canadian Peritonitis Debate, 1844–47." *Histoire sociale / Social History* 19, no. 28 (1987): 407–24.

– "The Guru and the Godfather: Henry E .Sigerist, Hugh Maclean and the Politics of Health Care Reform in 1940s Canada." *Canadian Bulletin of Medical History* 9, no. 2 (1992): 191–218.

– "A Hippocratic Triangle: History, Clinician-Historians, and Future Doctors." In *Locating Medical History: The Stories and Their Meanings*, edited by Frank Huisman and John Harley Warner, 432–49. Baltimore, MD: Johns Hopkins University Press, 2014.

– *History of Medicine: A Scandalously Short Introduction*. Toronto: University of Toronto Press, 1999. Reprinted in 2001, 2004, 2006, 2008, 2009; in 2000, for the United Kingdom and Europe by Macmillan Press; Korean translation 2007. A third edition is in preparation.

– "Hospitals of Rome in the Early Nineteenth Century: The Apostolic Visit of 1825." *Canadian Bulletin of Medical History* 33, no. 2 (2016): 517–33.

– "Infiltrating the Curriculum: An Integrative Approach to History for Medical Students." *Journal of Medical Humanities* 16, no. 3 (1995): 155–74.

– "Infiltrating the Curriculum: Triumphs and Disasters in Bringing History to Future Doctors." In *Students Matter: The Rewards of University Teaching*, edited by J. Kevin Dorsey and P.K. Rangachari, 74–92. Springfield: Southern Illinois University School of Medicine, 2012.

- "In Memoriam: Mirko Drazen Grmek, 9 January 1924–6 March 2000." *Bulletin of the History of Medicine* 74, no. 3 (2000): 561–5.
- "In View of the Body of Job Broom: A Glimpse of the Medical Knowledge and Practice of John Rolf." *Canadian Bulletin of Medical History* 7, no. 1 (1990): 9–30.
- "Laennec: entre la PA et la clinique." Thèse de doctorat du 3e c. Paris-I-Sorbonne, 1985.
- "'La mauvaise herbe': Unwanted Biographies Both Great and Small." In *The History and Poetics of Scientific Biography*, edited by Thomas Söderqvist, 185–97. Burlington, VT: Ashgate, 2007.
- *Langstaff: A Nineteenth-Century Medical Life.* Toronto: University of Toronto, 1993.
- "Lighting Candles, Making Sparks, and Remembering Not to Forget." In *Women in Medical Education: An Anthology of Experience*, edited by Delese Wear, 33–46. Albany: SUNY Press, 1996.
- *Lovers and Livers: Disease Concepts in History.* Toronto: University of Toronto Press, 2005.
- *Medical Miracles: Doctors, Saints, and Healing in the Modern World.* Oxford, UK: Oxford University Press, 2009.
- "Medical Miracles and the longue durée." *History and Philosophy of the Life Sciences* 27 (2005): 81–99.
- "The Medical Philosophy of R.T.H. Laennec (1781–1826)." *History and Philosophy of the Life Sciences* 8 (1986): 195–219.
- *Medical Saints: Cosmas and Damian in a Postmodern World.* New York: Oxford University Press, 2013.
- "Miracles and Wonders: Finding Canadian Medical History in the Vatican Archives." *Historical Studies* 77 (2011): 41–58.
- "Mirko Grmek, mon maître." In *Médecine, science, histoire. Le legs de Mirko Grmek*, edited by Pierre-Olivier Méthot, 239–58. Paris: Editions Matériologiques, 2019.
- "On Humanities in Medical Education." *Dermanities* 4, no. 1 (2003): a2.
- "OP-ED: Pondering Miracles, Medical and Religious." *New York Times*, 5 September 2015.
- "Parallels between Medicine and Religion through the Canonization Miracles, 1800–2000." In *Médecine et Religion: Compétitions, collaborations, conflits (XIIe–XXe siècles)*, edited by Luc Berlivet, Sara Cabibbo, Maria Pia Donato, Raimondo Michetti, and Marilyn Nicoud, 339–58. Rome: Ecole Française de Rome, 2013.
- "Poisoning the Spindle: Serendipity and Discovery of the Anti-Tumor Properties of the Vinca Alkaloids." *Pharmacy in History* 44 (2002): 64–76, 93–128.
- "The Queen's Jews: Religion, Race, and Change in Twentieth-Century Canada." *Canadian Journal of History* 49, no. 3 (2014): 369–94.

– "A Rural Practice in Nineteenth-Century Ontario: The Continuing Medical Education of James Miles Langstaff." *Canadian Bulletin of Medical History* 5 (1988): 3–28.
– "Salerno, Saints, and Sutton's Law: On the Origin of Europe's 'First' Medical School." *Medical Hypotheses* 73 (2009): 265–7.
– "Sick Doctors: Bayle and Laennec on Their Own Phthisis." *Journal of the History of Medicine and Allied Sciences* 43 (1988): 165–82.
– "Sweating Blood: History and Review." *Canadian Medical Association Journal (CMAJ)* 189, no. 42 (2017): E1315–E1317.
– "'They Fed Me; Fed My Horse': The Practice of James Miles Langstaff." *Canadian Family Physician* 36 (1990): 2189–93.
– *To See with a Better Eye: A Life of R.T.H. Laennec.* Princeton, NJ: Princeton University Press, 1998.
– "Vitalism and Organicism in the Philosophy of R.T.H. Laennec." *Bulletin of the History of Medicine* 62 (1988): 525–45.
– "What Goes Around, Comes Around: A History of Medical Tuition." *Canadian Medical Association Journal* 164, no. 1 (2001): 50–6.
– "Why Does Cirrhosis Belong to Laennec?" *Canadian Medicine Association Journal (CMAJ)* 137, no. 5 (1987): 393–6.
– "Why History of Medicine in the Undergraduate Curriculum." *University of Toronto Medical Journal* 88, no. 3 (2011): 127–8.
Duffin, Jacalyn, and Lola Cuddy. "Music, Memory, and Alzheimer's Disease: Is Music Recognition Spared in Dementia and How Can It Be Assessed?" *Neurology and Cognitive Disorders* 6, no. 1 (2006): 17–21.
Duffin, Jacalyn, and Leslie A. Falk. "Sigerist in Saskatchewan: The Quest for Balance in Social and Technical Medicine." *Bulletin of the History of Medicine* 70, no. 4 (1996): 658–83.
Duffin, Jacalyn, and Meryn Stuart. "Feminization of Canadian Medicine: Voices from the Second Wave." *Canadian Bulletin of Medical History* 29, no. 1 (2012): 83–100.
Duffin, Jacalyn, and Arthur Sweetman, eds. SARS *in Context: Memory, History, Policy.* Montreal, QC, and Kingston, ON: McGill-Queen's University Press, 2006.
Duffin, Jacalyn, and Mark Weisberg. "Evoking the Moral Imagination: Using Stories to Teach Ethics and Professionalism to Nursing, Medical, and Law Students." *Change, The Magazine of Higher Learning* 27, no. 1 (1995): 20–7.
Duffin, Jacalyn, and Jessica Duffin Wolfe. "The Annotated Vesalius." *Canadian Medical Association Journal (CMAJ)* 186, no. 11 (2014): 856–7.
Eom, Gina, Paul Grootendorst, and Jacalyn Duffin. "The Case for an Essential Medicines List for Canada." *Canadian Medical Association Journal (CMAJ)* 188, no. 17–18 (2016): E499–E503.
Eustace, Nicole. "When Fish Walk on Land: Social History in a Postmodern World." *Journal of Social History* 37, no. 1 (2003): 77–92.

Fass, Paul S. "Cultural History / Social History: Some Reflections on a Continuing Dialogue." *Journal of Social History* 37, no. 1 (2003): 39–46.

Fee, Elizabeth, and Theodore M. Brown. "Using Medical History to Shape a Profession: The Ideals of William Osler and Henry E. Sigerist." In *Locating Medical History: The Stories and Their Meanings*, edited by Frank Huisman and John Harley Warner, 139–64. Baltimore, MD: Johns Hopkins University Press, 2004.

Hunt, Lynn. *History: Why It Matters*. Medford, MA: Polity Press, 2018.

Jones, David S., Jeremy A. Greene, Jacalyn Duffin, and John Harley Warner. "Making the Case for History in Medical Education." *Journal of the History of Medicine and Allied Sciences* 70, no. 4 (2014): 165–94.

Klein, Alexandre. "Quelle place pour Mirko D. Grmek, élève de Georges Canguilhem dans l'historiographie médicale française?" In *Médecine, science, histoire. Le legs de Mirko Grmek*, edited by Pierre-Olivier Méthot, 65–77. Paris: Editions Matériologiques, 2019.

Linker, Beth. "Resuscitating the 'Great Doctor': The Career of Biography in Medical History." In *The History and Poetics of Scientific Biography*, edited by Thomas Söderqvist, 221–39. London: Routledge, 2007.

Méthot, Pierre-Olivier. "Mirko Grmek's Investigative Pathway." In *Pathological Realities: Essays on Disease, Experiments, and History by Mirko D. Grmek*, edited and translated by Pierre-Olivier Méthot, 1–28. New York: Fordham University Press, 2018.

Mosa, Adam, and Jacalyn Duffin. "The Interwoven History of Mercury Poisoning in Ontario and Japan." *Canadian Medical Association Journal (CMAJ)* 189, no. 5 (2017): E213–E215.

Mulder, Daniel J., Angela J. Nobel, Christopher J. Justinich, and Jacalyn Duffin. "A Tale of Two Diseases: The History of Inflammatory Bowel Disease." *Journal of Crohn's and Colitis* 8, no. 5 (2014): 341–8.

Numbers, Ronald L. "The History of American Medicine: A Field in Ferment." *Reviews in American History* 10, no. 4 (1982): 245–63.

Söderqvist, Thomas. "'No Genre of History Fell under More Odium than That of Biography': The Delicate Relations between Scientific Biography and the Historiography of Science." In *The History and Poetics of Scientific Biography*, edited by Thomas Söderqvist, 241–62. Burlington, VT: Ashgate, 2007.

Taylor, S., David Lillicrap, Jacalyn Duffin, et al. "Characterisation of the Original Christmas Disease Mutation Cysteine 206 to Serine: From Clinical Recognition to Molecular Modeling." *Journal of Thrombosis and Haemostasis* 67 (1991): 63–5.

Vanstone, A.D., Lola Cuddy, Jacalyn Duffin, and E. Alexander. "Exceptional Preservation of Memory for Tunes and Lyrics: Case Studies of Amusia, Profound, Deafness, and Alzheimer's Disease." *Annals of the New York Academy of Sciences* 1169 (2009): 291–4.

An Oral History with Jacalyn Duffin

Delia Gavrus and Susan Lamb

As editors of this volume, our choice to collect new scholarship on the history of medical education in honour of Jacalyn Duffin was inspired by what we see as the interrelationships between medicine and history exemplified in her work and methods. Over the course of two days in May 2019, in Kingston, Ontario, we conducted several lengthy interviews with Jackie, our fellow historian of medicine, in which she reflected on her life and career. This final case study is a curated Oral History that draws on those conversations to illuminate the themes of this volume. It also serves as a primary source, then, to study processes of learning, teaching, and belonging in her two professions, medicine and history, from the 1970s to the present. In order to enhance clarity and readability, with Jackie's approval we have edited and reordered parts of the text. The full verbatim transcript of the interviews has been deposited in the Queen's University Archives to be part of the existing Jacalyn Duffin fonds. Additional information and context for the discussion that follows can be found in chapter 20 of this volume.

Could you tell us the story of what led you to the history of medicine?

Like many historians of medicine, I didn't plan on it. Most of us fall backwards into the field. I had always been interested in history. It was something that was featured in my home growing up, and all through high school, I thought I wanted to become an archaeologist. I grew up with a map of ancient Egypt on my bedroom wall. It wasn't until my last year of high school that a guidance teacher, trying to encourage me, said, "Well, you know, you could do anything you want, and archaeology is not all that useful, and maybe you should think about doing something useful, like medicine." I found that surprising. The teacher also suggested law. I thought about it, and I decided maybe I could do medicine and should do medicine.

To back up a little bit, my father had died when I was twelve, and my mother had raised us on her own; she worked as a secretary at the university, and there wasn't a lot of money in our home. I had been working at the University of

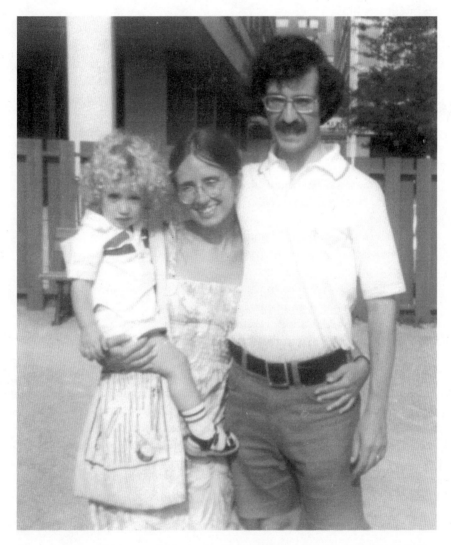

Figure 21.1 | Duffin and her first husband, Dr Lance Lipton, seen here with their son in Toronto in the late 1970s, just before their move to Thunder Bay where they each opened a specialty practice. A nephrologist, Lipton opened the city's first dialysis clinic before he was killed in an accident. Dr Josh Lipton-Duffin, their son, is today a physicist and professor. (Photograph courtesy of J. Duffin)

Western Ontario library, not only in the summers, but also on the weekends and at nights during the week, saving my money toward university all that time. I was very lucky to get accepted into the pre-med program at University of Toronto and went right through the six years and ended with my MD at twenty-three years old. I realized I was largely ignorant and maybe dangerous. The academic system sucks you in, and I just went forward into residency with a straight internship in internal medicine, because it seemed like the best way to prolong my medical education without hurting someone while deepening what I knew.

I discovered that I liked hematology and ended up specializing in it; however, the whole time I felt that I was pulling further and further away from the things I really liked. Not that I didn't like medicine. But the arts, the humanities ... when you're in medical school, it doesn't offer you a lot of time to pursue those things.

Then I got married to Hugh Lansing (Lance) Lipton and had a son (Figure 21.1). We moved to Thunder Bay where my husband was the only kidney doctor, and he started a dialysis unit. And I was the only blood doctor. A year to the day of our moving to Thunder Bay, he was killed in an accident. There I was, widowed. I had a good job, and I had my little boy. We carried on and the community was very supportive. I got a chance to marry again to an old friend, Robert David Wolfe (Figure 21.6), who had known my first husband, but we'd known each other from before I met Lance.

The one problem with this new husband was the fact that he was a diplomat, already on a posting to Paris when we decided to marry. I went directly from Thunder Bay to Paris with my little boy, and also, I went from being a pillar of the community, fulfilling an important role, to becoming the wife of a diplomat, which is a very strange occupation. My son went to school and spoke flawless Parisian French. My husband was an important person as a diplomat. And I was trying really hard to get a job.

Although I had letters from nice hematologists in Canada to French hematology luminaries, I couldn't work. They offered odd things, like translating for the *European Journal of Cancer*, and I did do some of that. They offered observing in the ORs for bone-marrow transplant procedures, because that was the hot thing at the time. They offered me to go back to medical school, which ... the thought! I just couldn't stomach it, because it wasn't all that long after I'd finished my medical and specialist training, and I didn't want to do that.

I started looking for something else to do. It was then, many years after I had entered medical school that I realized, well, you know, you always wanted to do history or archaeology or something. This is Paris – they must have everything here. Why don't you go to school and study something that you couldn't study in Canada? I can remember the specific moment when I got the idea because I had just received a letter rejecting me for yet another grant to work in research in bone-marrow transplantation. I was in a phone booth in the Fifth Arrondissement of Paris, talking to my husband at work, crying, because I had had another disappointment. As I hung up, I had this idea: you've got to do something else, or you're going to be miserable.

I went looking for history of medicine, and it took a very long time. My husband's father Roy Wolfe was an academic, a professor of geography at York University, and he happened to know another geographer in Paris who had just become the president of the Sorbonne. Through pulling various strings, I ended up having an interview with him. He sat in a huge office behind a massive desk that had nothing on it, and behind him was a great big image of the president of France. I explained that I wanted to find out where the history of medicine was taught in Paris. He turned to his *aide* and said: "You will find the history of medicine for Madame." It was all very formal, and I said thank you and scrapingly backed out the door and went home and waited. About five days later, the phone rang, and it was the *aide*, who said: "Madame, il n'y a pas d'histoire de la médecine en France." I said "merci beaucoup" and hung up, and thought, this can't be true!

I went into the medical schools, and I started looking in their libraries, where I found an article that had been published by Pierre Huard, who was a historian of surgery. Huard was also a surgeon who had served as the dean of the Hanoi Medical School. At the bottom of the article was an address in the Hôpital Cochin. I put on my nice clothes, and I went to the Hôpital Cochin. His office was in one of those long corridors where you turn on the light and the light goes out before you get to the end. I found the room, and I looked down; there seemed to be light under the door.

I knocked, and a voice said, *Entrez!* The door creaks open, and I go in, and there he is, Pierre Huard sitting at his desk, and behind him, light streams in from the window, illuminating him from behind so that his head is surrounded by glowing, white, fluffy hair, as if it was a halo. He was very old. He listened patiently to my little tale of woe, and then said, "You must find Grmek." I didn't know how to pronounce it, I'd never heard this name before. How do you write that?

Mirko Drazen Grmek gave me an appointment on Rue Colbert where there was a special rare book library at the Centre des synthèses. One of his first questions was, "How many languages do you speak?" When I replied, he said: "So few…" He puts his head down, wrinkles his brow, and thinks. Then he says: "You will study Laennec and you have time to complete a doctorate." I blurted out right away, "I don't want to study just one thing. I want to learn all of medical history! I want to take a course." He looked horrified and said "En France il faut avoir un sujet. Et en faisant bien votre sujet, vous allez comprendre toute l'histoire de la médecine." In other words, if you do your one subject well, you *will* learn all of medical history. I have thought back dozens of times to that moment, and how right he was.

Grmek viewed it as *fait accompli*, but I wasn't sure! From wanting to find a course in medical history to plunging into graduate studies like this? I went home and discussed it with my husband, and he said, "Well, why not?" I realized that I didn't have any other prospects in medicine that were going to make me any money. That is basically how I ended up doing a PhD in the history of medicine.

Would you tell us about your graduate training in History?

At that first meeting with Mirko Grmek, he told me time was short and that I had to go register at the Sorbonne. I just couldn't see how this would be right and immediately smelled a rat, thinking that he must have some personal project on this Laennec, whoever he was. He might be looking for an unpaid research assistant to do all the work! Then I asked this great historian of medicine and erudite: "Do you have any other students like me?" He looked very offended and said, "J'en ai plusieurs!"

He explained the process to me again: not only would I be studying Laennec, I would follow his seminar, which took place once a week, and I should also go to the seminar of historian of biology Jacques Roger. He was merrily listing all these things that I was going to do! But I had a child, and I wasn't sure what exactly he was planning for me. He assured me that I would be in France long enough to do a *doctorat de troisième cycle*. I wasn't sure what a *doctorat de troisième cycle* was (it's the "third cycle" after the bachelor). He said, "Votre sujet devrait être la conceptualisation de la maladie de René Théophile Laennec." There were a lot of new words going down! With the *doctorat de troisième cycle*, came *conceptualisation de la maladie* – what's *that*?

And then he said something else that was also very intriguing for its time of 1982. He knew that I was a doctor (and was giving me a lot of credit for that fact) and that I needed guidance into the discipline of history. First of all, he would write a letter for *les equivalences* so that my MD would be treated as if I had a master's degree already and I could be admitted to the *troisième cycle*.

Next Grmek asked me a question: "In medical history nowadays there are two kinds. There's one that's about people and events and politics, and there's one that's about ideas. Which do you prefer?" Because I hadn't had any formal training in history, I was throwing a dart at the wall. I remember sitting there and thinking. I couldn't tell which one he preferred, but sensed there was a right answer and a wrong one. I said, "I think I prefer ideas to events." He smiled. That was the beginning of a sometimes beautiful, sometimes horrible, relationship between us (Figure 21.4).

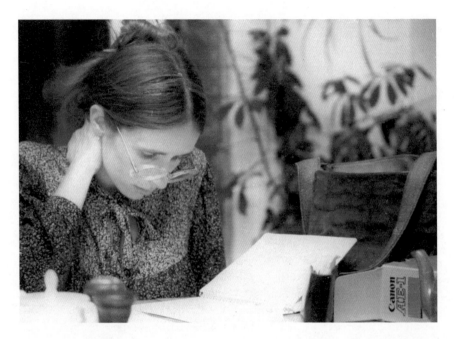

Figure 21.2 | Duffin completed a doctoral thesis in history and philosophy of science at the Université Paris-Sorbonne between 1982 and 1985. (Photograph courtesy of J. Duffin)

He also happened to inform me that he had just finished editing the cat-alogue to the manuscripts of Laennec. There were 10,000 pages of manu-scripts that had yet to be exploited, including many patient records. "Although you don't have Greek, and your Latin is minimal, and you don't speak Italian, and you don't have German," he said, "you have French, and you're a doctor, so you can read the clinical records and there are 700 patient records. So you have to go buy my catalogue *chez Masson*."

Grmek taught in the Ecole Practique des Hautes Etudes, which was physi-cally located in the Sorbonne building. His seminar happened every Thursday afternoon for two hours. One week he would cover a topic from antiquity, and the next week he would select a topic from modern medical history. He flipped back and forth, and I think he'd been doing that for a long time before I became his student.

My husband and I wanted to have another child, and it seemed a good thing to do while I was in Paris; our daughter was born in 1984. I took the baby to the opening seminar of the year. Grmek was shocked to see her. She was in a little "Snugli," a little carrier on my chest, and, for an hour, she was quiet and asleep, but then she started to get snuffly, as newborns do, so I took her out and sat in the empty hallway (Figure 21.5). I could hear him talking, and I nursed the baby, which was "not done" in those times. French women didn't nurse very long or in public, but I figured, Why not? I can do this here! When the seminar was over, Grmek and François Gallouin, a fellow graduate student, came rushing out and said, "Are you crazy? What are you doing here with a baby?" François handed me a lot of money, and said, "You must take a taxi back home. You should never be outside with that baby. How did you get here?" I said, "I took the metro." They said, "Absolutely impossible, there are germs!" France is the country of the *hygiaphone*.

We students were all writing our theses in the background of the seminars, each pretty much working alone (Figure 21.2). The research method for my PhD was given to me by Grmek, and I would say that his general overriding question has underpinned many of my other projects: that is, disease concepts. How do we know sick is sick? And how do we know normal is normal? Or, to use an older term, healthy is healthy? What is this distinction, and how is it that we incorporate science into our narrative about these things?

Grmek wanted me to explore Laennec's idea of what is a disease? He and his team had laboured over these manuscripts to prepare the catalogue, which runs to some 300 pages of what seems like very boring stuff. On each page there's a few key words, and the names of all the different archives that hold these records. There was no "disease concept" index entry. The collection included patient records, lecture notes, and loose notes to himself that Laennec had written during his last four years of life, while he taught at the College de France. By the end, he constructed all diseases in the same way, retaining and defending the life force. That idea was the richest source for my getting at his concept of disease.

Grmek told me: "You aren't going to work on his life. There's enough done about his life, and it's been romanticized. All the private letters are in the hands of family members, and they're hard to get at. Set the life aside. Just work on his disease concept with these scientific papers." I did as I was told, worked on Laennec's disease concepts, and wrapped up the thesis in three years.

Would you return to the period before the Sorbonne and tell us about your medical training?

I was accepted into the pre-med program at University of Toronto. They took 180 of us right out of high school into pre-med, and then they just threw the book at us; we had the hardest math course, the hardest physics course, the hardest chemistry course; and lots of labs. It was wall-to-wall classes, about thirty-five hours a week, which is just insane. Every single person in my class had been the valedictorian from their high school. They were all high achievers, but because these courses were so hard, deliberately hard, a lot of us started to get failing grades on some of the tests. There was huge pressure on us all the time.

It was the first time I'd lived away from home, and I can't say I was homesick so much as I was worried about my mother. Because money was tight, I didn't go home every weekend, but I tried to go home once a month.

The other thing about it, especially in pre-med, was that there was no residence for female medical students – we were 10 per cent of the class. I ended up living in Burton Hall, which was the nurses' residence for Women's College Hospital near Queen's Park. It was an ideal location. There were two other women medical students living with the nurses. The nurses were great, because they knew all kinds of medicine in a very practical way, and the other two medical women were one year and two years ahead of me. They would say, "Oh, don't worry about that exam. I failed that exam. You'll be okay. I failed this. I failed that." They were a little tiny support group in this insular nurses' residence. The next year, we three medical students moved to the nurses' residence at Mount Sinai Hospital – actually a school of nursing called Nightingale. It was a great move; newer rooms and fabulous, abundant food.

I had no life. I was studying all the time and worried about my mother. I ended up standing second in my class of pre-meds at the end of first year. (They used to send us our relative class standing with our marks.) Something happened to me over that summer. I realized that life was passing me by, and that I probably didn't have to study as much as I had done in my first year. I had developed the idea that, on top of the thirty-five hours of classes, I needed to study five hours every night – because if I didn't study five hours every night, I would fail. It became kind of like a sick obsession. But in the second year, I transferred the obsession into seeing how *little* I could study and still pass. I got rush tickets for the opera and seasons tickets for the ballet; I went to the symphony and to plays at obscure theatres. I was always bugging people to come out with me. That year, I stood seventh in the class, and figured that there was no point to studying at all. To be fair, the classes were much easier in the second year.

In the third year, my class was moving into medical school proper. Medical school in those days was "two and two" – two years of science in classrooms, and then two years of clinical in the hospitals. Toronto had six fabulous teaching hospitals. You could be assigned to any one of the six. Because I was without a vehicle, I tried to avoid having to do much at Sunnybrook, but I was in most of those hospitals for my training. The medical sciences building was brand new at the time. The labs were excellent. We had some charismatic laboratory instructors whom I've never forgotten, for anatomy, physiology, and pharmacology.

All the lectures were conjoined with labs. We worked in little pods. We had to dissect our own cadaver. That was a process that took a year. With me on the cadaver were three people: Beate Huber, Moshe Izsak, and Fred Hoy. We gave the large, male body a name, but I have forgotten it. We bonded a great deal over the cadaver. We had all come out of pre-med, hence we already knew each other well and had chosen to work together. We never talked about the war because our parents had all been killing each other in the past. Beate's father had been in the Luftwaffe. My father had been in the RCAF. Moshe's family was fleeing the Holocaust and ended up in Israel. Fred's family was interned in the Rockies by the Canadians. We had discovered this horror early in our knowing of each other, and it became something we completely avoided as a topic. We are still friends.

I became class president for one of the years. I was interested in the negotiation of our education with the faculty. You've got to remember that we started in '68, right? It was the time of student activism and the barricades in France. We didn't really see ourselves as radicals, but we felt emboldened to speak up for the things that we thought were right. We took the faculty to task. For example there was no nutrition in our curriculum, and we created an elective with the help of the Home Economics people at the University of Toronto. We created an elective in computers, because we thought computers were going to be important. No kidding! The faculty would come in to those meetings all angry, and then say, "Okay, sure, go do it." It turned out there could be a dialogue. Those were the pre-clinical years.

In the later clinical years, I had some amazing professors and some who were awful. I don't think that that's a feature of Toronto; I think that's a feature of just about everywhere. I have to say that I don't think that anyone was "awful" because they were sexist. It's important for me to say that because there were so few women in our class. The odd fellow in our class would tease us and say: "Well ... what are you doing here? You're just going to get married, and you're going to stop doing medicine." Never did any professor say that to me.

My professors were almost all men. I can't think of a woman professor, aside from a woman whom I found myself – because I liked her and I wanted to know more about obstetrics. She was Marjorie Moore, a wonderful obstetrician-gynecologist who was in private practice, but affiliated with Women's College Hospital. I think it was every Tuesday afternoon in our first year or second year, we were to do electives. I would hop on my bike and cycle up Avenue Road to her office on St Clair. It was a slog. I would spend the

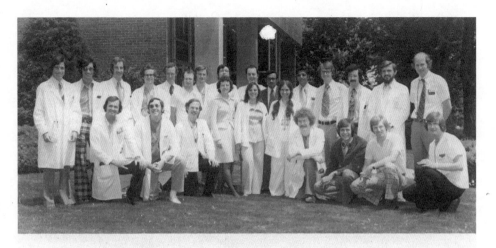

ST. JOSEPH'S HOSPITAL, LONDON, ONTARIO.   HOUSESTAFF 1974-75

Back Row (L to R) - R. Haig, A. Lam, K. Finnie, J. Harrison, P. Nichol,
                    J. MacKenzie, L. Olsson, P. Kyne, E. Francoeur,
                    Y. K. Siddiq, M. Mithoowani, D. Parsons, L. Lipton,
                    R. Hutchison, J. Simmons
Front Row (L to R) - J. Pook, R. Minielly, P. Dumont, M. Cumming, S. Boron,
                    J. Duffin, C. Hoch, A. Vance, G. Perkin, P. Larsen

Figure 21.3 | Duffin (standing right of centre, with long hair) with some fellow members of the house staff at St Joseph's Hospital, London, Ontario in 1975, including future husband Dr Hugh Lansing Lipton (standing in back row, third from right). (Photograph courtesy of J. Duffin)

afternoon in her clinic, and I learned how to do pelvic exams and got to feel tummies with babies inside. She was a most pragmatic, motherly, kind person; her husband had died when she was very young, and she raised their three daughters on her own. I was invited to her home and knew her daughters. She had a huge interest in medical history and knew a lot about it. She had read William Osler's biography when she was a high school student. Yet, her interest in science was outstanding. She had done part of her OB specialty in England, which, I think, had been a pragmatic, midwifery-type training that she was emulating in Canada. When she married another doctor, she modelled their honeymoon on that of William Osler and Grace Revere. I was so lucky to hang out with her. She remained a friend for the rest of her life. An incredible role model, not an official professor – but she was someone who was truly remarkable.

Why did you choose to specialize in hematology?

I had a great experience in residency. I loved what I was learning and had wonderful support. I loved the science and clinical side of hematology. I chose it because hematologists were the nicest people I knew with the best and most exciting science (Figure 21.3).

In my specialty training, I saw the advent of many new cures: for childhood leukemia (we cure about 50 per cent now, if not more) and for testicular cancers – both were invariably fatal when I started medical school; and bone-marrow transplants that revolutionized care. Outstanding science! The hematologists could deliver all of those outstanding things, but they never abandoned their patients. When they reached the end of the road, and there was nothing more to do, they didn't send the patients back to the family doctor, they kept them. They continued to look after them, accepting that comfort in dying was part of their work as well. I was just so full of admiration. I wanted to be like them.

Has medical education changed during your lifetime?

In lots of ways and yet not at all, because, in the end, the sick person is still the same sick person. One of the things I always say when I talk about the history of disease concepts is that the illness stays the same – for centuries, millennia – but the disease keeps changing. "Illness" is the subjective aspects of being sick, the symptoms; "disease" is how we talk about it through science. The science keeps changing, and medical schools have always had to adapt to the changing science. We end up changing the curriculum all the time, and everybody demonizes the old curriculum as if it was the worst thing ever known! But, if you've had the privilege, like I have, to teach in a medical school for three decades, you end up seeing that cycle happen several times. You remember when the now-demonized curriculum was actually the greatest thing since sliced bread.

The constant change in medical curriculum is as it should be, because medicine may not really be a science. I think it's more like an applied technology, but to be successful it has to adapt to the technologies that prevail and also to the diseases that prevail. Periodically, we do get some new diseases, but I'm not sure we get new illnesses.

Admission to medical education in my lifetime went from letting students in directly out of high school for pre-medicine, which was two years of intensive science. In effect, the first two years were a little bit like a hazing period rather than a true learning period. Now most schools require a degree. Teaching methods changed, possibly more than concepts. Some medical schools during my career plunged into problem-based learning. When I was a medical student, McMaster had just been founded, so we were tandem with the first graduates from McMaster medical school. We mercilessly made fun of them, claiming (wrongly) that they knew nothing and all their patients would die but they would never be sued because they were so nice. I don't know if I would have liked problem-based learning for myself at the time. I liked the touch-stone of the lecture hall, the discipline of note-taking, and the chance to go back and revisit the ideas with textbooks. Maybe it's because I'm a historian, and I like old-fashioned things. I found that old method to be ideal.

That said, "clinical skills" was and is always obligatory and should be, because it's probably the most important course in medical school. Some methods of delivery have changed, for example with standardized patients; yet, the manoeuvres in the clinical-skills course itself probably haven't changed much since I went to medical school. There's a few new instruments, for example, new kinds of stethoscopes. But the way you examine a patient is still the same. A few people out there are saying that the stethoscope is obsolete, and we'll all have hand-held ultrasound machines soon, making auscultation unnecessary. But we won't all have those machines, and the stethoscope is not yet obsolete. Clinical skills continues the same, as far as I know, and I do try to pay attention.

In 1985, Duffin returned from France with her young family to Ottawa, where her husband had a new posting, and she was awarded a post-doctoral fellowship under the direction of Toby Gelfand, the Hannah Chair in History of Medicine at the University of Ottawa.

You have practised history and medicine simultaneously. What insights have you accumulated about the dynamic between the two?

Having an MD and practising as an MD (even worse) was something to expiate with historians. I learned that really fast when I got back to North America. I wasn't trying to pretend that I was any better than anybody else, but I didn't think I was automatically worse! However, *many historians* did. If I had trouble making friends with historians, it was because of my MD. The fact that I chose to continue practising medicine was viewed as something to apologize for. I had tense words, for example, even with Toby Gelfand, who is one of my biggest supporters. I am eternally grateful to Toby, but we once had an argument in which he told me I had to choose between history and hematology. I couldn't do both, he said.

I found that massively upsetting. It was the second year of my three-year post-doc. The reason why it came up was that a Francophone hematologist, Dr Jeanne Drouin, at the University of Ottawa was going on sabbatical, and none of the other hematologists were able to speak French. She was leaving three outpatient clinics a week. Suddenly I was asked if I would help look after her patients. The others could do it, but it would have been a lot of extra work for them, and they weren't too happy about having to force these poor patients to speak English. I agreed, and it meant that I worked three half days a week as a hematologist.

First, I told Toby I didn't want to risk losing my clinical skills as a hematologist, because I wasn't convinced that I would find a job as a historian; there were so few. I could always go back to hematology, but only *if* I kept my skills up. That was really important for me. He just looked at all the time it was going to consume, and all the psychic energy, because, of course, there were calls at night and other things that go along with being a doctor for people who are super sick. I think he felt that he'd been helping me to become a historian, and here I was saying I was going to be a hematologist. I didn't see why I couldn't do both, given how little I was being paid: the post-doc didn't even cover the cost of daycare. It was a zero balance, a fair exchange. I would get a stipend for doing this coverage of Jeanne Drouin's clinics.

Even my friends wondered what I was doing trying to be both. Some of it was just pure survival. I had trained back when some people had said, "Oh, you'll just get married, and you'll stop practising" – and it was starting to come true! Giving up medicine wasn't ever something I'd planned or wanted. So I had to keep my clinical hand in. I admit that I didn't do as much historical research as I might have done in that time because I was also doing hematology. Teaching Toby's course was a great boot camp for discovering what can be done with undergrads. I learned a lot, because he was teaching material that I had never studied. I was only just a step ahead of the students at any given time. It was a great opportunity.

I was running around doing my own thing, and one day, Toby said, "We don't see enough of you." He and I booked into our schedule a lunch once a week, and we made peace. We are still friends, there's no doubt about it, and I owe him a lot.

While working as a hematologist in Ottawa hospitals, Duffin was asked to analyze and report on a set of bone marrows taken from a patient whom she did not know without being given any clinical information. It was an experience that eventually led her to do research in the Vatican Secret Archives on the role of medical miracles in canonization proceedings.

I put the bone marrow slides under the microscope, and right away there was the diagnosis: acute myeloblastic leukemia, the worst type we know. I could see the initials of the patient and the date, about seven or eight years earlier.

I thought, this patient is dead. The median survival with treatment at that time was about eighteen months. It turned out she *wasn't* dead. She'd had treatment and yet she was claiming that her recovery was a miracle worked through the intercession of Marie Marguerite d'Youville, who was a candidate for sainthood. Miracles are needed for canonization. Later, I had to testify and recognize my report before an ecclesiastical tribunal, held in order to prove that this case was extraordinary. No one asked me if it was a miracle, and I didn't have to say. Rather they asked if I could explain it and I couldn't. It was striking how scientifically respectful the process was, and how they were trying to square this recognition of a miracle with the canons of hematology. That really made me wonder: what were the other miracles? Were they medical too? And had anybody ever worked on it historically? That became a new research project, which eventually absorbed more than a decade of work and resulted in several articles and two books.

Could you tell us about your appointment in 1988 as the Hannah Professor in History of Medicine at Queen's University?

Just by training to be a doctor, you are an educator, because residents have clerks and other residents around, and we have to prepare rounds. I love the tradition of educating each other, the apprenticeship angle. While I was Toby's post-doctoral fellow, I taught his course, and I had residents and interns in clinics when I was replacing the hematologist. I hadn't been all that long detached from education, except for the three years in Paris.

Getting the job in the medical school was just fantastic for me. The Department of Medicine gave me a cross-appointment immediately – the hematologists thought it was great that I was a historian, which was bizarre. I was received in a wonderful way, because I had clinical credentials, and I was to be the school's historian.

The problem for me was that Sam Shortt had quit some years before, and there had been some argy-bargy over what would happen, and should he be replaced. Queen's apparently had tried to get an ethicist with the Hannah money, and Associated Medical Services, bless its heart, said, "No, the money is for *history* – good, go get ethics, but not from us – you can have the money if you have a *historian*." Queen's [medical school] said, "Well, historians are a pain in the neck, and we didn't have a great time with the last two, so you can keep your historian, and we'll just carry on."

Then Queen's medical school faced accreditation and was criticized for not having any humanities in its medical curriculum. The season was right, and they decided they'd better advertise for the Hannah position. Some things come around every year, like autumn and spring, and some things come once in a lifetime, like Halley's comet. That was a comet.

In my application letter, I said I'm bilingual … historian and physician … and blah, blah, blah! It was horrible, the whole process. I did get an interview. I went down to Kingston and, at the interview, of course, you end up learning who the competitors are. It was a short list of seven. I was the only physician on that short list. Correction: I was the only MD/PhD. There was one other physician without a PhD. And I was the only woman. The representatives of the Queen's History Department *refused* to meet me with the other members of the search committee, who were five physicians, and they did not attend my job talk. I learned later that they had ranked me last on this list of seven – and that the five doctors had ranked me first.

The strategy of the historians had been that everyone would go to the number-two candidate because it hadn't been unanimous. The expectation was that there ought to be a cross-appointment in the Arts and Sciences faculty so that the Hannah Professor could have grad students, which was viewed as appropriate to foster new scholarship. How can you do that if you're teaching in a medical school where the students are all going to be doctors? They were pretty sure that number two, a man with a PhD in History, would be picked.

These clever five doctors looked at my PhD and they took it to the new dean of medicine, Duncan Sinclair, and they said, "Look, it's History and Philosophy of Science. Forget the History Department, phone up Philosophy." They called the head of the Philosophy Department, Alistair MacLeod, who said: "What? Who? Where? She's here *today*?"

I went to lunch with a bunch of people from the Philosophy Department. It was lovely. We had a really nice time. They knew some of the people I knew, and I never for a moment pretended I was a philosopher. I said, "Yes, my degree is in history and philosophy of science, but it's way more history than philosophy." They said, "Yes, but you've done medical epistemology, and you understand about disease concepts, and that's really cool." They said, "We're trying to break into the medical school. We've been offering them ethics, but they won't have it." I went back to the dean's office, and, in the interval, he had had a phone call from the head of philosophy saying, "We offer her a cross-appointment." The doctors snubbed the History Department!

I was offered another history of medicine job in the same week, but I chose this one at Queen's because it was closest to my mother who was getting old and was still widowed, and my brother was no longer living in Canada. This one made a lot better sense. I thought family really comes first in absolutely everything. And Queen's was offering me, on a platter, history in a medical school and to be a hematologist. I could figure out the history department later.

Did you eventually figure out why the Queen's History Department had protested your recruitment?

Everybody tried to explain why they had rejected me. Three explanations came out early. First was gender: I was the only woman under consideration for the position, and that History Department had had a bad history with women professors. One of their female superstars had recently left in anger, after she was initially denied promotion even though she had won prizes for her scholarship. You might think that would make them say, "Well, let's have a cross-appointed woman, then we don't have to put up with her full time!" But no. Many faculty women told me that was the major issue.

Second, I was a practising physician. In the interviews, I was made to see the historians separately – they refused to interview me with the doctors! I had to go into a little room with two male historians, one was flipping through my thesis the whole time, telling me it was useless to have written it in French. He said that nothing important has ever been published in French (so I knew where he stood on Foucault!). He also said that "you can't be a physician and be credible on the history of your own discipline." He meant that doctors do really bad history, and my eagerly accepting the idea that I could continue to be a doctor would be a detriment to his students.

The third thing was that I had done my PhD in France at the Sorbonne, and that "wasn't a real university" (while Queen's was, to them, of course!).

So, these three explanations were out there in this aftermath between the offer and my acceptance. I thought, I need to take the bull by the horns. I went to see Jim Stayer, who was acting head of the History Department, because the head was on sabbatical. I asked: "In the whole process, I am now trying to decide if the history department is indifferent or hostile." He understood that I needed to know the truth before I accepted the offer. He said, "We viewed our role in this entire process of helping the medical school avoid the mistake of appointing a rank amateur, and since they have failed to heed our advice, we wash our hands of the entire affair." In other words, they were hostile.

My problem was not in the medical school. My problem was on campus in general, and when you are a young scholar, and you take on that kind of baggage, you start thinking everybody can see some flaw in you that is truly there. The funny thing was that the Philosophy Department is one floor above the History Department, and I became a very loyal member. I went to department meetings; I went to their weekly colloquium. It was a very healthy and happy department at the time, and they were nice to me. I found good friends in the Philosophy Department who are still my friends.

Gradually what happened is that grad students in the History Department would come to see me, and secretly say, "Don't tell anyone I've been here."

I helped them out, read their stuff, and gave suggestions and feedback. They would say, "I'm not going to name you in the acknowledgments" because they were afraid they'd get into trouble for having come to see me.

After seven biblical years of my not being a member of the History Department, the head at the time, Bob Malcolmson, asked me to lunch. Then the question came, would you be willing to accept a cross-appointment to History? I felt like saying "no." Because why should I? However, I realized that declining would be shooting myself in the foot. To mature as a scholar, you really do need to learn how to do supervisions. I knew that they were asking me because I was female, and that they needed better numbers of women and I didn't cost them a cent or even a position. They could have a girl, and save the real job for a boy. That's catty, but I think there really was a gender problem at the time. I went away and thought about it and then decided, yes, I should accept a cross-appointment. But I was not going to give up the cross-appointment in Philosophy. Later, I was given another in Education as well, and then Nursing gave me a cross-appointment, too. I had all these cross-appointments and no tenure![1]

Could you explain what you view as the complementary relationship between historical and clinical reasoning?

Doing a historical research project is a lot like approaching a patient clinically. The patient comes with a chief complaint, and the clinician takes a history, does a physical exam, comes up with a diagnosis, and then is guided by the diagnosis toward what to do next.

The historian begins with a question, which is a lot like the patient's chief complaint, and "takes a history" by looking at what other historians have published, the secondary sources, and then "does the physical exam" – in the sense that she researches for anything new or novel in terms of sources that have not been studied before – and then she comes to an interpretation, which mirrors a diagnosis. I think you could make the same analogy with a scientific research project, the aim, the materials, the methods, the discussion, etc.

I also think that this analogy between history and clinical work has the spinoff effect that is like learning a second language. When people learn a second language, it is much easier to acquire the third or the fourth; they understand the parts of speech: action words or verbs, adjectives and modifiers, etc. They know where to place these words intellectually, and, even if the grammar isn't identical, they understand that there will be rules to grammar. In a similar way, I think that learning historical research methods is useful for people who want to be clinicians or scientists.

What do you see as the utility of history to medical education?

Doctors have a terrible habit of thinking that history is the ultimate after-dinner speech. History as a kind of "edutainment." It's much, much more than that. Even if you're looking at antiquity, it has something to say about the present.

I have always thought that history belongs in medical school for two reasons. The first is to show that history is a research discipline like any form of science and that, as a research discipline, it has a role to play in current health care. Therefore, I did not think it was appropriate to give a separate course and have medical students look at names and dates and famous people. It's fun to know those things, but that wasn't what history in medical education was about. I wanted to infiltrate the curriculum so that they would learn history of anatomy while doing anatomy, and history of obstetrics while doing obstetrics, and that each history session would end with issues of the present. History can demonstrate how these problems arose, even if it doesn't show us what the solutions are.

The second reason is to make medical students skeptical about every single thing they're being taught. Information is not knowledge, and yet with all the information out there, students feel compelled to try to assimilate it all; they cram. I was a medical student once. I remember that urge. I wanted the information that I crammed to be true forever, because it was so much hard work getting it into my brain that I just didn't want anything to change, ever. I wanted it to be static.

History shows you that you'd better pay close attention because half of what you're being taught is not true; we just don't know which half it is. You have to be prepared to jettison that which you wanted to be true forever. We pay a great deal of lip service to lifelong learning and continuing medical education in medicine. History is an incentive, and inspiration to keep on learning.

History, perversely, is also a way of pushing the envelope about the scientific future. You can do that with the inspiring discoveries of the past, but you can do that with the terrible mistakes as well. When I was interviewed for the Hannah Chair, one of the medical professors on the committee was upset that I might teach about the mistakes. He said that all the students were depressed and "you need to inspire them, and they'll only be inspired by the good stuff – I don't want you to teach the bad stuff." I said, "Well, maybe I don't want to teach for you then if I have to leave out some of the past, or skew it, or pretend that it is something it's not." History is, or ought to be, an honest questioning of the past.

When you started at Queen's, you were confident that history should be integrated into medical education. What were the challenges and how did you go about it?

I had zero curriculum hours. I went around and met every single department head – there were twenty-five of them – and I asked them each for an hour. At first, I got an hour from only three different departments, which had a lot of hours: anatomy, pathology, and obstetrics. I was fortunate the heads of those departments actually were friendly toward history. When I gave my inaugural lectures – "the brass" from those respective departments showed up and sat in the front row, signalling to the students that this was important. Wonderful support.

Over time, I was able to add on one or two more classes each year from the other departments that eventually succumbed. When the school was accredited about three years into my tenure, other departments scrambled to have a history lecture because it looked good. Gradually, I had all the lectures I wanted. A few units actually asked for classes that I didn't want to give, but I gave them anyway. There were some sessions that, because of the changes in the curriculum, became redundant, so I killed them. I really don't like to teach things that don't map to the present medical learning.

There have been students whom I've taught who don't care at all about history, and I'm sure that I didn't reach all the students obliged to sit there. Queen's did let me have one question on every exam. Periodically medical student protests arose about the history question. How dare she have this question on the exam? I always made the case that they couldn't fail by getting that question wrong – they had to get a lot of the other questions wrong too. It was a motivator to try and get it right. Queen's tolerated my wanting to do those things. I've always said that if I've been successful, it's because Queen's let me. It gave me that core time.

I think the infiltrative method "worked" because it made history the servant of all of medicine in the sense that it pervaded the curriculum. It showed that history served and participated. I'd be preceded by a guy in a white coat, and followed by a guy in a white coat. History appeared to belong. I know my having an MD helped to draw the students' attention. They noticed when I too would put on a white coat and walk down Stuart Street to the hospital, and they'd see me as a "real" doctor. Sometimes I would show up to lectures with my stethoscope because I was coming from a clinic. The MD didn't make me a better historian. Not at all, but it focused their attention in a way that certainly helped advance my program.

I have been so lucky. I have been mostly well-supported by the faculty, and I have been very well-supported by the students. The students hand it on.

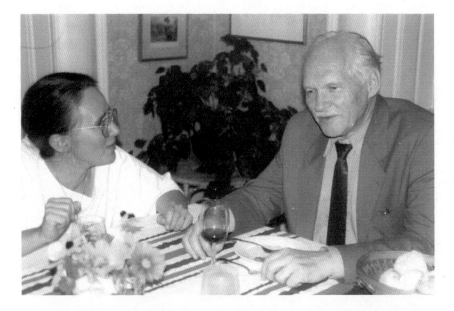

Figure 21.4 | In 1992, Duffin hosted historian of medicine Mirko Grmek, who was her doctoral advisor at the Sorbonne, at her Kingston home during his visit to Queen's University. (Photograph courtesy of J. Duffin)

They're in the school for four years, so there is an institutional memory that fosters interest in the younger cohort.

Truth to say, there have been opponents in the medical school. Some of them quite high up in the system. If I went away on sabbatical, I usually found someone to replace me, but there would be manipulations behind the scene, and I would return to discover that some or all history hours would be gone from the curriculum. I would have to work to get them all back again. Usually, I didn't have to go to all the department heads, and I was able to invoke students in order to help recover them. It was a constant warning to me that – even though things were going pretty well, and I was having a great time, and the deanery and students supported me – my program could be gone in a flash.

History was the most vulnerable thing in the medical school. You couldn't just arrive and design some sort of course and expect it never to change. If you want to be successful infiltrating, you have to understand what is going on in everything else being taught, and you have to deform your teaching methods and styles to match what the school wants.

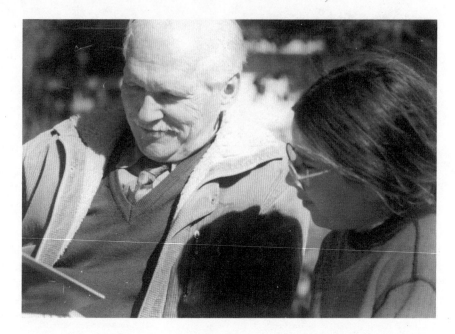

Figure 21.5 | Mirko Grmek and Duffin's daughter, Jessica Duffin Wolfe, during his 1992 visit to Kingston. She had attended his Sorbonne seminars as a babe in her mother's arms (to his astonishment) and today Dr Duffin Wolfe is a literary scholar and professor. (Photograph courtesy of J. Duffin)

I don't know that what I've done has gone much further than Queen's. If so, I would be honoured and pleased. But in the end, my last duty was to keep the local job alive, and to move over for a young scholar. It wasn't easy to convince them to replace me, and not spend the endowed money on something else. We're mortal, all of us, and you can't convince a university to replace you if you're dead. That was my final project.

Do physicians produce characteristic history?

Is there a kind of history done by physicians? I wrote that essay – "A Hippocratic Triangle" – and anyone who's interested can go read it. Basically, I talked myself out of the idea that physicians write a special type of history. I think there's only good history and bad. PhD historians have a tendency to "diss" the history that appears in some medical journals because it's derivative. Doctors rarely search further than an article – they forget that books exist, because

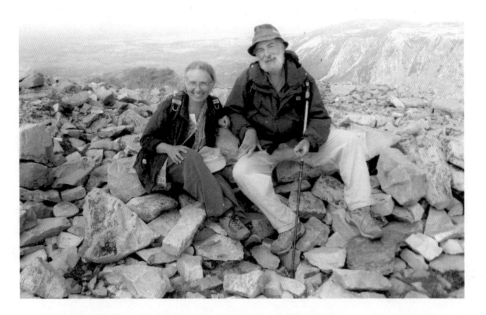

Figure 21.6 | In 2017, Duffin retired from the Hannah Chair in History of Medicine at Queen's University, where her long-time husband and supporter, Robert David Wolfe, is also an emeritus professor in policy studies. Photo taken at Gros Morne Mountain, Newfoundland, 2005. (Photograph courtesy of J. Duffin)

they're not indexed in PubMed or MEDLINE. So often the history they write is bad, but I would claim that it is not history at all.

One of the things that I'm proud of in my teaching is that, by playing the Heroes and Villains game, the medical students learn that MEDLINE does not index books.[2] Periodically, over the four years of their learning, I would fire a question at them: "What's wrong with MEDLINE?" The whole class would answer: "It doesn't index books!" Remind a bunch of doctors who want to do history to remember (or imagine) that someone's probably been there before you, and that they wrote *a book*. It is absolutely shocking when doctors miss books. For example, I am constantly being sent essays that present the history of the stethoscope without citing my book. The fault is not with the authors, because they are innocents – these are doctors who love history, true "amateurs." You blame the journal editors for not looking for the peer-review scholars who know about that period and can provide guidance to historical context.

So: there's only good history and bad, and it isn't fair to label all MD-written history as bad. When I examined scholarly histories written by doctors, I found little difference between them and those written by historians.

What achievements make you most proud?

Every book I wrote, I loved deeply as I was writing it. The process almost took over my life, and the books are like my children. I can't help but remember the phase of my life when I got the idea to do this book, or that book, and the pure pleasure in researching and writing them. There's a similar letting-go that you have to do as a parent and as an author. You move on to other things, because you must. Once published, the books have made their contribution. They're there for anyone who wants to find them, and I'm glad that I wrote them and acknowledge my responsibilities, but I let them go and turn to the next project, even in retirement. At least so far.

I'm also proud of some of the articles I've written. I continue to take pride in proving that Medicare enhanced MD income and in devising "carpenter hours" as a way of comparing finances. I understand that for a little while the Canadian Association of University Teachers started using it as a way of comparing salaries as well as tuitions. I am delighted with the work of utterly unknown collaborators in the slow but persistent project to crowd-source the translation of the Latin *consilia* of Paolo Zacchia. Lately, I am pleased with my recent article suggesting (with evidence) that clinical practice guidelines might be a cause of drug shortages.

But I'm more grateful than I am proud; grateful for the opportunities to be creative. The creativity was fun – designing the core curriculum, inventing games, debates, and events – like field trips. I'm grateful that Queen's let me, and I'm happy that it worked. It was an idea that did pay off, and, I suppose, I'm proud that I still hear from former students.

Would you offer some closing thoughts?

It wasn't a straight road to success; it was twisting and the destination was obscure. Most of the time somebody was there helping me. I don't feel like I can take too much credit for what happened because, in the end, what I did was what I wanted to do, and I got paid for it. That's just amazing. It's so rare and privileged.

NOTES

1   Before changes to the administrative structure of the AMS endowment in
    1999, the holder of the Hannah Chair was not eligible for tenure.
2   A research "game" devised by Duffin and described in her textbook *History of
    Medicine: A Scandalously Short Introduction*.

Contributors

ANNMARIE ADAMS is an architectural historian specializing in the intersections of medicine, gender, and the built environment. She holds the Stevenson Chair in the Philosophy and History of Science, including Medicine, at McGill University in Montreal. Adams is jointly appointed in the School of Architecture and Department of Social Studies of Medicine (SSoM). Her books include *Architecture in the Family Way* (MQUP, 1996); *'Designing Women'* (UTP, 2000); and *Medicine by Design* (UMP, 2007). She is currently writing a "spatial biography" of cardiologist and museum curator Maude Abbott, funded by SSHRC (Social Science and Humanities Research Council of Canada).

PRATIK CHAKRABARTI is the National Endowment for the Humanities and Cullen Chair in History and Medicine at the Department of History in the University of Houston. He has contributed widely to the history of science, medicine, and imperial history from the eighteenth to the twentieth centuries. His recent monograph is *Inscriptions of Nature: Geology and the Naturalization of Antiquity* (Johns Hopkins University Press, 2020).

MARIA PIA DONATO is a CNRS Research Professor at the Institut d'Histoire Moderne et Contemporaine in Paris and teaches the history of medicine and science at ENS and EHESS. She is a specialist in early modern culture and medicine, especially in Catholic contexts. Among her publications are *Sudden Death: Medicine and Religion in 18th-Century Rome* (2014) and *Medicine and the Inquisition in the Early Modern World* (ed., 2019).

DELIA GAVRUS is an associate professor in the History Department at the University of Winnipeg in Manitoba, Canada. She has published on topics in the history of the mind and brain sciences and medicine of the late

nineteenth century to the middle of the twentieth century. She is particularly
interested in models and theories of consciousness from a historical perspective, as well as in professional identity, surgical practice, epistemology, and
medical training, especially as these issues pertain to the first generations of
neurosurgeons. She is currently writing a series of biographical essays about
the Canadian neurosurgeon Wilder Penfield.

KIM GIROUARD holds a joint PhD (cotutelle) from the Université de
Montréal and the École Normale Supérieure de Lyon and is a specialist
in the history of medicine and health, and women and gender in modern
China. Her research program includes the medicalization of mother-
hood and the feminization of the medical profession in southern China's
Guangdong province in the early twentieth century. She is a Vanier Canada
Graduate Scholar and completed a post-doctoral fellowship at the Montreal
Centre for International Studies (CÉRIUM). Currently, she conducts
post-doctoral research in history of medicine at the University of Ottawa.

HEINI HAKOSALO, PhD, is a senior research fellow in history of sciences
and ideas at the University of Oulu, Finland, and associate professor in
history of science at the University of Turku, Finland. She specializes in the
history of modern and contemporary medicine and has published on the
histories of nineteenth-century brain sciences, women's medical education
in late-nineteenth- and early-twentieth-century Finland and Sweden, and
tuberculosis in twentieth-century Finland. Her most recent book is *Pursuit of
Healthy Environments: Lessons from Historical Cases on the Environment-Health Nexus*
(2021), co-edited with Esa Ruuskanen. Her current research interests include
the history of post–World War II epidemiology and the relationship of
infectious disease control and urban planning.

JENNA HEALEY is an assistant professor of history and the Jason A. Hannah
Chair in the History of Medicine at Queen's University, where she is responsible for integrating the humanities into the undergraduate medical curriculum. She received her PhD in the history of science and medicine from Yale
University in 2016. Her research interests lie at the intersection of gender,
race, and medical technology in the nineteenth and twentieth centuries. Her
current book project examines the relationship between aging and reproduction through a history of the biological clock.

JETHRO HERNÁNDEZ BERRONES is an associate professor and chair of
history at Southwestern University. His work examines the history of healing
practices in modern Mexico and Latin America. His articles and book

chapters, as well as his book manuscript "A Revolution in Small Doses," explore the change in models of medical science, medical institutions, and public health policies resulting from contesting understandings of the body, health, and disease. His work has been supported by the National Endowment for the Humanities, the American Association for the History of Medicine, the Robert Bosch Foundation Institute for the History of Medicine, and the Consejo Nacional de Ciencia y Tecnología, among other institutions.

GEOFFREY L. HUDSON, DPhil (Oxford), MA and BA Hons (McMaster), is an associate professor in the history of medicine in the Human Sciences Division at the Northern Ontario School of Medicine (currently Faculty of Medicine, Lakehead and Laurentian Universities). Hudson previously had stints as a research fellow at University College London (UK), and as the programs director at a research granting organization, the Hannah Institute for the History of Medicine / Associated Medical Services (Toronto). Just prior to his joining the Northern Ontario School of School as founding faculty in 2004, Hudson was acting director of the History of Health and Medicine Unit in the Faculty of Health Sciences at McMaster University. Hudson's areas of research and publication include the social history of medicine as well as the history of war and medicine, disability, and medical education.

FRANK HUISMAN is a professor in the history of medicine at the University Medical Center Utrecht, and staff member of the Descartes Center for the History and Philosophy of the Sciences and the Humanities of Utrecht University. He is series editor of *Clio Medica: Studies in the History of Medicine and Health* and founding editor of the *European Journal for the History of Medicine and Health* (to be published from 2021 onwards by Brill). His publications are on early-modern and modern Dutch health care. In English, he co-edited *Locating Medical History: The Stories and Their Meanings* (with John Harley Warner), *Health and Citizenship: Political Cultures of Health in Europe* (with Harry Oosterhuis), and *Blurring Boundaries: Towards a Medical History of the Twentieth Century* (with Joris Vandendriessche and Kaat Wils). He is now working on a monograph exploring the transformation of Dutch health care between the 1860s and the 1940s.

LORI JONES received her PhD in history from the University of Ottawa in 2017 after a two-decade career in international health and development. She is a sessional professor of the history of disease and medicine at Carleton University and the University of Ottawa. She has published numerous articles, book chapters, and podcasts on medieval and early modern plague treatises. She is also known for her work on detecting mislabelled plague images. McGill-Queen's University Press is publishing a monograph version of her dissertation in 2022; her two edited volumes related to disease in the medieval and early modern worlds are expected in 2022 as well. For three years she was a post-doctoral fellow in the Department of History at Carleton University (funded by the Social Sciences and Humanities Research Council of Canada and the Associated Medical Services).

LAURA KELLY is a senior lecturer in the history of health and medicine at the University of Strathclyde, Glasgow. Her research focuses on the social history of medicine in nineteenth- and twentieth-century Ireland. Her most recent book *Irish Medical Education and Student Culture, c. 1850–1950* was published by Liverpool University Press in 2017, and her previous book, *Irish Women in Medicine, c. 1880s–1920s: Origins, Education and Careers* was published by Manchester University Press in 2012. She is currently working on a major project on the history of contraception in modern Ireland, funded by a Wellcome Trust Research Fellowship in Medical Humanities.

M.A. MUJEEB KHAN, PhD (Cambridge), MS (Tokyo), AM (Harvard), BS (Stony Brook), is assistant professor of Japanese, Islamic studies, and comparative literary and cultural studies in the Department of World Languages and Cultures at the University of Utah. His research interests centre on comparative intellectual history and the intersection of culture, religion, science, and law in the premodern and modern periods, with a focus on East and West Asia. His publications include studies of Japanese medicine, Islamicate medicine, religion and medicine, and the role of text and interpretation in intellectual transmission. His current projects are a study of medicine in early Japan, an analysis of medical writing in the medieval Islamicate world, and a comparative project that expands his work in the present volume.

Co-editor and contributor SUSAN LAMB holds the Jason A. Hannah Chair in History of Medicine at the University of Ottawa and gratefully acknowledges AMS Healthcare for its ongoing support for teaching and research activities. Her current research is on the development of university medicine in North America within transatlantic contexts. She is the author of *Pathologist of the Mind: Adolf Meyer and the Origins of American Psychiatry* (Johns Hopkins University Press, 2014) and continues to study and collaborate on the significance of Meyerian psychiatry.

Medical anthropologist MARION MAAR, PhD (McMaster), MA (Trent), BSc (Guelph), is an associate professor and founding faculty at the Northern Ontario School of Medicine (NOSM), Human Sciences Division. Her teaching and research focus is in the area of culturally safe care, e-health, service evaluation, and Indigenous health and mental health. In her current work she collaborates with Indigenous knowledge-keepers to document the role of land-based activities on mental health and addictions recovery. She also promotes the use of art, photography, and film in the evaluation of First Nations culturally based programs. Prior to her faculty appointment at NOSM in 2005 Maar worked as a research and evaluation coordinator for an Indigenous Health Access Centre on Manitoulin Island in Northern Ontario for eight years with a focus on developing community-based participatory models for Indigenous health research and service evaluation.

DIANA MOORE is an adjunct assistant professor of history at John Jay College of Criminal Justice, City University of New York. Her research examines how women and other traditionally disenfranchised actors in nineteenth-century Europe utilized conservative, domestic, philanthropic, and religious discourses and practices to participate in various emancipatory movements. Her first book, *Revolutionary Domesticity in the Italian Risorgimento: Transnational Victorian Feminism, 1850–1890*, was published in July 2021 and offers a reevaluation of both Italian unification and nineteenth-century feminism. Her work has also been published in the *Journal of Women's History*, the *Catholic Historical Review*, and *Modern Italy*.

JEAN BAPTISTE NZOGUE is an associate professor of social history at the University of Douala (Cameroon). He has a strong interest in the history of medicine and health systems, and has worked on the effects of encounters between the Western world and Africa on contemporary African societies, from the slave trade to European colonial domination. His recent book, *L'alcool dans les rencontres entre l'Europe et l'Afrique noire* (co-authored with J.T. Sonfa Lela), was published in 2019 and deals with the role of alcohol in these encounters. He is currently working on a book project that examines the labour, trades, and careers of the Autochthonous in Cameroon under colonial rule (1884–1960).

SALLY P. RAGEP retired as a senior researcher at the Institute of Islamic Studies, McGill University, in 2020. She continues as an executive board member of the Islamic Scientific Manuscripts Initiative (ISMI), an international collaboration to make accessible online information on all Islamic manuscripts in the exact sciences (https://ismi.mpiwg-berlin.mpg.de/). Her research focuses on science teaching in pre-modern Islam, which includes the role of textbooks, commentaries, and institutional structures that sustained science in Islam for over a millennium. She also is engaged in cross-cultural comparisons of science teaching in Islam and other cultural areas, especially medieval and early modern Europe. Her publications include *Jaghmīnī's Mulakhkhaṣ: An Islamic Introduction to Ptolemaic Astronomy* (2016).

JONATHAN REINARZ is a professor of the history of medicine in the Institute of Applied Health Research at the University of Birmingham (UK). He has published extensively on the history of hospitals and medical education in provincial England in the nineteenth and twentieth centuries. His other research interests cover the history of the senses, alcohol, and accidents. His current AHRC-funded project, "Forged by Fire," run jointly with staff at Leeds Beckett University, is researching the history of burns injury in the UK, c. 1800–2000.

ANNA RUDDOCK is an independent scholar with a PhD in anthropology from King's College London. Her research interests concern the role of medical education in reproducing health inequalities, and critical feminist approaches to the experience of chronic illness. She is the author of *Special Treatment: Student Doctors at the All India Institute of Medical Sciences*, published by Stanford University Press.

MICHAEL STOLBERG is chair of history of medicine at the University of Würzburg in Germany. He is the author of *Experiencing Illness and the Sick Body in Early Modern Europe* (2011), *Uroscopy in Early Modern Europe, 1500–1800* (2015), and *History of Palliative Care, 1500–1970: Concepts, Practices and Ethical Challenges* (2017). His newest book, *Learned Physicians and Everyday Medical Practice in the Renaissance* (2022), draws on personal notebooks, practice journals, and letters to reconstruct the world of learned physicians in the sixteenth century. Since 2009, he has also directed a database project on early modern German-speaking physicians' correspondences (1500–1700) that currently offers access to the data of about 55,000 letters and provides a detailed summary for many thousands of them (www.aerztebriefe.de).

WHITNEY WOOD is Canada Research Chair in the Historical Dimensions of Women's Health in the Department of History at Vancouver Island University. She earned her PhD from Wilfrid Laurier University (part of the Tri-University Graduate Program) in 2016, and completed post-doctoral fellowships at Birkbeck, University of London, and the University of Calgary. Her research interests include the history of women's bodies, reproduction, and pain in nineteenth- and twentieth-century Canada, and her work has appeared in the *Canadian Bulletin of Medical History*, *Social History of Medicine*, and the *British Medical Journal: Medical Humanities*, in addition to a number of edited collections.

HARRY YI-JUI WU is an associate professor in the Cross-College Elite Program and the Department of Medical Humanities and Social Medicine, National Cheng-Kung University. Before arriving in Taiwan, he taught medical humanities in Singapore and Hong Kong. Harry's research mainly focuses on the transnational history of psychiatry and the role of the humanities in clinical sciences. He has published articles in various journals of history of medicine and medical education. His first book, *Mad by the Millions: Mental Disorders and the Early Years of the World Health Organization*, was published by MIT Press in 2021. Currently, besides writing his second monograph about the history of psychiatry in Hong Kong, he is using verbatim theatre to help various communities understand the burden of care.

AMS at 85: A History of Support for Patients, Historians, and Health Professions Education

Everyone involved in the publication of *Transforming Medical Education* is grateful to AMS Healthcare, which provided a publication grant to increase worldwide access to this volume.

For eighty-five years, AMS has been a catalyst for positive change in healthcare – first as a lifeline for patients, and later as a major funder of history of medicine, bioethics, and health professions education. Today, the organization is focused on helping to cultivate a Canadian healthcare system that is compassionate and at the forefront of technological innovation, in part by supporting the work of medical historians and promoting the value of history in medical education.

Founded by physician Jason Hannah in 1937, AMS was one of Canada's first not-for-profit prepaid health insurance organizations. Unlike plans that served membership groups, AMS provided healthcare coverage to individuals and families who did not otherwise qualify for private or group health insurance. In the midst of the Great Depression, the monthly subscription fee of $6.50 gave a family of four access to a family physician and covered costs for diagnostic tests, hospital care, surgery, and the fees of some medical specialists. By 1959, hundreds of thousands of Ontarians paid affordable monthly premiums to the organization for reliable medical and hospital care. In the 1970s, when the Ontario Health Insurance Plan assumed this responsibility, Dr Hannah reorganized AMS and its substantial financial reserves into a self-funded charitable organization to support research and teaching in the history of medicine.

Under Dr Hannah's leadership, AMS equipped and opened the Hannah Institute for the History of Medical and Related Sciences in Toronto, which provided a library and many other resources to support research and teaching. Shortly before Dr Hannah's death in 1977, AMS established five university chairs in Ontario faculties of medicine. Before AMS created this fundamental infrastructure, the discipline of history of medicine in Canada had no dedicated programs, institutions, or sources of funding. As a lasting tribute to his advocacy for history in medical education, today there is a Jason A. Hannah Chair in History of Medicine endowed by AMS at University of Calgary, McGill University (Hannah-Cotton), McMaster University, University of Ottawa, Queen's University, University of Toronto, and Western University. Most recently, in 2015, AMS established a Hannah Chair in the History of Indigenous Health and Indigenous Traditional Medicine at the Northern Ontario School of Medicine (NOSM).

Dr Jacalyn Duffin, whose contributions to history of medicine and to medical education this volume celebrates, held the AMS Hannah Chair in History of Medicine at Queen's University from 1988 to 2017. For over forty years, AMS has invested in the history of medicine in Canada as both a scholarly discipline and a meaningful component of health professions education with comprehensive funding for library and museum collections, research and teaching grants, graduate bursaries, postdoctoral fellowships, the Hannah Medal book prize, symposia, a bilingual Nursing History Research Unit (University of Ottawa), the Janus and Phoenix projects for healthcare practitioners, and continued support for the Canadian Society for the History of Medicine and its journal, the *Canadian Journal of Health History* (formerly *CBMH/BCHM*). In addition, AMS supports scholarly publication by providing subventions for books published in the Studies in the History of Medicine, Health, and Society series at McGill-Queen's University Press – an investment that has paid dividends of over fifty books, including this one, on health history and social policy. The editors and contributors of this volume are proud and grateful to be part of this series and of the rich legacy of AMS.

LEARN MORE ABOUT AMS

AMS website: https://www.amshealthcare.ca

Studies in the History of Medicine, Health, and Society series at McGill-Queen's University Press: https://www.mqup.ca.

"AMS 80th Anniversary: The Past and Future of Canadian Healthcare" (YouTube): https://youtu.be/fKytWLNHZ8I.

"Jason A. Hannah and the Hannah Chairs for the History of Medicine." *Bulletin of the History of Medicine* 52, no. 1 (1978): 125–7.

G.R. Paterson. "The Hannah Institute: Promoting Canadian History of Medicine." *CMAJ* 128 (1983): 1325–8.

Hissan Butt and Jacalyn Duffin. "Educating Future Physicians for Ontario and the 1986 Doctors Strike: The Roots of Competency-Based Medical Education." *CMAJ* 190, no. 7 (2018): E196–E198.

Index

Page numbers in italics refer to tables and figures.

Index